W9-CBA-881

SPRINGER SURGERY ATLAS SERIES

Series Editors: J.-S. P. Lumley · J.-R. Siewert

J.S.P. Lumley · J. J. Hoballah (Eds.)

Vascular Surgery

With 291 Color Figures,
in 345 separate Illustrations

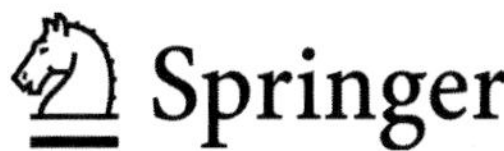

Springer

J.S.P. Lumley, MS, FRCS
Professor
St. Batholomews Hospital
5th Floor, King George V Block
West Smithfield
London, EC1A 7BE
UK

Jamal J. Hoballah, MD, MBA, FACS
Professor and Chairman
Division of Vascular Surgery
The University of Iowa
Iowa City, IA 52241
USA

ISBN 978-3-540-41102-4
Springer-Verlag Berlin Heidelberg New York

Library of Congress Control Number: 2005938808

Springer is a part of Springer Science+Business Media
springer.com

Wissenschaftliche Zeichnungen: Dr. Michael von Solodkoff, Christiane von Solodkoff, Neckargemünd, Heidelberg, Germany
Production: LE-TeX Jelonek, Schmidt & Vöckler GbR, Leipzig
Cover: Frido-Steinen-Broo, EStudio, Calamar, Spain
Typesetting: K. Detzner, 67346 Speyer, Germany

Printed on acid-free paper 21/3100YL 5 4 3 2 1 0

Preface

The second half of the twentieth century saw vascular surgery develop from a necessity for hemostasis to a mature reconstructive art. However, this was accompanied by increasing patient expectations and the introduction of the alternative techniques of dilatation and stenting. These factors have helped surgeons to focus attention on the need for clinical audit and to define clearly the limitations and standards of excellence that should be achieved in the specialty.

Vascular disease remains an extensive problem in developed countries and is of increasing importance in developing areas; therefore, the search for surgical excellence continues, in both patient selection and technical expertise. To achieve the latter, there is no substitute for practical involvement, first as an observer and then assisting and subsequently undertaking supervised and independent practice; finally it is crucial to maintain lifelong skills and search for lasting solutions.

This text is not a substitute for these essential measures, rather it is a support for good clinical practice. It brings together experts across the whole spectrum of vascular surgical practice, with a wealth of clinical experience, to illustrate standard and less common procedures, providing technical tips and practical know-how. It presents information in clearly defined illustrations and meaningful text; it aims to become a companion not only for the surgeon in training, but also for practicing surgeons, who may agree or disagree, but will be stimulated to question their surgical management and explore possible alternatives.

The only certainty of the future is that it will bring change. An essential requirement for facing that change is multidisciplinary teamwork, and within that framework to define the roles of endovascular and invasive procedures, as well as the place of medical management in the prevention and modification of vascular disease.

Although vascular surgery has come a long way, there are still problems to solve, particularly when and when not to operate. New techniques are likely to be minimally invasive, using hybrid techniques that combine open and endovascular skills, possibly using stapling devices and improving perioperative imaging. New methods of tissue and organ preservation are required, as are the means of improving the immediate and long-term results of small grafts. Adjuvant products are needed to reduce the thrombogenicity of vascular surfaces, particularly in the venous system and in grafts.

Vascular surgery remains one of the most rewarding surgical specialties, with the potential to save lives and limbs, and prevent debilitating disease.

October 2008
J. S. P. Lumley, London, UK
J. J. Hoballah, Iowa City, USA

Contents

List of Contributors

Mark A. Adelman
University Vascular Associates,
530 1st Ave., Suite #6F
New York, NY 10016
USA

Stephen J. Annest
Vascular Institute of the Rockies
1601 E. 19th Avenue, Suite 3950
Denver, CO 80218
USA

Jeffrey L. Ballard
Staff Vascular Surgeon
Vascular Institute, St. Joseph Hospital
and
Clinical Professor of Surgery
University of California, Irvine
Orange, CA

Colin D. Bicknell
Regional Vascular Unit
Imperial College School of Medicine
St. Mary's Hospital
London, W2 1NY
UK

Christopher T. Bunch
Duluth Clinic
400 East Third St.
Duluth, MN 55805
USA

Ruth L. Bush
Division of Vascular Surgery
and Endovascular Therapy
Michael E. DeBakey Department of Surgery
Baylor College of Medicine
Houston, TX 77030
USA

Keith D. Calligaro
Section of Vascular Surgery, Pennsylvania Hospital
700 Spruce St., Suite 101
Philadelphia, PA 19106
USA

Benjamin B. Chang
The Vascular Group, PLLC
The Institute for Vascular Health and Disease
47 New Scotland Avenue (MC 157)
Albany, NY 12208
USA

Nicholas J.W. Cheshire
Regional Vascular Unit
Imperial College School of Medicine
St. Mary's Hospital
London
UK

Michael S. Conners III
7777 Hennesey Blvd., Suite 108
Baton Rouge, LA 70808
USA

David C. Corry
Associates in General & Vascular Surgery
525 N. Foote Ave., #202
Colorado Springs, CO 80909
USA

R. Clement Darling III
The Vascular Group, PLLC
The Institute for Vascular Health and Disease
47 New Scotland Avenue (MC 157)
Albany, NY 12208
USA

Alun H. Davies
Department of Vascular Surgery
Charing Cross Hospital
Fulham Palace Road
London, W6 8RF
UK

Tina R. Desai
Department of Surgery, University of Chicago
5841 South Maryland Avenue, MC 5029
Chicago, IL 60637
USA

Matthew J. Dougherty
Section of Vascular Surgery
Pennsylvania Hospital
Philadelphia, PA 19106
USA

Anthony L. Estrera
Department of Cardiothoracic
and Vascular Surgery
The University of Texas at Houston Medical School
Memorial Hermann Hospital
Houston, TX 77030
USA

Julie A. Freischlag
Department of Surgery
The Johns Hopkins Medical Institutions
720 Rutland Avenue, Ross 759
Baltimore, MD 21205
USA

Joseph J. Fulton
Department of Surgery
University of North Carolina
2115 Bioinformatics Building, CB# 7050
Chapel Hill, NC 27599-7050
USA

Patrick J. Geraghty
Section of Vascular Surgery
Washington University Medical School
660 S. Euclid Avenue, Campus Box 8109
St. Louis, MO 63110-1094
USA

Bruce L. Gewertz
Department of Surgery, University of Chicago
5841 South Maryland Avenue, MC 5029
Chicago, IL 60637
USA

Joseph S. Giglia
Department of Surgery
Division of Vascular Surgery
University of Cincinnati
231 Albert Sabin Way
Cincinnati, OH 45267-0558
USA

Nicholas J. Goddard
Department of Orthopaedics
Royal Free Hospital
London, NW3 2QG
UK

Peter K. Henke
Section of Vascular Surgery
Department of Vascular Surgery
University of Michigan Medical School
Ann Arbor, MI 48109
USA

Jamal J. Hoballah
Division of Vascular Surgery
University of Iowa Hospitals and Clinics
200 Hawkins Drive
Iowa City, IA 52242-1086
USA

Blair A. Keagy
Department of Surgery
University of North Carolina
2115 Bioinformatics Building, CB# 7050
Chapel Hill, NC 27599-7050
USA

Paul B. Kreienberg
The Vascular Group, PLLC
The Institute for Vascular Health and Disease
47 New Scotland Avenue (MC 157)
Albany, NY 12208
USA

Timothy F. Kresovik
Division of Vascular Surgery
University of Iowa Hospitals and Clinics
200 Hawkins Drive
Iowa City, IA 52242-1086
USA

Brajesh K. Lal
Department of Surgery
Division of Vascular Surgery
UMDNJ-New Jersey Medical School
185 S. Orange Avenue, MSB-H570
Newark, NJ 07103
USA

John S. Lane
San Francisco General Hospital
1001 Potrero Ave., Ward 3A
San Francisco, CA 94110
USA

Peter H. Lin
Division of Vascular Surgery
and Endovascular Therapy
Michael E. DeBakey Department of Surgery
Baylor College of Medicine
Houston, TX 77030
USA

John Lumley
Honorary Consultant Surgeon
Great Ormond Street Children's Hospital
Great Ormond Street
London, WC1N 3JH
UK

Alan B. Lumsden
Michael E. DeBakey Department of Surgery
Baylor College of Medicine
6550 Fannin St., Suite 1661
Houston, TX 77030
USA

Manish Mehta
The Vascular Group, PLLC
The Institute for Vascular Health and Disease
47 New Scotland Avenue (MC 157)
Albany, NY 12208
USA

Louis M. Messina
Division of Vascular Surgery, School of Medicine
University of California at San Francisco
San Francisco, CA 94121
USA

Samuel R. Money
Section of Vascular Surgery
Ochsner Clinic Foundation
1514 Jefferson Hwy.
New Orleans, LA 70121
USA

Jonathon C. Nelson
Division of Vascular Surgery
and Endovascular Therapy
Michael E. DeBakey Department of Surgery
Baylor College of Medicine
Houston, TX 77030
USA

Lyssa N. Ochoa
Division of Vascular Surgery
and Endovascular Therapy
Michael E. DeBakey Department of Surgery
Baylor College of Medicine
Houston, TX 77030
USA

Kathleen J. Ozsvath
The Vascular Group, PLLC
The Institute for Vascular Health and Disease
47 New Scotland Avenue (MC 157)
Albany, NY 12208
USA

Peter J. Pappas
Division of Vascular Surgery
UMDNJ-New Jersey Medical School
Newark, NJ 07107-3001
USA

Philip S.K. Paty
The Vascular Group, PLLC
The Institute for Vascular Health and Disease
47 New Scotland Avenue (MC 157)
Albany, NY 12208
USA

Eric K. Peden
Division of Vascular Surgery
and Endovascular Therapy
Michael E. DeBakey Department of Surgery
Baylor College of Medicine
Houston, TX 77030
USA

Kingsley P. Robinson
Douglas Bader Unit
Queen Mary's Hospital
Roehampton Lane
London, SW15 5PN
UK

Sean P. Roddy
The Vascular Group, PLLC
The Institute for Vascular Health and Disease
47 New Scotland Avenue (MC 157)
Albany, NY 12208
USA

Hazim J. Safi
Department of Cardiothoracic
and Vascular Surgery
The University of Texas at Houston Medical School
UTH Medical Center
6410 Fannin Street, Suite 450
Houston, TX 77030
USA

Rajabrata Sarkar
Division of Vascular Surgery, School of Medicine
University of California at San Francisco
4150 Clement Street (112G)
San Francisco, CA 94121
USA

Dhiraj M. Shah
The Vascular Group, PLLC
The Institute for Vascular Health and Disease
47 New Scotland Avenue (MC 157)
Albany, NY 12208
USA

Melhem J. Sharafuddin
Department of Surgery
University of Iowa Hospitals and Clinics
200 Hawkins Drive
Iowa City, IA 52242-1077
USA

W. John Sharp
Division of Vascular Surgery
University of Iowa Hospitals and Clinics
200 Hawkins Drive
Iowa City, IA 52242-1086
USA

Gregorio A. Sicard
Division of General Surgery
and Section of Vascular Surgery
Washington University Medical School
660 S. Euclid Avenue
St. Louis, MO 63110-1094
USA

Paul Srodon
St. Mary's Hospital
Imperial College London Ealing
London, W2 1NY
UK

James C. Stanley
Department of Surgery
University of Michigan Medical School
University Hospital, 2210-THCC
1500 East Medical Center Drive
Ann Arbor, MI 48109-0325
USA

Alan Y. Synn
Vascular Institute of the Rockies
1601 E. 19th Avenue, Suite 3950
Denver, CO 80218
USA

Robert W. Thompson
Section of Vascular Surgery
Washington University School of Medicine
9901 Wohl Hospital
4960 Children's Place
St. Louis, MO 63110
USA

Patricia E. Thorpe
Department of Radiology
University of Iowa College of Medicine
200 Hawkins Drive
Iowa City, IA 52242
USA

Ronnie Word
Division of Vascular Surgery
University of Iowa Hospitals and Clinics
200 Hawkins Drive
Iowa City, IA 52242-1086
USA

John W. York
2704 Henry Street
Greensboro, NC 27405
USA

Part I Head and Neck

CHAPTER 1

Carotid Endarterectomy

John Lumley, Paul Srodon

INTRODUCTION

Cerebrovascular disease is a leading cause of death and disability worldwide. In the United States there are approximately 730,000 strokes per year, and the annual management cost of these, and the 4 million survivors, is approximately $40 billion.

In the United Kingdom, stroke-related disease accounts for 13% of bed usage in National Health Service hospitals, and 25% in private nursing homes.

Reduction of stroke risk can be achieved by control of hypertension, lipid lowering agents, antiplatelet agents, appropriate management of myocardial infarction and auricular fibrillation, stopping smoking, and avoiding obesity and excess alcohol consumption.

Carotid endarterectomy reduces the stroke risk sevenfold in patients with transient ischemic attacks, and has an absolute risk reduction of 5.0% over 5 years in asymptomatic patients with 60–90% stenosis of the origin of the internal carotid artery. Further studies are required of the stroke risk of coronary artery bypass grafting in patients with carotid artery disease, and the relation of carotid atheromatous plaque morphology to stroke morbidity.

Carotid endarterectomy carries a stroke morbidity and mortality of 3–5%, and in spite of extensive research over the last 50 years, it is not known whether this is primarily due to perioperative ischemia, embolism or thrombosis. The highest incidence of perioperative stroke, associated with severe bilateral carotid artery stenosis, may be due to precapillary cerebral spasm post-revascularization, the resultant stasis predisposing to thrombosis over the highly thrombogenic endarterectomized segment.

The operation is usually undertaken with the patient under general anesthesia with tracheal intubation. This provides control of the airway and adequate oxygenation, together with painless insertion of lines for monitoring and maintenance of blood pressure and anesthesia. However, monitoring of cerebral function has to be undertaken by indirect measures such as internal carotid artery back flow, stump pressures, EEGs, isotope studies and transcranial monitoring by Doppler or other means. When selective shunting, rather than routine shunting or avoidance of shunts, is being undertaken, an alternative approach is to use regional or local anesthesia monitoring contralateral grip strength. The patient is asked to squeeze an audible device in a rhythmic fashion throughout the period of clamping, shunting being initiated if the grip becomes defective. Sedation must be sufficient to allay anxiety without inhibiting the gripping sequence.

Figure 1

The patient is positioned supine with his/her head up to reduce cervical venous pressure, and feet up to stabilize on the operating table. The head is placed on a ring, with a sandbag under the shoulders. The head is rotated and flexed to the non-operated side, exposing the full length of the sternomastoid muscle. Anesthetic tubing is preferably taken superiorly, away from the operative field: the hair is dampened and brushed posterosuperiorly away from the ear.

Skin preparation crosses the midline and passes laterally to include the tip of the shoulder. Superiorly it includes the lower jaw and all the ear, particular care being taken to prepare the back of the lobe and the mastoid process. Inferiorly it passes to the nipple. A head towel is used, enclosing the anesthetic apparatus, the chin and half the ear. The square towels expose the length of the sternomastoid, the upper manubrium sternum and the medial half of the clavicle. The skin incision can be marked together with transverse lines for subsequent realignment.

A sterile drape serves to retain towels and also the ear lobe, retracted anterosuperiorly away from the mastoid process. The incision passes from the mastoid process along the anterior border of the sternomastoid muscle for two-thirds of its length. It may pass more transversely, with slight improvement of the subsequent scar, but this incision does not provide good access for a low bifurcation of the common carotid artery.

Figure 2

The incision is deepened on to the anterior border of the sternomastoid muscle. Superiorly the dissection passes behind the parotid gland: a number of small divided vessels may need diathermy. The external jugular vein is mobilized and ligated. Anterior cutaneous nerves of the neck are divided, as is the arteria branch of the great auricular nerve if this cannot be mobilized free of the incision. (The patient should be warned of possible postoperative, non-recoverable anesthesia of the ear lobe.) The dissection is carried around the anterior border of the sternomastoid muscle to allow insertion of a self-retaining retractor. Small vessels to the anterior border are diathermied, as are any further veins that are encountered.

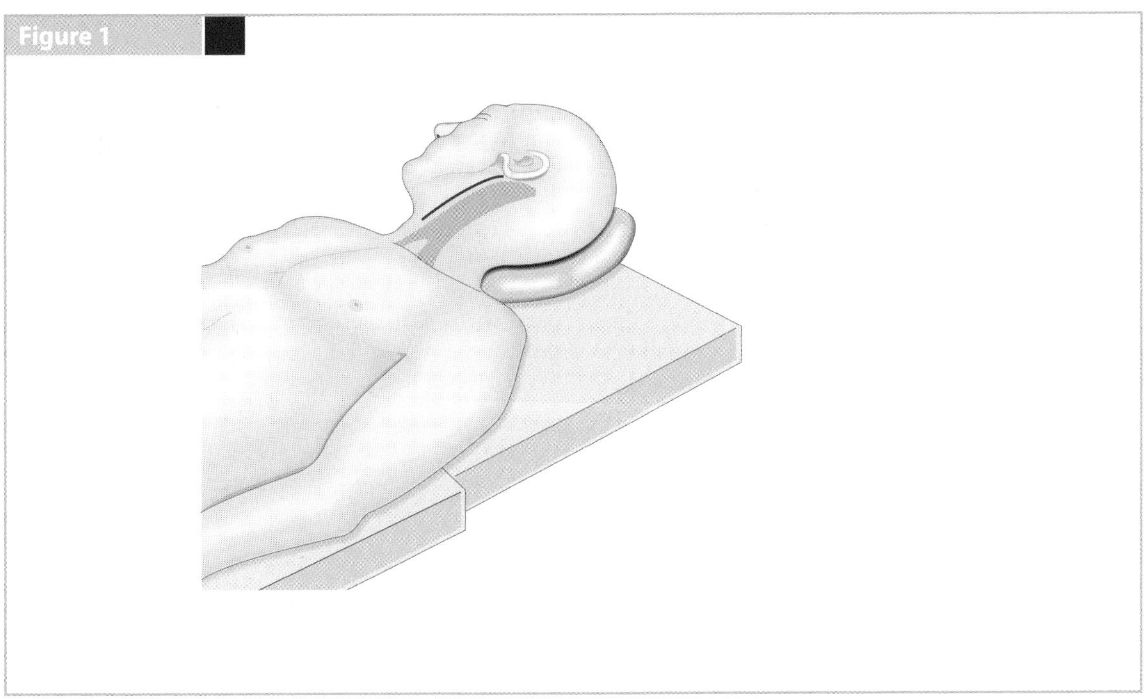

Figure 1

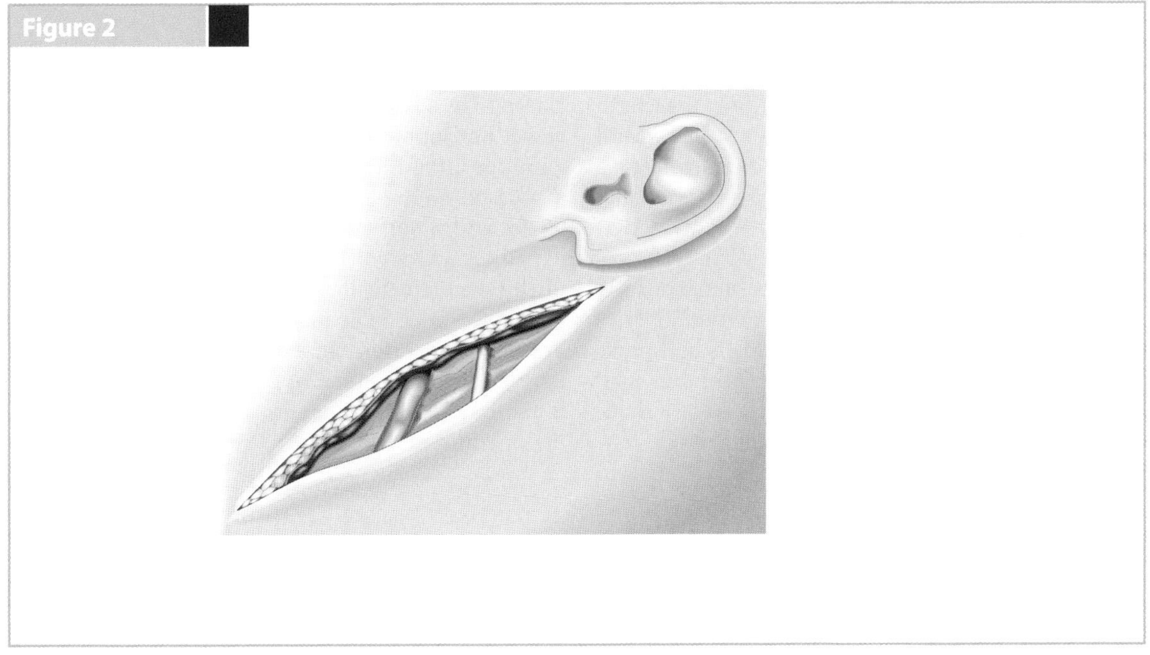

Figure 2

Figure 3

The dissection is deepened on to the internal jugular vein and its common facial branch: the latter is divided to expose the underlying common carotid artery. Superiorly the dissection is carried down to the posterior belly of the digastric muscle, passing behind the lower pole of the parotid gland. Bleeding is common in this area and is treated with diathermy. Inferiorly the middle thyroid vein may require ligation and the omohyoid muscle may have small vessels passing along its upper border, requiring division and diathermy, when further exposure is required. A variable number of lymph nodes lie anterior to the internal jugular vein, covering the carotid bifurcation, common facial vein, hypoglossal nerve and its descendens hypoglossi branch. The nodes are dissected anteriorly, small vessels requiring diathermy. A bloodless field ensures good visualization of the hypoglossal nerve, which may be adherent to the deep surface of the common facial vein, and additional pharyngeal veins may be encountered deep to the posterior belly of the digastric muscle.

Figure 4

The hypoglossal nerve is mobilized as it crosses the internal and external carotid arteries. Its descendens hypoglossi branch (ansa cervicalis) follows the length of the internal and common carotid arteries within the operative field. This is mobilized and retracted medially and the self-retaining retractor gradually deepened. The ansa cervicalis may be divided if needed to entrance the exposure. The ansa cervicalis may be divided if needed to entrance the exposure. The common, internal and external carotid arteries are mobilized by sharp dissection. This is undertaken away from the bifurcation where thrombus may be present over the atheromatous disease. By holding the vessel's adventitia and adjacent tissue, tension can be applied and the plane developed close to the vessel wall, mobilizing each side in turn until the two planes meet. This allows the jaws of the vascular clamp to be subsequently passed on either side of the vessel and approximated for temporary occlusion. Once the circumferential plane has been established, a pointed suture passer can be placed around the vessel and a soft sling drawn through. This is not usually required of the internal carotid artery and must be avoided if the dissection is adjacent to suspected thrombogenic material. The superior thyroid branch of the external carotid artery is gently mobilized and a double loop of the thread applied so that it can be tightened to control backbleeding later in the operation.

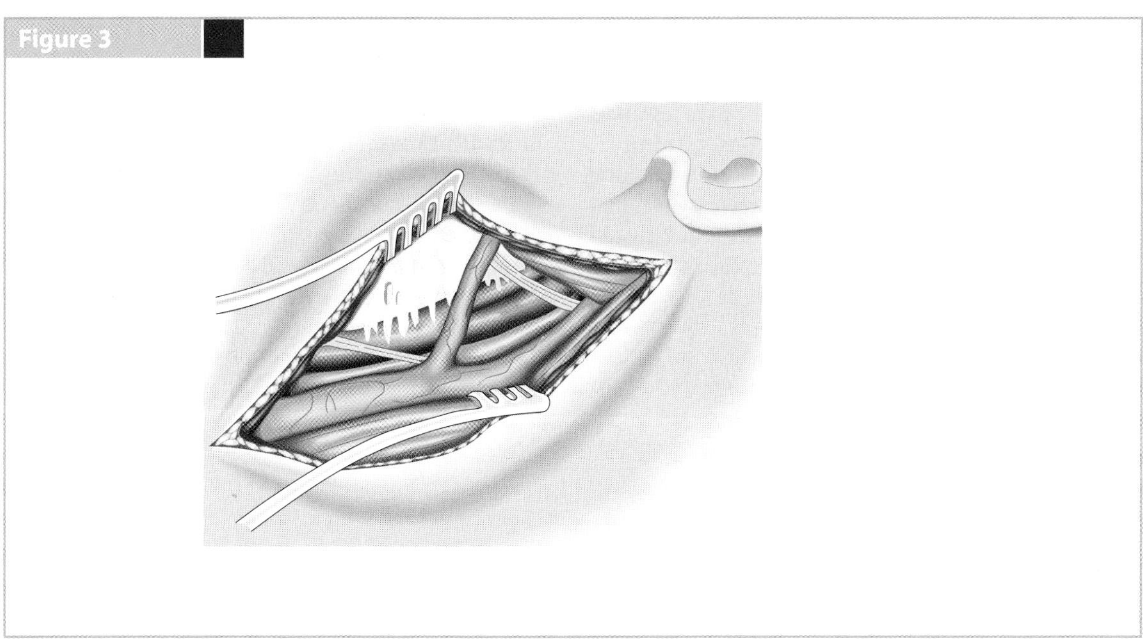
Figure 3

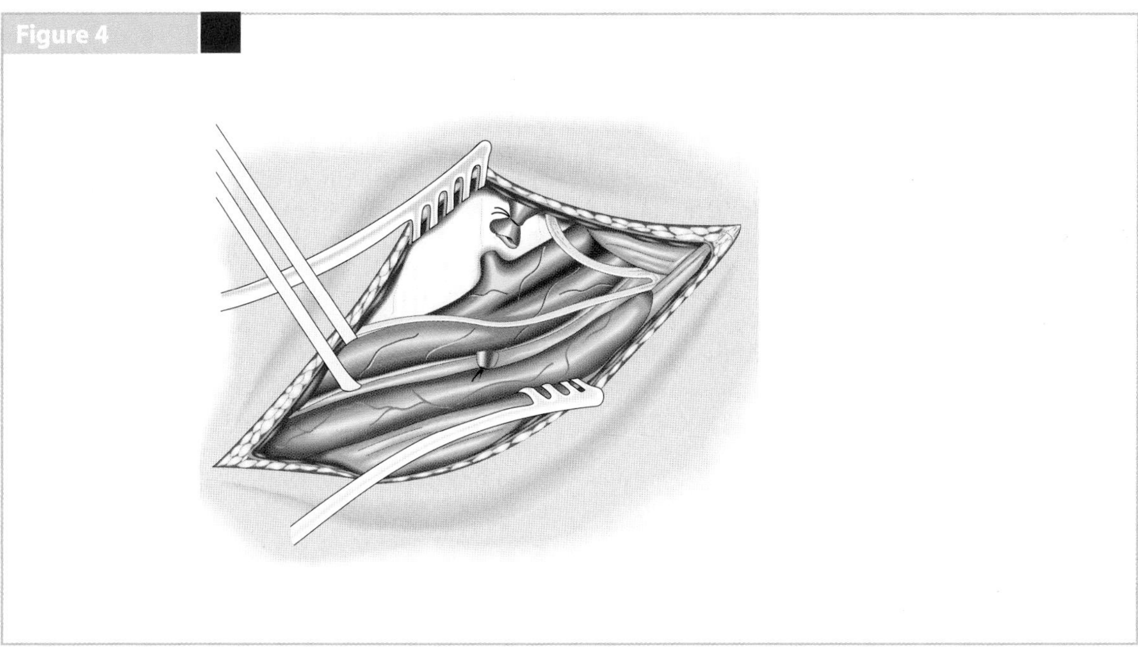
Figure 4

Figure 5

Surgeons vary in their use of heparin. Blood should not clot in the normal vessel away from the bifurcation during the time of clamping but systemic heparinization does provide some security against this eventuality. Heparinized saline should be used for flushing the interior of the vessel during endarterectomy.

Lightweight vascular clamps are used; clamping starts with the internal carotid artery to reduce the risk of embolization through this vessel during the clamping procedure. A sling around the common carotid artery allows gentle manipulation of the vessel once the internal carotid artery has been secured to ensure that the proximal clamp is appropriately applied.

Figure 6

Once the three carotid arteries have been clamped and the double loop around the superior thyroid artery tightened, an incision is made along the anterolateral aspect of the carotid bifurcation. The point of a No. 11 scalpel blade is inserted obliquely with the cutting edge outwards so that once the lumen is entered, the blade can be drawn outwards to commence a longitudinal arteriotomy.

Figure 5

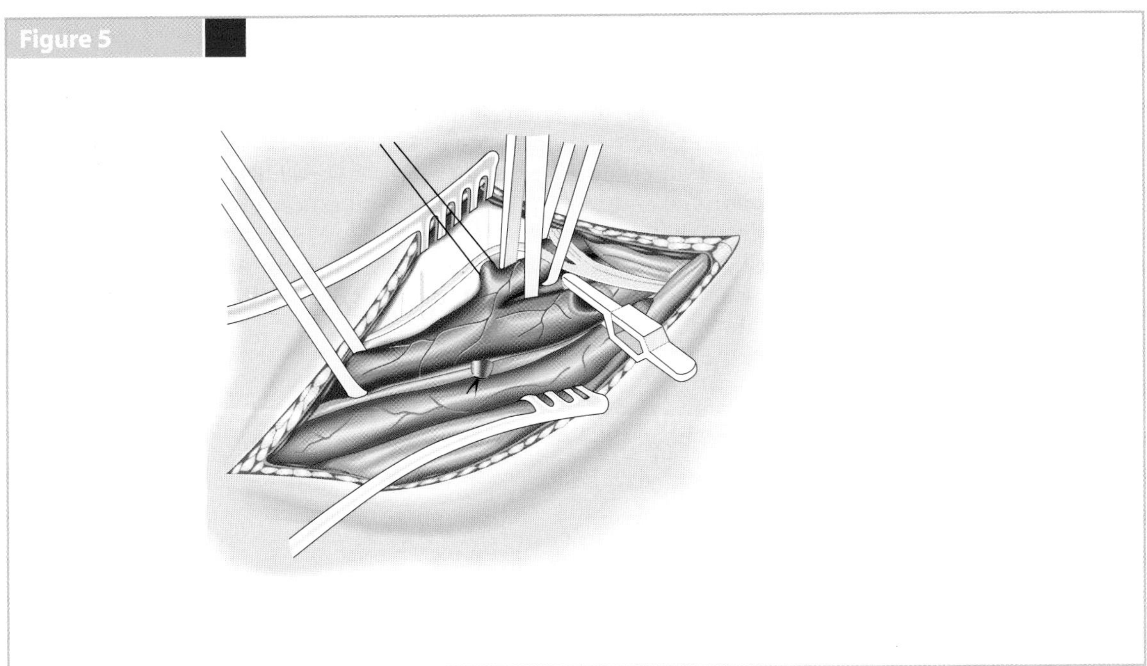

Figure 6

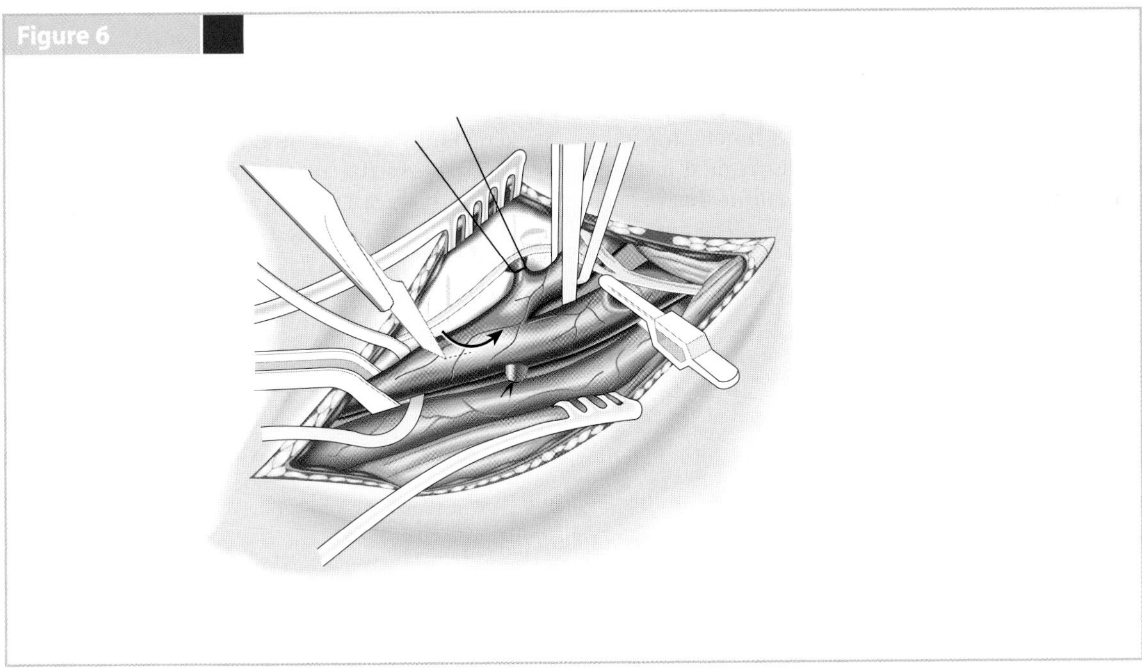

Figure 7

Once the lumen is entered, one blade of a pair of Potts angle scissors is inserted and the longitudinal arteriotomy extended in each direction beyond the diseased segment. The arteriotomy follows an anterolateral course in both common and internal carotid arteries. Proximally, the disease is continuous to the level of the aorta, but the severe irregular thickening is usually confined to the distal centimeter of the common carotid; otherwise the vessel is palpated to find a target area of lesser disease where the endarterectomy can be stopped. Distally the arteriotomy on the anterolateral aspect of the internal carotid is taken beyond the severe disease, this being usually within 1–2 centimeters of its origin (shunting is considered in chapter 5).

Figure 8

A dissector is used to define the plane for endarterectomy, there being usually two distinct planes of cleavage. The inner is a thickened, irregular longitudinal length of atheroma with the intima that may be ulcerated and covered with thrombus. The outer layer is yellow and uniform in thickness: it is a layer of thickened intimomedial fibers that may peel off easily as a circular strip, but which can also be left in situ if firmly adherent to the wall. The two layers may peel together off the underlying pinkish medial wall.

Figure 7

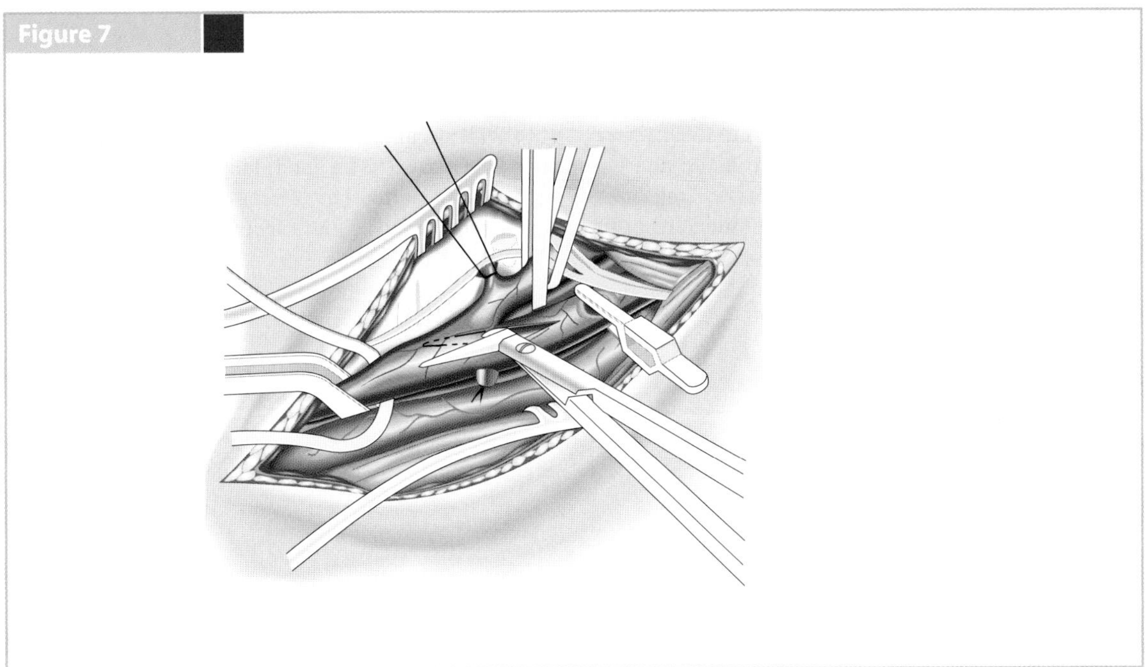

Figure 8

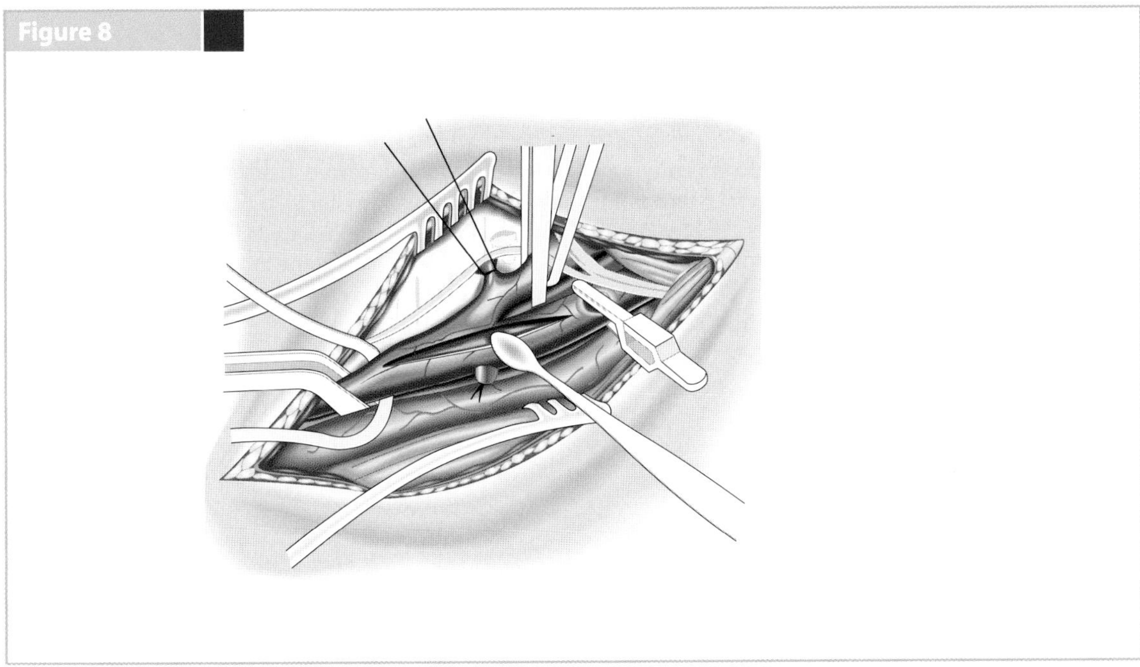

1

Figure 9

The inner core of atheroma is gently mobilized along its length until an end point is reached in the internal carotid artery: here it thins down to a transparent thin layer of intima. This is gently pulled free but a clean end point must be seen and obtained either by cutting the adherent intima close to the wall, or by pulling it down to tear it without residual frills. It may be necessary to extend the incision to obtain such an end point. The absence of any residual frills is tested by flushing and careful excision.

Figures 10, 11

Proximally, obtaining a satisfactory end point may be more difficult. The core of atheroma is gently mobilized from each side towards the chosen end point and then cut flush with the artery obliquely so there is a chamfering with a smooth end point circumferentially. On rare occasions it may not be possible to obtain a good end point in the common carotid artery, in which case a longitudinally placed vascular suture may be inserted from outside the vessel to gently pin down any loose intimal edge. This is even more uncommon in the internal carotid artery, where it is advisable to follow the atheroma until it reaches its thin end point.

Figure 9

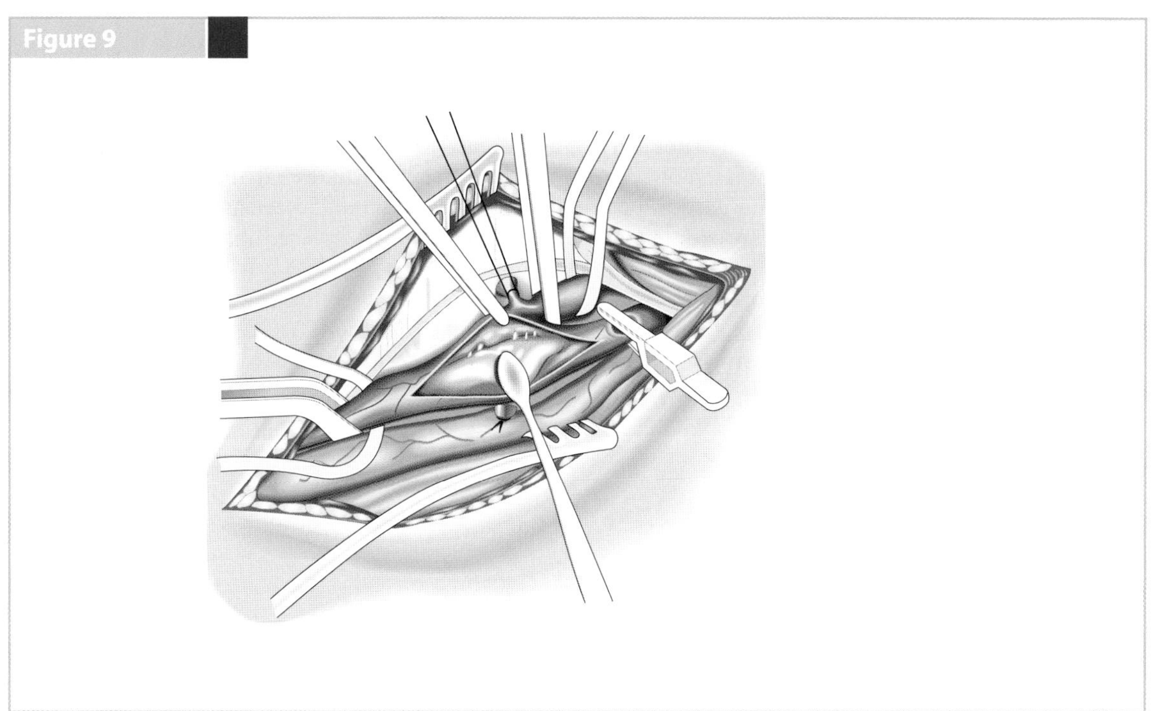

Figure 10

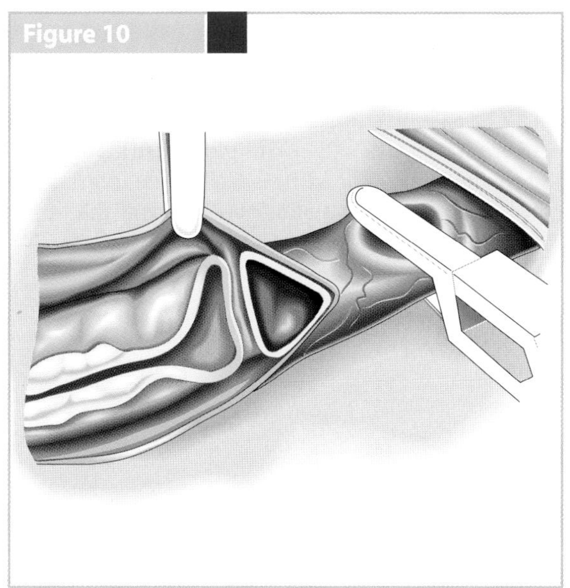

Figure 11

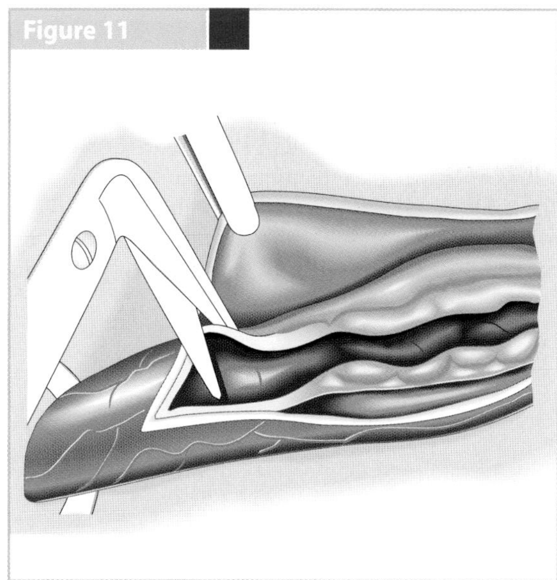

Figure 12

The atheromatous core extends into the external carotid artery, usually for 5–10 mm. It is mobilized around the origin so it can be gently teased out. The clamp on the external carotid artery is used to push the origin of the vessel forwards, and by countertraction on the cut wall the origin may thus be everted in "nipple-link" fashion, allowing the core to be visualized to the point where it thins out and can be gently pulled away leaving a thin adherent intimal edge. If this is not satisfactorily obtained, the forceps and clamp are pulled in opposite directions to allow the surgeon to look along the length of the lumen and use forceps to withdraw residual atheroma up to the level of the clamp. On the rare occasion when a good end point is not obtained, an additional longitudinal arteriotomy may be placed distally in the external carotid artery to withdraw residual thick atheromatous plaque. Copious flushing is used to identify residual fronds of atheroma requiring removal, these being usually transverse strips of the outer atheromatous layer.

Figure 13

When the endarterectomy is complete and good end points have been obtained in all three carotid vessels with a smooth endarterectomized wall, either through the pinkish medial layer or smooth residual outer atheromatous covering, the clamps are briefly removed on each vessel in turn to ensure good forward- or backbleeding. Residual clot is flushed away. Closure starts with a distal simple suture incorporating the normal full thickness wall of the internal carotid artery above the endarterectomy at the upper extreme of the incision.

Figure 12

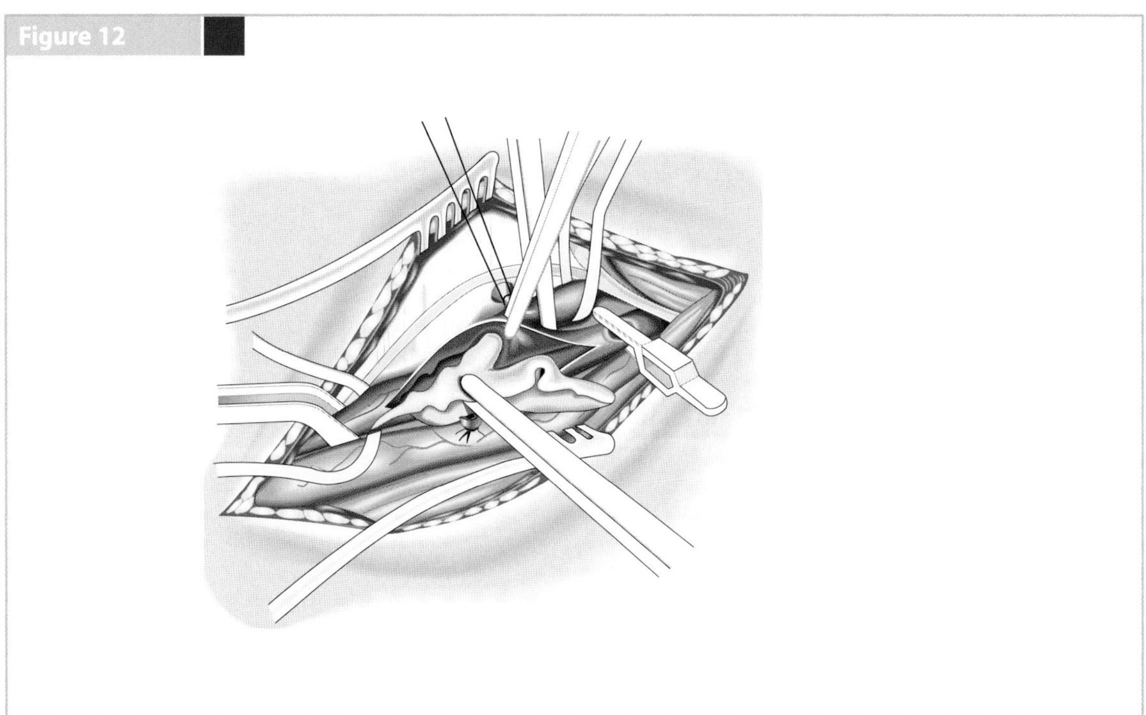

Figure 13

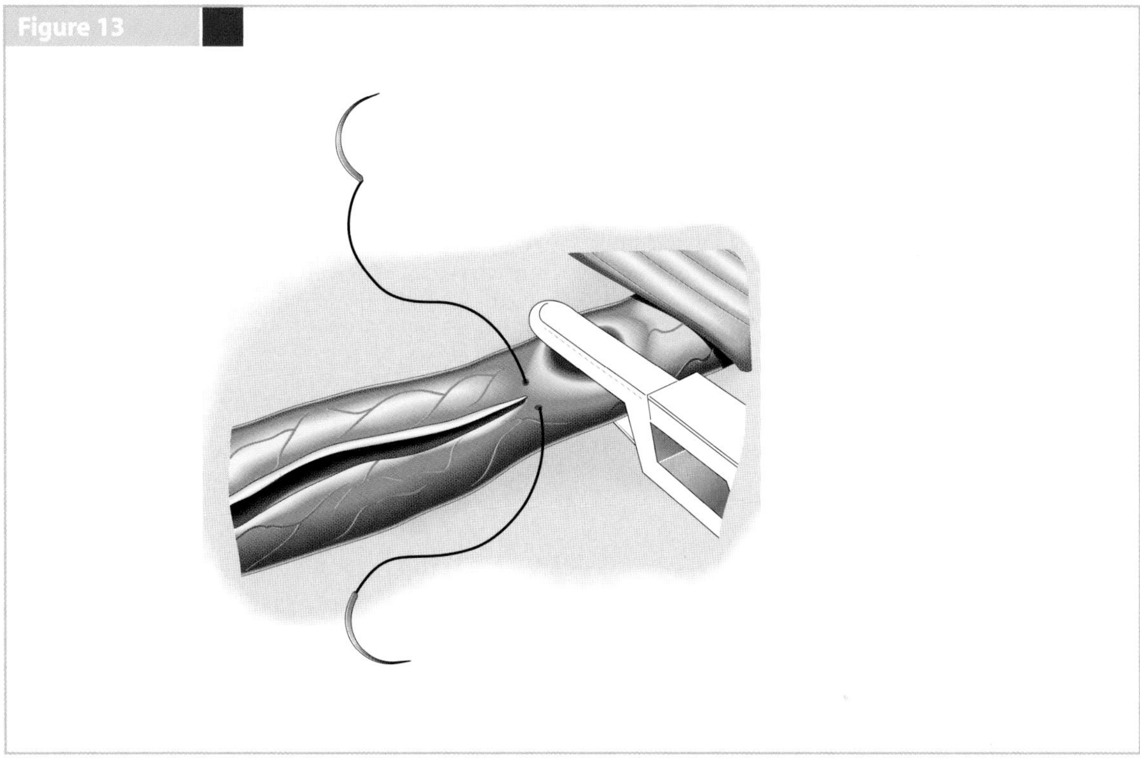

1

Figure 14

A continuous suture of a 6/0 vascular suture is used. Another suture is started in the common carotid artery, and tied to the first where they meet.

Figure 15

If the proximal atheromatous layer is not adherent to the wall, a second suture may be used to pin this down at the proximal limit of the arteriotomy, to ensure that the stitch can be seen to hold the atheroma in place rather than be the blind end tie of a single suture. As the suture line is almost complete, further flooding of the segment with heparinized saline solution is undertaken to remove any residual debris and to fill the segment with fluid, removing any air bubbles. At this stage the loop may be released around the superior thyroid artery to allow blood to fill the segment, flushing out any remaining bubbles. When a single suture is used for closure, it must carry on into the full thickness of the proximal vessel beyond the arteriotomy to ensure sound closure: an additional loop is applied for tying. The internal carotid artery clamp is removed first to ensure that there are no leaks, then the external. Finally, digital pressure is applied across the origin of the internal carotid artery while the common carotid artery clamp is released. This ensures that any residual debris selectively passes into the external rather than the internal carotid system. When all clamps have been removed, a swab is retained over the anastomosis for a few minutes.

Figure 14

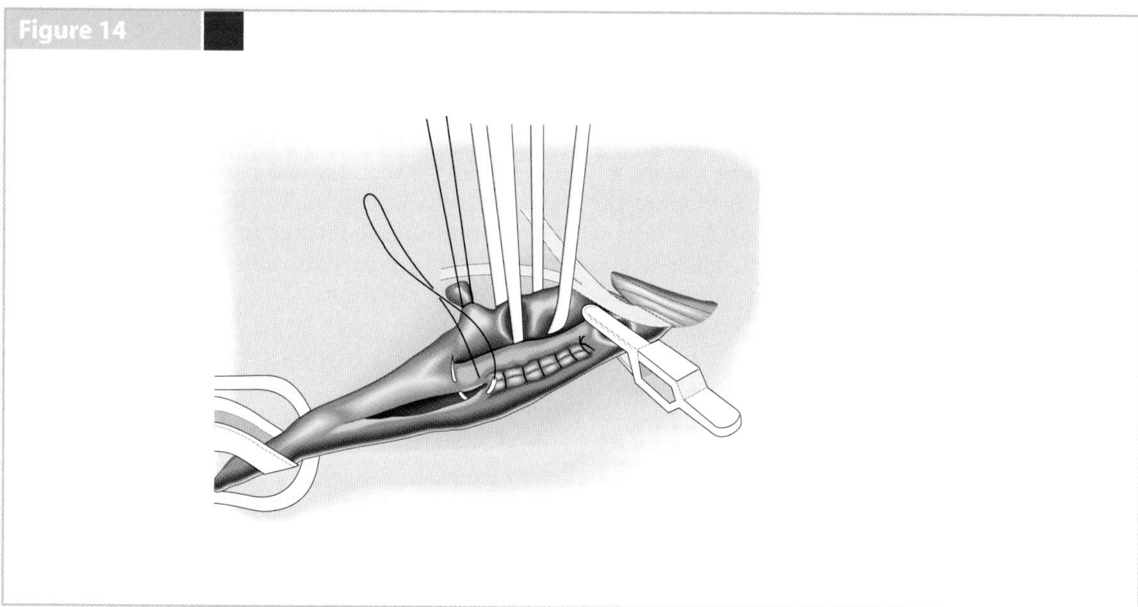

Figure 15

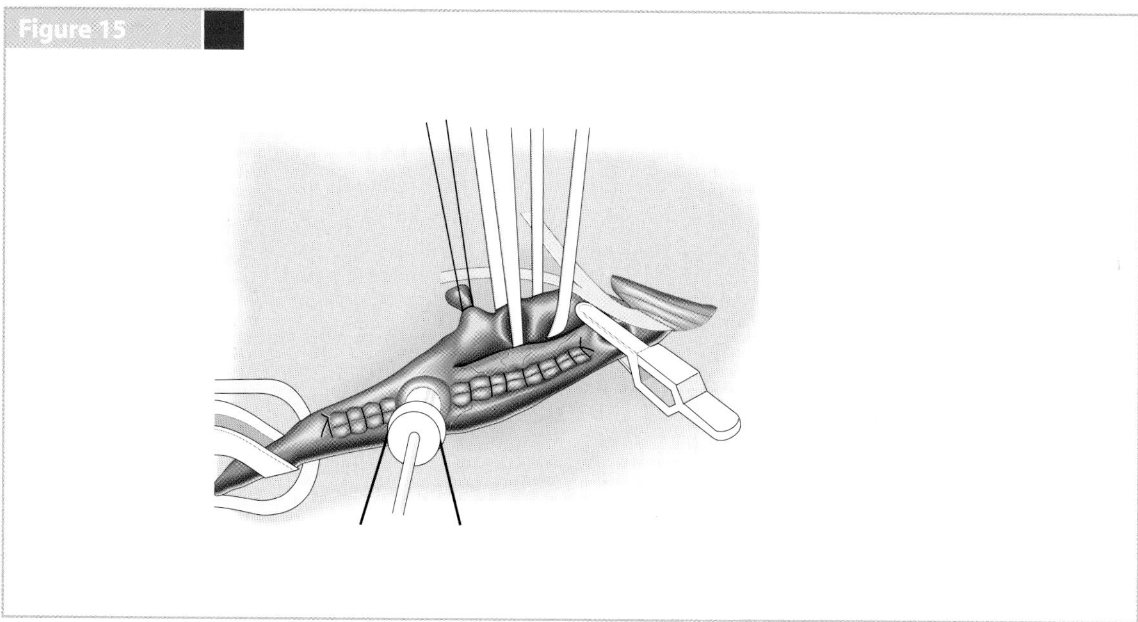

Figure 16

A patch is inserted in patients with small or damaged vessels, women or patients with recurrent carotid disease. Closure with a patch has gained wider acceptance in the US, with many surgeons adopting the policy of routine patching. There has also been a shift toward using a prosthetic patch rather than a venous one. Vein patches carry a small risk of rupture, especially with ankle saphenous veins. In addition to decreasing the availability of venous conduit for future use as a bypass, the inconvenience of having to harvest the vein and the patient's complaints about the leg wound make prosthetic patches more attractive. Current prosthetic patches have a lower chance of aneurysmal dilation, but still carry a small risk of patch infection.

Figure 17

Secure hemostasis must be achieved before closure, particular attention being given to venous bleeding. Large veins need to be ligated and the ends of smaller veins accurately diathermied. A suction drainage tube is laid along the length of the dissected carotid sheath and brought out laterally through the skin adjacent to the lower end of the incision and secured with a skin suture. A subcutaneous absorbable suture includes the divided platysma muscle in the lower half of the wound. Skin sutures or clips are applied along with a dry dressing.

Initially quarter-hour observations include monitoring for an adequate airway, pulse, blood pressure and neurological observations that, on regaining consciousness, include: limb and facial movements, hand grips and pupillary responses.

Hemorrhage is identified by bleeding through the dressing, neck swelling, with or without tracheal compression, and blood collected in the drainage bottle. As heparin is not usually reversed, some hemorrhage can be expected through the dressing and in the drainage bottle, but this should subside within 2 h. Continued hemorrhage of greater than 100 ml/h and/or tracheal compression may require reexploration, evacuation of the hematoma and securing hemostasis.

Hypotension unrelated to blood loss is common, this being related to reactivation of baroreceptors, which usually takes 6–8 h to reset volume replacement and rarely the use of vasopressor drugs may be needed.

Whereas controlled hypotension is rarely followed by neurological sequelae, hypertension is more serious as it may both indicate and accentuate cerebral ischemia. It must be treated by a careful titration of a rapid reacting hypotensive agent to maintain normotension, avoiding overcorrection which may be harmful in this situation.

A stroke that is present on regaining consciousness is probably a peroperative event and its presence may have been anticipated if there had been technical problems with suspected embolization or failure of backbleeding from the internal carotid artery. In these circumstances, reoperation is unlikely to improve the situation. The onset of a stroke after initial full recovery must be immediately identified and if severe and more than transient, requires immediate reexploration of the endarterectomized vessel.

Although non-invasive studies, such as transcranial Doppler monitoring, may facilitate the diagnosis, they should in no way delay the reexploration, since the usual finding is thrombosis of the endarterectomized origin of the internal carotid artery. At the operation there is rarely any unsuspected local flap or other technical abnormality to explain the thrombosis. The possible explanation is slowing of cerebral blood flow within the ipsilateral hemisphere, with consequent thrombus formation within the thrombogenic endarterectomized segment. This reperfusion syndrome is usually seen in tight stenosis, and it is postulated that the reestablishment of the normal blood flow in a previously poorly perfused area produces a reactive precapillary spasm, with resultant stasis. A calcium channel blocker may reduce this incidence and following reexploration it is advised

Figure 16

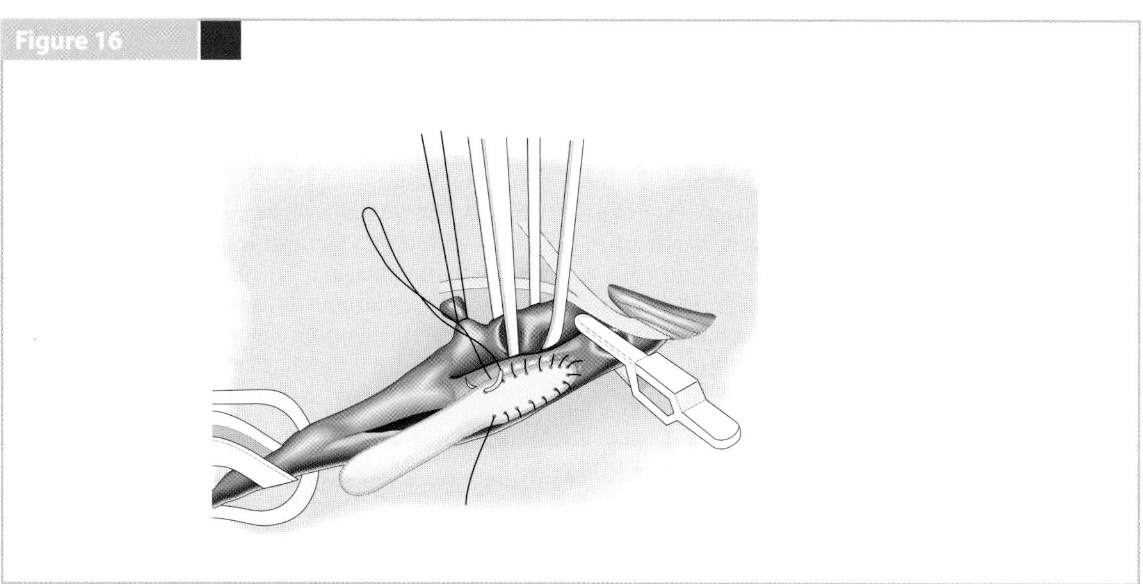

Figure 17

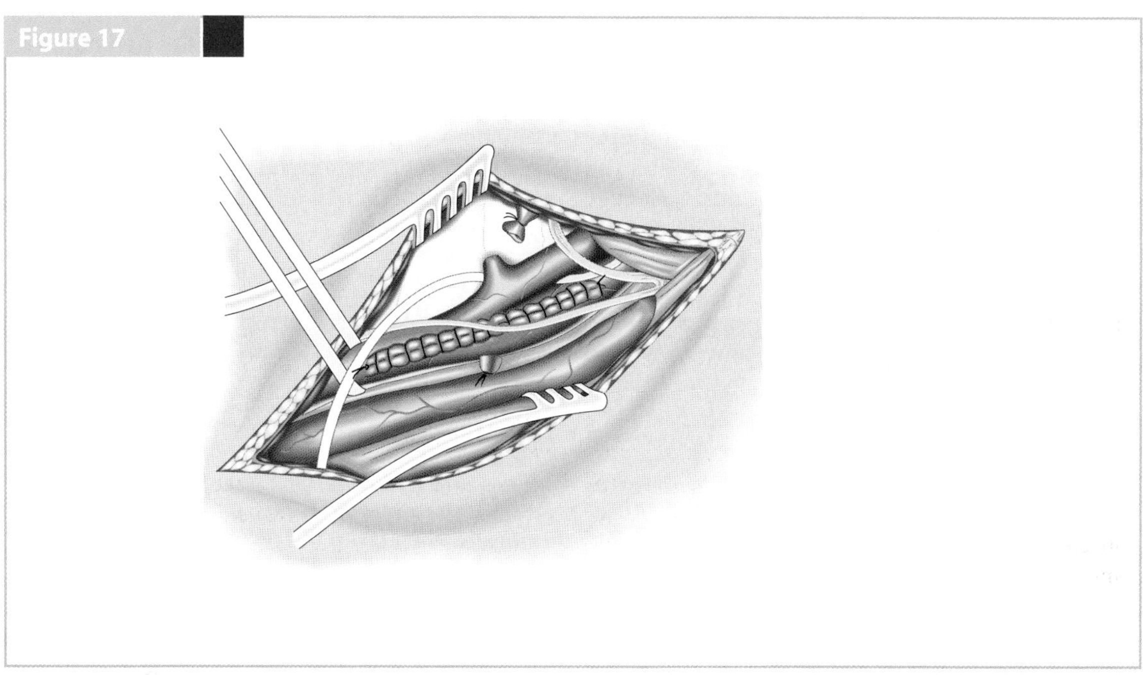

Figure 17 (Continued)

that the patient is ventilated over the next 12 h to ensure precise control of airway and blood pressure.

The epidural cannula and drain are removed after 12 h, or when they are no longer required; skin clips are removed on the fourth and fifth postoperative day.

Restenosis of an endarterectomized vessel is probably in the region of 10%, due to atheroma proximal or distal to the endarterectomy rather than further disease across the operative segment. However, the precise Figure is not known since TIAs and strokes are unusual post carotid endarterectomy, and routine postoperative imaging of these vessels is not widely reported. Occasionally reported is a small number of patients with a smooth fibrotic reaction across the endarterectomy which can produce tight stenosis within 1–2 years. Re-endarterectomy is difficult in these vessels and graft interposition between the common and internal carotid arteries may be appropriate.

CONCLUSION

The high incidence of death and disability from stroke demand the continued search for safe and effective preventive measures. Identification of individuals at risk is usually a history of transient ischemic attacks and amaurosis fugax, but screening of high-risk populations, particularly in cardiac and peripheral vascular units, produces a high incidence of patients with internal carotid artery stenosis. Epidemiological studies have demonstrated that stenoses of greater than 70% and echolucent plaques have the highest stroke risk. Intervention must produce minimal operative stroke risk and provide long-term stroke prophylaxis. The current risk of death and severe stroke morbidity of 3–5% following carotid endarterectomy has not changed over the last quarter of a century, and research for safer operative techniques and better cerebral protection must continue. Each unit undertaking these procedures should maintain a strict audit, to document all aspects of their practice, searching for ways of improving the management of this devastating disease.

SELECTED BIBLIOGRAPHY

Barnett HJ, Taylor DW, Eliasziw M, Fox AJ, Ferguson GG, Haynes RB, Rankin RN, Clagett GP, Hachinski VC, Sackett DL, Thorpe KE, Meldrum HE (1998) Benefit of carotid endarterectomy in patients with symptomatic moderate or severe stenosis. North American Symptomatic Carotid Endarterectomy Trial Collaborators. N Engl J Med 339:1415–1425

MRC European Carotid Surgery Trial (1998) Randomised trial of endarterectomy for recently symptomatic carotid stenosis: final results of the MRC European Carotid Surgery Trial 1998. Lancet 351:1379–1387

North American Symptomatic Carotid Endarterectomy Trial Collaborators (1991) Beneficial effect of carotid endarterectomy in symptomatic patients with high-grade carotid stenosis. N Engl J Med 325:445–453

Executive Committee for the Asymptomatic Carotid Atherosclerosis Study (1995) Endarterectomy for asymptomatic carotid artery stenosis. JAMA 273 1421–1428

European Carotid Surgery Trialists' Collaborative Group (1991) MRC European Carotid Surgery Trial: interim results for symptomatic patients with severe (70–99%) or with mild (0–29%) carotid stenosis (1991). Lancet 337:1235–1243

CHAPTER 2

Eversion Carotid Endarterectomy

R. Clement Darling III, Sean P. Roddy, Manish Mehta, Philip S.K. Paty, Kathleen J. Ozsvath, Paul B. Kreienberg, Benjamin B. Chang, Dhiraj M. Shah

INTRODUCTION

Several randomized trials have validated the use of carotid endarterectomy (CEA) for management of hemodynamically significant symptomatic and asymptomatic carotid artery stenosis (Executive Committee for the Asymptomatic Carotid Atherosclerosis Study 1995; North American Symptomatic Carotid Endarterectomy Trial Collaborators 1991). Classically, CEA has been accomplished through a longitudinal arteriotomy either primarily closed or with a patch comprising autogenous or prosthetic material (Hertzer et al. 1987).

The incidence of recurrent stenosis following standard longitudinal CEA ranges from 2% to 30% (Healy et al. 1989). Patch angioplasty closure requires either vein harvest or the use of a prosthetic, which may increase the incidence of bleeding and infection (Archie 1986; Hertzer et al. 1987; Lord et al. 1989). Furthermore, closure of a longitudinal carotid arteriotomy, even with patch, may not reduce restenosis of the distal internal carotid artery (ICA), where it is most narrow. In order to successfully negotiate these technical hurdles and minimize restenosis, occlusion, and stroke, some surgeons have turned to the alternative technique of eversion CEA (Darling et al. 2000; DeBakey et al. 1959; Kasparzak and Raithel 1989).

Eversion CEA has a history almost as old as CEA itself. A report by DeBakey et al. in 1959 illustrated the use of an everting technique in which the distal common carotid artery (CCA) was transected and the atheroma removed by everting the bifurcation while the internal and external carotid arteries remained attached (DeBakey et al. 1959). Both branches were left connected, with limited cephalad plaque exposure and visualization of the distal end point. Hence, this technique was considered unreliable in patients whose disease extended beyond the bifurcation, and the eversion technique never gained acceptance. For many years, the most effective application of the eversion endarterectomy technique involved its use in the external iliac and common femoral arteries, where surgeons were able to visualize the end points and perform autogenous arterial reconstructions with excellent results (Darling et al. 1993).

Separately, Berguer et al., and Kasparzak and Raithel in 1989, revised the DeBakey eversion CEA technique by transecting the ICA at the carotid bulb and reported their results of decreased recurrent stenosis and occlusion (Kasparzak and Raithel 1989). The primary advantage of eversion CEA is that the ICA is divided at the largest part of the two vessels, and the subsequent anastomosis onto the CCA is easier with less potential for a closure related restenosis (Darling et al. 2000). This avoids a distal ICA suture line where the artery is narrow and its closure is prone to restenosis. Furthermore, the improved visualization facilitates plaque extraction, and management of the end points. These two seemingly small advantages in experienced hands result in reduced carotid cross-clamp time, total operative time, the incidence of carotid restenosis, and stroke mortality rates.

The technique of standard CEA has been performed with excellent results over the past 3 decades. Most surgeons are reluctant to change but there is always room for improvement. The eversion CEA technique offers just that by displacing the anastomosis from a narrow distal ICA to a larger carotid bulb and proximal ICA.

Surgeons adopting eversion CEA need not change the majority of their technique. The anesthetic choice as well as methods of cerebral monitoring and protection can be the same for both eversion and standard longitudinal CEA. We prefer eversion CEA under cervical block anesthesia, with selective shunting only in patients who develop neurological deterioration during cross-clamping (Chang et al. 2000).

As currently conceived, eversion CEA can be used to treat almost all cases of primary carotid bifurcation disease and selective cases of recurrent stenosis. This technique is ideal for treatment of carotid arteries with kinks or loops, as shortening of the ICA can be incorporated within the process of eversion.

The extent of disease at the bifurcation may affect one's ease in performing CEA by any method. Disease limited to or near the bifurcation is much easier to treat than disease that extends distally into the ICA. External visualization is used to adequately evaluate the distal extension of the atherosclerotic plaque prior to division of the ICA. Transition from a yellow atheromatous abnormal plaque to a smooth purplish pliable normal distal ICA usually signifies the type of disease that is easily correctable via eversion endarterectomy. Treatment of extensive disease in the ICA up to or beyond the level of the digastric muscle can be more difficult: such cases should be reserved until ample experience with eversion CEA is gained.

2

Figure 1

Exposure of the carotid artery is identical with either method of endarterectomy. Although circumferential dissection of the ICA along its length is a necessary part of the eversion technique, this is best managed after clamping and division of the ICA. Thus, only sufficient dissection to accommodate the clamps need be performed initially. Following carotid artery exposure, the ICA should be externally examined. The plaque end point is visualized as the transition from the yellowish diseased artery to the normal bluish artery. Ideally the clamp should be placed across the normal artery well above the transition zone as this makes eversion of the ICA and examination of the end point easier. When the plaque extends cephalad to what is attainable by the usual measures of division of the ansa cervicalis, mobilization of the hypoglossal nerve and division of the digastric muscle, an endarterectomy is difficult by any technique. In such cases, the operator should use whatever method is more familiar. The patient is systemically anticoagulated (30 u/kg body weight of intravenous heparin) and the carotid arteries are clamped. The ICA is obliquely divided at the carotid bulb. The line of transection should be in the range of 30–60 degrees from the horizontal and extend on to the CCA, encompassing most of the plaque. It is important for the line of transection to end in the crotch of the carotid bulb and not higher up into the internal or external carotids; failure to do so is not necessarily catastrophic but can increase the complexity of the anastomosis.

Figure 2

After division, cephalad and lateral traction on the ICA helps with circumferential mobilization. This consists of the carotid sinus tissue medially and the looser areolar tissue posteriorly, in which the vagus nerve usually resides. Dissection close to and along the divided ICA mobilizes the remaining length of artery while avoiding injury to the adjacent structures.

Once freed from the surrounding tissue, some ICA redundancy is generally recognized in relation to the CCA. This redundancy may range from a very few millimeters to several centimeters in cases presenting with carotid kinks or loops. The heel of the ICA (side formerly adherent to the carotid body) is divided longitudinally such that it lines up with the upper end of the common carotid arteriotomy. The anterolateral border of the CCA is extended proximally to match the length of internal carotid arteriotomy. The resultant opening of the carotid arteries is usually 15–30 mm in length; this is important as the extra length allows a wider anastomosis which is easily performed with a lower chance of restenosis. Patients with extensively redundant ICAs require oblique *resection of a segment of ICA* excision of the ICA to match the common carotid arteriotomy. When CCA plaque cannot be adequately removed by eversion, the arteriotomy should be extended proximally to facilitate complete endarterectomy. Closure of the additional common carotid arteriotomy may be accomplished by "pulling down" the ICA and using it as a patch over the common carotid arteriotomy. Alternatively, the proximal common carotid arteriotomy may be closed primarily. The latter results in a Y-shaped suture line where the linear common carotid closure meets the circumferential CCA–ICA suture line.

Figure 1

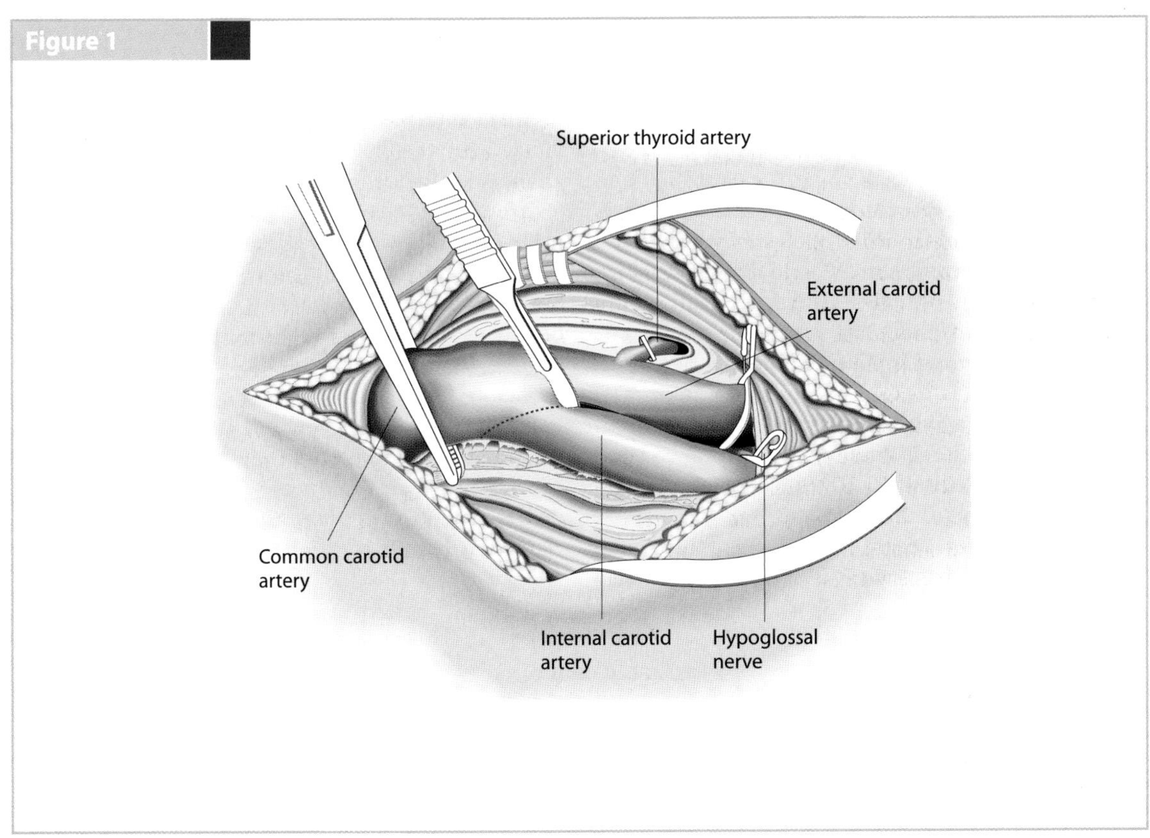

Figure 2

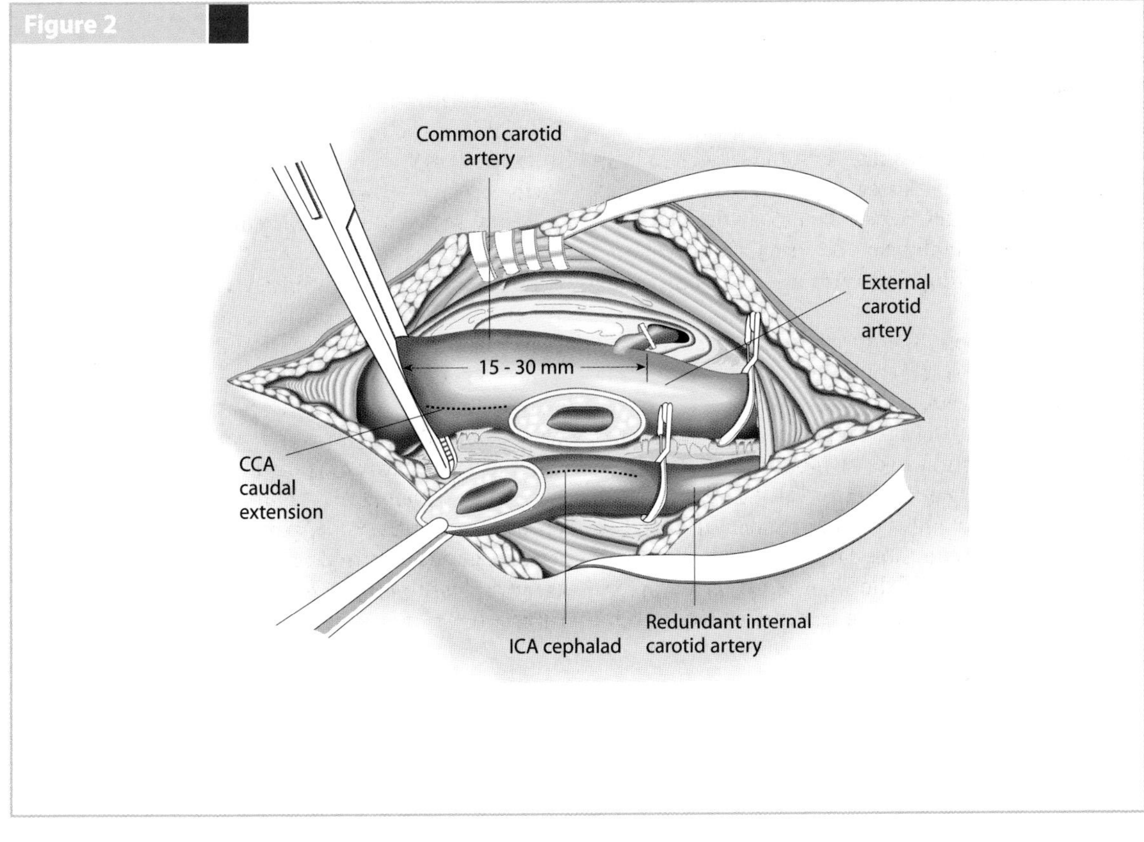

Figure 3

Removing the bulk of the ICA plaque is a simple maneuver that usually can be accomplished expeditiously. The standard CEA plane is established and the adventitia is elevated from the plaque circumferentially. The adventitia is everted along the entire length of the atherosclerotic plaque until a distal intimal end point is observed similar to rolling up a sleeve. One forceps holds the plaque in place while the other provides cephalad traction on the adventitia. If the plaque is merely pulled out without fully everting the artery, the end point is poorly visualized. If the adventitia is merely pushed cephalad and not everted, the redundant adventitia obstructs adequate visualization of the end point.

As the end point is reached, the bulk of the plaque usually separates from the distal intima relatively cleanly. Alternatively, the plaque may be sharply divided with either fine scissors or a scalpel. Loose atherosclerotic debris can be shaved off of the wall. If a carotid shunt is needed, it can be inserted either prior to or following the endarterectomy.

The superior visualization of the endpoint prior to arterial closure of the artery is one of the advantages of this technique, as compared to conventional endarterectomy. This is the most critical step of the procedure and the operator should take the time to make the end point as perfect as possible. Gentle irrigation of the end point with heparin saline solution can also facilitate removal of loose atherosclerotic debris. *The external carotid endarterectomy is carried out using the eversion technique.*

Figure 3

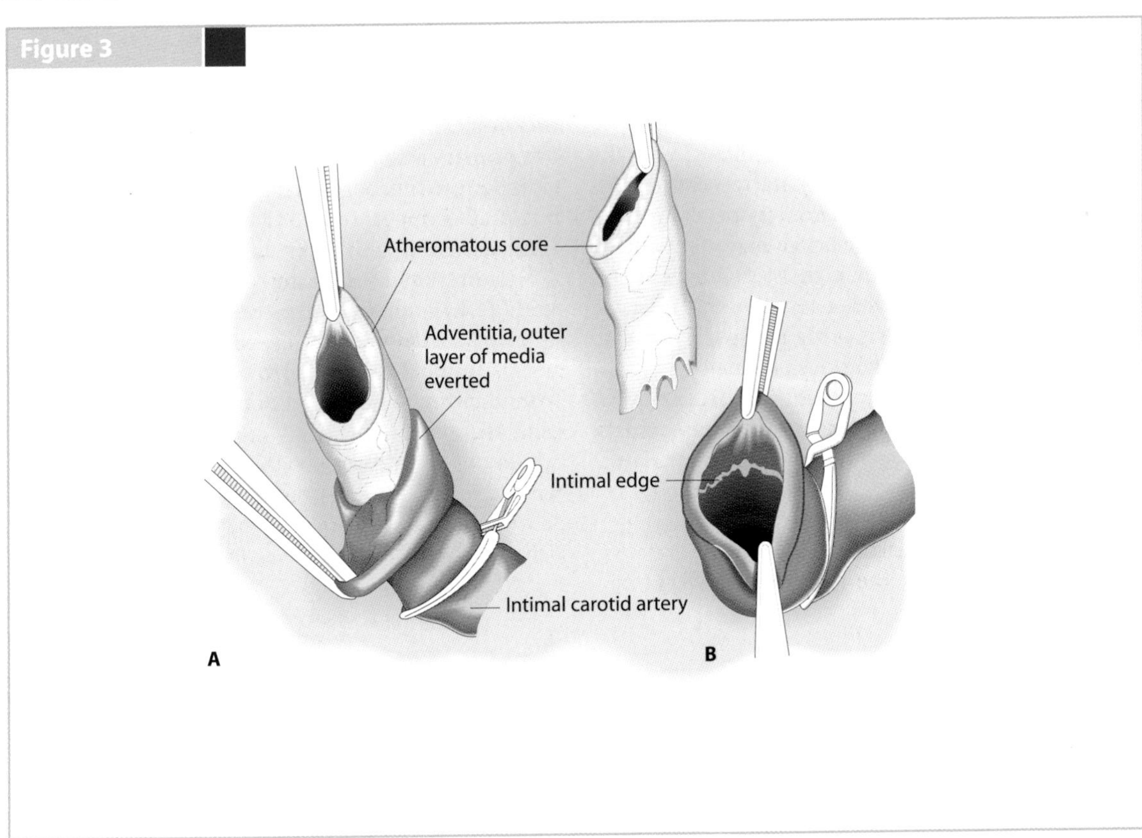
Atheromatous core
Adventitia, outer layer of media everted
Intimal edge
Intimal carotid artery
A
B

Figure 4A, B

A fine monofilament nonabsorbable suture (i.e., 6-0 polypropylene) is used to reattach the ICA to the distal CCA. The suture is usually started at the most cephalad ends of both arteriotomies and completed using a parachuted technique. The major advantage of eversion endarterectomy is that the common and internal carotid arteriotomies (15–30 mm) are used to "patch" each other. It is fairly straightforward to sew the arteries together without producing a stenosis. Because one of the major technical issues of CEA is resolved by simplifying the arterial anastomosis, eversion CEA obviates the need for patching or tedious primary closure of the distal ICA. The anastomosis is done in the more accessible center of the wound, not in the upper reach. Clamps are released in a similar fashion to that in standard longitudinal CEA; flow is first established into the external carotid artery (ECA) and subsequently into the ICA. Flow is assessed by Doppler ultrasound and the awake patients monitored for neurologic changes. Type of wound closure and use of drains is at the discretion of the surgeon.

Figure 4A

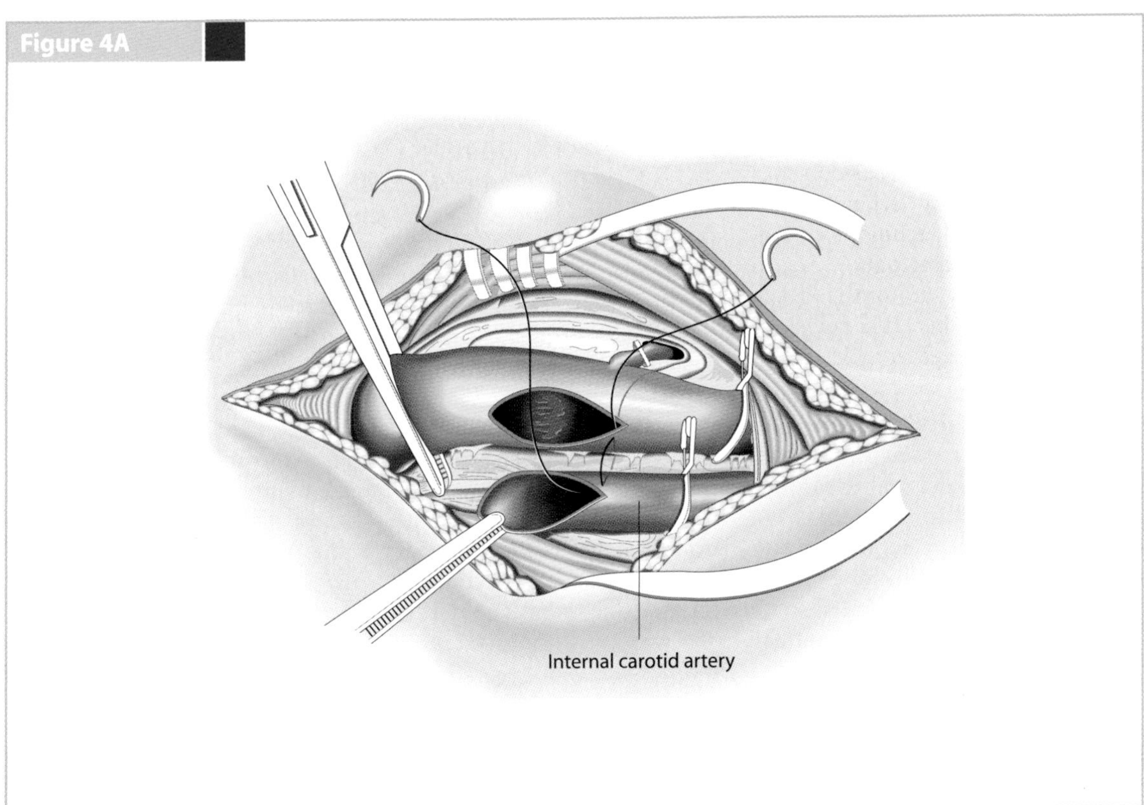

Figure 4B

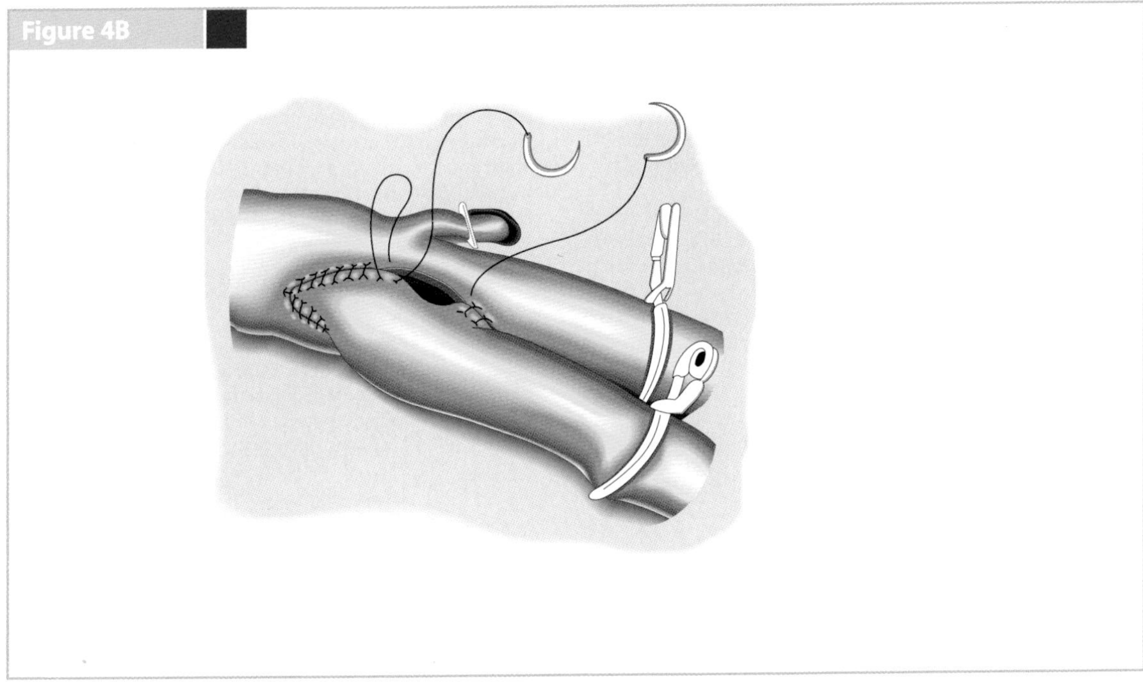

CONCLUSION

Carotid endarterectomy by the eversion technique has proven to be a durable method that encompasses the entire scope of normal carotid surgeries. Although it is uniquely useful for the treatment of redundant ICAs, it can be used for treatment of almost all symptomatic and asymptomatic carotid stenosis. The major advantage of this technique is that the closure of the artery is no longer a technical challenge. Instead, by using the arteries to patch each other, there is little chance of producing a substantial recurrent stenosis. Furthermore, vein or prosthetic materials are not needed. Eversion technique can also be used on smaller caliber carotid arteries. This is further evidenced for the fact that female patients undergoing CEA are more likely to require patch closure or have a higher rate of restenosis in long-term follow-up. As elaborated in this chapter, the eversion technique may be routinely used with or without shunts. Our results with this technique demonstrate a recurrence rate in women that is less than 1%, identical to their male cohorts.

Management of the end point requires the surgeon to learn how to evert the ICA. This is not technically challenging and requires a minimum of effort to learn. In many cases, visualization of the end point is superior to standard techniques, thereby simplifying the other major technical issue facing the operative surgeon. However, ICAs with long-running plaques are difficult to manage regardless of the technique. We discourage indirect visualization of the end point via angioscopy in favor of direct visualization and complete removal of the plaque.

Although it is always difficult to improve on a well-accepted technique, we believe that eversion endarterectomy is truly an advance in carotid surgery and one that we have adopted enthusiastically with improved results.

REFERENCES

Archie JP (1986) Prevention of early restenosis and thrombosis-occlusion after carotid endarterectomy by saphenous vein patch angioplasty. Stroke 17:901–905

Berguer R (1993) Eversion endarterectomy of the carotid bifurcation. In: Veith FJ (ed) Current critical problems in vascular surgery, vol 5. Quality Medical Publishing, St. Louis, pp 441–447

Chang BB, Darling RC III, Patel M, Roddy SP, Paty PSK, Kreienberg PB, Lloyd WE, Shah DM (2000) Use of shunts with eversion carotid endarterectomy. J Vasc Surg 32 :655–662

Darling RC III, Leather RP, Chang BB et al. (1993) Is the iliac artery a suitable inflow conduit for iliofemoral occlusive disease? An analysis of 514 aortoiliac reconstructions. J Vasc Surg 17:15–19

Darling RC III, Shah DM, Chang BB, Paty PSK, Kreienberg PB, Lloyd WE, Roddy SP (2000) Carotid endarterectomy using the eversion technique. Semin Vasc Surg 13(1):4–9

DeBakey ME, Crawford ES, Cooley DA et al. (1959) Surgical considerations of occlusive disease of innominate, carotid, subclavian and vertebral arteries. Ann Surg 149:690–710

Executive Committee for the Asymptomatic Carotid Atherosclerosis Study (1995) Endarterectomy for asymptomatic carotid artery stenosis. JAMA 273:1421–1428

Healy DA, Zierler RE, Nicholls SC et al. (1989) Long-term follow-up and clinical outcome of carotid restenosis. J Vasc Surg 10:662–669

Hertzer NR, Beven EG, O'Hara PJ, Krajewsksi LP (1987) A prospective study of vein patch angioplasty during carotid endarterectomy: three year results for 801 patients and 917 operations. Ann Surg 206:628–635

Kasparzak PM, Raithel D (1989) Eversion carotid endarterectomy: Technique and early results. J Cardiovasc Surg 30:495

Lord RSA, Raj B, Stary DL et al. (1989) Comparison of saphenous vein patch, polytetrafluoroethylene patch and direct arteriotomy closure after carotid endarterectomy. Part I. Perioperative results. J Vasc Surg 9:521–529

North American Symptomatic Carotid Endarterectomy Trial Collaborators (1991) Beneficial effect of carotid endarterectomy in symptomatic patients with high-grade carotid stenosis. N Engl J Med 325:445–453

CHAPTER 3

Carotid Artery Stenting

Brajesh K. Lal, Peter J. Pappas

INTRODUCTION

Stroke is the third most common cause of death and the leading cause of disability in the United States. Management of identifiable risk factors and careful selection of patients for revascularization of extracranial carotid artery stenosis constitute the current approach toward reducing the morbidity and mortality associated with stroke. The controversy over proper management of carotid stenosis prompted several randomized controlled multi-institutional trials during the past 2 decades. They have provided statistically reliable results that form the basis of current management recommendations. Carotid endarterectomy (CEA), performed with a low peri-procedural complication rate, is the only form of mechanical cerebral revascularization for which level 1 evidence of clinical effectiveness in preventing stroke has been reported (Barnett et al. 1998; Executive Committee for the Asymptomatic Carotid Atherosclerosis Study 1995).

Recently, anecdotal reports, case series and single institutional registries demonstrated the feasibility of carotid artery stenting (CAS) as a possible alternative to CEA. Its popularity is due, at least in part, to the perceived advantages of a less invasive treatment for extracranial carotid occlusive disease. Two randomized trials have now compared CAS and CEA. The SAPPHIRE (Stenting and Angioplasty with Protection in Patients at High Risk for Endarterectomy) investigators randomized 334 high-risk patients to CAS or CEA (Yadav et al. 2004) and reported no difference in the composite stroke, death and myocardial infarction rate. The European CAVATAS (Carotid and Vertebral Artery Transluminal Angioplasty Study) investigators reported similar results (CAVATAS 2001). Both studies concluded that CAS was not inferior to CEA. These trials were not powered to identify superiority between CAS and CEA. The NIH-supported CREST (Carotid Revascularization Endarterectomy versus Stent Trial) is currently underway to make that determination but the lead-in phase of the trial has yielded low complication rates with CAS (combined stroke and death: 5.6% for symptomatic, 2.4% for asymptomatic patients) (Hobson et al. 2004). These results have encouraged the Food and Drug Administration in the United States to approve the use of CAS in selected high-risk individuals. In addition, the NIH has expanded CREST to investigate asymptomatic patients in addition to the symptomatic patients already being recruited.

On the basis of the recommendations of a multidisciplinary panel (Veith et al. 2001) specific subgroups of patients (high-risk patients with significant medical co-morbidities and patients with carotid restenosis after previous CEA, anatomically inaccessible lesions above C2, and radiation-induced stenoses) are generally considered candidates for CAS. Furthermore, the FDA has permitted the use of CAS in patients with neurological symptoms (stroke, TIA, AF) in association with severe medical co-morbidities. Meanwhile, the NIH-sponsored CREST is currently underway to obtain level 1 data on the efficacy and risks of CAS compared to CEA.

The procedure requires advanced catheter-guidewire skills that have recently been outlined in a consensus document published by the Society for Vascular Surgery (Rosenfield 2005). While a fixed imaging unit with a large image intensifier may be ideal, the procedure has been safely performed in the operating room with a mobile table and portable C-arm. Patients are placed on aspirin 325 mg QD and clopidogrel 75 mg BID at least 2 days prior to the procedure (failing which, a loading dose of 300 mg is given on the day of the procedure). The procedure is performed with the patient supine on the table. The head is placed on a ring, cradle or similar stabilizing support. Care is taken to traverse all EKG wires away from the chest, neck and head to avoid interference with aortic arch, cervical and intracranial angiography. The preferred site for vascular access is the femoral artery. The groin is prepped and draped with four sterile towels to delineate a square area encompassing the palpable femoral pulse. A large drape is then placed over the entire body leaving the face uncovered. Access into the femoral artery is usually gained with a single wall puncture needle and a 0.035-inch guidewire under fluoroscopic guidance. A 5F short sheath is then positioned into the artery. If the femoral arteries are occluded, brachial access may be utilized. The right brachial artery is the preferred approach to a left carotid stenosis and a left brachial access to treat right carotid lesions.

The procedure is performed under local infiltration anesthesia with the patient awake. Generally, the patients are not sedated. There must be constant contact with the patient and the patient is usually asked to squeeze an audible device with the contralateral arm to assess gross neurological function during all maneuvers involving instrumentation of the carotid artery. Continuous EKG, oxygen saturation and invasive blood pressure monitoring are mandatory since bradycardia and hypotension may occur during instrumentation of the carotid bulb. Atropine, dopamine, nitroglycerin, oxygen and IV fluids must be readily available in the room. In vivo studies using transcranial Doppler and ex vivo models have demonstrated that carotid stenting releases atheroembolic particles. To reduce the incidence of embolization and possible neurological complications, one of several antiembolic protection devices is recommended. They fall under three major categories: distal filters, distal occlusive balloons, or proximal occlusion and flow reversal systems. Of these, the former two have been most commonly used. Post-procedure, the patients are placed on aspirin 325 mg and clopidogrel 75 mg once daily for at least 4 weeks; aspirin is then continued indefinitely. A baseline duplex ultrasound (DU) examination is performed prior to discharge home. Patients are currently being followed clinically and with a DU at 3, 6, and 12 months, and annually thereafter (Lal et al. 2003).

Figure 1: Assessment of Arch Anatomy

A 5F diagnostic catheter (pigtail) is advanced over the 0.035-inch guidewire and the tip positioned in the ascending aorta. A power injector set at 900 psi and the image intensifier rotated to a left anterior oblique view allows an appropriate view of the aortic arch branches. A flush arch aortogram is extremely useful in identifying arch anatomic variations, which determines the type of catheter to be used for common carotid cannulation. In most circumstances, this will also allow determination of the extent of carotid stenosis. Once a decision to proceed has been made, the patient is loaded with 100 units/kg of heparin. This is supplemented through the duration of the procedure to maintain an ACT of 250–300 s. Figure 1 is an example of an arch angiogram demonstrating the origins of arch branches as well as a high-grade left internal carotid artery stenosis

Figure 1

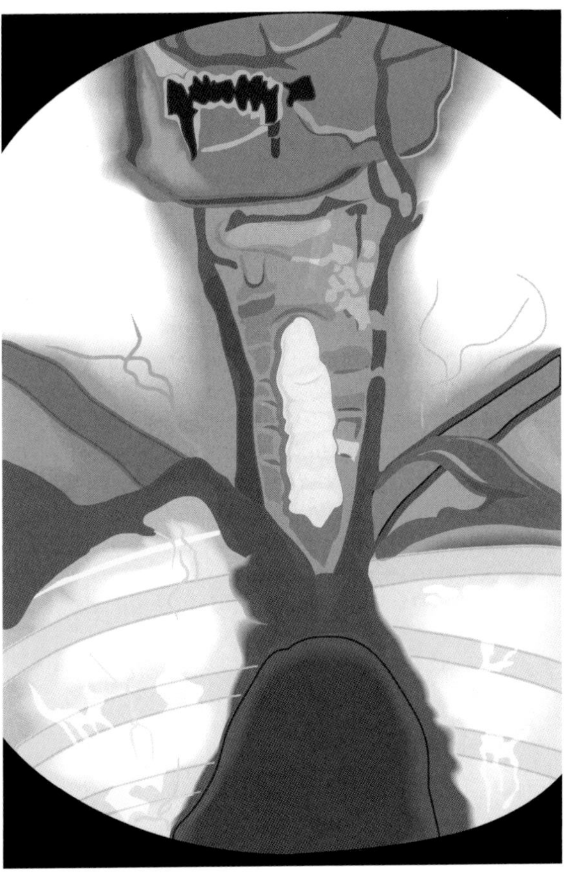

Figure 2A, B: Cannulation of Common Carotid Artery

The most important factor in achieving technical success in a CAS procedure involves the ability to gain access to the CCA through a long introducer sheath. A 5F angled glide catheter (non-reverse curve, Cook Inc., Bloomington, IN) or a 5F Vitek catheter (reverse curve, Cook Inc., Bloomington, IN) will allow successful cannulation of most carotid arteries. Several 0.035-inch guidewires can be used for cannulation, the most common ones being an angled glidewire, a Wholey modified guidewire (Mallinckrodt, St. Louis, MO) or a Connors guidewire (Meditech/Boston Scientific, Natick, MA). Two approaches can be used for cannulation. The first involves cannulation of the CCA with the 5F catheter over the guidewire and then exchanging the catheter for a long 6F sheath (Cordis Inc., Miami, FL) advanced over the guidewire and dilator into the CCA. When one is more comfortable with the procedure, the wire, catheter and sheath can be advanced as one into the arch. This can be followed by sequential cannulation of the CCA with the wire, catheter and sheath. One major reason for procedural failure in CAS is an inability to advance the catheter into the CCA. To move the catheter forward into the artery, a technique involving a slow push and pull on the catheter and wire can be used. The wire is best positioned in the external carotid artery. This allows improved purchase to support passage of the long sheath, without having to cross the stenosis with a large caliber wire. If access to the CCA has not been achieved in approximately 30–45 min, it is suggested that surgical therapy be considered. Multiple prolonged maneuvers within the aortic arch and near the CCA carry a significant risk for atheroembolic complications. Figure 2A demonstrates cannulation of the innominate artery with a Vitek catheter and a 0.035-inch Wholey wire being advanced into the common carotid artery. In Fig. 2B, the catheter has been exchanged for a 6F long sheath that is being advanced into the right common carotid artery

Figure 2A

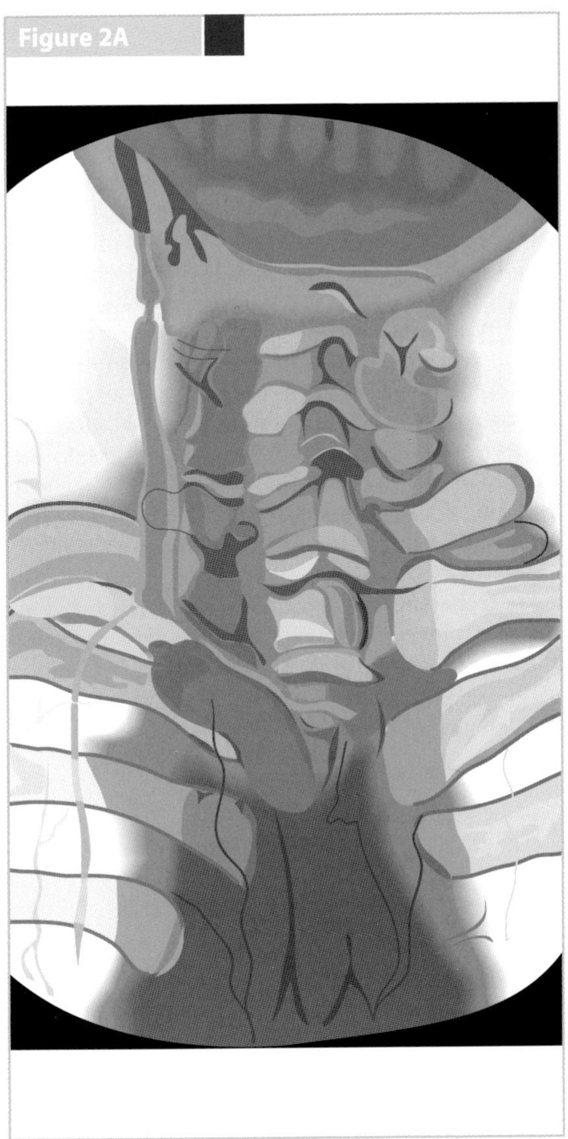

Figure 2B

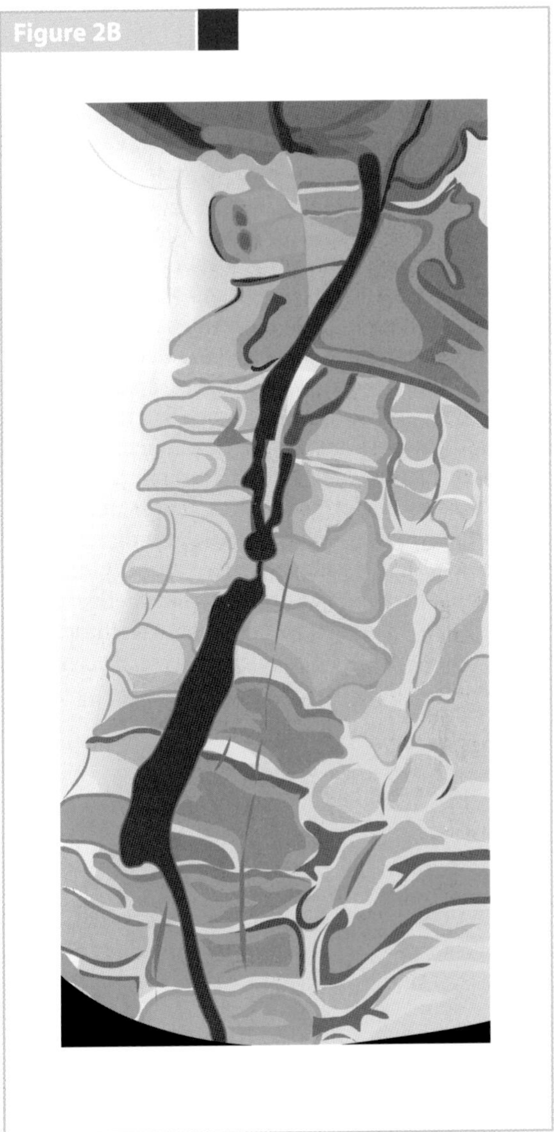

3

Figure 3A–D: Antiembolic Devices

Distal occlusive balloons were the first antiembolic devices (AED) used. One such balloon, Percusurge/Guardwire (Medtronic Vascular, Santa Rosa, CA), is housed on a 0.014-inch guidewire which is inflated through a small side port. Once a long sheath has been positioned in the distal CCA, the 0.014-inch wire is advanced across the stenosis and the balloon is inflated 2–3 cm distal to the lesion. Balloon devices are the smallest in profile (2.2F), which thereby enhances flexibility and ease of traverse across tortuous or highly stenosed carotid arteries. However, it is not possible to perform angiograms during the inflation. Additionally, 6–10% of individuals will not tolerate total occlusion of the ICA. Filter devices are made of a metallic skeleton overlaid with a polyethylene net with 80–200 μm pores. The device is attached to the distal end of a 0.014-inch delivery wire with "strings" that can be used to sheathe or unsheathe the device. The device is delivered across the stenosis sheathed by a delivery catheter. Filter devices have a larger profile (3–4F) and, on occasion, predilation with a 2–3 mm coronary balloon (Boston Scientific, Natick, MA) is required when the stenosis is too tight to pass the filter. After being positioned 2–3 cm distal to the lesion, the catheter is withdrawn to unsheathe the device, which opens up like an umbrella. Care must be taken to immobilize the wire and all AEDs. Undue movement may result in intimal trauma to the distal internal carotid artery with subsequent spasm and/or thrombosis. In both types of devices, the 0.014-inch delivery wire is subsequently used to advance the balloon and a stent to treat the lesion. Figure 3A and B demonstrate two commonly used antiembolic devices: the Guidant Accunet filter, and the Medtronic Percusurge balloon, respectively. Figure 3C demonstrates a filter device deployed in the internal carotid artery distal to the stenosis (Fig. 3D).

Figure 3A

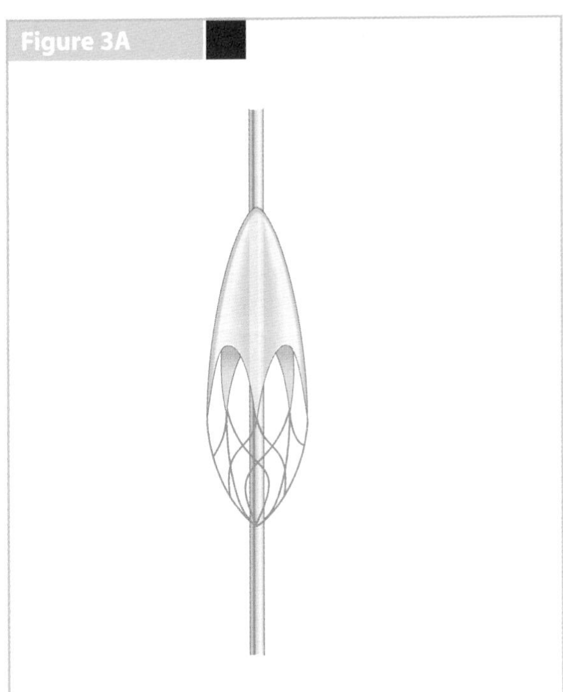

Figure 3B

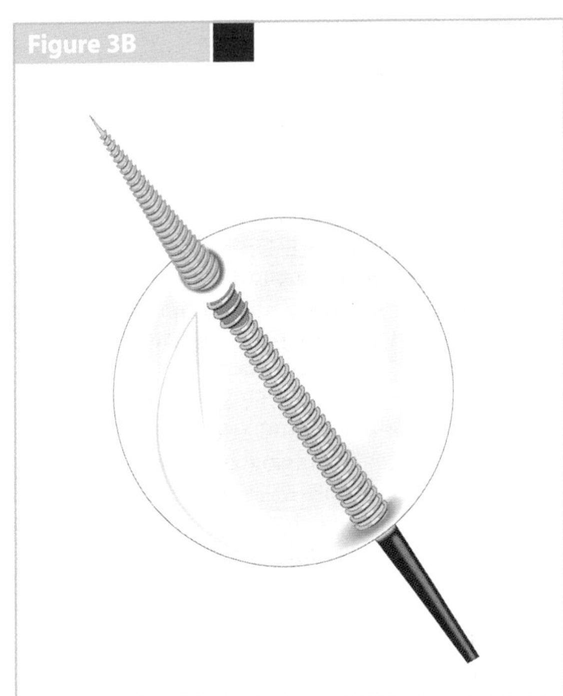

Figure 3C

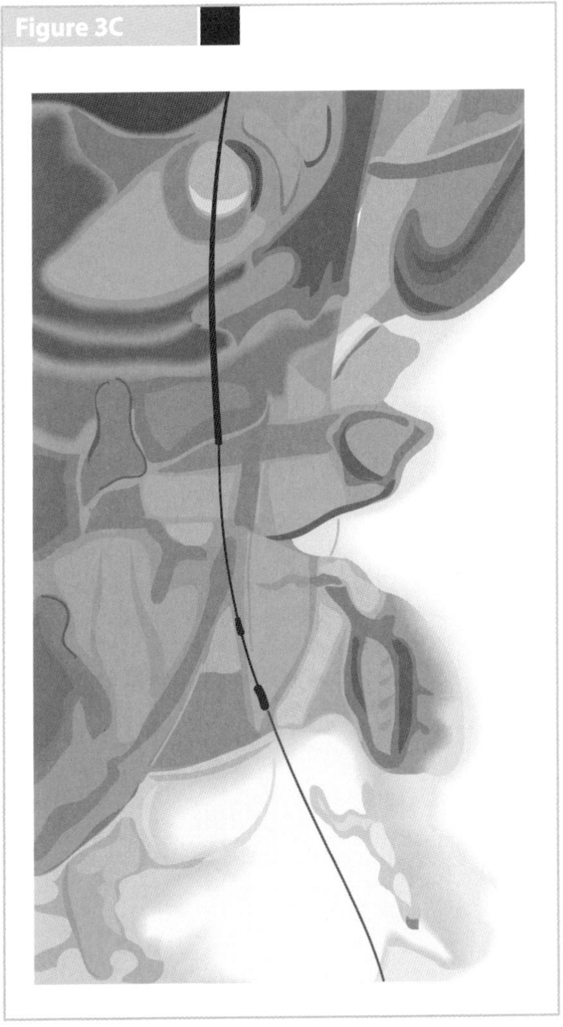

Figure 3D

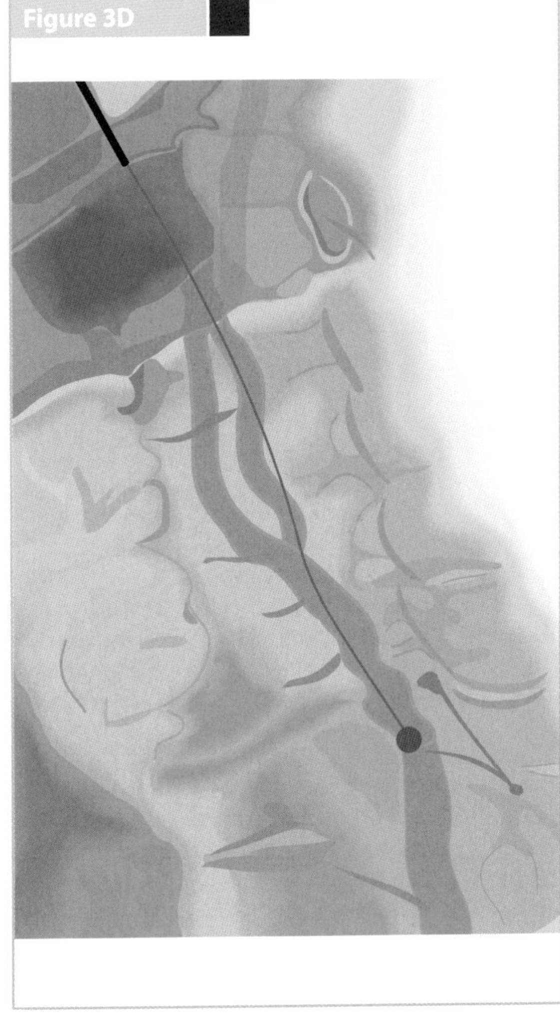

Figure 4A–C: Carotid Stenting

Unlike several other vascular beds, short- and long-term results with primary stenting of the carotid have been better than with angioplasty and selective stenting. The one exception to this is intervention for post-CAS restenosis, in which case angioplasty alone may suffice. When the stenosis is extremely high-grade, a 3.5–4 mm coronary balloon may be used to pre-dilate the lesion. In most instances the stent spans the carotid bifurcation extending from the ICA into the CCA; in these situations, a tapered stent (6–8 mm or 7–10 mm, Acculink, Guidant, Menlo Park, CA) has been preferred. However, 6–10 mm tubular stents (e.g., WallStents, Boston Scientific, Natick, MA) sized according to the distal CCA have also been used extensively. Caging the external carotid artery does not usually result in occlusion as evidenced by follow-up duplex ultrasonography and angiography in multiple studies. On the less frequent occasion where the lesion can be addressed with a stent located within the ICA alone, a tubular configuration is preferred. All stents must be sized and deployed to cover the entire lesion; this usually necessitates stent lengths of 30–40 mm. The use of self expanding stents is preferred because of greater resilience against cervical motion, kinking and deformation. Self expanding nitinol stents are characterized by higher radial strength, and higher adaptability to tortuous arteries. Stents based on a rapid exchange monorail system allow for more comfortable and precise delivery of the stents. Figure 4A demonstrates predilation of an extremely high-grade stenosis after filter deployment. This allows comfortable positioning of the stent across the lesion (Fig. 4B) and subsequent deployment of a Guidant Acculink stent (Fig. 4C)

Figure 4A

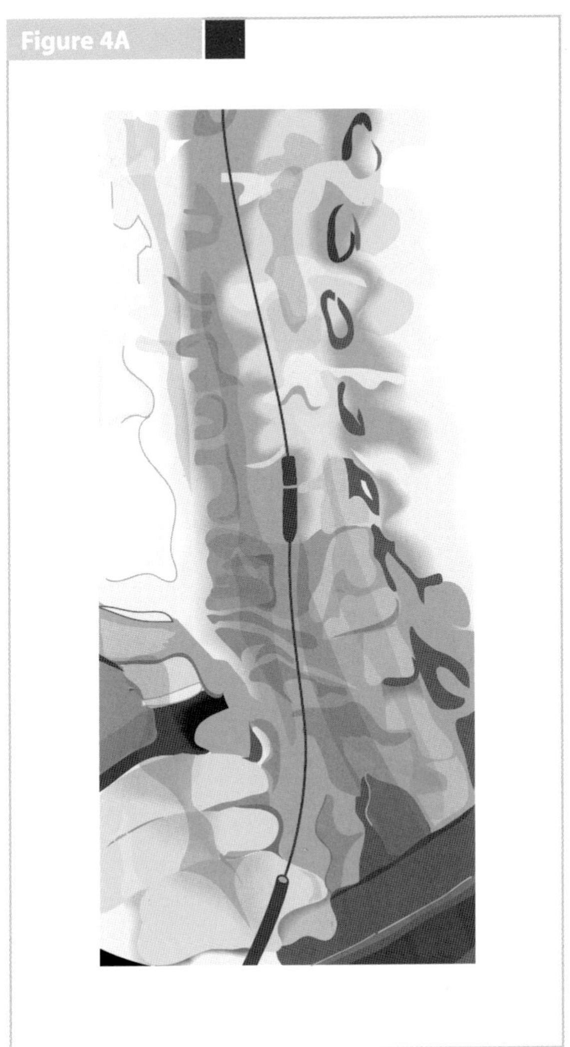

Figure 4B

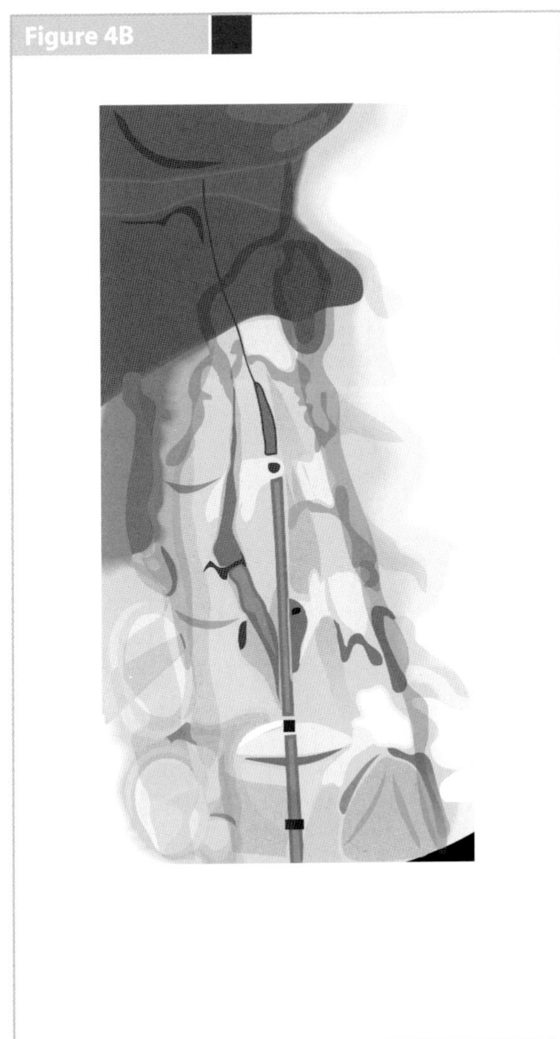

Figure 4C

Figure 4C

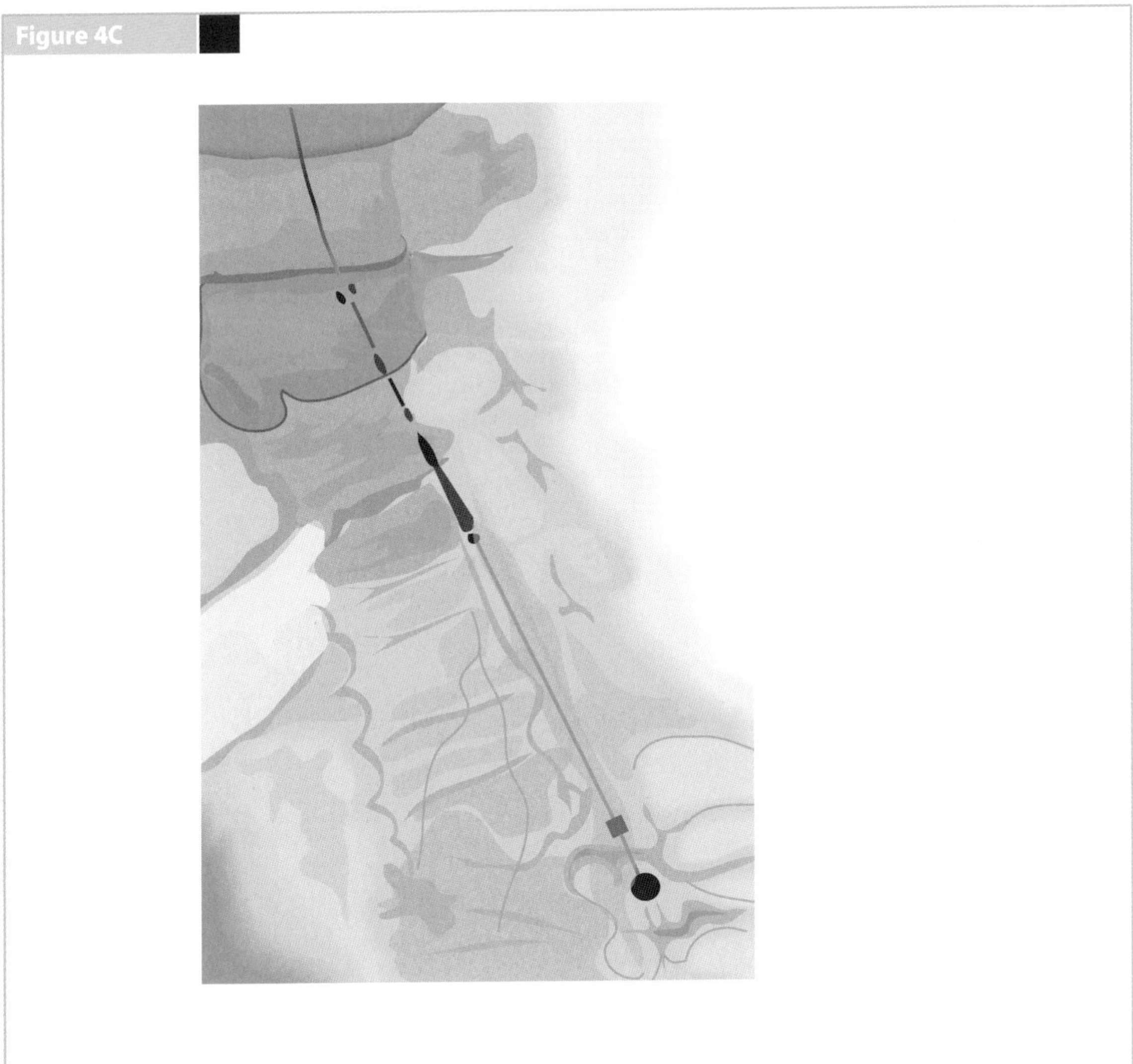

Figure 5A, B: Poststenting Dilation

Once the stent has been deployed, the delivery system is withdrawn and a hand injected angiogram is performed to study the result. In most instances, postdelivery dilation is with a 5–6×20-mm balloon (e.g., Ultra-soft balloons, Boston Scientific) inflated to 8–10 atm. A period of 10–30 s is necessary. Poststenting dilation has been demonstrated to release significant atheroemboli. Despite the presence of an AED, we attempt to reduce this embolic load by undersizing the balloon with respect to both the arterial diameter and the stent length. Unlike coronary stenting, we do not attempt to obtain residual stenoses of 0%; post-CAS residual stenoses up to 20–30% are adequate results. This avoids the risk of dissection and/or arterial rupture. Additionally, there is data emerging that continued expansion of self-expanding stents may result in positive remodeling over time. A completion angiogram is performed; a residual lumen 20% as compared to the distal ICA where the walls become parallel is considered a technical success. In Fig. 5A, poststenting balloon dilation is being performed with a 5.5 coronary balloon. Figure 5B demonstrates adequate technical resolution of the stenosis on a completion angiogram

Figure 5A

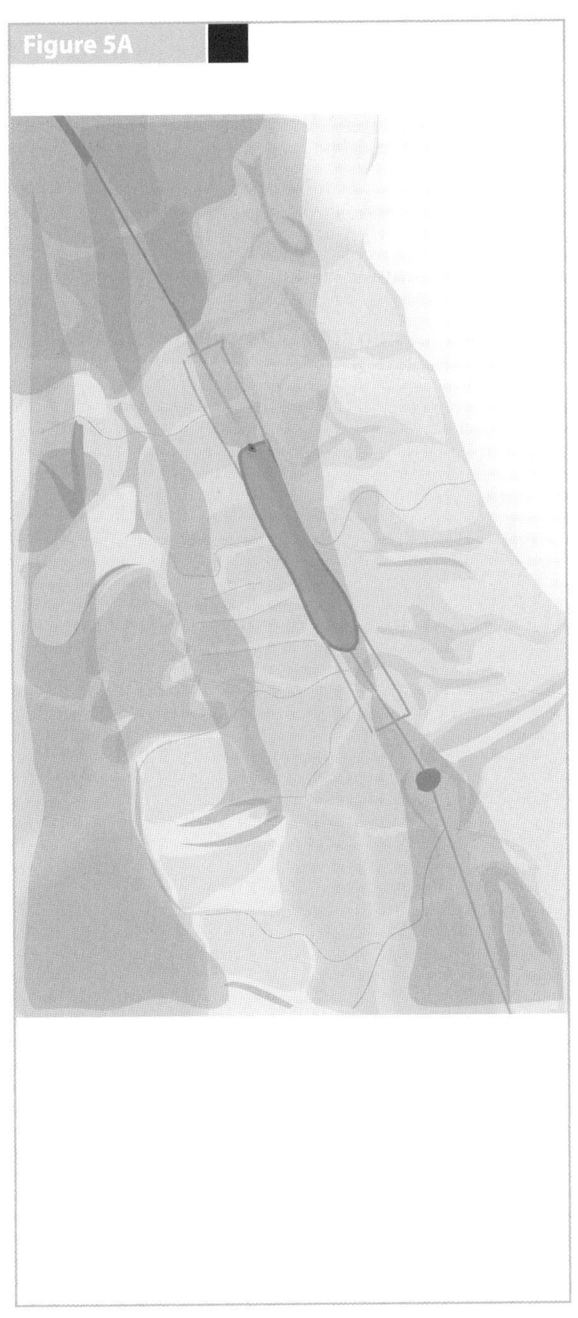

Figure 5B

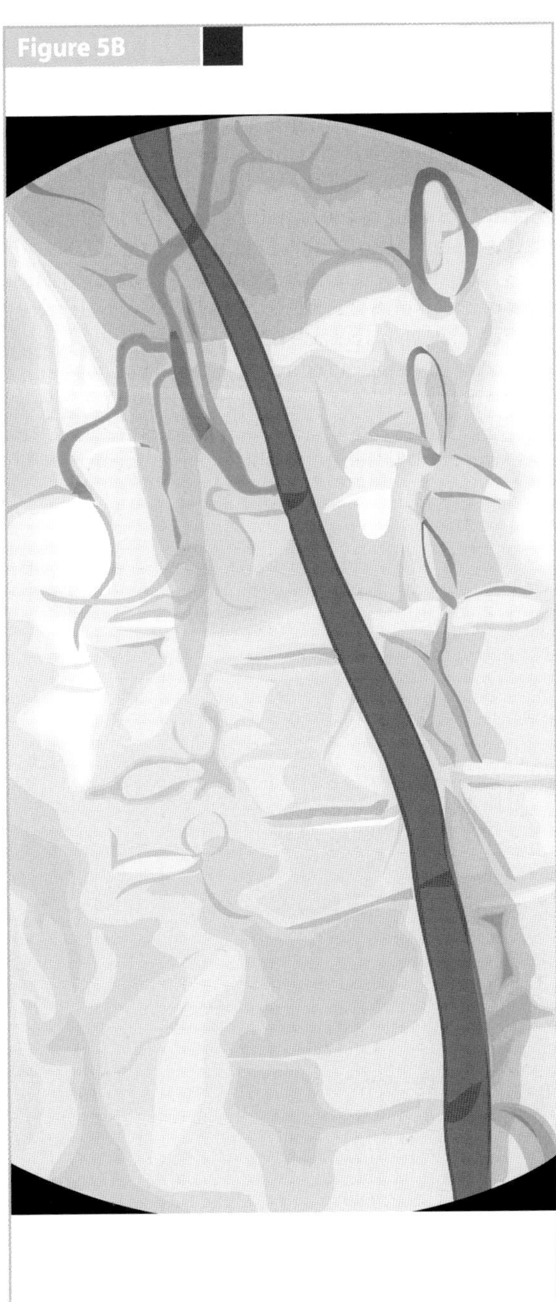

Figure 6A, B: Capture and Retrieval of AED

Once the procedure is considered complete, the AED must be retrieved. If a distal balloon occlusion device was used, then a catheter is inserted over the wire and the column of blood contained in the occluded ICA is aspirated. This will remove any debris released during the stenting procedure. The balloon is then deflated and the guidewire withdrawn. If a distal filter device was used, it is closed by advancing a retrieval catheter and withdrawn. On occasion, spasm may be noted upon completion of the procedure and removal of the AED. This results from movement of the device against the distal ICA. This can be successfully treated with an intra-arterial injection of nitroglycerin (100 μg) delivered directly into the ICA through the sheath. Figure 6A demonstrates spasm in the distal internal carotid artery at the area where the filter device had been deployed. This resolved 2 min after nitroglycerin was delivered to the site through the sheath (Fig. 6B).

Figure 6A

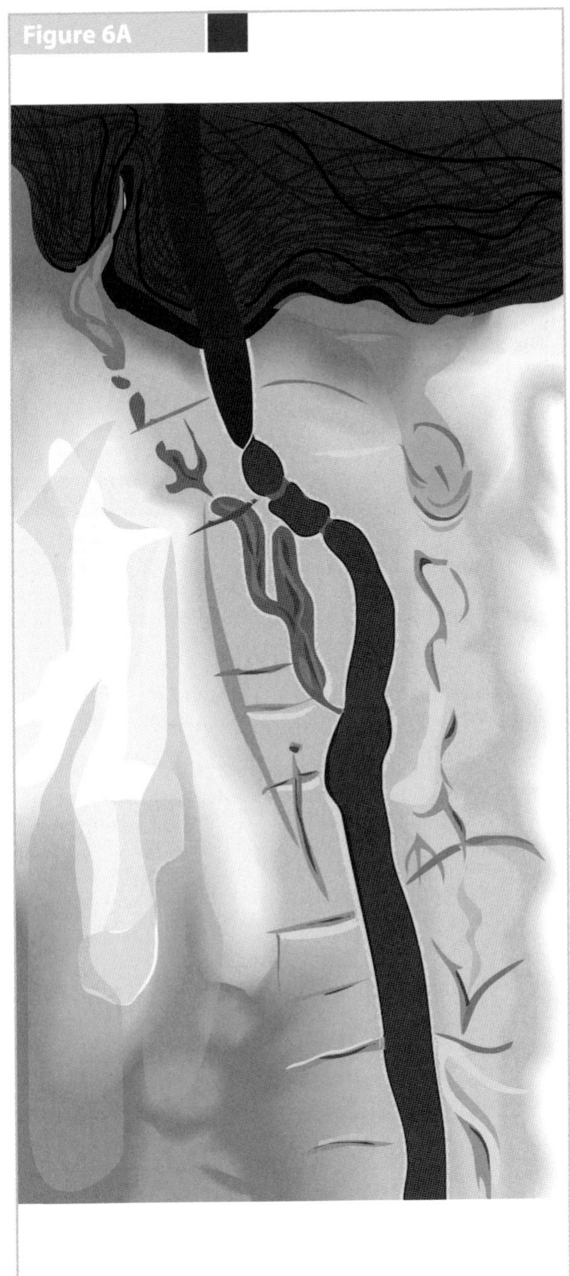

Figure 6B

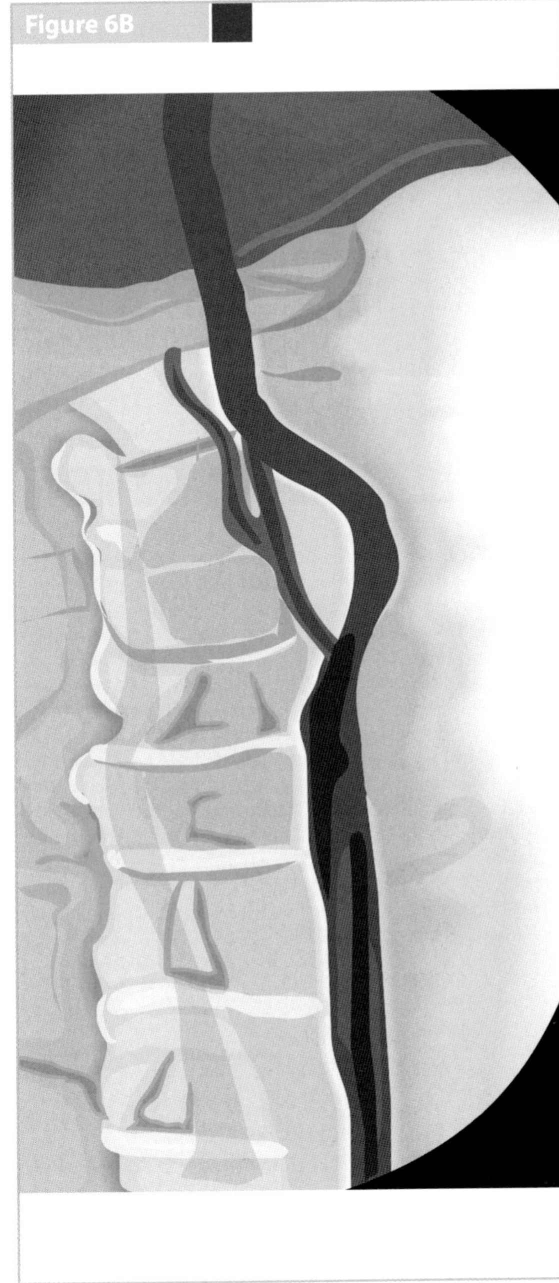

3

CONCLUSION

A prerequisite for successful CAS involves adequate catheter-guidewire skills and familiarity with invasive imaging and selected pharmacotherapy. Above all, sound judgment regarding indications and limitations of each technique are essential. CAS is being performed in an increasing number of patients. Technical success rates are high in well-selected cases while 30-day peri-procedural and longer-term results may indicate equivalence with CEA. In patients at high risk for surgery, CAS may be favorable compared to CEA. However, CAS must be practiced with caution in low-risk and asymptomatic patients, especially in the context of limited large-scale long-term efficacy data. Conversely, technological advances are constantly offering an increasing number of innovative device improvements that are enhancing the efficacy and safety of the procedure. Therefore for those performing CAS, there is an ongoing responsibility to maintain familiarity with advances in the field.

REFERENCES

Barnett HJ, Taylor DW, Eliasziw M et al. (1998) Benefit of carotid endarterectomy in patients with symptomatic moderate or severe stenosis. North American Symptomatic Carotid Endarterectomy Trial Collaborators. N Engl J Med 339(20) : 1415–1425

Carotid and Vertebral Artery Transluminal Angioplasty Study (2001) Endovascular versus surgical treatment in patients with carotid stenosis in the Carotid and Vertebral Artery Transluminal Angioplasty Study (CAVATAS) (2001): a randomised trial. Lancet 357(9270):1729–1737

Executive Committee for the Asymptomatic Carotid Atherosclerosis Study (1995) Endarterectomy for asymptomatic carotid artery stenosis. JAMA 273(18):1421–1428

Hobson RW 2nd, Howard VJ, Roubin GS et al. (2004) Carotid artery stenting is associated with increased complications in octogenarians: 30-day stroke and death rates in the CREST lead-in phase. J Vasc Surg 40(6):1106–1111

Lal BK, Hobson RW 2nd, Goldstein J et al. (2003) In-stent recurrent stenosis after carotid artery stenting: life table analysis and clinical relevance. J Vasc Surg 38(6):1162–1168; discussion 1169

Rosenfield KM (2005) Clinical competence statement on carotid stenting: training and credentialing for carotid stenting – multispecialty consensus recommendations. J Vasc Surg 41(1):160–168

Veith FJ, Amor M, Ohki T et al. (2001) Current status of carotid bifurcation angioplasty and stenting based on a consensus of opinion leaders. J Vasc Surg 33(2 Suppl):S111–116

Yadav JS, Wholey MH, Kuntz RE et al. (2004) Protected carotid-artery stenting versus endarterectomy in high-risk patients. N Engl J Med 351(15):1493–1501

CHAPTER 4

Carotid Body Tumor

Paul Srodon, John Lumley

INTRODUCTION

Carotid body tumors are rare neoplasms of the carotid chemoreceptors, which lie in the adventitia of the carotid bifurcation. They may be non-secreting chemodectomas of cells of neural crest origin, or neuropeptide secreting apudomas. Most are sporadic, but 10% are familial, with autosomal dominant inheritance. Bilateral tumors occur in 32% of familial cases, but in only 5% of the remainder (Parkin 1981). Tumors are usually benign, but 5% eventually show invasive malignant characteristics and metastasize (Padberg et al. 1983). They typically occur in the 40–60 year age group, with equal incidence in males and females.

Patients usually present with a hard painless lump in the carotid triangle, which gradually enlarges over 5–10 years. Larger or more invasive tumors produce symptoms from compression of the last four cranial nerves, or transient ischemic attacks and stroke. Sensitivity of the carotid sinus may cause syncope, bradycardia or hypotension. The tumor may have slight lateral mobility, but is fixed longitudinally; there may be expansile pulsation and an overlying bruit.

Assessment by Duplex ultrasound demonstrates a well-vascularized lesion, splaying the carotid bifurcation. CT or MRI scanning helps to delineate the extent of local invasion, and may identify contralateral tumors. The Shamblin classification (Shamblin et al. 1971) gives: Type I – well localized resectable tumor; Type II – tumor adherent to vessels, or partly surrounding vessels; Type III – tumor surrounds carotid arteries. Four-vessel angiography demonstrates the tumor as a vascular "blush," with splaying of the carotid bifurcation; it may identify contralateral tumors and delineates the intracerebral circulation. Most tumors are surgically resectable, although long-standing small tumors in patients with significant co-morbidity may be managed by observation. Invasive tumors may have to be resected together with the carotid bifurcation, and a vein graft inserted between the common and internal carotid arteries. In bilateral cases, where there have been complications from surgery on one side, the second tumor is best observed. Radiotherapy may be appropriate where an invasive tumor cannot be resected, or where there is residual tumor at the skull base. Preoperative radiological embolization has been used to reduce the vascularity of large invasive tumors, prior to resection.

A glomus vagale tumor, arising from the ganglion of the vagus nerve, may be difficult to differentiate from a carotid body tumor. It may cause vagal, hypoglossal or glossopharyngeal nerve dysfunction, and tinnitus. On CT and MRI, these tumors will nearly always displace the internal carotid artery anteromedially. The tumor can be resected in a similar manner to a carotid body tumor.

4

Figure 1

The procedure is performed with the patient under general anesthesia. The patient is positioned, prepared and draped in a similar manner to that for carotid endarterectomy, with provision of bipolar diathermy, to reduce nerve injury. An incision is made over the anterior border of sternomastoid – from the mastoid process to the medial end of the clavicle, and continued through platysma, with division of the external jugular vein and if necessary, the anterior branch of the great auricular nerve (as described in chapter 1). Dissection is continued to expose the tumor, carotid bifurcation and internal jugular vein – progress may be slow as in large and invasive tumors normal tissue planes are lost. Dissection starts in the lower zone with mobilization of the common carotid artery and the vagus nerve, and both are encircled with Silastic slings. Superficially the posterior belly of the digastric muscle is separated from the tumor mass. In the upper anterior zone the following are identified, and may be controlled with Silastic slings or silk ties: the external carotid artery, the overlying hypoglossal nerve, the underlying superior laryngeal nerve, and the mandibular branch of the facial nerve. In the upper posterior zone lie the glossopharyngeal, vagus, spinal accessory and hypoglossal nerves.

In Fig. 1 the internal carotid artery and internal jugular vein have been mobilized proximally, but there are still dense adhesions between these vessels and the tumor at the level of the carotid bifurcation; also between the tumor and the posterior belly of the digastric muscle. Line A is the approach taken to mobilize the posterior belly of the digastic muscle and the hypoglossal nerve, and line B is the approach taken to mobilize the internal jugular vein. The internal carotid artery can be palfated within the surface of the tumor along line C, and the tumor tissue over the artery is divided by a mixture of the sharfs and delicate blient dissection. If no plane of dissection is found, this segment of artery is replaced by a venous graft.

Figure 2

A plane of separation is created between the tumor, and the carotid vessels – this is best sought at the lateral surface of the tumor, where it is adherent to the internal carotid artery. The artery is embedded in the lateral surface of the mass and a plane of dissection is developed around it. Mosquito forceps are introduced and gently opened in the periadventitial plane, ligating or applying bipolar diathermy to the separated vascular tumor tissue and the adventitia. A leash of small veins at the bifurcation require diathermy. If creating a plane on the lateral aspect of the tumor proves difficult, one alternative is to move toward the medial aspect of the tumor and to try to develop a plane between the tumor and the external carotid artery. Branches from the external carotid artery typically feed the tumor, and ligation and division of such branches may decrease the tumor's vascularity and bleeding during the resection. Furthermore, the external carotid artery may be more forgiving should an inadvertent arteriotomy occur during the dissection due to excessive adherence of the tumor. If a plane cannot be found, or if the carotid arteries are inadvertently opened, the vessels should be temporarily clamped, and a shunt placed through the common carotid artery. If the need to clamp the arteries is foreseen, 2500 units of heparin is given intravenously. The dissection process continues until the tumor is completely separated from surrounding structures – or, if the tumor cannot be separated from them, the vessels and involved nerves are resected with it. The ends of resected internal jugular vein can be ligated with non absorbable. If the carotid bifurcation has been resected, a suitable length vein is harvested for use as an interposition graft – long saphenous vein is appropriate, and in this location should not be reversed. After flushing the vein with heparinized saline, end-to-end anastomoses are fashioned using 5/0 Prolene – from common carotid artery to vein, and vein to internal carotid artery. The external carotid artery is ligated with ligature. Suction drains are placed, and the wound closed in a similar manner to carotid endarterectomy. Postoperative care is similar to that for carotid endarterectomy.

In Fig. 2 the internal carotid artery has been mobilized in the tumor throughout its length. Note the external burns from the bipolar managment of the extensive number of fine-bleeding vessels encountered during the dissection and spasm of the artery. The hypoglossal nerve and internal jugular vein have also been mobilized for dense, but less vascular, adhesions. The external carotid and its branches have not yet been mobilized, and a decision is being made as to whether it is safer to sacrifice this vessel by ligating the adherent segment.

Figure 1

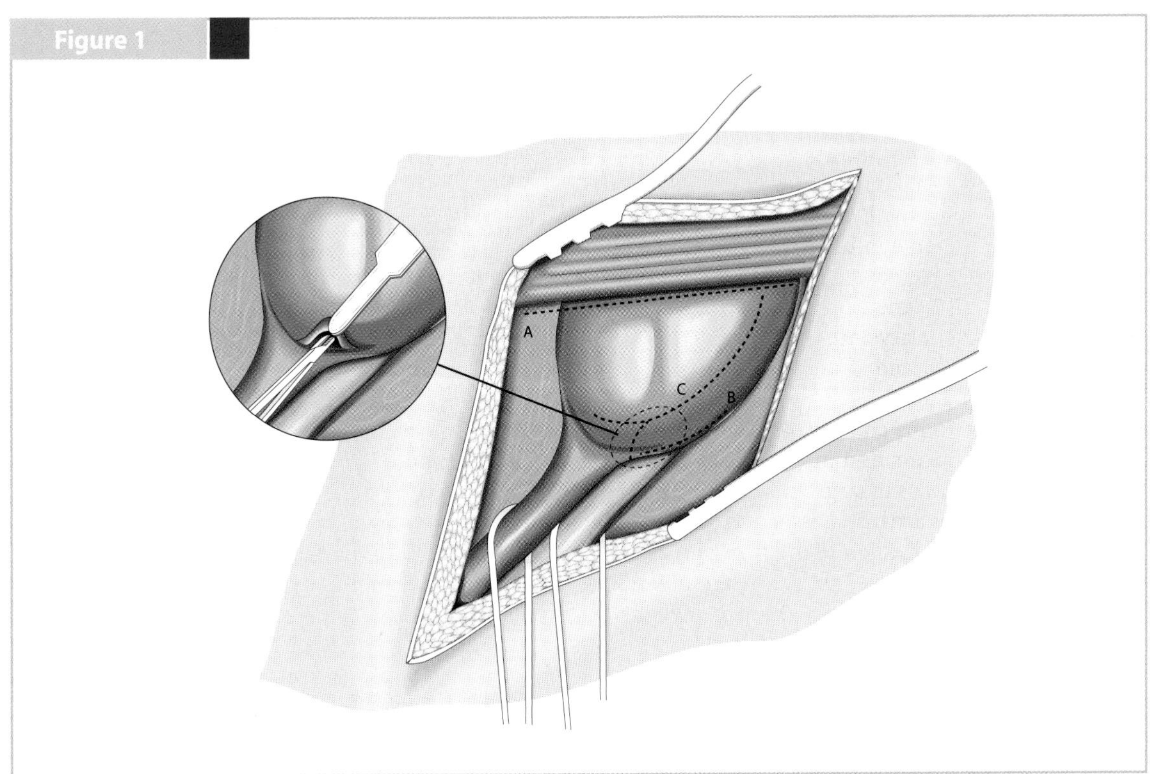

Figure 2

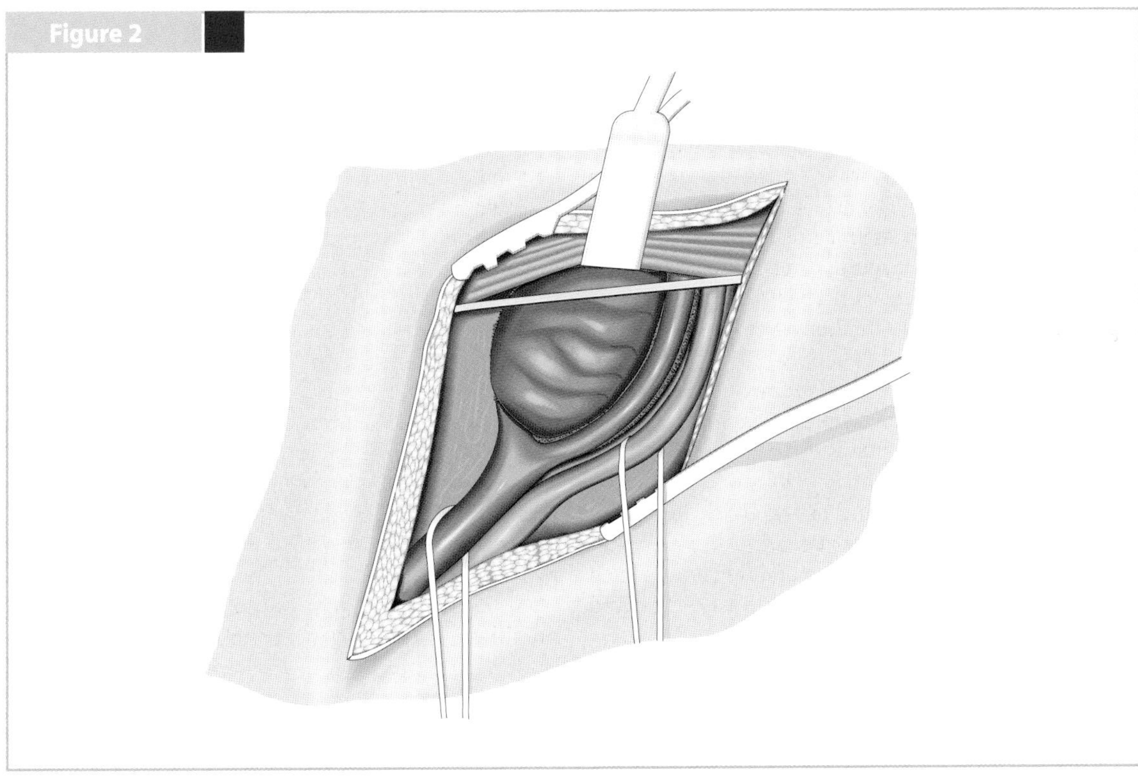

CONCLUSION

The majority of carotid body tumors can be resected, with a perioperative stroke rate of 2% and a mortality of 2%. Cranial nerve injury is common: 20% of patients have temporary hypoglossal or mandibular nerve palsy, and permanent cranial nerve deficit occurs in 20%. Recurrence occurs in 6% and metastasis in 2% after resection; subsequent survival is equivalent to that of age and sex matched controls (Nora et al. 1988).

REFERENCES

Nora JD, Hallett JW, O'Brien PC, Naessens JM, Cherry KJ, Pairolero PC (1988) Surgical resection of carotid body tumours: long-term survival, recurrence, and metastasis. Mayo Clin Proc 63:348–352

Padberg FT Jr, Caddy B, Persson AV (1983) Carotid body tumour (chemodectoma). Am J Surg 145:526–528

Parkin JL (1981) Familial multiple glomus tumours and phaeochromocytomas. Ann Otol Rhinol Laryngol 90:60–63

Shamblin WR, ReMine WH, Sheps SG, Harrison EG (1971) Carotid body tumour: clinicopathological analysis of ninety cases. Am J Surg 122:732–739

CHAPTER 5

Carotid Aneurysms

John Lumley

INTRODUCTION

The general features of aneurysmal surgery are considered with abdominal aortic aneurysms. Carotid aneurysms are relatively uncommon but they present in diverse etiological patterns. Congenital aneurysms often present as thin-walled saccular lesions near the origin of the internal carotid artery. The origin may also be fusiformly dilated and associated with congenital loops of the vessel. Some poststenotic dilation is not uncommon with focal atheromatous lesions at this site.

Post-traumatic false aneurysms are among the commonest in the carotid territory. This results from the superficial situation of the bifurcation, tonsillar, pharyngeal and laryngeal surgery and the practice in some vascular units of using a synthetic patch across the arteriotomy of carotid endarterectomy. The latter has not been our practice and none of the internal carotid aneurysms seen has been secondary to endarterectomy. Inflammatory nodes and suppuration of the oro- and nasopharynx, together with radiotherapy and infiltrating neoplasia, may give rise to aneurysms around the carotid bifurcation. In the past, syphilitic aneurysms were common and Astley Cooper's first carotid operations were undertaken for this condition.

Figure 1

Carotid aneurysms may present as an asymptomatic pulsatile swelling or with neurological symptoms from emboli or thrombosis. Surgery is usually required as enlargement is progressive, although prominence is sufficient to bring the patient to a doctor before rupture. Prominence of the distal innominate at the origin of its branches can bring hypertensive patients to the surgeon and the condition must be recognized as a generalized dilation and tortuosity, carrying no local risk and requiring conservative management.

Arteriography is essential before carotid surgery is contemplated to demonstrate the position of vessels distal to the aneurysm and also the intracranial circulation. Currently magnetic resonance angiography or computerized axial tomographic angiography have replaced digital subtraction angiography due to their noninvasive nature. With aneurysms caused by local infection or mycotic problems, adequate antibiotic therapy must precede surgery.

The initial exposure is as described for carotid endarterectomy in Chapter 1. Saccular aneurysms sometimes extend to the base of the skull and angiographic workup is essential before any form of surgery (Fig. 1). Control proximal and distal to the aneurysm is necessary, although the distal artery may be obscured by the aneurysm. In this situation, the aneurysm may need to be mobilized and retracted caudally to identify the artery distal to the aneurysm. Before manipulation of such aneurysms, which potentially contain thrombus, the patient should be systemically heparinized and the internal carotid artery temporarily clamped while distal mobilization is undertaken to identify the position of the distal vessel. It may be necessary to open the sac in order to identify the distal artery, so that a Fogarty catheter can be used to control bleeding or a shunt inserted, if there is difficulty in mobilizing the aneurysmal sac and reconstruction is likely to take more than 8–10 min.

Figure 1

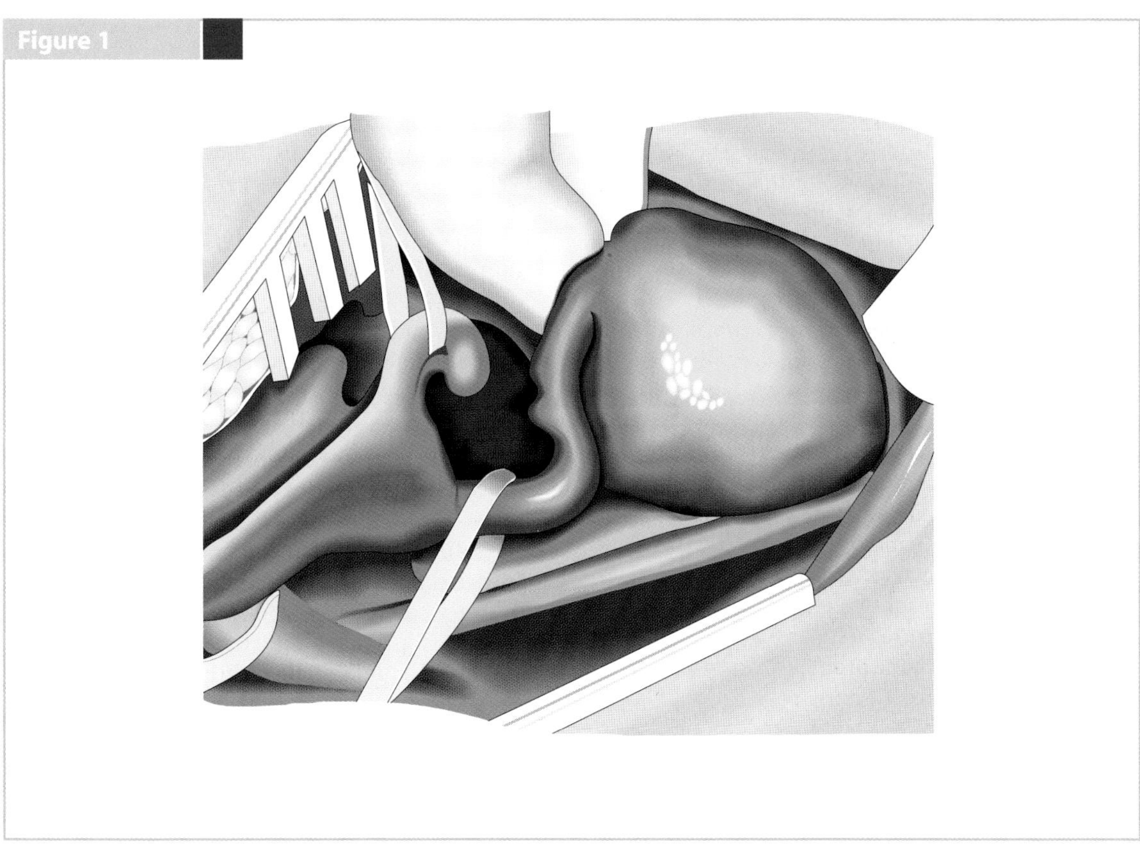

Figures 2, 3

Proximal control of carotid aneurysms is not usually a problem, but high internal carotid aneurysms may be difficult to mobilize distally. If this is not possible without a good deal of manipulation, the patient should be systemically heparinized and the common and external carotid arteries clamped to reduce the likelihood of distal embolization. The ICA can then be expeditiously mobilized and a shunt inserted (Fig. 2). If a challenging distal control is anticipated preoperatively, nasotracheal intubation can enhance the exposure. Increased exposure can be obtained by dividing the posterior belly of the digastric muscle, by mandibular subluxation or by dividing the sternomastoid muscle near its attachment to the base of the skull. Other maneuvers have also been described, such as fracturing the styloid process laterally or dividing the neck of the mandible. These various maneuvers are rarely necessary, but the dissection must pass on to the anterior surface of the mastoid process and extend along the entire anterior upper border of the sternomastoid muscle. Shunts are advisable for lengthy procedures, as cerebral collateral blood flow is not as prominent as in atherosclerotic occlusive disease. Insertion of the distal end of a shunt into the internal carotid artery may, however, not be possible until a late stage in an operative procedure. The figure shows a balloon shunt; the shunt is particularly valuable in this patient because the distal internal carotid artery has not been mobilized sufficiently to place an external ring around the cannulated artery.

It is essential that all vascular surgeons be skilled in the insertion of shunts, as they may be used in many situations. Although not advised for routine use in severe stenotic carotid artery disease, a shunt should always be available, as the procedure may unexpectedly require prolonged clamp time. Shunts should also be available in all cases of severe vascular trauma.

The shunt is cross-clamped in the middle, and the larger proximal end is inserted first and fixed into position by balloon and ring clamp. The clamp on the shunt is partially released to fill it with the patient's blood and remains ready for release (with a bubble free system) and is introduced into the distal vessel and the clamp on the latter opened simultaneously. Be on the look out for any dispant of vessel and shunt size, or other reason why shunt insertion may be difficult! Figure 3 shows the reconstruction.

Figure 2

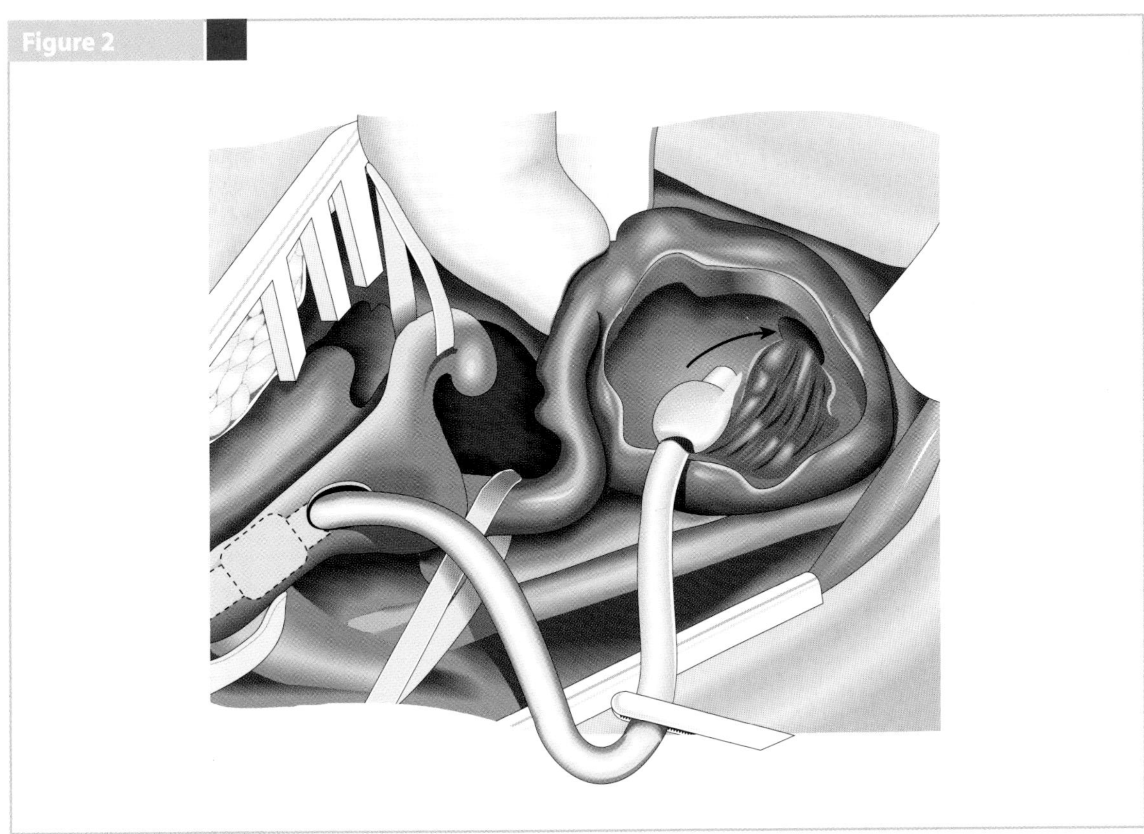

Figure 3

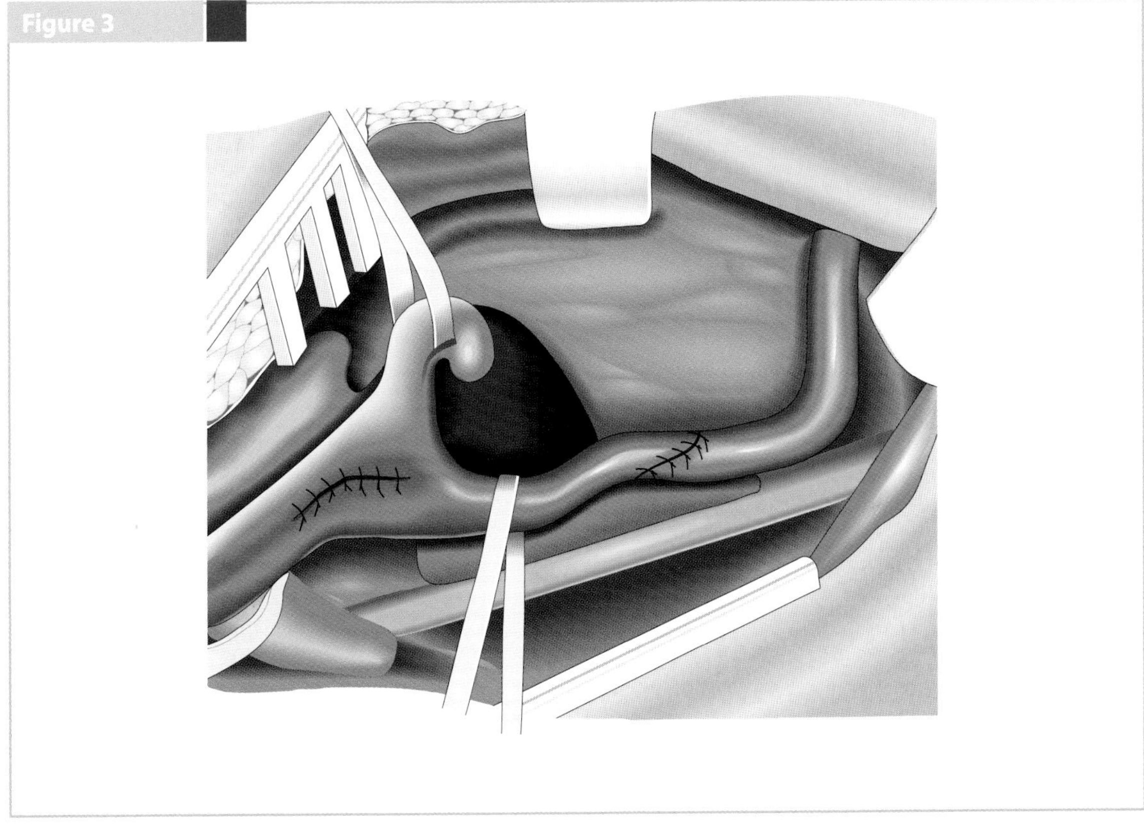

Figures 4, 5

Many aneurysms can be resected with an end-to-end anastomosis, particularly of the internal carotid artery, or resection of the carotid bifurcation. If this is not possible, a vein graft replacement is preferred, although occasionally Dacron or Polytetrafluorethylene may be more appropriate in size or for inlay procedures. Indurated areas resulting from infection, radiotherapy or neoplasia are best bypassed with end-to-end anastomoses away from the diseased site.

Aneurysms of the internal carotid artery near the base of the skull, within the carotid canal, or within the cranial cavity may require balloon occlusion or ligation of this vessel and this may be accompanied by a transcranial bypass.

Atheromatous aneurysms may have a marked surrounding inflammatory reaction (Fig. 4), as may mycotic aneurysms. Normal proximal and distal vessels must be identified and mobilized where possible before incision of the sac. In Fig. 4 a probe has been passed into the internal carotid artery origin from within the sac. The external carotid artery origin is involved in the aneurysmal wall and occluded.

Occasionally in such irregular aneurysms an inlay technique can be used (Fig. 5), as more fully described for the abdominal aorta. This is dependent on identifying a rim of reasonably normal arterial tissue proximally and distally for circumferential suture. This was possible in this patient, where a length of 8 mm Dacron has been inlaid within the aneurysmal sac.

Figure 4

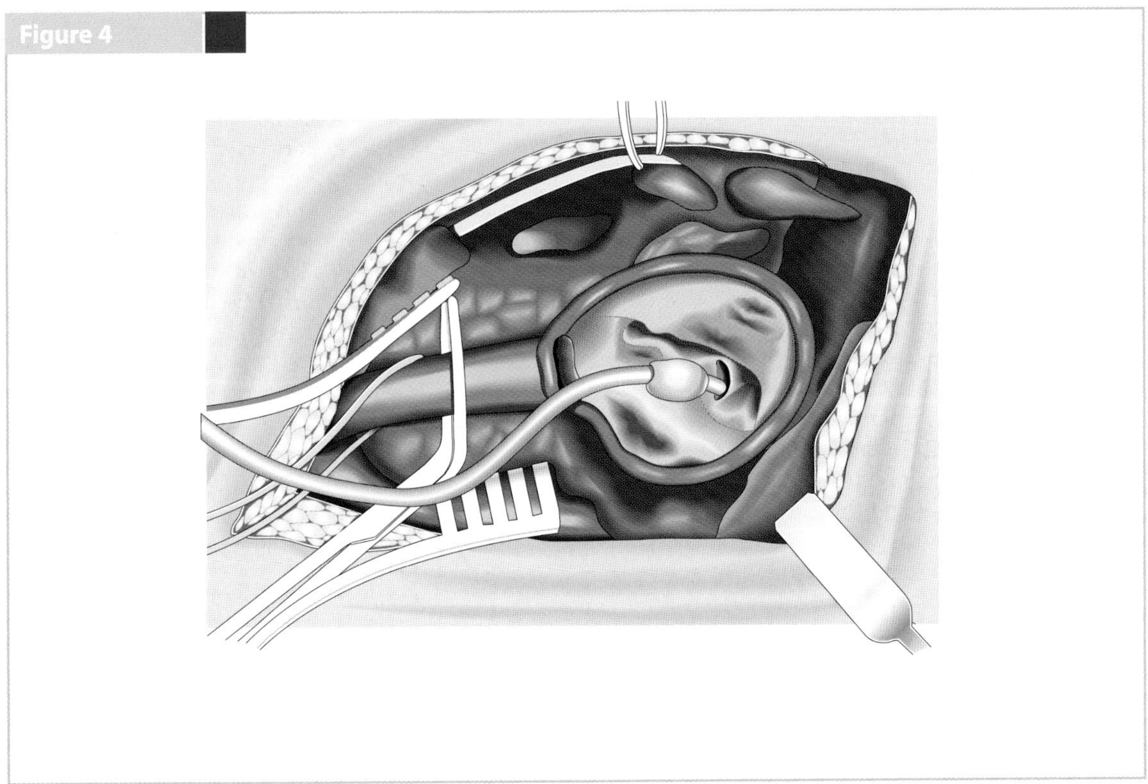

Figure 5

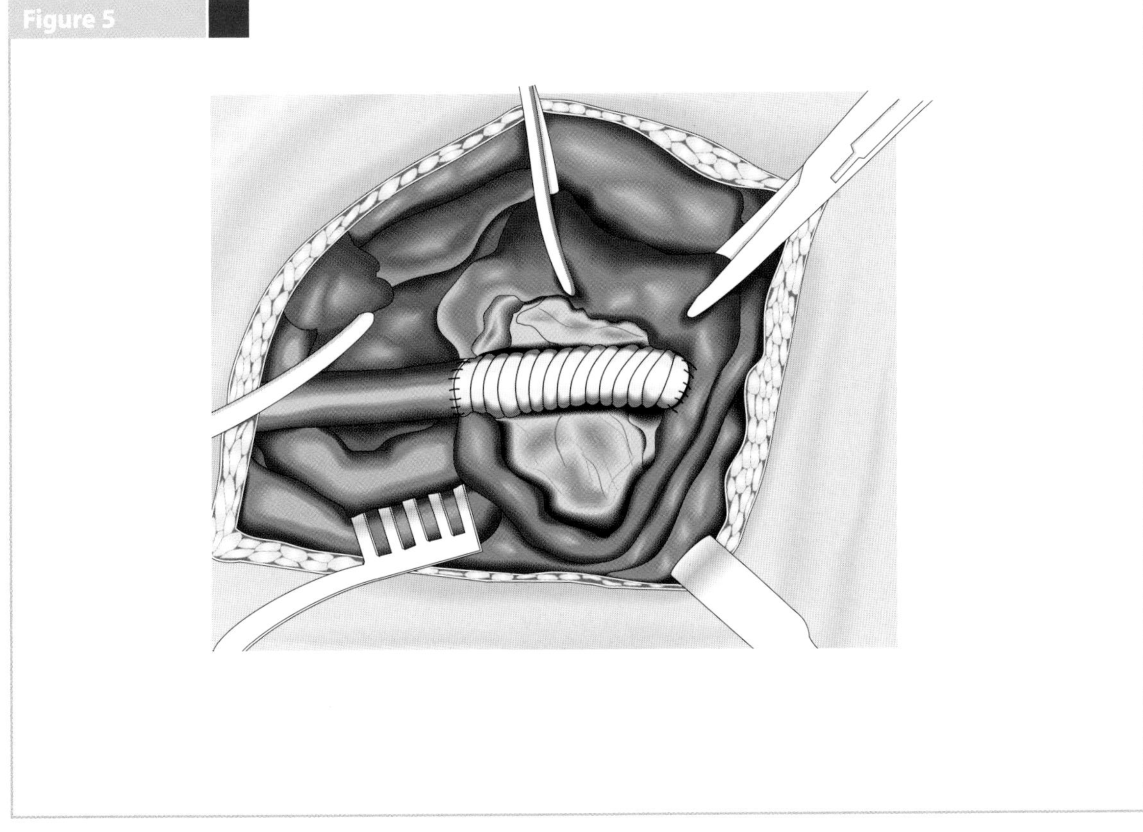

Part II

Upper Thorax, Root of Neck, and Upper Limb

CHAPTER 6

Surgical Reconstruction for Innominate Artery Occlusive Disease

Jeffrey L. Ballard

INTRODUCTION

The incidence of occlusive disease affecting the innominate artery is unknown because severe atherosclerotic lesions remain undetected by commonly employed screening modalities such as duplex ultrasound. Furthermore, symptoms are frequently minimal and clinical examination findings are subtle. However, abnormalities of the aortic arch branch vessels are increasingly encountered in patients with severe peripheral vascular disorders (Ballard 2001; Chang et al. 1997; Owens et al. 1995; Sakopoulos et al. 2000; Twena and Ballard 2000). In addition, the atherosclerotic process tends to occur in the proximal one-third of these arteries. This makes upper mediastinal access ideal for surgical reconstruction of innominate artery occlusive disease (Owens et al. 1995; Twena and Ballard 2000). The mini-sternotomy technique described in this chapter maximizes direct surgical reconstruction options such as aorto-innominate artery bypass and, less commonly, innominate artery endarterectomy. Alternatively, extrathoracic bypass procedures utilizing the subclavian and/or axillary arteries may be advisable for prohibitive surgical risk patients or if the planned sternotomy would be a complex re-do procedure.

The most common surgical indication for innominate artery reconstruction in our practice is a symptomatic stenosis >50%. Some patients with an incidentally discovered asymptomatic stenosis >70% or a deep ulcerated plaque lesion associated with >50% stenosis are also considered for surgical reconstruction. This approach for treatment of asymptomatic innominate artery occlusive disease is due to the potential sequelae associated with untreated atheromatous lesions such as transient ischemic attack, stroke or upper extremity embolism.

Figure 1

Direct surgical reconstruction of the innominate artery is performed under general anesthesia with the patient in supine position. It is wise to turn the head to the left in case the exposure requires extension into the right supraclavicular fossa. The neck and anterior chest are prepped and draped in standard fashion to facilitate a midline skin incision made from the sternal notch to the third intercostal space. This incision is deepened to the sternum with electrocautery. An oscillating blade mounted on a (redo) sternotomy saw (Stryker, Kalamazoo, MI) is used to make a sternal incision from the notch to the third intercostal space. The sternal incision is "T'd" at the third intercostal space to expose the upper mediastinum. Care is taken to not injure the internal mammary vessels, which are adjacent to the sternum. Hemostasis should be obtained at the periosteal edges before placement of a pediatric sternal retractor to separate the upper sternum.

Figure 2

The two lobes of the thymus gland are separated in the midline, and entry into either pleural space can be avoided by observation of the pleural bulge during inspiration. Nutrient vessels to the thymus gland are ligated and divided to maintain a dry field. These vessels arise from the internal thoracic artery and drain into the internal thoracic or brachiocephalic veins. The upper pericardium is then opened vertically and the edges are sewn to the skin with silk suture. The left brachiocephalic vein should be dissected circumferentially and isolated with a Silastic vessel loop. This maneuver improves exposure of the ascending aorta, which is gently mobilized from surrounding tissue, with care not to injure adjacent pulmonary or surrounding neurolymphatic structures. Bypass grafts should originate from a disease free portion of the right anterolateral ascending aorta proximal to the innominate artery. We prefer to use the intrapericardial ascending aorta as the anastomotic site of graft origin. In addition, it is wise to use a secure partial occluding clamp on the ascending aorta, such as the Cooley All-Purpose clamp. This will ensure that the clamp will not dislodge or move once applied on the ascending aorta.

Figure 1

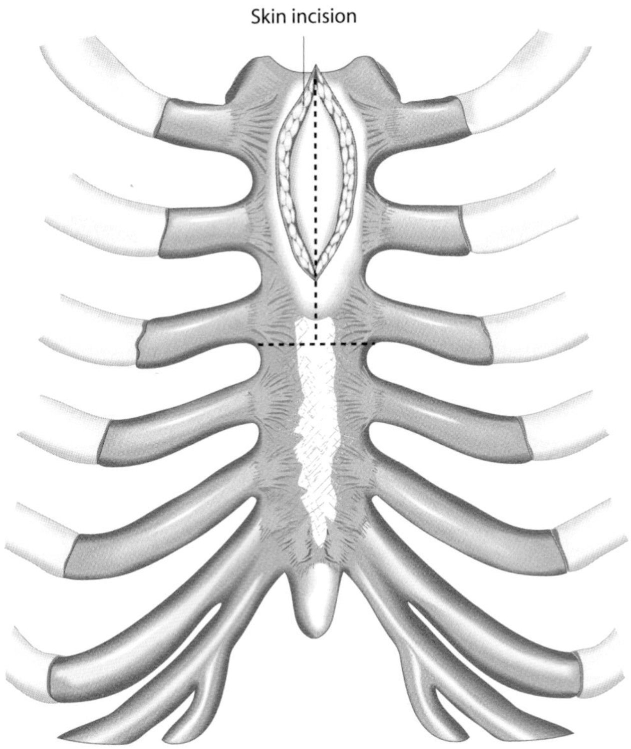

Skin incision

Figure 2

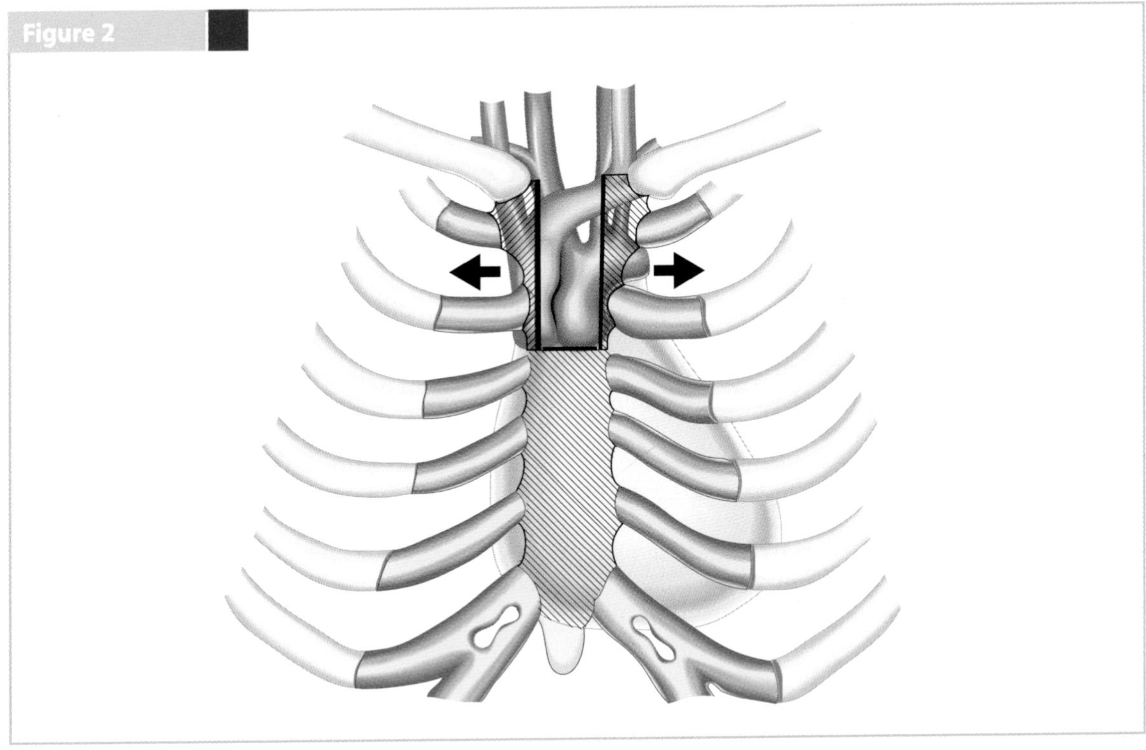

Figure 3

The innominate artery is identified and circumferentially dissected to its bifurcation into the right subclavian and common carotid arteries. The origin of each of these arteries is exposed and then controlled with a Silastic vessel loop. The recurrent laryngeal nerve, which wraps around the proximal subclavian artery from anterior to posterior, should remain undisturbed during this dissection. Occasionally, more extensive exposure of each vessel is required to facilitate a durable bypass. In particular, experience has demonstrated that subclavian atherosclerotic plaque may extend beyond the exposure of a sternotomy, and for this reason the subclavian artery can be a troublesome site in which to achieve unimpeded outflow. If the subclavian artery atheroma extends too far distal to achieve a sound endpoint, and reconstruction is not mandatory, a staged carotid-subclavian artery reconstruction may be appropriate on rare occasion. Otherwise, the exposure can be extended in a supraclavicular fashion to improve distal subclavian artery exposure and to achieve a satisfactory plaque endpoint where the bypass graft can safely terminate.

Extension of the mini-sternotomy incision above and parallel to the clavicle facilitates extended exposure of the right subclavian artery. The right sternohyoid and sternothyroid muscles are divided, followed by exposure of the scalene fat pad. Branches of the thyrocervical trunk are divided and the dissection is deepened to expose the anterior scalene muscle. The phrenic nerve is identified and protected as it courses from lateral to medial across the surface of the anterior scalene muscle to pass into the superior mediastinum. The subclavian artery comes into view with division of the anterior scalene muscle just above its insertion on the first rib.

Figure 4

Aorto-innominate artery bypass begins with an aortotomy created in the right anterolateral aspect of the intrapericardial ascending aorta. This incision is best made with a #11 blade and lengthened appropriately with angled Potts scissors. A Dacron tube graft sized to match to distal innominate artery is anastomosed in an end-to-side fashion to the ascending aorta using a running 4-0 Prolene suture. This proximal anastomosis should be created with a rounded graft toe. This configuration is facilitated by cutting a graft limb off the body of a bifurcated graft or by cutting a tube graft with a curve on the back wall. It is wise to reinforce the suture line with a strip of Teflon felt, particularly if the ascending aorta appears friable.

Secure hemostasis of the graft-to-ascending aorta anastomosis should be confirmed before proceeding on to proximal innominate artery ligation and the distal anastomosis. Applying an atraumatic clamp on the proximal aspect of the graft, so that the side-biting clamp on the ascending aorta can be released, facilitates this maneuver. The bypass graft should ideally be routed anterolaterally and under the left brachiocephalic vein so that the overlying sternum or clavicular head of sternocleidomastoid muscle does not compress it. Despite this precaution, bony compression of the graft may occur near the sternoclavicular joint. The posterior elements of this joint can be safely removed with a rongeur to widen the space and allow for an uncompromised graft route.

Vascular occluding clamps are applied to the proximal innominate, right subclavian and common carotid arteries. The innominate artery is transected distally and oversewn proximally using two separate layers of 4-0 Prolene suture. Then to facilitate a sound end-to-end anastomosis at the level of the distal innominate artery, the Dacron tube graft should be cut with a slight obliquity. The anastomosis is created using a running 5-0 Prolene suture. Just prior to completion of the anastomosis, the right subclavian and common carotid arteries are allowed to backbleed and the bypass graft is flushed to clear all air and debris from the lumens. Antegrade blood flow is first established to the subclavian artery followed by the right common carotid. Immediate intraoperative duplex ultrasound is used to confirm a widely patent innominate artery reconstruction.

Figure 3

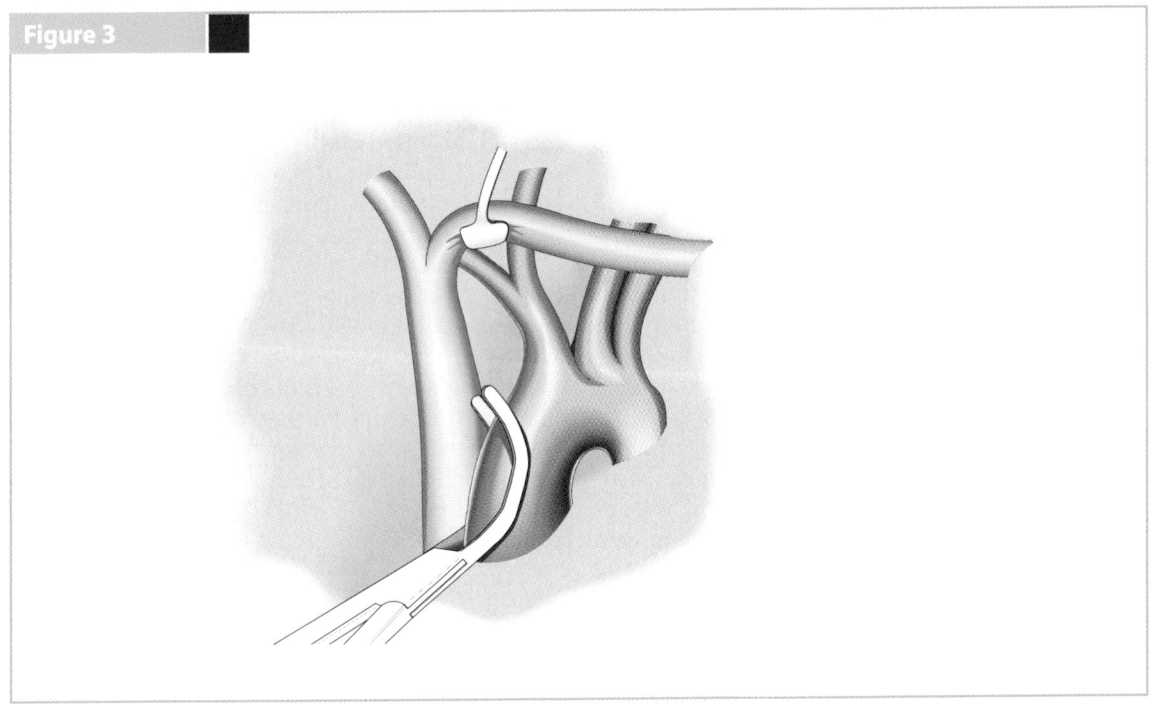

Figure 4

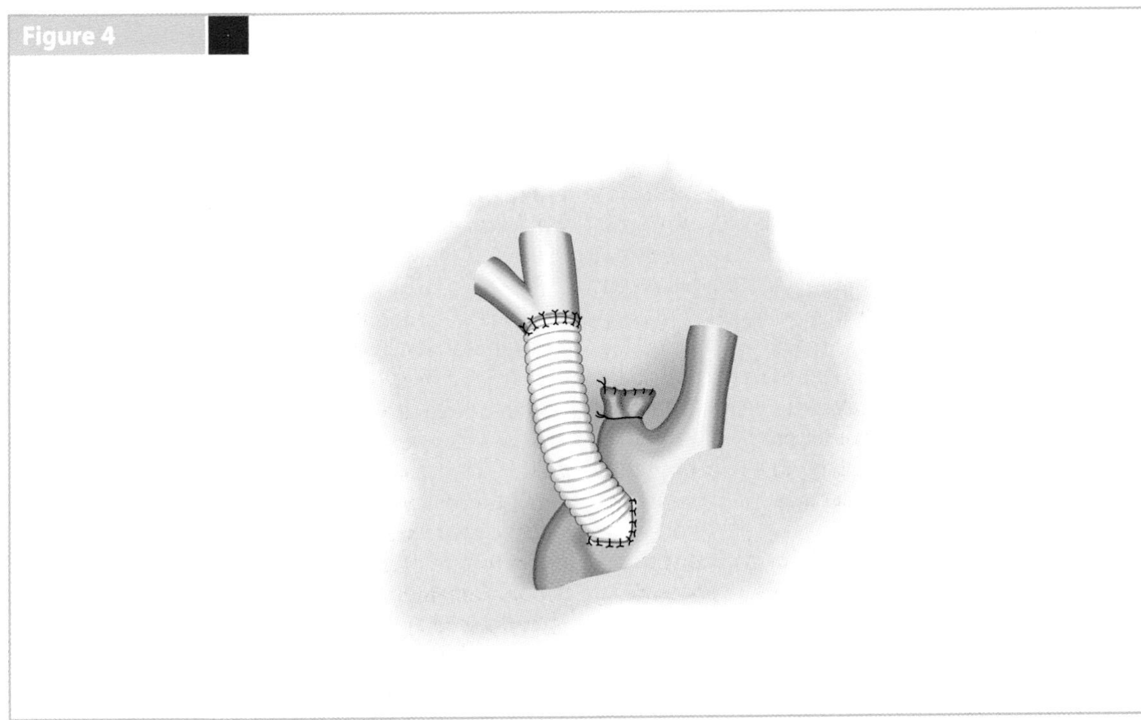

Figure 5

It is wise to use a single-limb graft with an added side limb if the left common carotid artery also requires reconstruction. This reduces overall graft size compared to a bifurcated graft and there is a decreased chance of graft limb kinking with sternal closure. Optimal placement of added side arm grafts can be ascertained by releasing tension on the sternal retractor. The left brachiocephalic vein may be divided or the bypassed innominate artery resected to ensure graft routes free of impingement or compression.

Upon completion of the vascular procedure, heparin is reversed with protamine sulfate and hemostasis is obtained throughout the upper mediastinum. A 19F Blake drain (Johnson & Johnson, Cincinnati, OH) is placed within the pericardium and brought out through a separate stab incision made in the second intercostal space. The drain should be secured at the skin exit site using a 3-0 nylon suture and connected to a Heimlich valve grenade suction device. Chest tubes are not required. Two wires are utilized to bring the upper and lower sternal edges of the "T" together while two more are placed in the manubrium. If needed, another wire placed as a "Figure-of-eight" at the level of the second intercostal space completely rejoins the divided upper sternum. After approximating the muscular and subcutaneous planes in two layers, the skin is closed in a subcuticular fashion. The patient is awakened in the operating room and noted to have a normal neurological examination before proceeding to the recovery room.

Figure 5

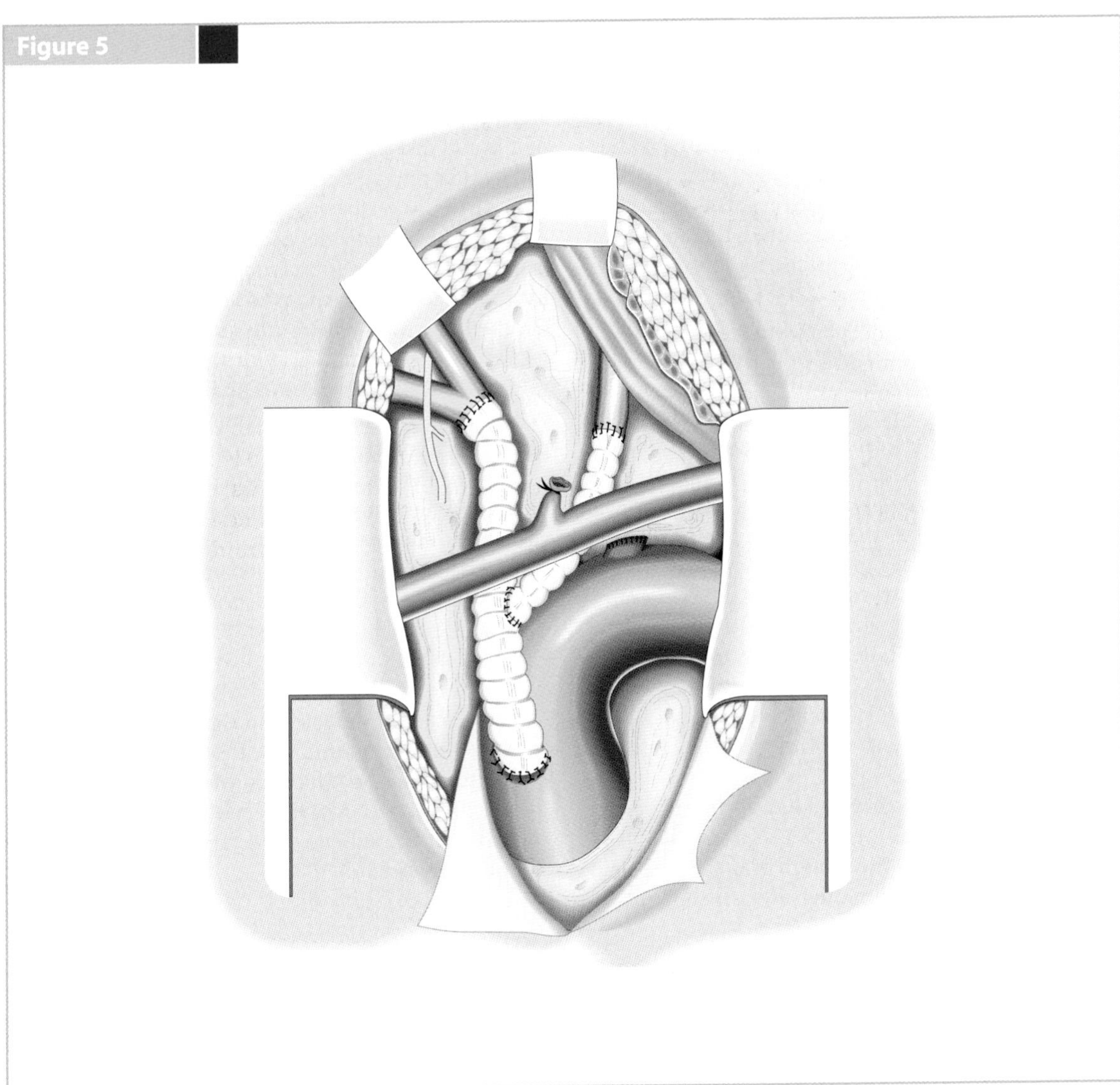

Figure 6: Subclavian to Subclavian Artery Bypass

Occasionally direct surgical reconstruction of the diseased innominate artery is precluded by patient co-morbid factors or the complexity of a potential re-do sternotomy. In this situation extrathoracic bypass can be performed using either the subclavian and/or axillary arteries for graft origin and destination. Subclavian-subclavian artery bypass is preferred because graft patency is better and the graft can be routed above the sternal notch instead of across the sternum as for axillary-axillary bypass grafts. In addition, supraclavicular exposure of the right subclavian artery facilitates ligation of the very distal innominate artery to exclude a potential embolic source. Alternatively, the subclavian artery can be ligated proximal to the vertebral artery origin if exposure of the distal innominate artery is hazardous. To maintain antegrade cerebral perfusion in this setting, the right common carotid artery can be transposed to a more lateral position on the subclavian artery or bypassed with a graft limb extension from the subclavian-subclavian artery bypass graft. Distal innominate artery ligation is unnecessary if the vessel is occluded.

Exposure of the second portion of the subclavian artery is accomplished through a supraclavicular incision, beginning over the tendon of the sternocleidomastoid muscle and extending laterally for 8–10 cm. The platysma muscle is divided and the scalene fat pad mobilized superolaterally. Thyrocervical vessels are ligated and divided as encountered, with exposure of the anterior surface of the anterior scalene muscle. The phrenic nerve can be seen coursing from lateral to medial over this muscle and should be gently mobilized and preserved during the dissection. On the left side, the thoracic duct must also be protected at its termination with the confluence of the internal jugular, brachiocephalic and subclavian veins. Unrecognized injury may result in a lymphocele or lymphocutaneous fistula.

The anterior scalene muscle is divided just above its point of insertion on the first rib to facilitate exposure of the subclavian artery. Division of this muscle should be done under direct vision and without cautery as the brachial plexus is immediately adjacent to the lateral aspect of the anterior scalene muscle. The origin of the left vertebral artery arises from the medial surface of the subclavian artery medial to the anterior scalene muscle and behind the sternoclavicular joint. The internal thoracic artery, which originates from the inferior surface of the subclavian artery opposite the thyrocervical trunk, should be protected as the subclavian artery is dissected free of surrounding tissue.

Figure 7

A subcutaneous tunnel created above the sternal notch connects the two subclavian artery exposures so that the bypass graft (6- or 8-mm Dacron tube graft) lies low in the neck and courses just above the clavicles. Each end-to-side anastomosis should originate from the subclavian artery distal to the vertebral artery origin. A broken-back (Pilling Weck) or similarly shaped vascular occluding clamp can be nestled around the subclavian artery by gently pulling up on a previously placed Silastic vessel loop and sliding the clamp down along the sides of the artery. Care should be taken to ensure that no nerve tissue courses between the closing clamp and artery. An arteriotomy is created with a #11 blade and lengthened appropriately with angled Potts scissors. 5-0 Prolene suture is used to complete the end-to-side anastomosis. Brief clamp release just prior to its completion facilitates appropriate backbleeding.

Figure 6

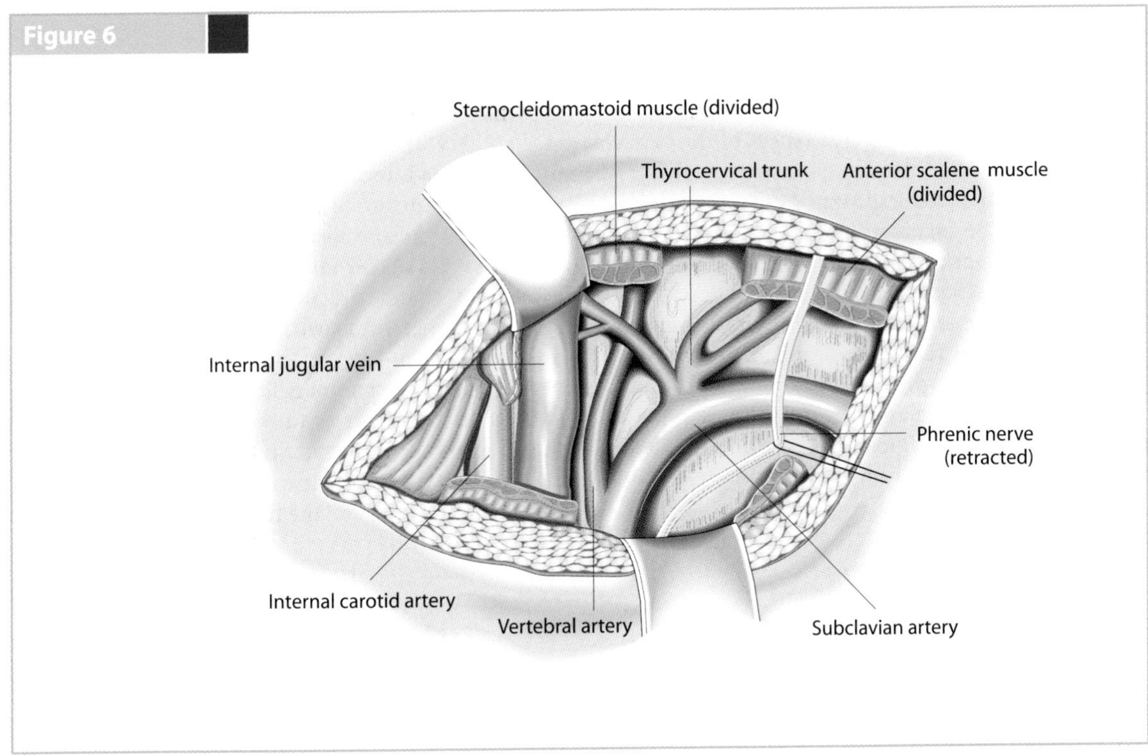
Sternocleidomastoid muscle (divided)
Thyrocervical trunk
Anterior scalene muscle (divided)
Internal jugular vein
Phrenic nerve (retracted)
Internal carotid artery
Vertebral artery
Subclavian artery

Figure 7

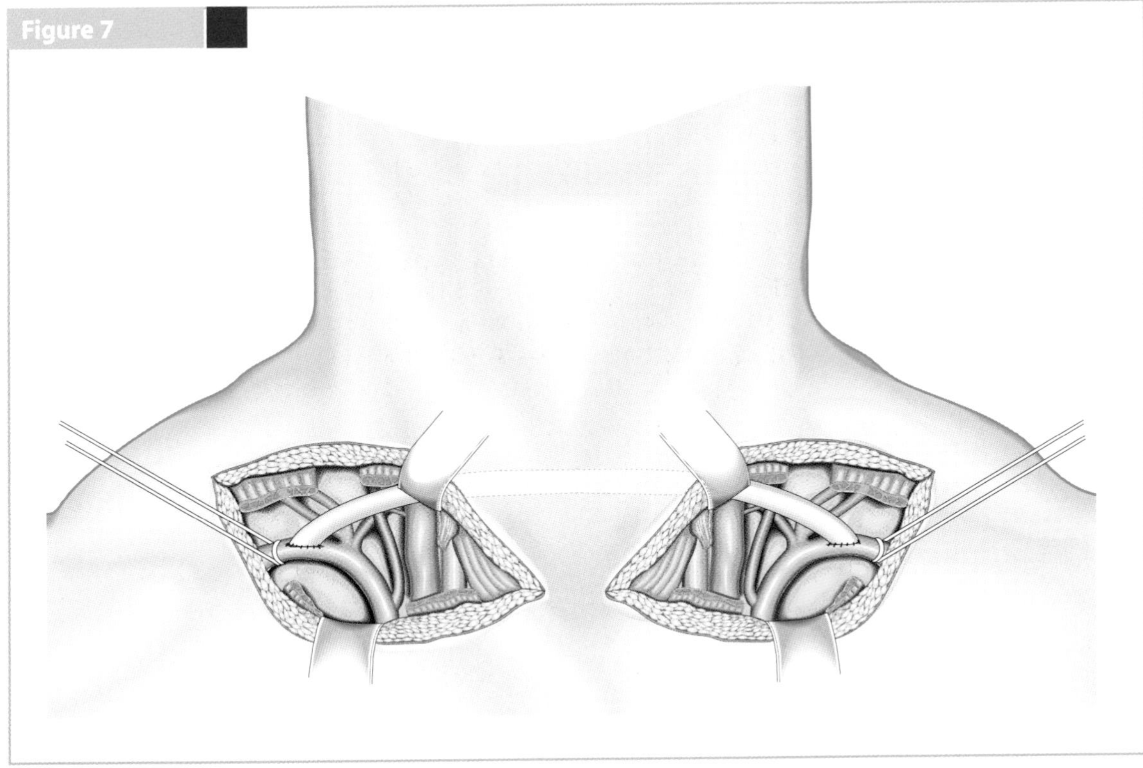

Figure 8: Axillary – Axillary Artery Bypass

A short infraclavicular incision made approximately 1.5 cm below the mid-to-lateral aspect of the clavicle and parallel to the pectoralis major muscle fibers facilitates dissection and exposure of the proximal axillary artery. The incision is deepened between the clavicular and sternal portions of the pectoralis major muscle to expose the clavipectoral fascia. This fascia is incised sharply to reveal underlying adipose tissue. Within this tissue are branches of the thoracoacromial vessels, which require ligation and division to expose the axillary vein first and then the axillary artery above and posterior to the vein. Dissection medial to the pectoralis minor muscle provides appropriate exposure of the axillary artery for axillary-axillary artery bypass graft origin. Division of the pectoralis minor muscle is rarely required to improve exposure of the axillary artery. However, if additional exposure is required laterally, a portion of the pectoralis minor muscle can be divided near its insertion into the coracoid process of the scapula.

The bypass graft is usually routed in a subcutaneous plane at the level of the first interspace and superficial to the sternum. Alternatively, a retrosternal graft route can be created, although potential complications are greatly increased using this graft path.

Figure 8

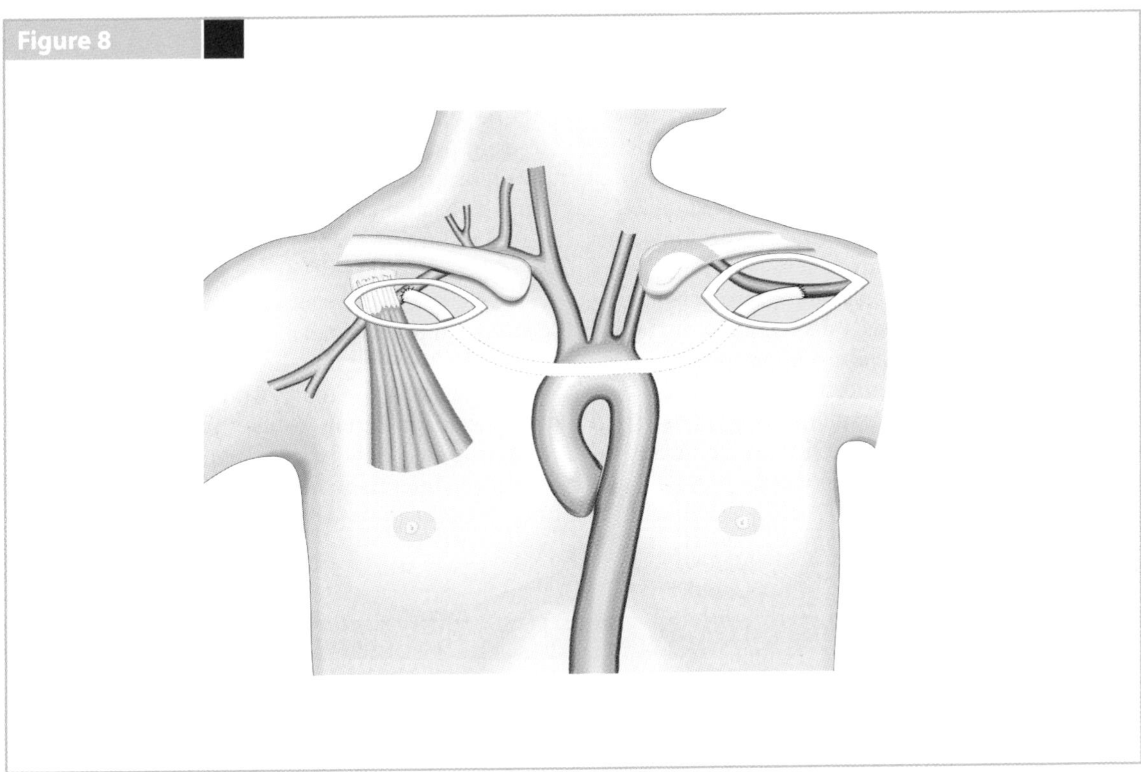

CONCLUSION

Results of transthoracic reconstruction of the innominate artery are excellent. This is particularly true for good-risk patients with extensive pathology or multivessel disease. Long-term symptom relief is maintained in 87–90% of patients. The long-term graft patency rate ranges from 94% to 98% at 5 years and from 88% to 96% at 10 years. As expected, morbidity and mortality rates are decreased for extrathoracic bypass procedures; however, graft durability is decreased as is maintenance of symptom free survival. Poor-risk surgical patients with single vessel disease or with prior sternotomy are better served with extrathoracic bypass procedures.

Perioperative vascular complications include bleeding, pseudoaneurysm, distal embolization, graft thrombosis or infection, and ischemia of the hand or brain. Nonvascular complications are predominately related to local nerve injury. The right recurrent laryngeal nerve, phrenic nerve, brachial plexus and sympathetic chain are all vulnerable during the dissections. Supraclavicular dissections in particular expose the thoracic duct on the left and other lymphatic channels to injury with the potential for a lymphocele or lymph fistula. Other less common complications include pneumothorax, aortic arch dissection, internal mammary artery injury, mediastinal bleeding and mediastinitis.

REFERENCES

Ballard JL (2005) Anatomy and surgical exposure of the vascular system. In: Moore WS (ed) Vascular surgery: A comprehensive review, 7th edn. WB Saunders, Philadelphia, pp 46–68

Chang JB, Stein TA, Liu JP, Dunn ME (1997) Long-term results of axillo-axillary bypass grafts for symptomatic subclavian artery insufficiency. J Vasc Surg 25:173–178

Crawford ES, DeBakey ME, Morris GC, Howell JF (1969) Surgical treatment of occlusion of the innominate, common carotid, and subclavian arteries: a 10-year experience. Surgery 65:17–31

Owens LV, Tinsley EA Jr, Criado E et al. (1995) Extrathoracic reconstruction of arterial occlusive disease involving the supraaortic trunks. J Vasc Surg 22:217–222

Sakopoulos AG, Ballard JL, Gundry SR (2000) Minimally invasive approach for aortic arch branch vessel reconstruction. J Vasc Surg 31:200–202

Twena MF, Ballard JL (2000) Surgical approach to lesions of the subclavian, axillary and brachial arteries. In: Dyet JF, Ettles DF, Nicholson AA, Wilson SE (eds) Textbook of endovascular surgery. WB Saunders, Philadelphia, pp 174–183

CHAPTER 7

Carotid-Subclavian Transposition and Carotid-Subclavian Bypass

John S. Lane, Julie A. Freischlag

INTRODUCTION

Carotid-subclavian transposition (CST) and carotid-subclavian bypass (CSB) are performed for symptomatic stenosis of the proximal subclavian artery. These procedures are more commonly performed on the left subclavian artery (70%), as opposed to the right subclavian artery. This is due to the relative size of the arteries and the more frequent and significant involvement of the left subclavian with atherosclerotic disease at the aortic arch.

The term "subclavian steal syndrome" was first introduced in 1961 and was described as the reversal of flow in the vertebral artery associated with a proximal subclavian stenosis. The true incidence of the subclavian steal syndrome is unknown as the majority of cases are asymptomatic. Symptomatic subclavian steal occurs in conjunction with concomitant stenosis of the contralateral vertebral artery or in conjunction with stenosis of the anterior (carotid) circulation. Otherwise, with an intact communicating circulation, reversal of flow in the vertebral artery rarely causes vertebrobasilar symptoms.

Symptoms initiating investigation into proximal subclavian disease are usually vertebrobasilar in nature and include visual disturbances, vertigo, ataxia, syncope, dysphagia, dysarthria, transient hemiparesis or hemisensory disturbances. However, in rare instances (<5%) upper extremity ischemic symptoms may occur, including fatigue on exertion, rest pain or stigmata of microembolic disease. Rarely, a patient who has undergone coronary artery bypass using a left internal mammary artery (LIMA) graft will present with a "coronary steal syndrome." This occurs when left arm exertion causes reversal of flow in the LIMA graft precipitating anginal symptoms. Any combination of vertebrobasilar and upper extremity symptoms should stimulate investigation into proximal subclavian disease.

A thorough history and physical exam should be performed, including auscultation for supraclavicular bruits. Blood pressure should be measured in both arms, with a differential of >20 mmHg considered significant. A duplex ultrasound can be performed to confirm the reversal of flow in the vertebral artery and may identify the area of stenosis in the proximal subclavian. This should be performed at rest and with exercise or with reactive hyperemia. It should be emphasized that finding of reversal of flow within the vertebral is not pathognomonic of subclavian steal, as the majority of these cases are asymptomatic. Confirmatory radiological tests can localize the area of stenosis and include arch aortography, computerized tomography or magnetic resonance angiography. No selective subclavian catheterization should be performed, as it often misses proximal lesions and may traumatize existing plaques. The carotid circulation should also be evaluated by means of duplex ultrasound or angiography. As previously mentioned, concomitant lesions in the anterior circulation often exist. In our experience, significant carotid stenosis should be surgically addressed first. By re-establishing adequate carotid perfusion, vertebrobasilar symptoms may be redressed. Other standard preoperative screening tests should be performed, including an assessment of cardiorespiratory fitness.

The use of clopidogrel should be discontinued at least 2 weeks prior to operation, while the use of aspirin should continue until the night prior to operation.

CAROTID-SUBCLAVIAN TRANSPOSITION

Carotid-subclavian transposition (CST) is the procedure of choice for the treatment of symptomatic proximal subclavian stenosis in our institution (see "Conclusion"). Advantages of this approach include the need to perform only one vascular anastomosis, no prosthetic material is necessary, and the source of any potential emboli (from the proximal subclavian) is removed from the circulation. Disadvantages include the need for more extensive mobilization of the subclavian artery, proximal to the vertebral origin, to allow the vessel to be transposed. If this is not technically feasible, or if the proximal subclavian artery is extensively involved with atherosclerotic disease, this approach is contraindicated and a carotid-subclavian bypass should be performed.

Figure 1: Patient Preparation and Incision

Routine use of electroencephalographic (EEG) monitoring is performed in our institution to assess the need for intraoperative carotid shunting. EEG electrodes are placed preoperatively, and baseline brain-wave activity is recorded.

After the induction of general anesthesia, the patient is positioned supinely on the operating table, with the shoulder elevated by a roll of sheets, allowing full extension of the neck. The head is rotated away from the side of interest, and is supported with a soft ring. Skin preparation includes the area bordered by the earlobe superiorly, the nipple inferiorly, the corner of the mouth medially and the shoulder laterally. Sterile drapes are applied and the skin is covered with an adherent, iodine-impregnated plastic barrier. Intravenous antibiotics are administered to cover skin flora, usually cefazolin or vancomycin.

A transverse supraclavicular incision is placed 2.0 cm above the clavicle. The incision extends laterally from the border of the sternocleidomastoid for a distance of approximately 10.0 cm. The subcutaneous tissue and the platysma are divided with electrocautery. Additional exposure may be gained medially by dividing the lateral (clavicular) head of the sternocleidomastoid or the omohyoid muscle if necessary. These muscles should be reapproximated during closure to prevent unwanted cosmetic effects. The scalene fat pad is then encountered and should be separated from its attachments to the clavicle inferiorly and retracted superiorly. The scalene fat pad should not be excised to prevent the appearance of a sunken supraclavicular space.

Figure 2: Anterior Scalene Muscle Division

Below the scalene fat pad, the anterior scalene is visible. This muscle must be divided to provide a "gateway to the subclavian artery." The phrenic nerve is situated on the anterior surface of the anterior scalene, as it courses from lateral to medial. This nerve must be carefully dissected and retracted laterally. It should be laterally to prevent injury and subsequent diaphragmatic dysfunction. The thoracic duct on the left may also be encountered at this level as it courses from beneath the clavicle to join the confluence of the subclavian and jugular veins. It is our practice to doubly ligate and divide the thoracic duct to prevent inadvertent injury and subsequent chylous leak.

The anterior scalene muscle is divided with electrocautery and retracted to gain exposure to the subclavian artery.

Figure 1

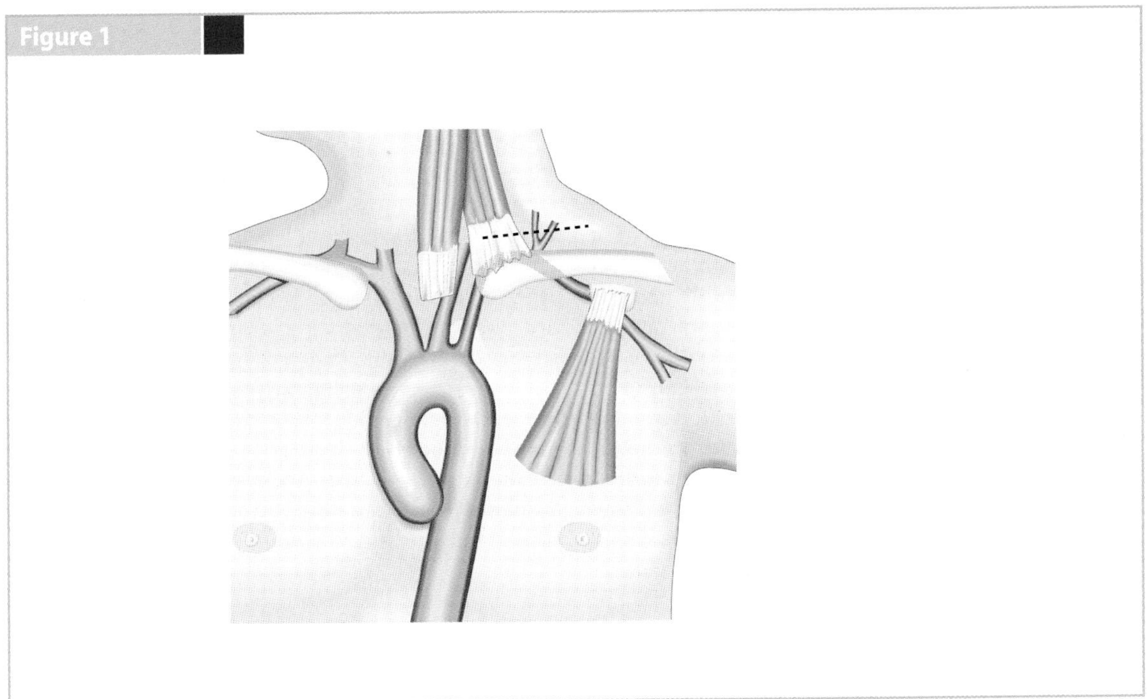

Figure 2

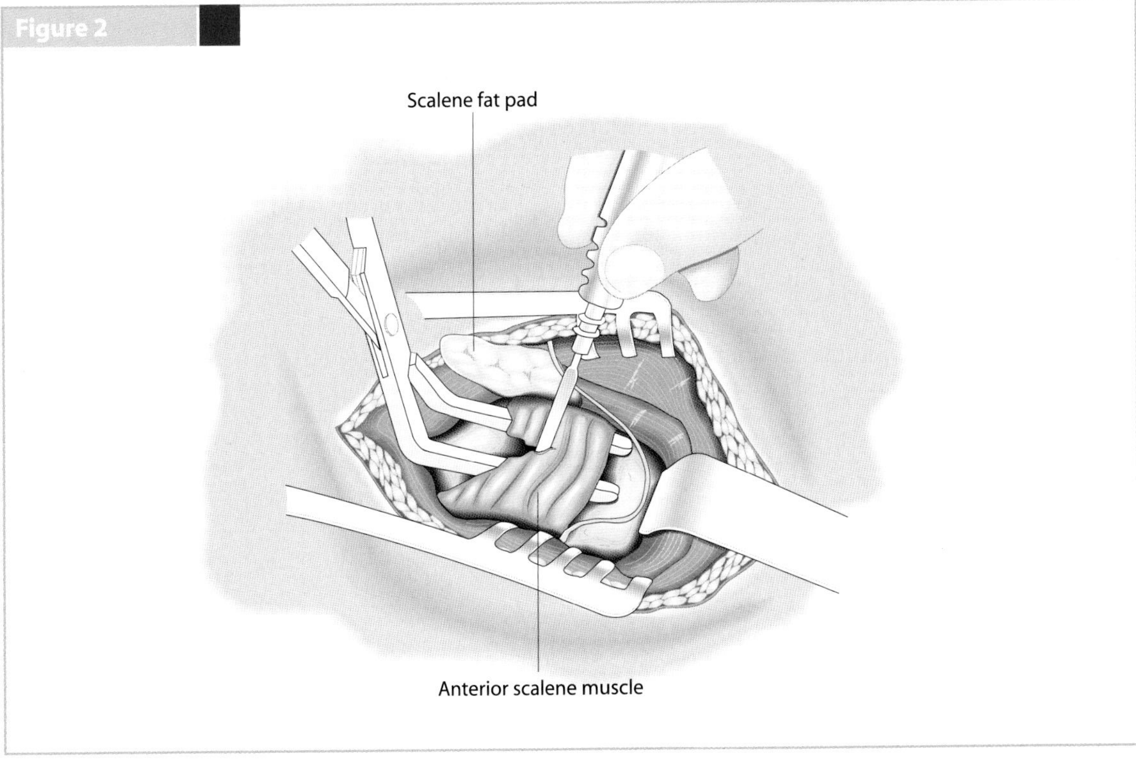

Figure 3: Subclavian Artery Exposure

The subclavian artery lies deep to the anterior scalene. At this level the artery is situated superiorly to the subclavian vein. The lower cords of the brachial plexus are found deep to the subclavian artery and should be carefully handled during the placement of retractors. The branches of the subclavian artery include the thyrocervical and costocervical trunks, the internal mammary artery and the vertebral artery. These branches should be controlled with vessel loops or heavy silk sutures during the dissection and mobilization of the subclavian artery. The costocervical thyrocervical trunk and/or the internal mammary artery may be sacrificed to gain needed mobility of the subclavian artery to facilitate transposition to the carotid artery. However, we prefer not to sacrifice the internal mammary artery and will resort to a carotid-subclavian bypass if a transposition is not anatomically feasible. Dissection of the subclavian artery is carried medially until 1.0–2.0 cm of subclavian artery is accessible proximal to the vertebral artery. The vessel is palpated to assess the extent of atherosclerotic disease. If clamping of the vessel is not possible at this level, transposition is aborted and a carotid-subclavian bypass is performed. If control of the subclavian artery is lost near its origin, it is extremely difficult to regain and a thoracotomy may be required.

The subclavian artery is encircled with a vessel loop proximally to the vertebral and attention is turned to the carotid artery.

Figure 4: Common Carotid Artery Exposure

The carotid sheath is located in the medial part of the field beneath the sternocleidomastoid muscle. The carotid sheath is opened with care not to injure the vagus nerve, which runs between the artery and the vein. The internal jugular vein is retracted anteromedially, gaining exposure to the common carotid artery. The carotid artery is dissected for a distance of 3.0–4.0 cm and is encircled with moistened umbilical tapes. Visual inspection or measurement of the available length of subclavian artery should be performed to determine whether transposition is possible.

Once the decision is made to proceed, intravenous heparin is administered (5000 units).

Figure 3

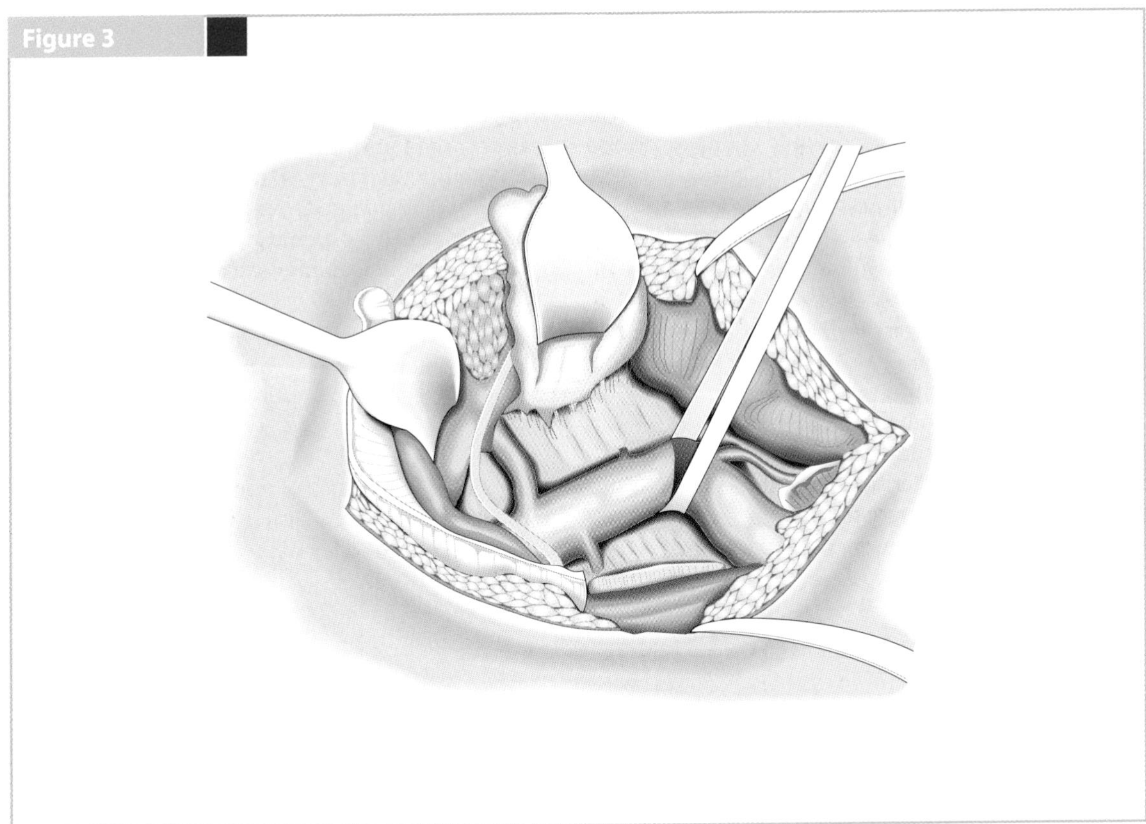

Figure 4

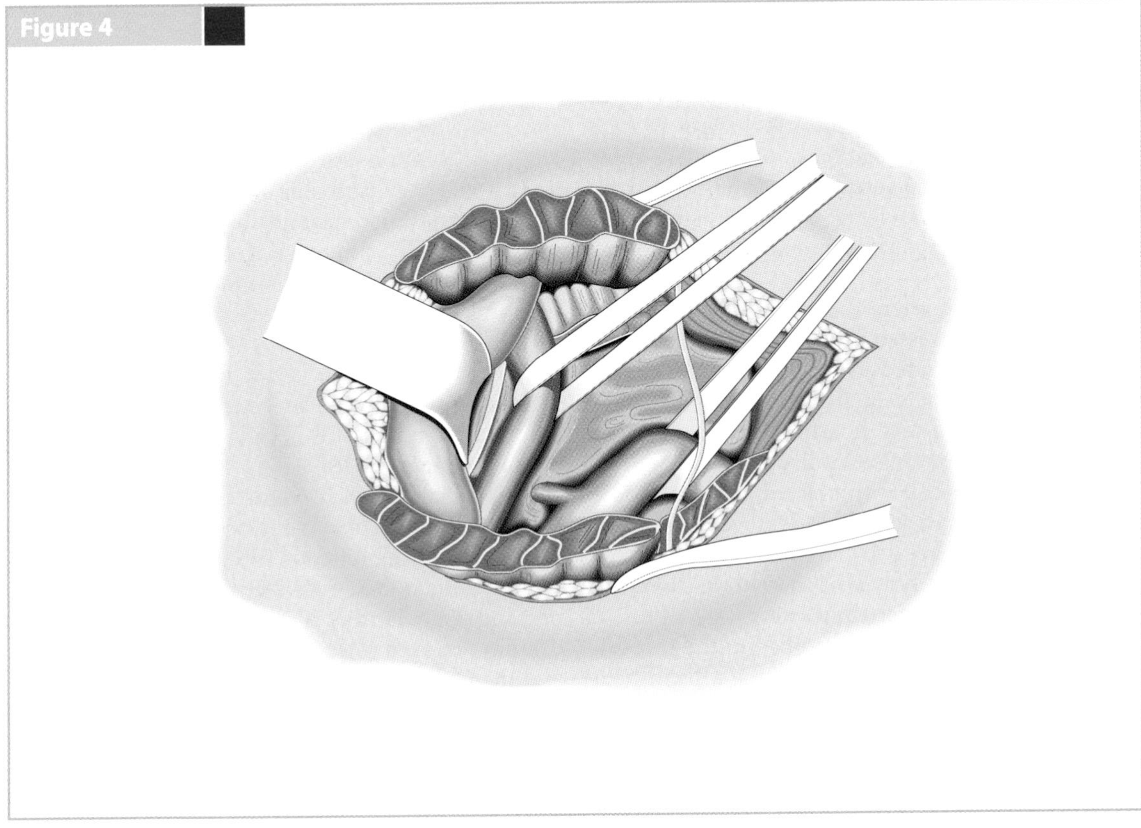

Figure 5: Division of the Subclavian Artery

The branches of the subclavian artery are controlled and the subclavian artery is doubly clamped proximally to the vertebral artery. The subclavian artery is divided between the clamps using a surgical scalpel. The proximal stump of the subclavian artery is oversewn using two rows of 4.0 polypropylene sutures in a horizontal mattress fashion. The proximal clamp is carefully removed and hemostasis is assessed.

The distal subclavian artery is swung superiorly to an appropriate position on the common carotid artery. Rotating the artery 90 degrees reduces kinking while affording adequate length. The artery is tunneled deep to the phrenic nerve and the internal jugular vein to the common carotid artery.

Figure 6: Carotid-Subclavian Anastomosis

The common carotid artery is controlled using two angled vascular clamps or a single side-biting clamp. Attention must be directed toward changes in EEG activity during this portion of the operation, as antegrade flow to both the vertebral and the carotid artery is interrupted. If changes in EEG activity are noticed, the surgeon must be prepared to place a carotid shunt.

Once the carotid artery is controlled, a longitudinal arteriotomy is created using a #11 scalpel and the arteriotomy is extended using Potts scissors. Stay sutures are placed to facilitate exposure of the arterial lumen. An end-to-side arterial anastomosis is performed using running 6.0 polypropylene sutures. Before the anastomosis is completed, the arteries are back-bled and forward-bled to remove all air and debris. The sutures are tied and the subclavian artery clamp removed. The flow is opened to the common carotid artery and the vertebral artery last.

Assessment of flow is determined in the carotid, subclavian and vertebral arteries using a hand-held Doppler probe or using color flow duplex imaging. A completion angiogram is not routinely performed in our institution, unless there is a question as to the technical result if an endarterectomy of one of the vessels had been performed.

Hemostasis is achieved in the operative field and a Silastic, closed-suction drain is placed to the supraclavicular fossa. The scalene fat pad is returned to its anatomic location and secured to the clavicle using interrupted 3.0 absorbable sutures. The lateral head of the sternocleidomastoid is also reapproximated using absorbable sutures, if it had been divided. The platysma is closed using running 3.0 absorbable suture and the skin is closed using a 5.0 subcuticular suture.

Reversal of heparin is not routinely performed. The patient is allowed to emerge from anesthesia, and neurological status is carefully assessed. In the absence of neurological deficit, the patient is allowed to recover and then brought to the surgical ward. Neurological function is reassessed every 4 h overnight. Swallowing function is determined by observing the patient swallow water on postoperative day one and a regular diet is started. The closed-suction drain is removed when the output is <30 cc over 24 h and the patient is tolerating a regular diet without a chylous leak. Aspirin is restarted on postoperative day one and the patient is usually discharged on the second postoperative day.

Figure 5

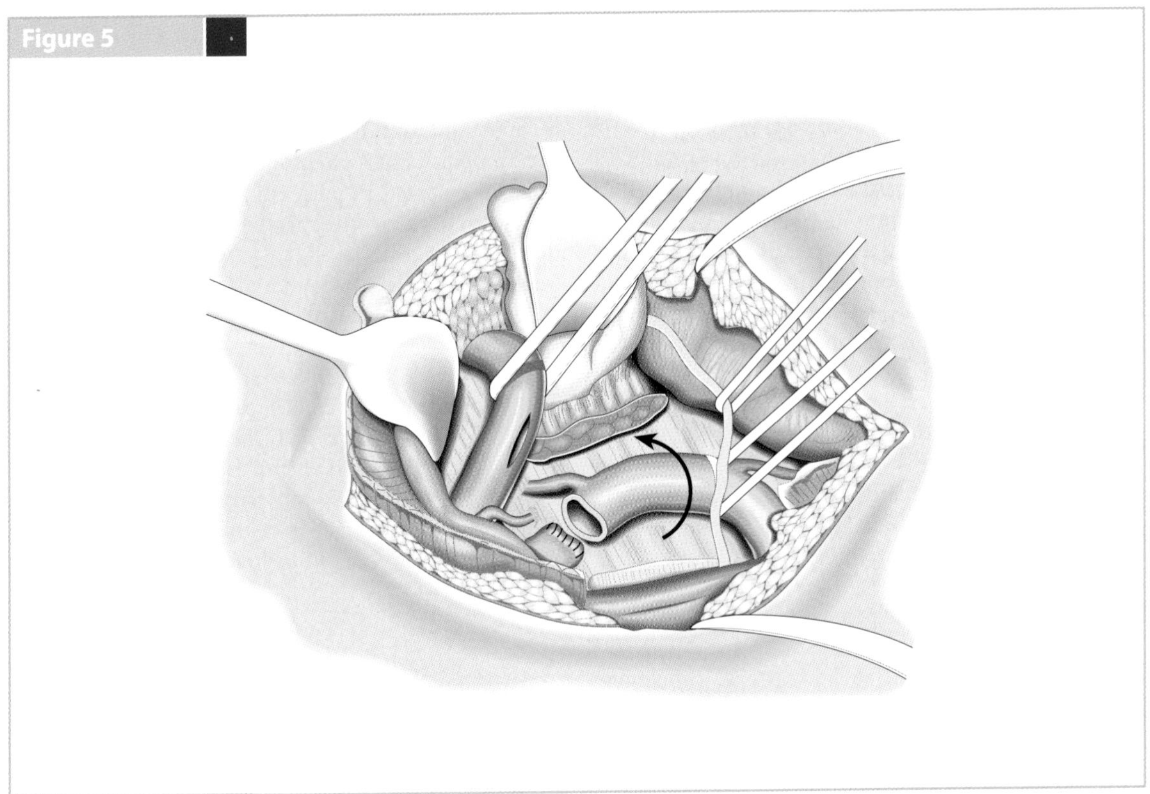

Figure 6

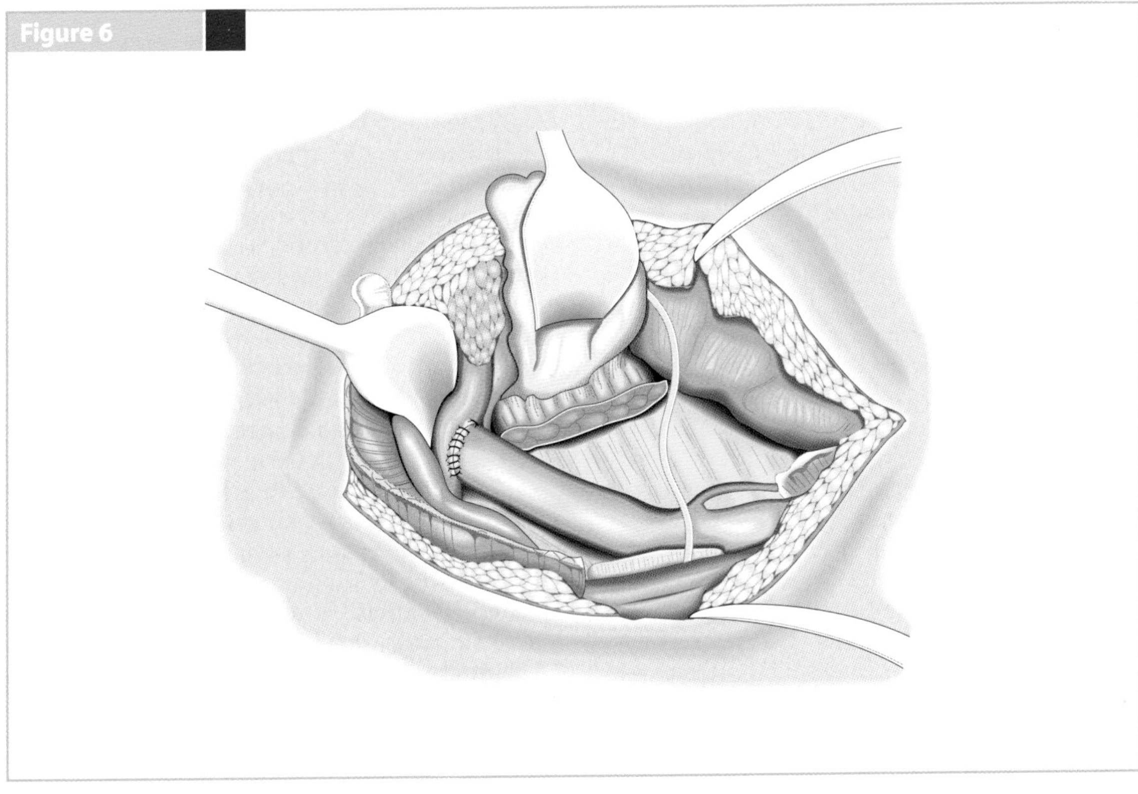

CAROTID-SUBCLAVIAN BYPASS

Carotid-subclavian bypass (CSB) is a more versatile operation than carotid-subclavian transposition and may be performed when a transposition is not possible due to technical considerations. This includes a "hostile neck," secondary to previous operations, radiation changes, anatomic variations or extensive atherosclerotic disease. In these instances, a convenient location on the subclavian artery can be selected to perform the distal anastomosis in an end-to-side fashion. However, in situations in which embolization into the vertebral or brachial circulation is present, the source of emboli is not excluded from the circulation. In this case, the subclavian artery must be ligated proximally to the vertebral artery to prevent continued embolization while maintaining retrograde flow to the vertebral artery.

■ **Exposure.** Surgical exposure for CSB is similar to CST, including a supraclavicular approach and control of the common carotid artery, subclavian artery and its branches. However, a less extensive dissection of the subclavian artery is required and a convenient location is selected for the performance of the distal anastomosis. Exposure of the vertebral artery is not necessary unless a concurrent vertebral endarterectomy is to be performed. The subclavian artery is encircled with vessel loops and the common carotid artery is controlled with moist umbilical tapes.

Figure 7: Distal Anastomosis

The distal anastomosis is first performed to minimize the amount of time the common carotid artery is clamped. A convenient location on the subclavian artery is selected to perform the distal anastomosis, which would allow the minimal amount of graft material to be used. After systemic heparinization (5000 units), the subclavian artery is clamped using vascular clamps. Visualization of the luminal surface is facilitated by the placement of 6.0 polypropylene stay sutures. We utilize 6.0- or 8.0-mm polytetrafluoroethylene (PTFE) prosthetic grafts (non-ringed) as our conduit of choice (see discussion). The graft is spatulated and an end-to-side anastomosis is performed using 6.0 polypropylene in a running fashion. The graft is clamped near the anastomosis and flow is re-established to the upper extremity.

Figure 8: Proximal Anastomosis

The site for the proximal anastomosis is selected on the common carotid artery so as to minimize the amount of graft material used. The graft is tunneled deep to the phrenic nerve and the internal jugular vein. The common carotid is clamped with vascular clamps or a single side-biting clamp while close monitoring of the EEG is maintained. Carotid shunting is selectively performed on the basis of changes in EEG activity. Stay sutures are also placed to facilitate exposure of the luminal surface. The graft is trimmed and spatulated appropriately. An end-to-side anastomosis is performed using 6.0 running polypropylene suture. The graft is back-bled and forward-bled to remove air and debris. Flow is first opened into the upper extremity circulation before re-establishing flow to the carotid and vertebral circulation. Hemostasis is meticulously achieved. Drain placement and wound closure is performed as in CST. Intravenous antibiotics are continued for 24 h postoperatively.

Figure 7

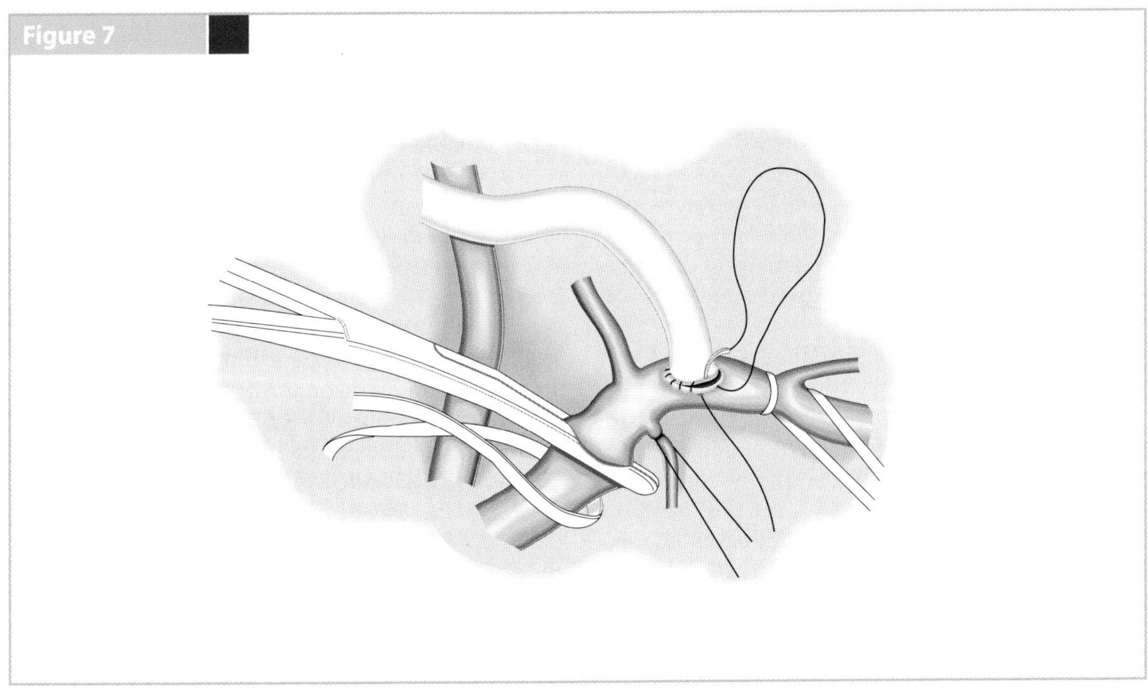

Figure 8

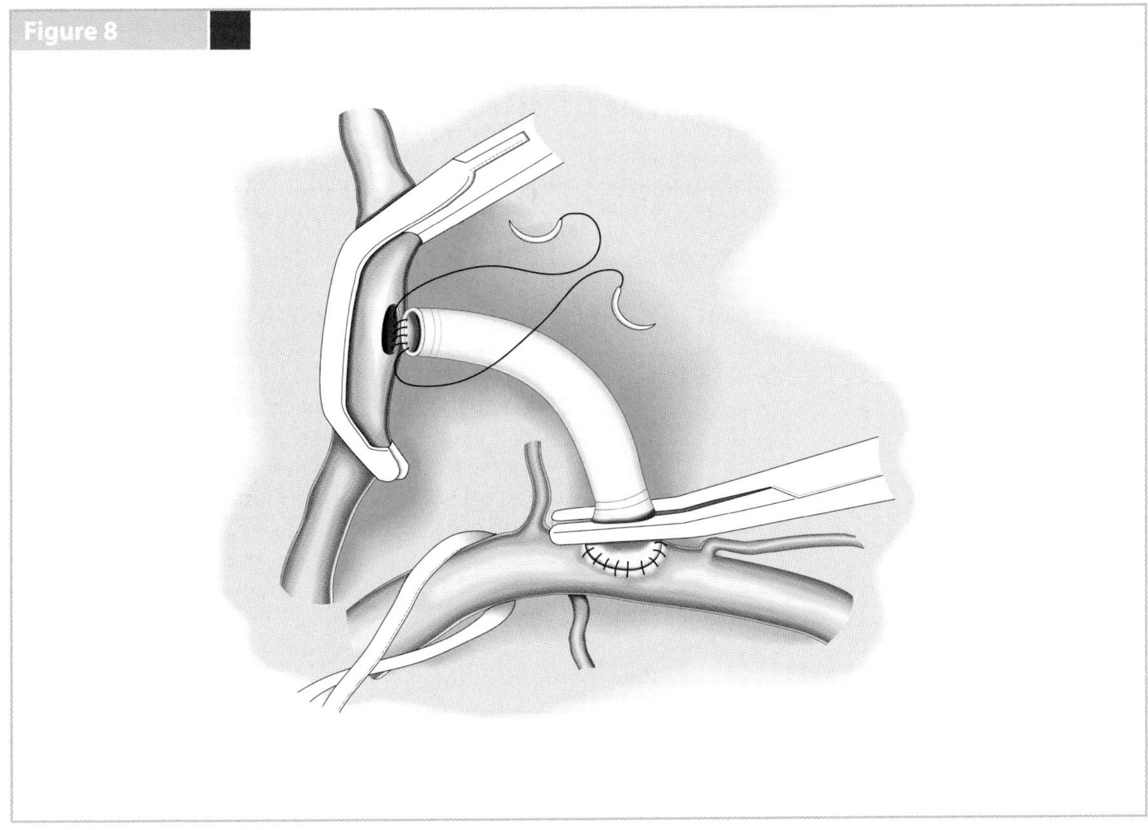

CONCLUSION

Carotid-subclavian transposition (CST) and carotid-subclavian bypass (CSB) are known to be safe and durable procedures for the treatment of symptomatic subclavian occlusive disease. However, we prefer to perform a transposition, when technically feasible, for reasons of ease of performance, the omission of graft material and improved long-term patency.

Cina and colleagues reviewed the results of all CST and CSB procedures reported in the literature between 1966 and 2000. They found CST allowed for improved patency over CSB at 5-year follow-up (99% vs. 84%). In addition, CST yielded a superior freedom from symptoms at 5 years over CSB (99% vs. 88%). These improved results are thought to be secondary to a reduced rate of thrombosis. SCT reduced the relative risk of thrombosis by 74% and the absolute risk of thrombosis by 2.6% over SCB. There may also be hemodynamic advantages to CST which maintains physiological, antegrade flow in the subclavian and vertebral arteries. In CSB, the vertebral artery is supplied by retrograde flow and there may be areas of stagnant flow in the proximal subclavian. These findings support the use of CST over CSB when possible.

The use of different prosthetic materials in the performance of CSB has been addressed by studies from our institution. We found that PTFE grafts showed a superior patency (95%) when compared to Dacron (84%) and autologous saphenous vein (65%). We attribute these differences to superior handling of PTFE, reduced kinking, and the tolerance of lower flow rates without thrombosis. We use PTFE preferentially when performing CSB.

Despite the differences in patency, both CST and CSB can be performed with minimal morbidity and mortality. In Cina's review, 30-day mortality was 1.2% for both procedures with no significant differences in stroke rates (6.6% CSB vs. 4.4% CST). Other complications were equivalent between procedures, including nerve injury, lymphatic leak and wound hematoma. Graft infection rate in CSB was 1.2%.

Overall, CST and CSB can be safely performed in carefully selected patients with symptomatic subclavian occlusive disease in the hands of experienced vascular specialists.

SELECTED BIBLIOGRAPHY

Cherry KJ (2000) Arteriosclerotic occlusive disease of brachiocephalic arteries. In: Rutherford RB (ed) Vascular surgery. WB Saunders, Philadelphia, pp 1140–1162

Cina CS, Safar HA, Lagan A, Arena G, Clase CM (2002) Subclavian-carotid transposition and bypass grafting: consecutive cohort study and systemic review. J Vasc Surg 35:422–429

Fisher CM (1961) A new vascular syndrome – "the subclavian steal." N Engl J Med 265:912–913

Law MM, Colburn MD, Moore WS, Quinones-Baldrich WJ, Machleder HI, Gelabert HA (1995) Carotid-subclavian bypass for brachiocephalic occlusive disease: choice of conduit and long-term follow-up. Stroke 25:1565–1571

Ziomek S, Quinones-Baldrich WJ, Busuttil RW, Baker JD, Machleder HI, Moore WS (1986) The superiority of synthetic arterial grafts over autologous veins in carotid-subclavian bypass. J Vasc Surg 3:140–145

CHAPTER 8

Vertebral Artery Reconstruction

Mark A. Adelman, David C. Corry

INTRODUCTION

Vertebrobasilar insufficiency is a somewhat uncommon manifestation of cerebral vascular disease. Symptomatic patients present with the hallmark signs of posterior fossa hypoperfusion: these symptoms are cranial nerve, pontine or cerebellar ischemia. Typically patients present with diplopia, dysarthria, ataxia, perioral numbness or drop attacks. Oftentimes patients will lose the ability to stand or ambulate but remain fully conscious during these drop attacks. The circle of Willis provides good collateral circulation to the posterior fossa in most patients. The posterior communicating arteries provide collateral flow from the carotid arteries to the vertebral basilar distribution. Most patients with vertebrobasilar insufficiency and carotid stenosis are easily treated by repairing the anterior (carotid artery) lesion first, allowing collateral flow to alleviate any posterior brain arterial insufficiency. In patients who have concomitant anterior and posterior lesions, 10–40% remain symptomatic after anterior revascularization (Berguer et al. 2000; Blaisdell et al. 1969; Humphries et al. 1965). These patients require vertebral artery reconstruction.

In order to facilitate appropriate reconstruction, proper imaging of the vertebrobasilar system must be performed. Imaging starts with duplex ultrasound evaluation of the extracranial cerebrovasculature, where flow-limiting lesions in the carotid arteries may be easily identified. The duplex ultrasound is also excellent at determining subclavian artery flow disturbances and direction of blood flow through the vertebral arteries. If the subclavian flow disturbance exists and retrograde flow is seen in a vertebral artery, this is ultrasonographic evidence of subclavian steal syndrome. Clinically, these patients have a diminished blood pressure along with a diminished or absent radial pulse in the ipsilateral arm. If a patient has symptoms of vertebrobasilar insufficiency concomitant with either duplex ultrasound criteria for vertebrobasilar insufficiency or diminished blood pressure in one upper extremity, further imaging evaluation is warranted.

Since the vertebral vasculature arises from the great vessels, imaging of the aortic arch, great vessels, vertebral arteries, and basilar system are imperative prior to reconstruction. In the past, contrast arch aortography with cerebrovascular runoff has been the gold standard in vertebral basilar imaging. Special vertebral artery views must be obtained, as a simple anterior-posterior view will not allow visualization of the vertebral artery origins as they derive from the superior-posterior aspect of the subclavian artery. Occasionally, patients will have a normal appearing angiogram of the extracranial cerebrovasculature, but have persistent posterior fossa symptoms. Oftentimes these symptoms may be elicited by head turning or axial loading. In these situations, dynamic vertebral angiography (with head turning to each side and axial loading) may be necessary to visualize kinking of the vertebral arteries.

More recently, advances in magnetic resonance angiography (MRA) and computed tomographic angiography (CTA) have led to exceptionally good images of the vertebrobasilar system. These images may be formatted using multiplanar reconstructions to easily visualize the vertebral artery origins. Associated lesions such as carotid artery disease can be seen as well. Time-of-flight MRA of the intracranial cerebrovasculature is done without contrast and delineates collateral blood flow to the vertebrobasilar circulation. It will also visualize the basilar artery and its branches. In addition, time-of-flight MRA is sensitive to retrograde vertebral artery flow. This may be helpful in making a diagnosis of subclavian steal syndrome. Imaging of the internal mammary artery (IMA) may be necessary in patients who have undergone coronary artery bypass grafting with IMA bypass graft.

Figure 1

Typically the vertebral arteries arise from the superoposterior aspect of the subclavian arteries. However, occasionally anomalies occur where the vertebral arteries arise directly from the aortic arch. As the vertebral arteries ascend, they can be divided into four segments. The first segment (V1) encompasses the region from the subclavian artery to the investment of the vertebral arteries in the bony vertebral canal. This typically occurs at the level of the sixth cervical vertebra but can occasionally occur at the level of the seventh. The second segment (V2) is the region of its bony investment. This segment is very difficult to access surgically: It requires bony resection of the transverse processes. At the level of the second cervical vertebrae, the vertebral artery exits its bony canal and forms a loop prior to going through the transverse process of the first vertebral body. This loop forms the third segment (V3) and is easily accessible by the vascular surgeon. Once intracranial, the V4 segments of the vertebral arteries join to form the basilar artery, which provides circulation to the posterior fossa. In the absence of subclavian steal syndrome, normal antegrade perfusion of one vertebral artery provides adequate perfusion to the contents of the posterior fossa.

Disease affecting posterior fossa perfusion may occur in the subclavian artery proximal to the vertebral origin or within segments V1 through V3 of the vertebral artery on either side. When a paucity of antegrade flow through both vertebrals exists, symptoms occur (of note, most patients can remain asymptomatic with only one vertebral artery patent). Patients with intrinsic basilar artery disease also present with posterior symptoms. It is therefore critical that adequate preoperative imaging of the entire vertebrobasilar system be performed prior to reconstruction, since proximal vertebral reconstruction will not be helpful in treating posterior fossa ischemia if a patient has intrinsic basilar disease.

Proximal subclavian stenosis can cause posterior fossa hypoperfusion if a subclavian steal syndrome is present. Here, proximal subclavian artery reconstruction may be warranted to increase vertebral artery perfusion.

PROXIMAL VERTEBRAL ARTERY RECONSTRUION

Exposure of the vertebral arteries is performed with the patient under general anesthesia. An arterial catheter is placed in the radial artery contralateral to the side of reconstruction as the ipsilateral subclavian vessel may be clamped. An endotracheal tube is placed with the ventilator tubing running to the top of the bed. The patient is placed in a supine position with a roll under the shoulders to allow neck extension. The head is turned to the contralateral side and the neck is extended. The bed is placed in a beachchair position (back flexed, foot down). The operating table may be rotated to the contralateral side to allow better visualization for the assistant. Standard vascular surgical instrumentation is used. However, a blunt tipped pediatric tonsil suction may be helpful as the surgical field is small. In addition, a monopolar electric cautery is used for the subcutaneous tissues. However, once working in proximity to the brachial plexus and cranial nerves, bipolar electric cautery is advised.

A curvilinear skin incision is made from the lateral border of the medial head of the sternocleidomastoid muscle, approximately 1 cm above and parallel to the clavicle see Chap. 7, "Carotid-Subclavian transposition". The skin incision should be carried for a distance of approximately 5–6 cm. It is not necessary to divide the lateral head of the sternocleidomastoid muscle, as this muscle may be easily retracted and superior cosmesis will result if left intact. If a vertebral-carotid artery transposition is considered, the skin incision may need to be carried to the midline. In this case, division of the sternocleidomastoid muscle may be necessary to provide adequate exposure.

After the skin incision, the platysma muscle is divided with electrocautery. Two Weitlaner retractors are placed below the level of the platysma muscle, and the deep cervical fascia is entered to expose the scalene fat pad.

The scalene fat bed is encountered and divided medially and inferiorly. This fat pad may be retracted laterally and placed under the Weitlaner retractors. Do not remove this tissue, as it will provide good soft tissue coverage of the phrenic nerve prior to wound closure. The phrenic nerve is encountered along the anterior surface of scalenus anticus muscle. The sternocleidomastoid muscle is usually kept intact and retracted medially, unless further exposure is required for vertebral artery transposition, where it is transected (as shown).

Figure 1

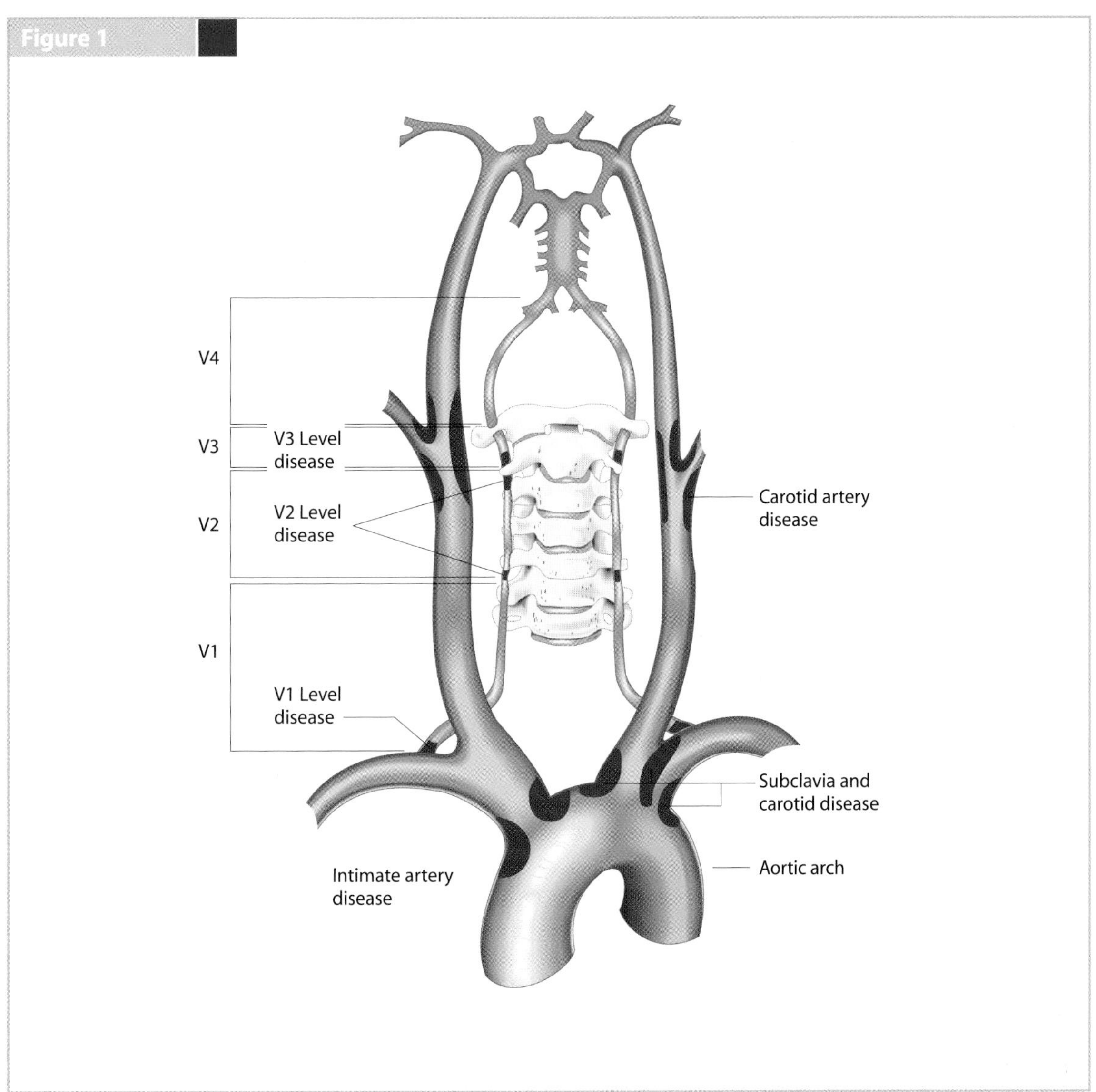
V4
V3
V3 Level disease
V2
V2 Level disease
V1
V1 Level disease
Carotid artery disease
Subclavia and carotid disease
Aortic arch
Intimate artery disease

Figure 2

The phrenic nerve is gently mobilized from the scalenus anticus muscle taking care to avoid traction injury. The pediatric tonsil sucker is a helpful instrument to assist with phrenic nerve mobilization without placing excess traction on the nerve. Once mobilized, the scalene fat pad is useful as a sling to retract the phrenic nerve (as shown). Use of vessel loops on the nerve is avoided to prevent an inadvertent stretch injury. The sternocleidomastoid muscle is mobilized, kept intact (as previously described) and retracted medially along with the internal jugular vein.

When performing surgery on the left vertebral artery, the thoracic duct should be identified. It is typically seen traversing laterally along the posterior aspect of the jugulosubclavian junction. The duct should be avoided entirely. However, if an injury is suspected the duct must be identified and ligated directly.

The distal subclavian artery is found emerging laterally from the posterior aspect of the scalenus anticus muscle. Once the phrenic nerve is mobilized the medial and lateral borders of the scalenus anticus muscle are seen. Division of the scalenus anticus muscle maximizes surgical exposure, greatly facilitating reconstruction of the proximal vertebral artery. The muscle is carefully divided in stages to avoid nerve injury, using a right angle clamp, and to pinpoint monopolar electrocautery. Once divided, it should be noted that the proximal vertebral artery is located at the medial edge of the inferior scalenus anticus muscle.

Figure 3

Exposure of the vertebral artery origin is easiest by working from the distal subclavian to the proximal. First, the costocervical and thyrocervical trunks are encountered. As exposure extends medially, the vertebral origin is often seen opposite the internal mammary artery. Care should be taken to avoid injuring or clamping the left internal mammary artery if a patient has had this vessel used during coronary artery bypass grafting. The inferior thyroid artery is seen crossing the vertebral artery and vertebral vein. This should be divided between ligatures. Superficial venous tributaries, including the vertebral veins, will be encountered superficial to the vertebral artery and should be divided between ligatures.

After division of the vertebral veins, the vertebral artery is encountered distal to its origin. A vessel loop is placed and exposure is extended proximally. At this point, the origin of the vertebral artery as well as the midsection of the first segment of the vertebral artery is seen. Oftentimes, the stellate ganglion is seen over the proximal portion of the V1 segment of the vertebral artery. With vessel loops on the artery, the vertebral artery may be freed without division of the stellate ganglion. Nevertheless, most patients will have a transient Horner's syndrome after this vertebral artery exposure.

Once the vertebral artery is completely mobilized, it is typically redundant. In many patients, the region of stenosis is a kink at the vertebral artery origin. With a redundant vertebral artery, vertebral artery angioplasty and vein patch may be performed as described by Imparato.

Following complete exposure and mobilization of the V1 segment of the vertebral artery, a "keyhole" arteriotomy is planned as shown. Full systemic heparinization is administered. The vertebral artery is clamped distally. Clamps are subsequently placed on the proximal and distal subclavian arteries, followed by clamping of the internal mammary artery. Caution should be exercised if the patient has received coronary revascularization via the IMA and vertebral artery transposition should be considered instead of plication. The arteriotomy along the anterior aspect of the vertebral artery is completed, excising the patch of subclavian artery encompassing the thyrocervical trunk.

Figure 2

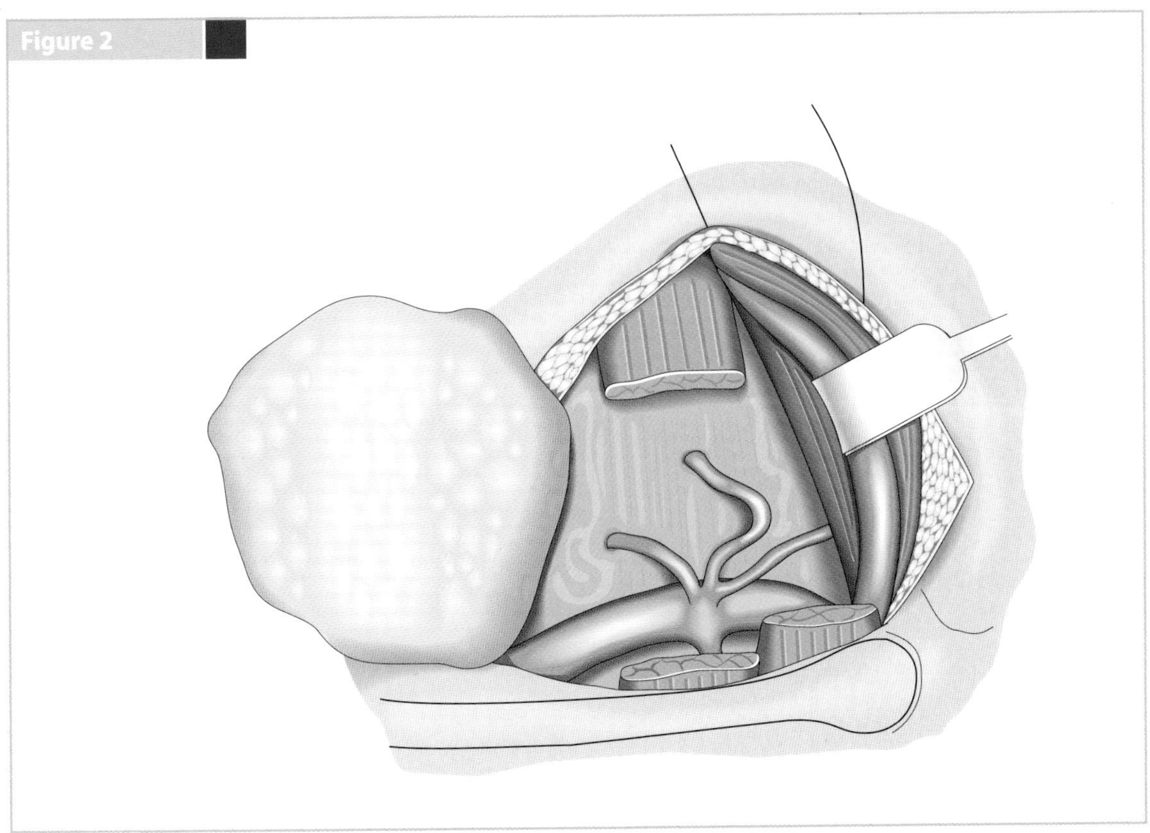

Figure 3

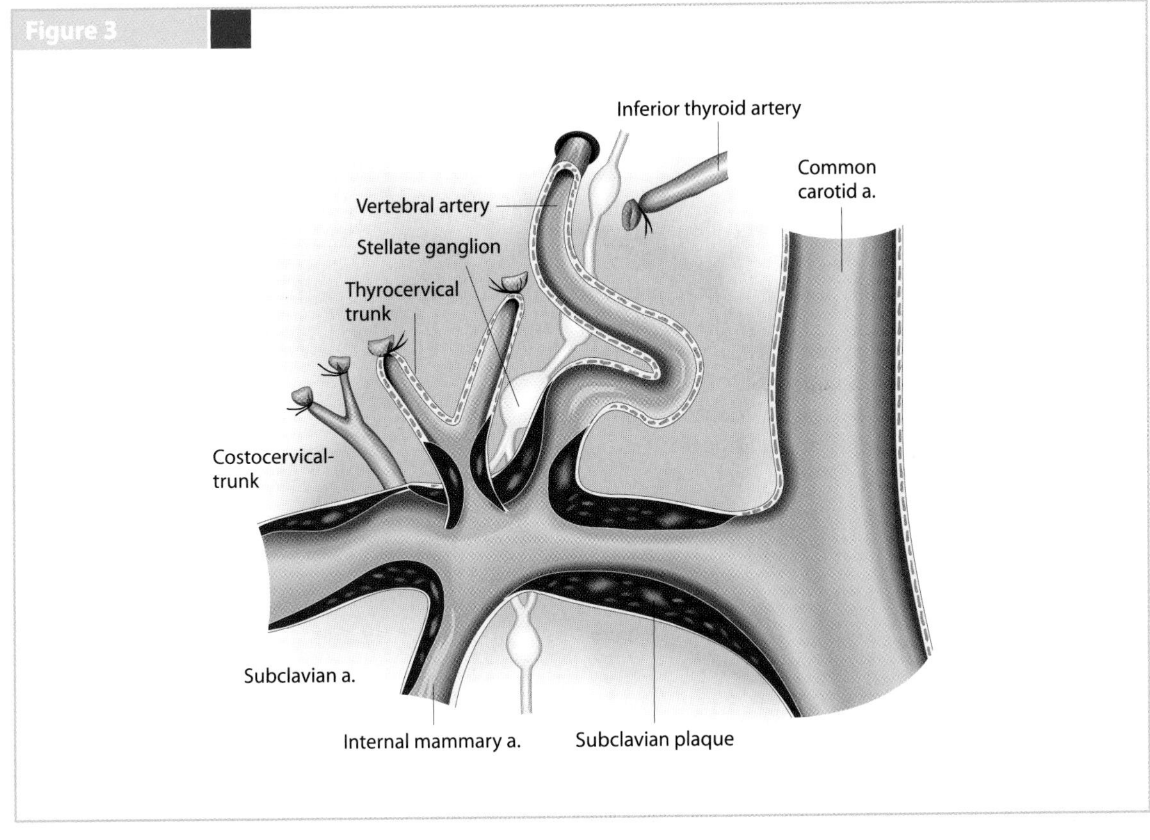
Inferior thyroid artery
Common
carotid a.
Vertebral artery
Stellate ganglion
Thyrocervical
trunk
Costocervical-
trunk
Subclavian a.
Internal mammary a.
Subclavian plaque

Figure 4

A plication angioplasty of the vertebral artery is constructed to reduce the redundant portion segment of V1. The plication is constructed with interrupted monofilament sutures as shown, where point A is approximated to point A1, point B is approximated to point B1, and so forth.

8

Figure 5

The sutures are tightened and tied posteriorly to appose the distal portion of the vertebral artery arteriotomy to the subclavian artery. This maneuver both excludes the diseased portion of the vertebral artery and eliminates its redundancy, thereby providing unimpeded straight-line flow (as seen in the cross-section view).

If needed, further sutures (interrupted or running monofilament) are placed to complete the posterior suture line. The "dog ears" are oversewn to eliminate their edges as a source of possible bleeding.

Figure 6

The segment of saphenous vein or cervical vein has been harvested and is sewn as a vein patch angioplasty over the vertebral artery origin, thus completing the reconstruction anastomosis.

Figure 4

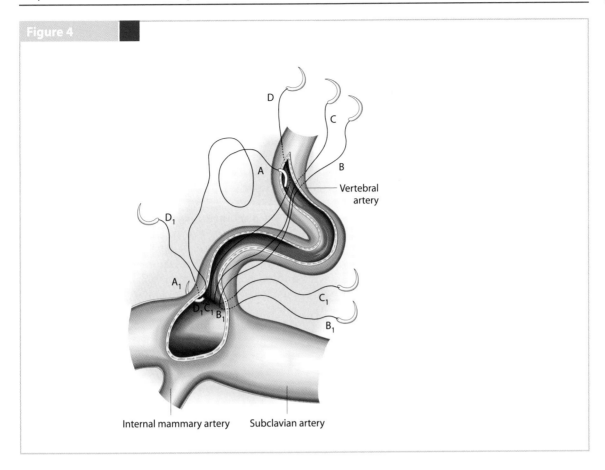

D
C
B
A
Vertebral artery
D_1
A_1
D_1 C_1 B_1
C_1
B_1
Internal mammary artery
Subclavian artery

Figure 5

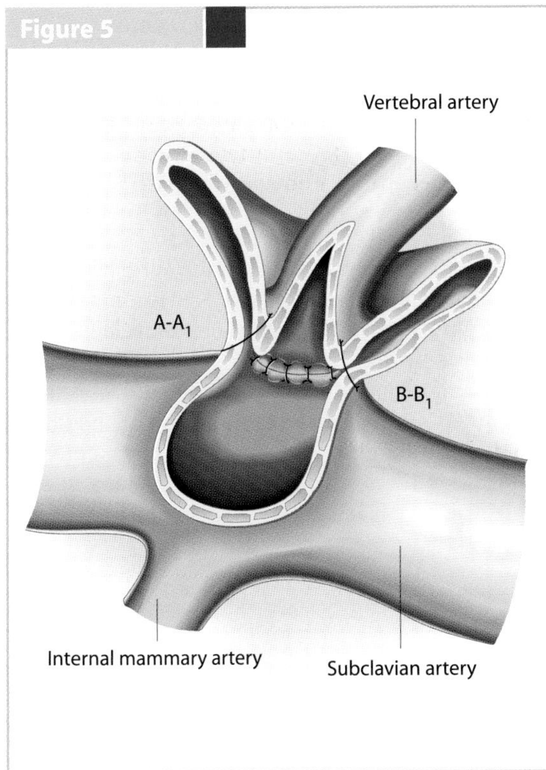

Figure 6

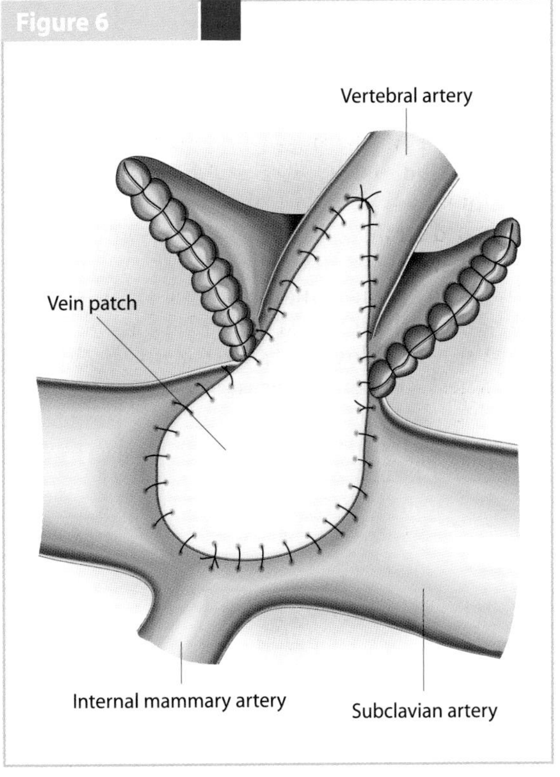

VERTEBRAL TO COMMON CAROTID TRANSPOSITION

Alternatively, should operative conditions dictate, a vertebral artery to common carotid artery transposition may be performed. The incision and exposure are the same as detailed above, except the retraction of the carotid sheath is changed to release the common carotid artery (see Fig. 2). The common carotid artery is then mobilized for a distance of approximately 5 cm.

The patient is systemically heparinized. The vertebral artery is clamped proximally and distally and divided just distal to its origin off of the subclavian. The stump of the vertebral artery is closed with 6-0 Prolene in running fashion.

Once the vertebral artery is divided, the transposition anastomosis can be constructed. Since the vertebral artery lies posterior to the common carotid artery, it is critical to plan the anastomosis in three dimensions. Therefore, a posterolateral arteriotomy on the common carotid artery and reciprocal anteromedial arteriotomy on the vertebral artery will be necessary to create an anastomosis without kinking.

The vertebral artery is brought to the common carotid artery under minimal tension. Typically, it will be approaching the common carotid artery from its posterolateral region. The anteromedial vertebral arteriotomy is extended upwards from its transected edge for approximately 6–8 mm. Once the vertebral artery arteriotomy has been made, a mark should be made on the posterolateral aspect of the common carotid artery, marking the heel and the toe of the anastomosis.

The proximal and distal common carotid artery is clamped using two small angled patent ductus clamps. The artery is approached from the lateral position such that the clamp handles may be rotated anteriorly. This rotation of the posterolateral common carotid artery into a more lateral position improves exposure of the required posterolateral arteriotomy and facilitates suturing of the anastomosis. An 11 blade is used to make a small arteriotomy, and a 5–6 mm aortic punch used to remove an ellipse of the common carotid artery.

Figure 7

A 7-0 Prolene continuous suture line is begun along the midpoint of the posterior wall of the anastomosis. The suture line is continued superiorly and inferiorly along the posterior wall, thereby completing the anterior anastomosis closure in a running fashion. After backbleeding from the vertebral carotid arteries to remove any accumulated thrombus and flushing of the anastomosis with heparinized saline, the suture line is completed. The proximal carotid clamp is released first to allow egress of air trapped in the anastomosis through the suture line while loosely tying the suture. The knot is then slowly tightened and secured, using care to avoid 'purse-stringing' the suture line. The vertebral artery clamp is removed during the above-mentioned de-airing procedure. Lastly, the distal common carotid artery clamp is removed, restoring antegrade circulation to the carotid bifurcation. Heparin effect is reversed with protamine as needed.

If the common carotid artery is particularly thick-walled, a longer arteriotomy may be made and then closed with a vein patch. Then, a venotomy is performed and the vertebral artery is sutured directly to the vein patch in a similar fashion to primary vertebral-to-carotid artery transposition, as described above.

Prior to final wound closure a 7-mm closed suction drain is placed deep in the wound. The drain should not directly abut the anastomosis and can be brought out of the skin through the surgical wound. The scalene fat pad is placed over the drain, and over the phrenic nerve. The platysma muscle is reapproximated using absorbable suture. The skin is closed using absorbable subcuticular suture. A single interrupted 5-0 nylon suture is placed at the lateral aspect of the skin incision where the drain emerges. The drain is removed on postoperative day #1 providing drainage is less than 30 cc per shift.

Figure 7

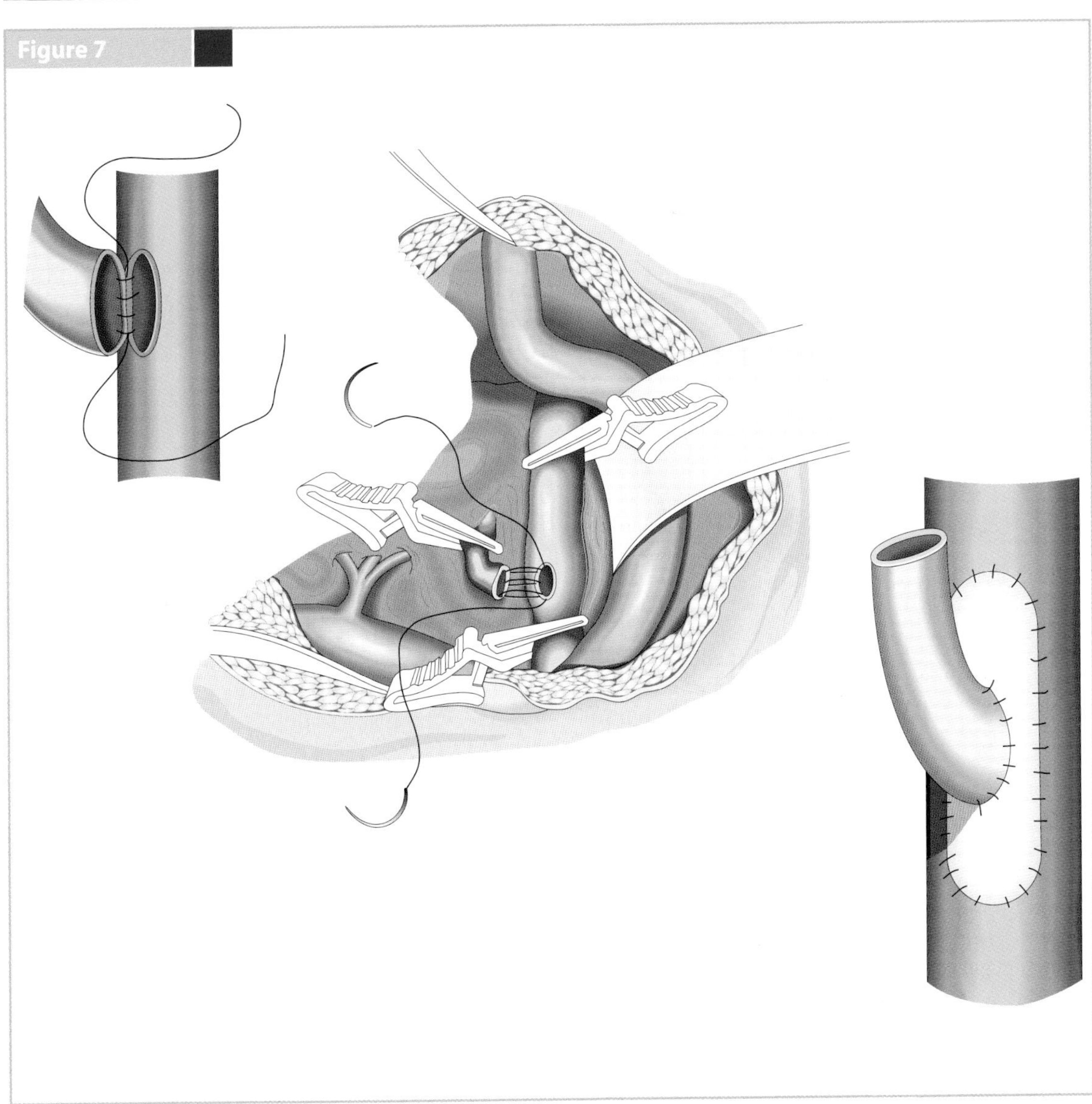

DISTAL VERTEBRAL ARTERY RECONSTRUCTION

If arterial occlusive disease of the vertebral arteries includes the V1 or V2 segments, distal reconstruction may be necessary. Here, the V3 segment of the vertebral artery is easily accessible between the first and second cervical vertebrae as the artery makes a loop at this level. A bypass graft from the common carotid artery to the third segment of vertebral artery is performed using a reverse saphenous graft.

Positioning for this procedure is the same as for carotid endarterectomy. An incision is made along the anterior border of the sternocleidomastoid muscle extending up posterior to the earlobe. The proximal extent of this incision should be planned about 4 cm proximal to the carotid bifurcation.

Attention is first turned toward carotid artery exposure. After reflecting the sternocleidomastoid muscle laterally (see exposure of carotid bifurcation), the common carotid artery is identified just medial to the jugular vein. The artery is cleaned for a distance of approximately 3–4 cm and care is taken to avoid the carotid bifurcation, where atheromatous disease may be present.

8

Figure 8

Attention is then turned to the superior aspect of the incision for identification of the spinal accessory nerve. Typically, the nerve is found 2 cm below the mastoid tip and posterior to the anterior edge of the sternocleidomastoid muscle. The nerve is identified and mobilized. Care is taken to avoid a nerve traction injury. Once the nerve is identified and mobilized, palpate the transverse process of the first cervical vertebrae. The vertebral artery lies just inferior and deep to the transverse process of the C1 vertebra.

Figure 9

The soft tissue overlying the levator scapulae muscle is divided. This soft tissue lies just deep to the spinal accessory nerve. A right-angled clamp is used to divide this muscle in layers using scissors to divide the levator scapulae muscle from its attachments to the first cervical vertebra. Electrocautery should not be used here. The anterior ramus of the second cervical nerve is seen just deep to the levator scapulae muscle. The vertebral artery lies just deep to the anterior ramus of C2. Therefore, the nerve is dissected free and cut, thereby exposing the vertebral artery.

Once the vertebral artery is identified, a plexus of vertebral veins is typically intimately associated. These veins should be carefully dissected free using sharp scissors. The veins are then divided between ligatures and broad based veins may be divided between suture ligatures. A vessel loop is placed around the vertebral artery and it is mobilized for a distance of approximately 2 cm. To prepare the V3 segment for clamping prior to the distal anastomosis, the surgeon should carefully locate the small side branches that may stem from the vertebral artery in this location. If these branches are torn, troublesome bleeding may be encountered; they should therefore be meticulously ligated with small hemoclips. Removal of the transverse process of C2 (±C3) anterior to the vertebral artery (i.e. shaded areas of Fig. 9) may be needed to improve access.

Attention is first turned to the proximal anastomosis. A 10-cm segment of greater saphenous vein is harvested from the thigh, taking care to match the size of the saphenous vein to the vertebral artery. (A size mismatch with a large greater saphenous vein and a small vertebral artery will make for a technically inferior distal anastomosis; see Fig. 7.) After heparinization, the common carotid artery is clamped proximally distally and a small ellipse of common carotid artery is removed with sharp scissors or an aortic punch. An end-to-side anastomosis of vein into common carotid artery is then performed with 6-0 Prolene in a running fashion. Prior to tying the suture, forward- and backbleeding of the common carotid artery is performed to remove any thrombus or debris. The anastomosis is then completed and flow is restored first through the external carotid first, followed by the internal carotid. A tunnel is constructed posterior to the jugular vein and anterior to the vagus nerve such that the vein graft approximates the lateral aspect of the distal common carotid artery. The saphenous graft is pulled into position next to the exposed V3 vertebral artery segment.

Figure 8

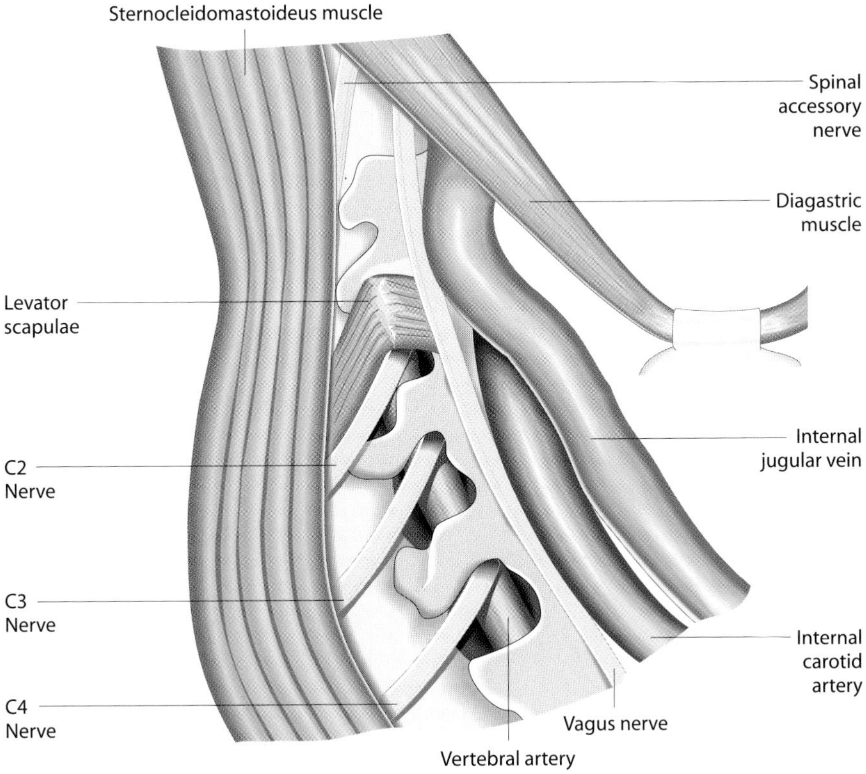

Sternocleidomastoideus muscle
Spinal accessory nerve
Diagastric muscle
Levator scapulae
C2 Nerve
C3 Nerve
C4 Nerve
Internal jugular vein
Internal carotid artery
Vagus nerve
Vertebral artery

Figure 9

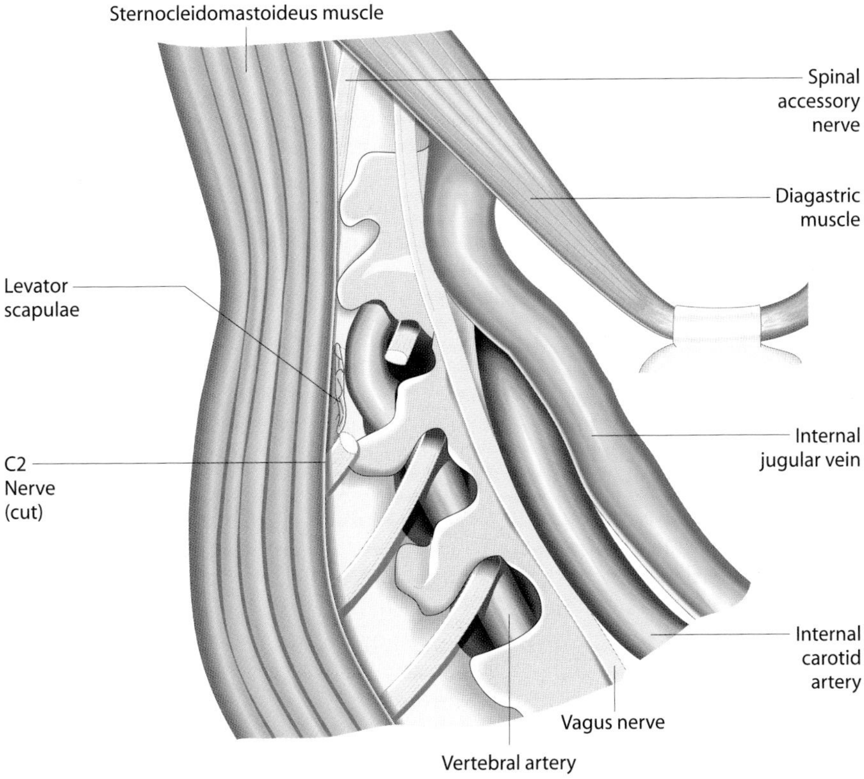

Sternocleidomastoideus muscle
Spinal accessory nerve
Diagastric muscle
Levator scapulae
C2 Nerve (cut)
Internal jugular vein
Internal carotid artery
Vagus nerve
Vertebral artery

Figure 10

Attention is then turned to the distal anastomosis. The saphenous graft is trimmed to the appropriate length and the distal end of the vein is spatulated for an end-to-side anastomosis. Soft bulldog clamps are placed at the proximal and distal extent of the mobilized vertebral artery. A small (4–6 mm) arteriotomy is created in the vertebral artery. Running 7-0 Prolene is used to complete the bypass into the V3 segment of the vertebral artery. Again, before the anastomosis is tied, forward- and backbleeding is allowed to flush debris and air, after which forward flow is initiated through the saphenous bypass graft. The graft should be seen to lie without kinks and without tension on either suture line. Postoperatively, this graft may be monitored using duplex ultrasound evaluation.

Figure 10

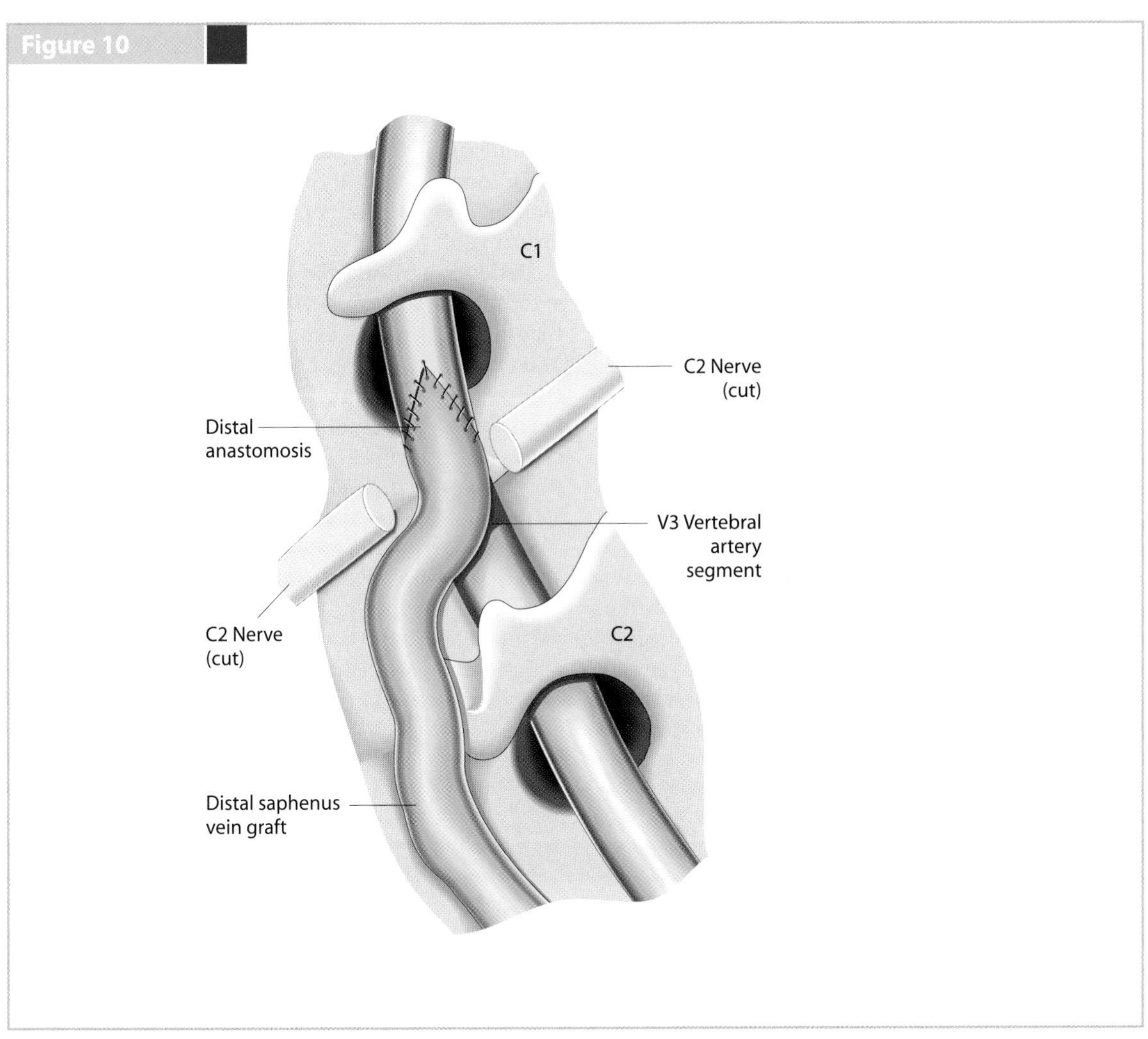
C1
C2 Nerve
(cut)
Distal
anastomosis
V3 Vertebral
artery
segment
C2 Nerve
(cut)
C2
Distal saphenus
vein graft

CONCLUSION

Vertebrobasilar artery occlusive disease is oftentimes occult and usually unilateral; only after patients become symptomatic is it identified. Symptomatic patients most often have bilateral disease, and only after developing symptoms do they require revascularization. Sixty to 90% of patients with vertebrobasilar insufficiency and concomitant carotid artery disease will resolve their symptoms after carotid artery reconstruction. Thus, vertebral artery reconstruction should only be considered in patients who are symptomatic and only after all anterior lesions have been appropriately treated.

A thorough knowledge of cervical anatomy is paramount to avoiding complications from these infrequently performed procedures. Surgeons must be careful to avoid unrecognized injury of the thoracic duct, and injury to the stellate ganglion, phrenic nerve, and vagus nerve. They must be cognizant of patients with a left internal mammary artery bypass graft to a coronary artery and protect its circulation. Right-sided reconstructions may be complicated by injury to a recurrent laryngeal nerve, as it recurs around the right subclavian artery. The surgeon must be cautious in identifying and preserving this nerve while gaining exposure near the proximal subclavian artery.

Patients typically have immediate relief of their symptoms and long-term results of these surgical reconstructions are excellent, with 5-year survival and patency rates approaching 70–80%, respectively (Imparato 1985; Berguer et al. 2000). Patients should be monitored annually with duplex scanning, and subsequently with MRA or standard angiography if flows become difficult to interpret or if symptoms return.

■ **Acknowledgements.** The authors wish to express their appreciation to Dr. Anthony Imparato for providing detailed intraoperative diagrams and photos, which were an invaluable reference for the illustrations represented in this chapter.

REFERENCES

Berguer R, Flynn LM, Kline RA, Caplan L (2000) Surgical reconstruction of the extracranial vertebral artery: Management and outcome. J Vasc Surg 31:9–18

Blaisdell WF, Clauss RH, Galbraith JG, Imparato AM, Wylie EJ (1969) Joint study of extracranial arterial occlusion. IV: A review of surgical considerations. JAMA 209:1889–1895

Humphries AW, Young JR, Beven EG, Le Fevre FA, deWolfe VG (1965) Relief of vertebrobasilar symptoms by carotid endarterectomy. Surgery 57:48–53

Imparato AM (1985) Vertebral arterial reconstruction: a nineteen-year experience. J Vasc Surg 2:626–634

Imparato AM, Riles TS (1994) Vertebral artery reconstruction. In: Jamieson C, Yao JST (eds) Rob and Smith's operative surgery: vascular surgery, 5th edn. Chapman & Hall Medical, London, pp 105–122

Ruotolo C, Hazan H, Rancurel G, Kieffer E (1992) Dynamic arteriography. In: Berguer R, Caplan L (eds) Vertebrobasilar arterial disease. Quality Medical Publishing, St. Louis, pp 116–123

CHAPTER 9

Transaxillary Thoracic Outlet Decompression

Alan Y. Synn, Stephen J. Annest

INTRODUCTION

Thoracic outlet syndrome (TOS) is the symptomatic compression of the neurovascular structures that traverse the thoracic outlet. Three distinct types exist. Compression of the nerves is by far the most common (95%), while venous (4%) and arterial (1%) remain less frequent. Each of the three types is due to distinct structural causes and presents with different clinical syndromes.

The typical anomalies that result in arterial TOS include a cervical rib and an elongated C7 transverse process with a fibrous extension to the first rib. The consequent rigid extrinsic compression upon the adjacent subclavian artery initially results in its narrowing and occasional upper extremity fatigue. Later, poststenotic dilation with intimal injury results in distal embolization and the presentation of a threatened limb.

In contrast, venous TOS is commonly due to a forward displaced anterior scalene muscle insertion with a taut fibromuscular band that runs under the subclavian vein as it attaches to the costal cartilage. In addition, enlargement of the subclavius muscle tendon may compress the subclavian vein from the opposite side. Initial complaints of chronic swelling and ill defined aching are typical. However, acute thrombosis is heralded by more severe symptoms of pain, swelling, discoloration and venous engorgement.

The causes of neurogenic TOS are more varied. The structural anomalies that compress the brachial plexus in the thoracic outlet have been categorized by Roos into those predominately affecting the upper and middle trunk distribution of the brachial plexus in distinction to those affecting the lower trunk distribution. Congenital anomalies such as a scalene minimus muscle and fibromuscular bands that bridge the inner curvature of the first rib may compress the lower trunk of the brachial plexus and its contributing nerve roots. Whereas the various anomalies of the anterior and middle scalene muscles have differing effects upon the upper, middle and lower trunks due to the proximity of these muscles to all levels of the brachial plexus. The variety of structural causes of neurogenic TOS underlies a diversity of clinical presentations involving pain, paresthesia, weakness and coolness. Nevertheless, general patterns of clinical presentation can be ascribed to each of the upper/middle trunk, lower trunk and combined involvements.

The diagnosis of arterial and venous TOS is confirmed by contrast studies of the involved blood vessels. However, neurogenic TOS remains a clinical diagnosis. The patient usually has experienced some form of hyperextension injury or repetitive stress injury as the inciting event. The symptoms are consistent and reproducible upon elevation of the arms in a stress position. Findings of arterial compression by physical examination or on vascular laboratory studies are irrelevant to the diagnosis of neurogenic TOS. Standard electrodiagnostic studies and radiologic tests are neither sensitive nor specific in the diagnosis of neurogenic TOS. Their principal use is in the identification of alternative diagnoses such as cervical disc disease, spinal stenosis, shoulder impingement, carpal tunnel syndrome and cuboid tunnel syndrome. Physical therapy involving nerve glide techniques and Feldenkrais postural training are useful in reducing the symptoms of neurogenic TOS. However, severe refractory symptoms may not improve without surgical decompression.

The transaxillary approach is versatile, providing access for the complete excision of the first and cervical ribs as well as direct excision of the structures compressing the C7, C8 and T1 nerve roots, lower trunk, subclavian artery and vein. Extrapleural thoracic sympathectomy and localized repair of the artery and vein may be performed with this approach. Additionally, *total disinsertion* of the anterior scalene muscle from the scalene tubercle and adjacent Sibson's fascia is best accomplished through a transaxillary exposure. This allows the retraction of the anterior scalene muscle into the neck and release of the tension within that muscle. Since upper/middle plexus symptoms are predominantly due to tight muscular bands originating from the anterior scalene, this release of tension may improve these symptoms as well. The supraclavicular approach is reserved as part of a more complex vascular reconstruction or in the setting of residual or recurrent neurogenic TOS symptoms. In the latter case, plexus neurolysis is performed.

Figure 1

General anesthesia is accomplished without paralytics in order that later nerve stimulation remains unimpaired. After intubation, the patient is placed in the lateral position with the back moved towards the edge of the table. A soft roll is placed under the dependent axilla and the head is padded in axial alignment. The position is secured with Stahlberg padded hip bolsters. The sterile field is prepared to include the axilla, arm, anterior chest across the sternum, and neck to the level of the mandible. The surgeon wears a headlight and stands to the patient's back, with the first assistant across the table and the second assistant cephalad to the surgeon. A mechanical arm holder is preferred and secured to the side bar of the bed at the level of the patient's mouth. When one is unavailable, the second assistant supports the arm in a double wristlock technique.

The incision is made from the anterior edge of the latissimus dorsi muscle to the posterior edge of the pectoralis major muscle just below the axillary hairline. In females, the axillomammary fold (demonstrated by pushing the shoulder downward and the breast upward towards the axilla) is cosmetically preferred.

Figure 2

The incision is carried to the chest wall inferior to the axillary lymph nodes. Two Gelpi retractors are placed. A tunnel is then developed under direct vision towards a cul-de-sac of thin fascia separating the axilla from the contents of the thoracic outlet. Within this tunnel, three consistent structures are encountered. The lateral thoracic artery and thoracoepigastric vein are encountered first in the midaxillary line, and require ligation and division. Next, the intercostobrachial nerve (sometimes duplicated) bridges the second or third intercostal space and axillary fat. This nerve provides sensation to the axilla and medial brachium. Despite the most meticulous technique to protect this nerve, contusion and stretching during the course of the operation is common as is the resultant numbness. Since burning dysesthesia may result from more severe injury, it is reasonable to divide the nerve in cases of severe contusion. The third and more inconstant structure is the supreme thoracic artery and vein bridging from their axillary vessel origins to the first intercostal space. When identified, ligation and division is necessary in order to avoid later troublesome bleeding.

Gentle spreading of scissors to identify the subclavian vein, anterior scalene muscle, subclavian artery, lower trunk of the brachial plexus and T1 nerve root opens the cul-de-sac overlying the thoracic outlet. The assistant's positioning a lighted mammary retractor along the pectoralis major muscle facilitates exposure of these deep structures. The arm holder is elevated enough to visualize the structures but not so much as to place the nerves on tension.

The first rib is clearly identified. The anterior scalene muscle insertion at the tubercle of the first rib is circumscribed with a right angle hemostat, pulled laterally towards the wound, and divided with scissors under direct vision. In this fashion, the phrenic nerve is avoided.

Figure 1

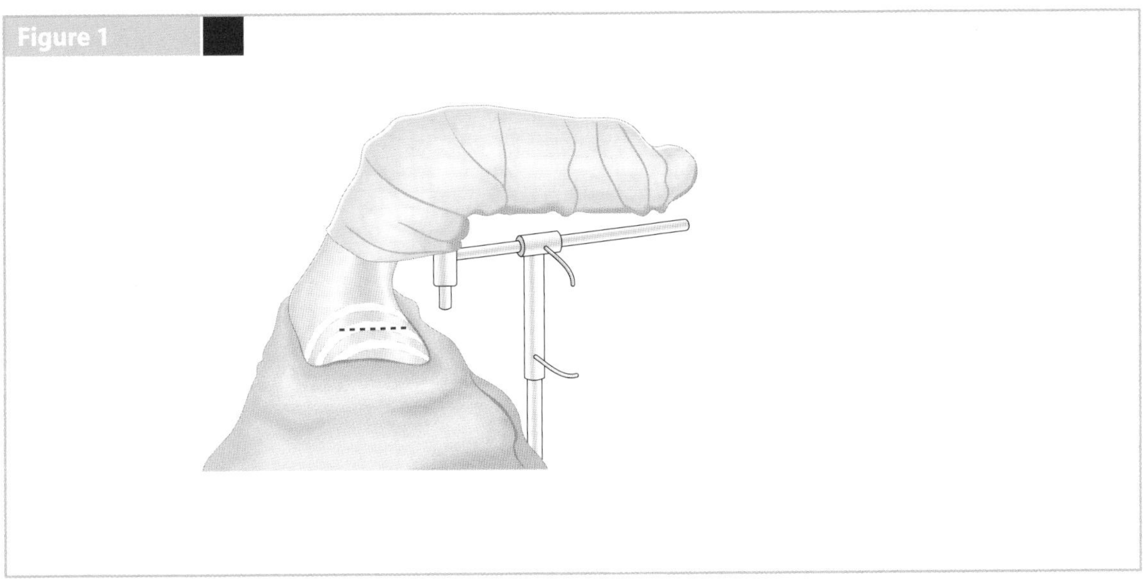

Figure 2

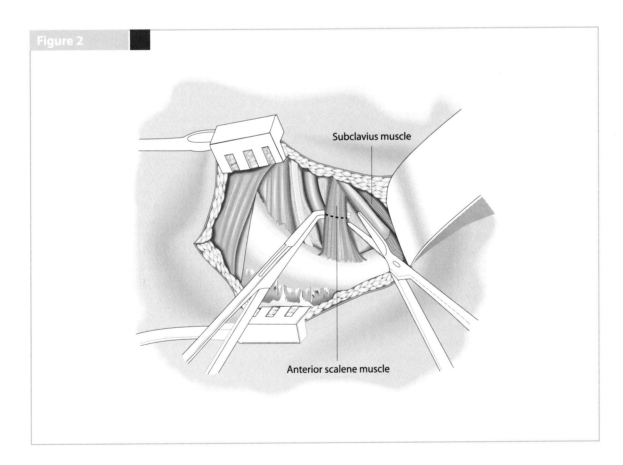

Subclavius muscle

Anterior scalene muscle

Figure 3A, B

An extraperiosteal excision of the first rib is performed next under direct vision. It is necessary to remove the periosteum with the rib in order to prevent residual periosteum from forming new bone and subsequent scarring to the brachial plexus. The subclavius muscle tendon is divided with a Matson elevator using a side-to-side motion, with the posterior adjacent vein under direct vision. The same instrument is used in a pushing motion to separate the intercostal muscles from the outer edge of the first rib. The middle scalene muscle is similarly detached from the posterior lateral surface of the first rib with the T1 nerve root under direct vision. Staying on the rib during this muscle detachment prevents injury to the long thoracic nerve. The right angle hook of an Overholt #1 raspatory is passed under the rib from its outer edge to separate the undersurface of the rib from the adherent Sibson's fascia and pleura. The right angle hook is then passed along the inner edge of the rib from the neck of the rib posteriorly to the costocartilage anteriorly. The pleura is now free of the first rib and will fall to the level of the second rib.

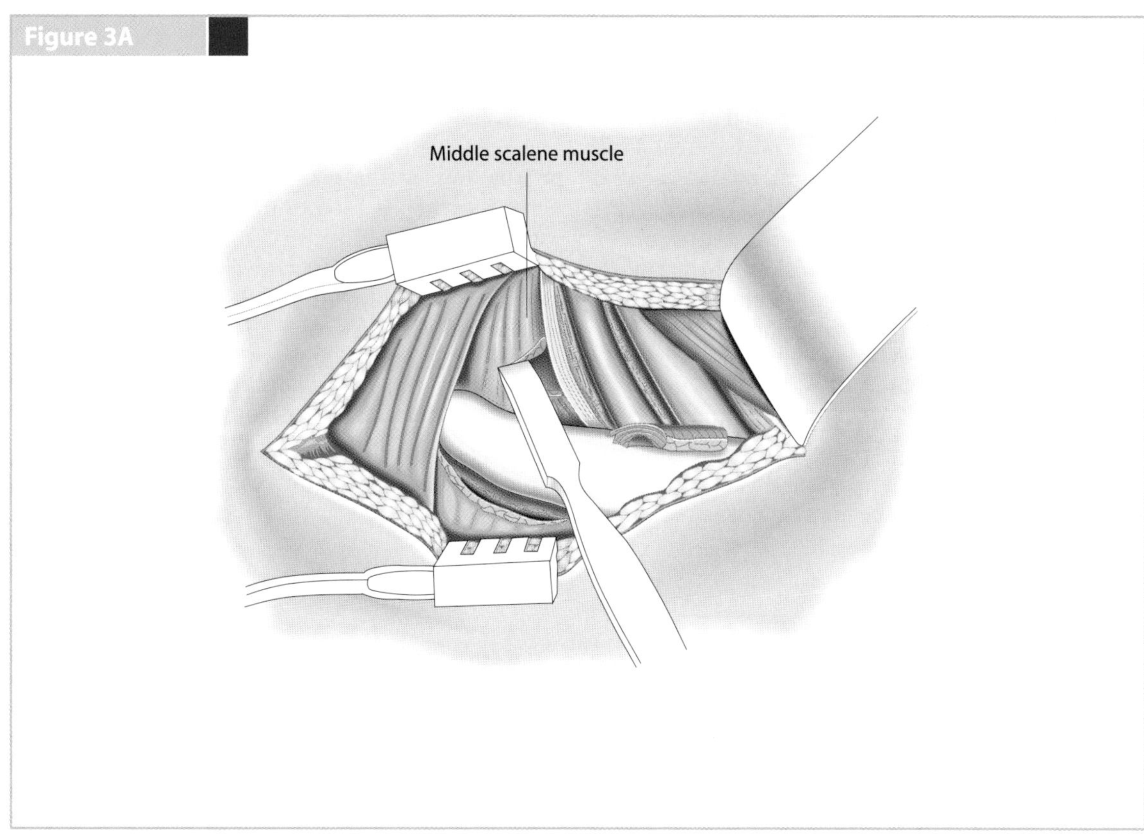
Figure 3A
Middle scalene muscle

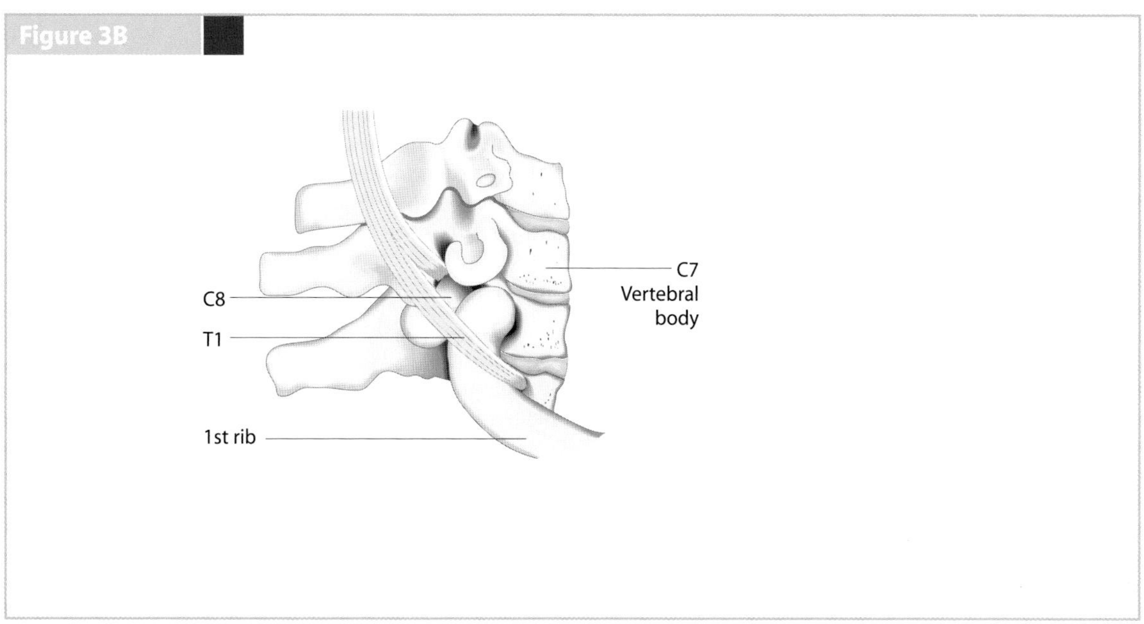
Figure 3B
C7
Vertebral
body
C8
T1
1st rib

Figure 4

Excision of the first rib requires special attention to protecting nearby neurovascular structures. Both lowering and positioning the arm holder forward improves the exposure of the neck of the rib. This draws the T1 nerve root towards the center of the operative field and under less tension. Furthermore, a deep Wylie retractor is positioned along the posterior outer edge of the first rib for enhanced visualization. In order to prevent injury to the long thoracic nerve with resultant winged scapula, the nerve is identified with the use of a nerve stimulator along the anterior edge of the posterior scalene muscle. Additionally, the surgical assistant is careful to avoid pulling posteriorly with the Wylie retractor, which would otherwise compress the long thoracic nerve. The T1 nerve root passes beneath and in close approximation to the neck of the first rib. A paddle nerve retractor is used to protect the T1 nerve root while the rib is divided with a right-angle rib shear. The anterior rib is then divided with a 60-degree angled rib shear while the paddle nerve retractor protects the subclavian vein. The rib is delivered off the field and a box rongeur is used to shorten the residual stumps. The rib is cut to the level of the costocartilage anteriorly and to within 1 cm of the transverse process posteriorly. A double-action bone rongeur is a useful tool to smooth out residual bony spicules.

9

Figure 5

Though the anterior scalene muscle has been separated from its insertion onto the first rib, residual anterior scalene muscle fibers cross beneath the subclavian artery and insert onto Sibson's fascia. These fibers prevent the total disinsertion of the anterior scalene muscle at the base of the thoracic outlet. Reoperations performed for recurrent neurogenic TOS typically reveal a scarred anterior scalene muscle adherent to the nerves at this location. In order to mobilize the anterior scalene so that it may retract freely back into the neck, long scissors are used to dissect the residual slips of muscle from the undersurface of the subclavian artery. Circumferential control of the artery with a vessel loop allows for easier handling. Careful attention to the presence of arterial branches is required.

The presence of residual congenital anomalies compressing the brachial plexus is next explored. The C7, C8, and T1 nerve roots, as well as the lower and middle trunks of the brachial plexus, are accessible through this exposure. Scalenus minimus muscle slips that attach to Sibson's fascia, fibrous bands of the middle scalene muscle, and musculofibrous tissue crossing across Sibson's fascia are among the common anomalies. These must be excised with long scissors during the careful exploration of the nerves.

Minor wound bleeding comes under ready control by packing the wound and lowering the arm holder for 5 min. The wound is reevaluated and residual bleeding points controlled with a bipolar cautery. The wound is irrigated with saline and evaluated for any pleural leaks. The wound is drained at its depths with a 19F Silastic drain under closed suction. If a pleural leak is identified, the end of the drain is placed through the defect into the pleural space. A transcutaneous microcatheter is placed between the subclavian artery and the brachial plexus. Marcaine (0.25%) is continuously infused through this catheter for two days. The wound is closed in two layers with a subcutaneous layer of 3-0 Vicryl and a subcuticular layer of 4-0 Monocril. In the presence of a pleural leak, the anesthesiologist administers a maximal breath hold and the closed suction bulb is applied. The patient is extubated and a portable chest X-ray is obtained in the recovery room to assure full lung expansion and document the absence of a phrenic nerve palsy.

Figure 4

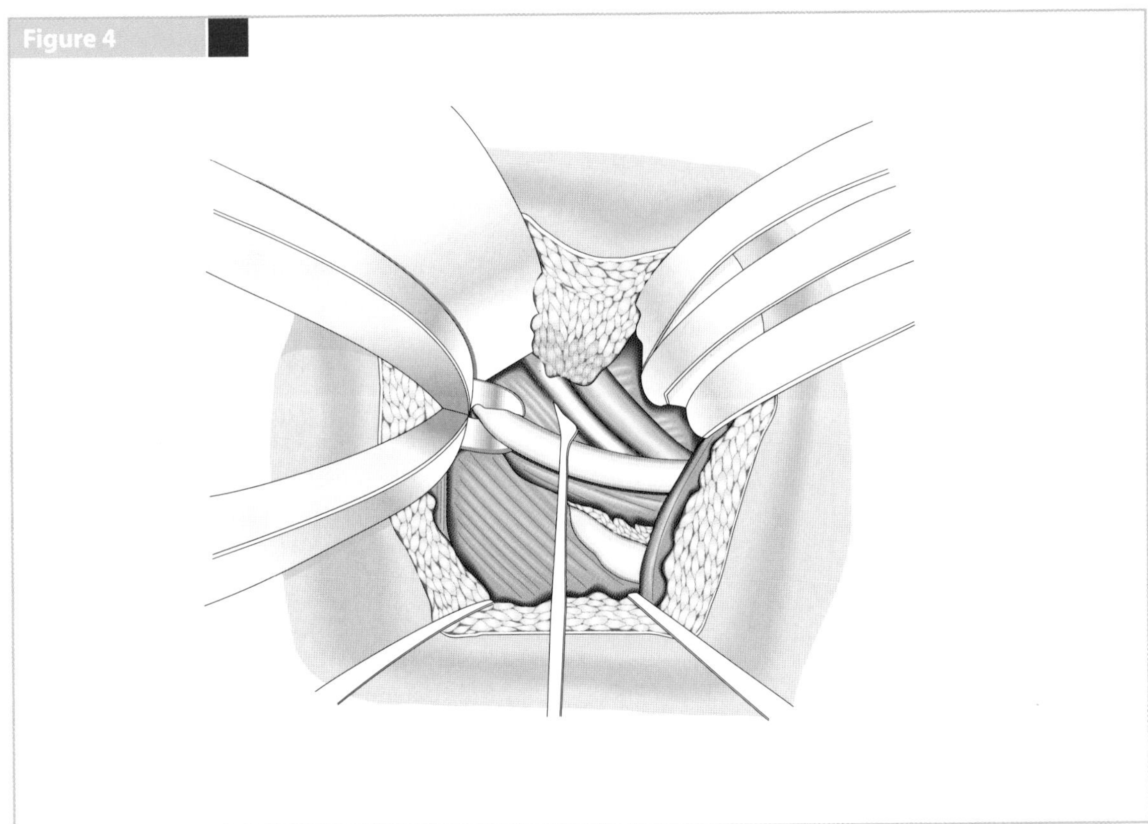

Figure 5

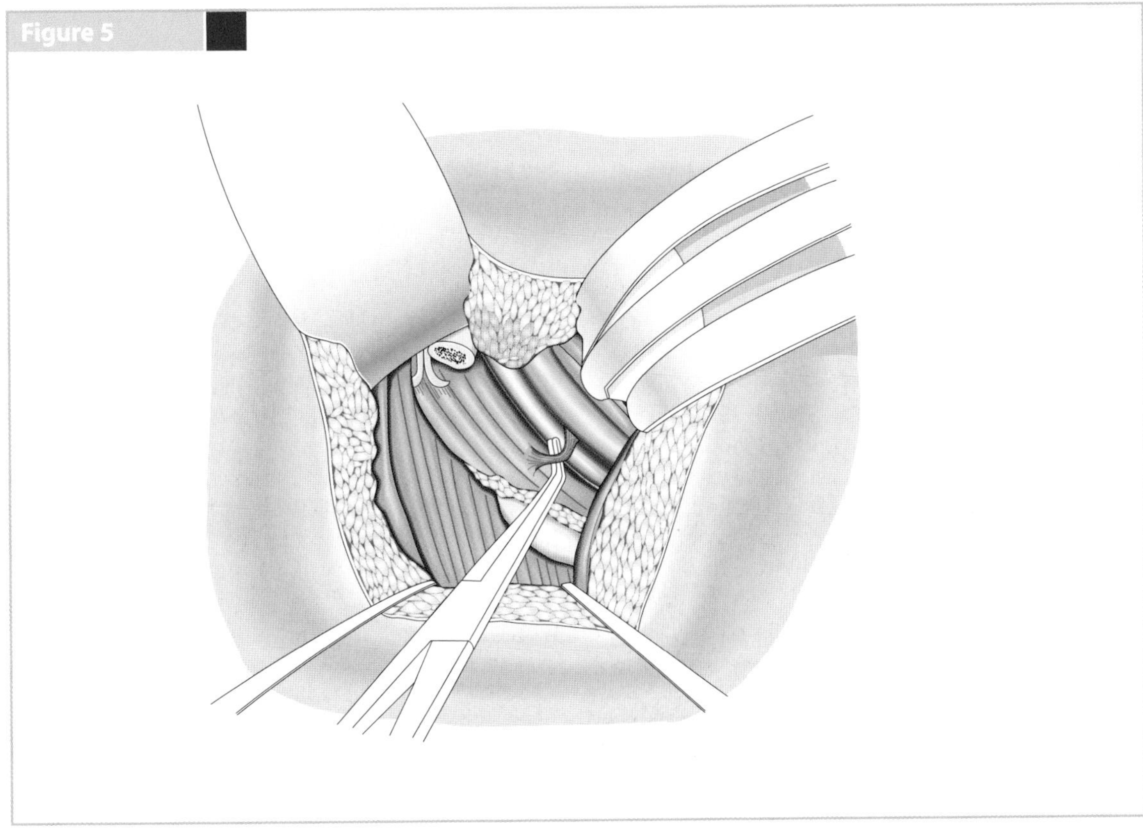

CONCLUSION

The transaxillary approach to the thoracic outlet provides a safe and excellent exposure for the treatment of TOS. A fundamental understanding of the expected structural anomalies responsible for the particular clinical situation is required. Direct visualization of the compressed neurovascular structures is enhanced by the use of an adjustable arm holder, a lighted retractor, a Vital View lighted suction device, a headlight and two surgical assistants.

Direct repair of the subclavian artery and vein is feasible through this incision, once the first rib has been excised. More extensive repairs may require surgical exposure above the clavicle and, in the case of distal emboli, into the arm.

The long-term benefits from the surgical treatment of neurogenic TOS remain limited by the problems of scar tissue adherence to the brachial plexus and resultant recurrence of symptoms. This remains unpredictable in any given case. We are aware of no effective barrier to such scar formation. Experience in the reoperative care of such patients has revealed that the anterior scalene muscle is frequently stuck to Sibson's fascia by thick bands of scar, with resultant entrapment of the lower plexus and tension within the muscle. The subclavian artery is similarly bound down by this scar tissue. When fully mobilized, the scar tissue is divided and the anterior scalene is free to retract into the neck. The *total disinsertion* of the anterior scalene muscle at the base of the thoracic outlet is the best method available for preventing this from occurring.

Others have advocated a supraclavicular approach to decompressing the brachial plexus. This approach provides ready access to the nerve roots and trunks. However, we have observed a greater problem with scar adherence to the brachial plexus following a supraclavicular approach when compared to a transaxillary approach. This is especially the case when a formal scalenectomy is included. Consequently, we resect only that amount of scalene muscle necessary to decompress the involved nerves or vessels. Furthermore, we have been impressed that *total disinsertion* of the anterior scalene muscle as part of a transaxillary first rib resection improves symptoms of upper/middle trunk compression as well by releasing the tension within that muscle.

The risks of transaxillary thoracic outlet decompression include nerve injuries. Intercostobrachial neuritis is exceedingly common, resulting in hypesthesia or dysesthesia to the axilla and medial brachium. More debilitating nerve injuries include the long thoracic nerve, the phrenic nerve, the stellate ganglion and the brachial plexus. When injured, the cause is usually a traction injury. Consequently, the surgeon must be cognizant of the location and force placed by the retractors and arm holder. Severe bleeding due to injury of the subclavian artery or vein is potentially life threatening. Exceptional care is employed during dissection around these vessels. Despite the potential severity of such complications, permanent brachial plexus nerve injury and subclavian vessel injury each occurs in less than 1% of cases.

Considerable attention is required for the postoperative care of the patient. The patient is provided with patient-controlled analgesia (PCA) until transitioned onto oral narcotics. A muscle relaxant, nonsteroidal anti-inflammatory medication, and sleeping agent are also provided. A cooling pad to limit swelling is placed anteriorly, while a shoulder heating pad is placed posteriorly at the patient's discretion. All patients are instructed preoperatively in nerve glide stretches so that they may apply these early in the postoperative course. They are admonished not to push these exercises to the point of discomfort.

Patients who undergo transaxillary thoracic outlet decompression for neurogenic TOS have severely limiting symptoms. When properly selected, 75–80% of patients are expected to improve.

SELECTED BIBLIOGRAPHY

Roos DB (1971) Experience with first rib resection for thoracic outlet syndrome. Ann Surg 173:429–442

Roos DB (1989) Thoracic outlet nerve compression. In: Rutherford RB (ed) Vascular surgery, 3rd edn. WB Saunders, Philadelphia, pp 858–875

Roos DB, Annest SJ, Brantigan CO (1999) Historical and anatomic perspective on thoracic outlet syndrome. Chest Surg Clin N Am 9(4):713–723

Roos DB, Annest SJ, Brantigan CO (2001) Transaxillary thoracic outlet decompression. In: Ernst CB, Stanley JC (eds) Current therapy in vascular surgery, 4th edn. Mosby, St. Louis, MO, pp 180–184

Sanders RJ (1996) Results of the surgical treatment for thoracic outlet syndrome. Semin Thoracic Cardiovasc Surg 8(2):221–228

CHAPTER 10

Treatment of Thoracic Outlet Sydromes and Cervical Sympathectomy

Robert W. Thompson

INTRODUCTION

The thoracic outlet is a unique anatomic region dominated by the first rib, the anterior and middle scalene muscles, and their associated neurovascular structures. Within this relatively confined space, the subclavian artery, subclavian vein, and nerve roots of the brachial plexus are all potentially subject to extrinsic compression. Whereas vascular lesions associated with thoracic outlet compression give rise to easily recognized syndromes, such as effort thrombosis of the subclavian vein or thromboembolism resulting from poststenotic aneurysms of the subclavian artery, the diagnosis of neurogenic thoracic outlet syndrome (TOS) often remains difficult, confusing and elusive. Nonetheless, it is possible to achieve excellent results for all forms of TOS by a comprehensive treatment approach, which includes a prominent role for surgical treatment in well-selected patients.

Neurogenic TOS is often associated with a history of previous trauma to the head, neck or upper extremity, followed by a variable interval before the onset of upper extremity symptoms. It is thought that post-traumatic spasm and inflammation of the scalene musculature can lead to delayed fibrotic reactions, eventually resulting in compressive neurologic symptoms. It is important to recognize that low-grade repetitive trauma can also contribute to this disorder and, conversely, that not all patients with TOS have their condition brought on by a specific traumatic event. Age-related postural changes superimposed upon congenital variations of scalene musculature, acting together, may also lead to extrinsic neural compression.

Symptoms of neurogenic TOS include hand or arm pain, dysesthesias, numbness and weakness. These complaints usually occur in a distribution distinct from that referable to a single peripheral nerve and are therefore difficult to classify. Headaches are also a common complaint in neurogenic TOS, most likely due to secondary spasm within the trapezius and paraspinous muscles. In almost all patients with neurogenic TOS the arm symptoms are reproducibly exacerbated by activities requiring elevation or sustained use of the upper extremity, such as reaching for objects overhead, driving, speaking on the telephone, shaving, and combing or brushing the hair, and prolonged typing or work at computer consoles. While the majority of patients with neurogenic TOS are affected to only a mild and tolerable degree, those consulting the vascular surgeon often exhibit progressively disabling symptoms that effectively prevent work or simple daily activities. In some cases, the symptoms of TOS may have progressed to resemble those of causalgia (i.e., reflex sympathetic dystrophy), with persistent vasospasm, disuse edema, hypersensitivity, and avoidance withdrawal from even light touch. A long history of physician consultations, partial or ineffective treatments, and medicolegal entanglements is also a consistent theme in this patient population.

Physical examination is directed towards eliciting the degree of neurogenic disability and to identify particular factors that exacerbate painful hand and arm complaints. The neck is examined to identify the extent of any local muscle spasm, and to localize specific areas that reproduce the individual patient's symptom pattern upon focal digital compression. The presence of such "trigger points," most often identified over the scalene triangle in the supraclavicular space, serves to reinforce the diagnosis of TOS. The Adson maneuver is used to identify any degree of subclavian artery compression, by detecting ablation of the radial pulse when the patient inspires deeply and turns the neck away from the affected extremity. Although this maneuver does not specifically reveal nerve root compression, positive findings are often associated with neurogenic TOS. It is important to recognize that a positive Adson sign is also quite common in the asymptomatic general population. This maneuver or similar tests in the vascular laboratory may therefore serve to support, but not prove, the diagnosis of TOS, and it is equally important to recognize that negative findings of arterial compression do not exclude a diagnosis of neurogenic TOS. Perhaps the most useful component of physical examination is the elevated arm stress test ("EAST"), in which the patient is asked to repetitively open and close the fists with the arms elevated in a "surrender" position. Most patients with authentic neurogenic TOS report the rapid reproduction of their typical upper extremity symptoms with EAST, often being unable to complete the exercise beyond 30–60 s. During physical examination, the surgeon should also seek evidence of arterial compromise to the upper extremity, such as sympathetic overactivity with vasospasm, digital or hand ischemia, cutaneous ulceration or emboli, forearm claudication, or the pulsatile supraclavicular mass and/or bruit characteristic of a subclavian artery aneurysm. Venous TOS, in contrast, is associated with hand and arm edema, cyanosis, enlarged subcutaneous collateral veins, and early forearm fatigue in the absence of arterial compromise.

No specific diagnostic test or imaging study can replace the clinical diagnosis of neurogenic TOS. Plain radiographs of the neck may be helpful in determining if an osseous cervical rib or abnormally wide transverse process of the cervical vertebrae is present, but the results of computed tomography, magnetic resonance imaging and electromyography/nerve conduction studies are usually negative. These studies are nonetheless useful to exclude other conditions that could be responsible for neurogenic symptoms, such as degenerative cervical spine disease.

For patients with features that suggest arterial TOS, contrast arteriography is necessary to exclude or prove the existence of a fixed arterial lesion. When venous TOS is suspected, contrast venography should be performed to verify subclavian vein occlusion, especially in the context of an "effort thrombosis" event; moreover, the initial treatment for this condition includes catheter-directed venous thrombolysis. It is helpful to utilize positional maneuvers during these vascular radiologic examinations, and to consider bilateral studies if there is any suggestion of contralateral symptoms. There is no role for balloon angioplasty and placement of intravascular stents in venous TOS, at least prior to surgical decompression, as indwelling stents in this situation are likely to become compressed and occluded.

Whereas early surgical decompression and vascular reconstruction is indicated for almost all patients with either arterial or venous forms of TOS, physical therapy serves as the initial and often only treatment necessary for neurogenic TOS. These therapeutic efforts are focused on relaxing the scalene muscles and strengthening the muscles of posture, combined with hydrotherapy and massage. Many patients with neurogenic TOS experience considerable symptomatic relief following physical therapy, and thereafter require only further conservative measures for maintenance. Nonetheless, physical therapy provides insufficient benefit for a subset of patients who are then considered for surgical treatment.

Figure 1A, B

The surgical anatomy of the thoracic outlet is centered upon spinal nerve roots C5 through T1, which interdigitate to form the brachial plexus as they cross under the clavicle and over the first rib. Several important cervical nerve branches also arise within the thoracic outlet region, including the long thoracic and phrenic nerves. Within the supraclavicular space the brachial plexus nerve roots pass through the "scalene triangle," an area bordered by the anterior and middle scalene muscles on each side and the first rib at the base. After entering the neck from the superior mediastinum, the subclavian artery also courses through the scalene triangle in direct relation to the brachial plexus nerve roots. The subclavian vein passes from the axilla to cross over the first rib immediately in front of the anterior scalene muscle, before joining with the internal jugular vein to form the innominate vein in the superior mediastinum. Each of these neurovascular structures is potentially subject to extrinsic compression by the musculoskeletal components of the scalene triangle, thereby giving rise to the various forms of thoracic outlet syndrome. Symptoms of TOS are often exacerbated by elevation of the arm, a position that places greater strain on the neurovascular structures that pass through the scalene triangle.

Figure 1A

C5

C6

C7

C8

T1

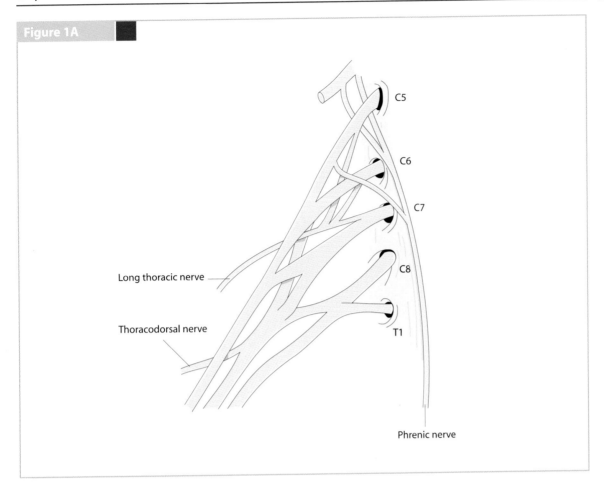

Long thoracic nerve

Thoracodorsal nerve

Phrenic nerve

Figure 1B

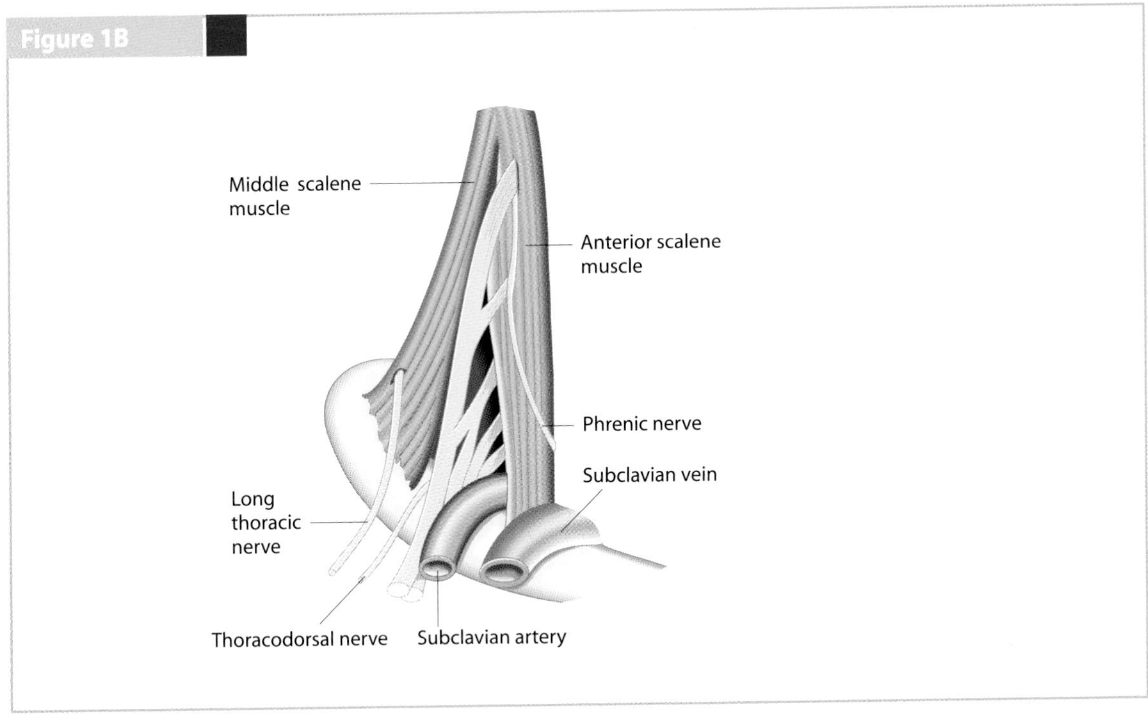

Figure 2

After induction of general endotracheal anesthesia, the patient is positioned supine with the head of the bed elevated 30 degrees. The hips and knees are flexed for comfortable positioning, and a small towel roll is placed behind the shoulders. The neck is extended and turned to the opposite side with skin preparation including the neck and upper chest, and the affected upper extremity is wrapped in stockinette. A transverse skin incision is made approximately 2 cm above the clavicle (*dashed line*), beginning at the lateral border of the sternocleidomastoid muscle, in order to center the surgical exposure over the scalene triangle. The incision is then carried through the platysma muscle layer to expose the scalene fat pad. Supraclavicular cutaneous nerves that cross the operative field may be divided if necessary for exposure, with recognition that this will result in an anesthetic area of skin over the shoulder and infraclavicular area.

Figure 3

After exposure of the scalene fat pad, a self-retaining retractor is placed in the wound and the omohyoid muscle is resected. Mobilization of the scalene fat pad begins at the lateral edge of the internal jugular vein, where several small veins and lymphatic channels must be ligated and divided (including the thoracic duct for operations on the left side). The scalene fat pad is progressively mobilized from its medial attachments to expose the anterior surface of the anterior scalene muscle. Great care is taken to identify and protect the phrenic nerve, which courses in a superolateral to inferomedial direction within the investing fascia of the anterior scalene muscle. The inferior and superior attachments of the scalene fat pad are then divided, often requiring further division of small blood vessels and lymphatics between ligatures, to allow full exposure of the anterior scalene muscle. After reflecting the scalene fat pad on a lateral pedicle (held in place with a stay suture), the underlying roots of the brachial plexus are exposed. The distal portion of the subclavian artery is also identified behind the lateral edge of the anterior scalene muscle, immediately inferior to the brachial plexus nerve roots.

Figure 2

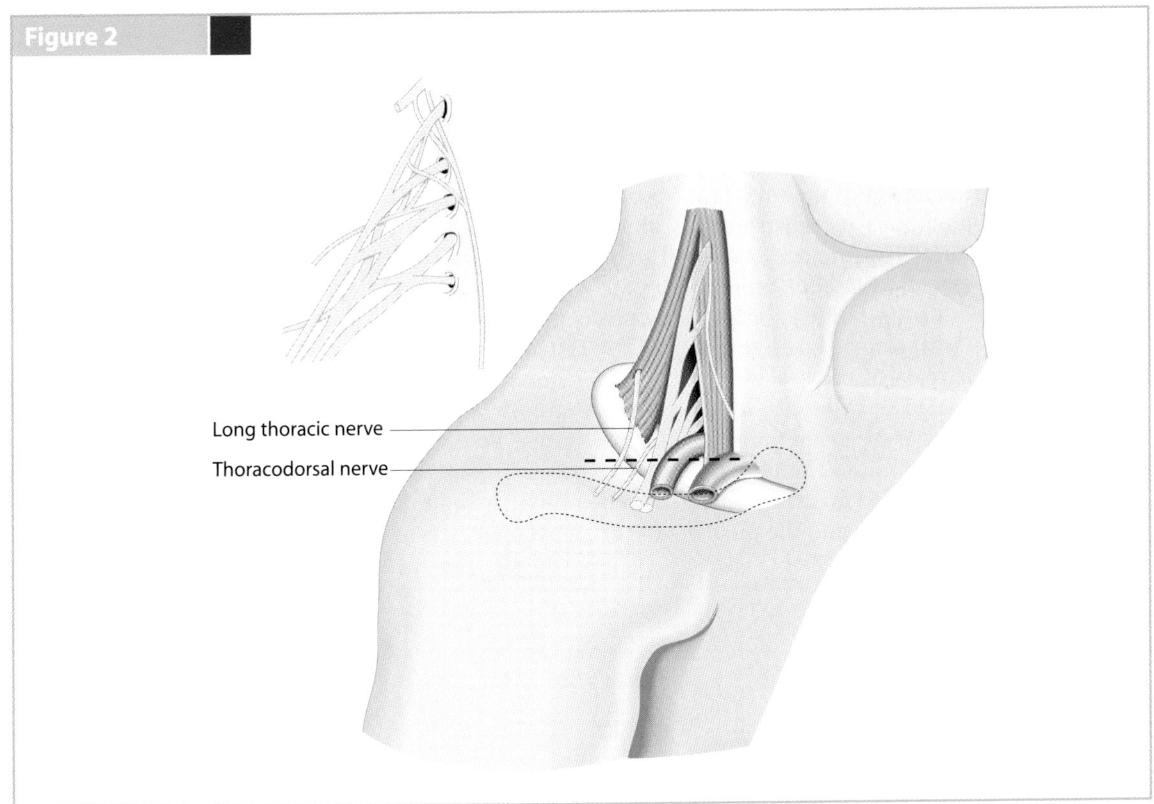

Figure 3

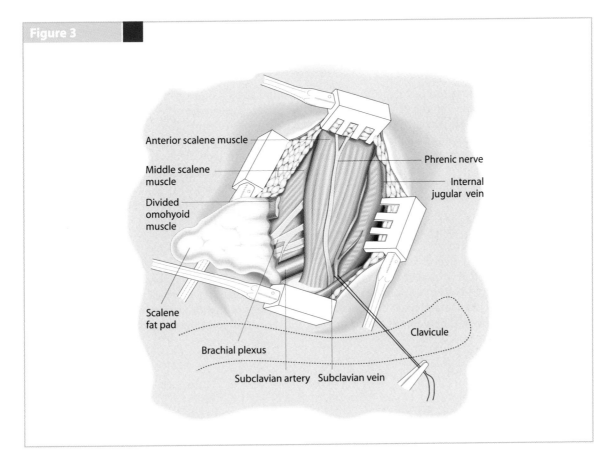

Anterior scalene muscle
Phrenic nerve
Middle scalene muscle
Internal jugular vein
Divided omohyoid muscle
Scalene fat pad
Clavicule
Brachial plexus
Subclavian artery
Subclavian vein

Figure 4

Exposure of the anterior scalene muscle is continued in a circumferential manner just above its insertion upon the first rib, in preparation for its division. The posterior aspect of the muscle is usually quite firm and tendinous in consistency, making this space anatomically restricted. Special effort is taken to avoid excessive traction on the phrenic nerve as it is separated from the anterior surface of the muscle. Care must also be taken to avoid injury to the uppermost roots of the brachial plexus (C5 and C6) and the subclavian artery, located at the lateral edge and posterior to the anterior scalene muscle during its mobilization. Similarly, the proximal portion of the subclavian artery must be well visualized and protected behind the medial edge of the anterior scalene. Once exposure is sufficient to pass a finger or right-angle clamp behind the anterior scalene muscle at the level of the first rib, the muscle and tendon are sharply divided from the edge of their osseous insertion. This is always done under direct vision with curved scissors rather than the cautery, using the surgeon's finger to prevent any unintended injury to the underlying neurovascular structures. In addition to the attachment of the anterior scalene muscle to the top of the first rib, there are often additional slips of muscle or tendon that must be divided more posteriorly, including direct attachments of the muscle to the thickened pleural lining behind the rib itself (Sibson's fascia).

Figure 5

Once the insertion of the anterior scalene muscle has been completely divided from the first rib, the muscle is lifted superiorly and detached from the additional structures underneath, including the pleural apex, the subclavian artery, and the brachial plexus nerve roots. The dissection is carried superiorly to the apex of the scalene triangle, where the anterior scalene muscle originates from the transverse process of the cervical vertebrae. At this level, muscle fibers are often found interdigitating with the proximal roots (C5 and C6) of the brachial plexus, requiring great care to avoid neural injury while these muscle fibers are divided. It is also common at this stage in the procedure to observe a scalene minimus muscle; this anomaly is characterized by fibers that originate in the plane of the middle scalene muscle (behind the C5 and C6 nerve roots) and then pass across or between the nerve roots to join the plane of the anterior scalene muscle, thereby serving as a potential source of neural compression and irritation. Once the anterior scalene muscle has been completely detached from its origins, it is removed and sent to the pathology laboratory for study. It is of interest that a high proportion of patients with neurogenic TOS exhibit myopathic changes in the anterior scalene muscle by light and electron microscopy, including fibrous thickening of the endomysium, fiber type redistribution to a predominance of type II ("slow-twitch") muscle fibers and even mitochondrial abnormalities otherwise associated with various forms of muscular dystrophy. The clinical significance of these alterations is unknown.

Figure 4

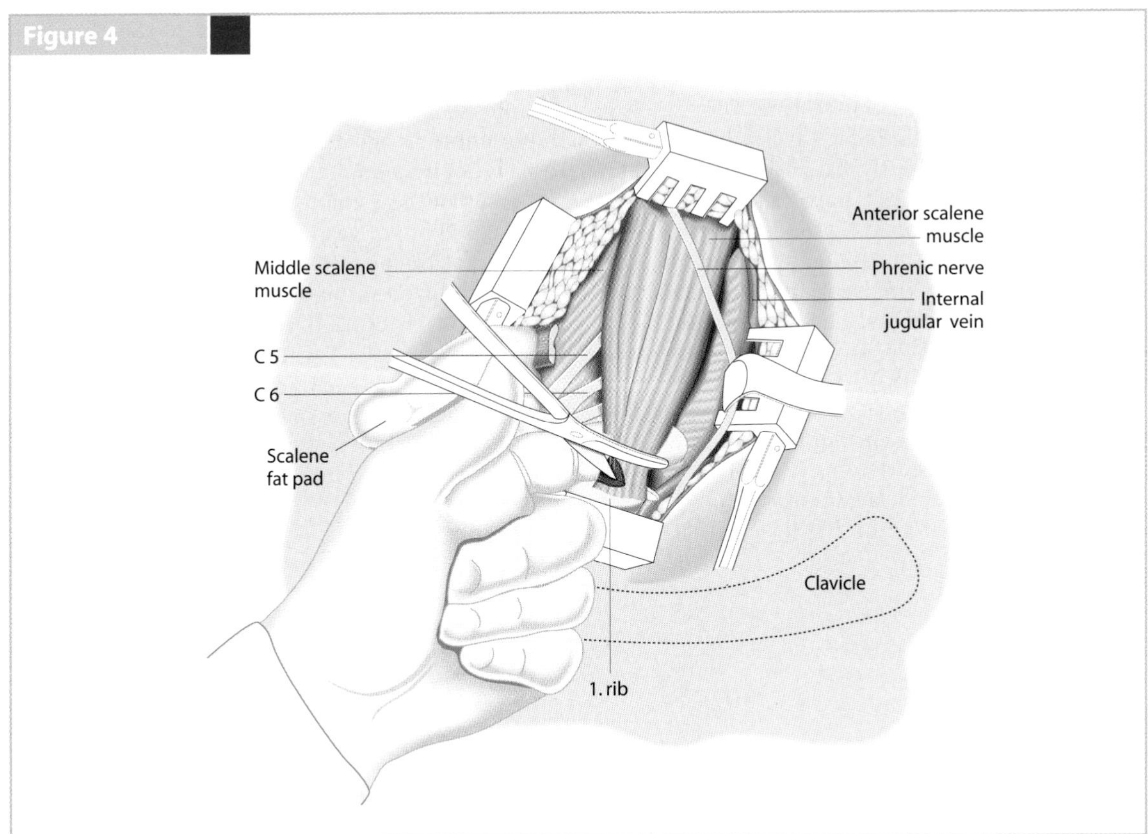
Anterior scalene muscle
Middle scalene muscle
Phrenic nerve
Internal jugular vein
C 5
C 6
Scalene fat pad
Clavicle
1. rib

Figure 5

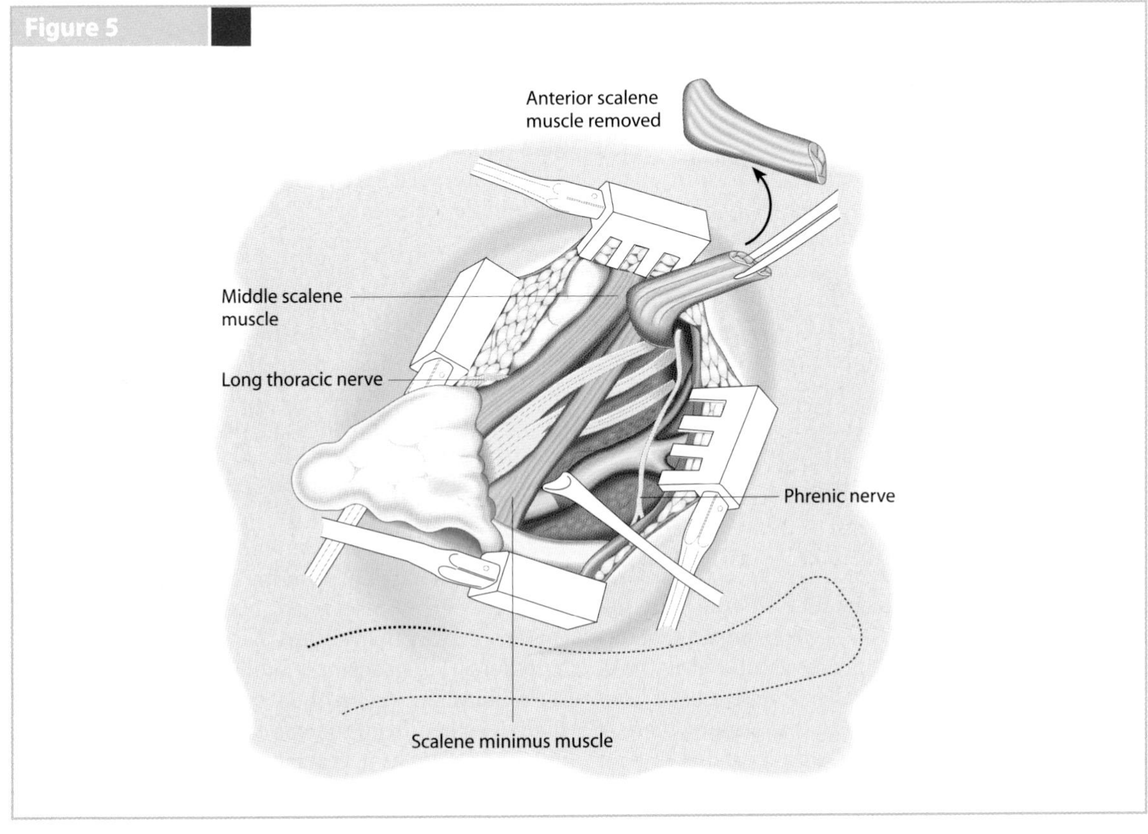
Anterior scalene muscle removed
Middle scalene muscle
Long thoracic nerve
Phrenic nerve
Scalene minimus muscle

Figure 6

Following complete anterior scalenectomy, each of the nerve roots contributing to the brachial plexus is identified and meticulously dissected free of any surrounding tissue. It is not uncommon to find the brachial plexus enveloped by moderately dense fibrotic tissue during this step in the procedure, especially in patients with long-standing neurogenic TOS where nerve root compression and irritation by inflammatory tissue may contribute to the generation of symptoms. Failure to perform an adequate brachial plexus neurolysis may therefore be one cause of persistent symptoms despite otherwise adequate decompression. During this phase of the dissection it is important to recognize that anatomic fusion of nerve roots is not uncommon (i.e., C5 with C6 and C8 with T1), and that these connections must not be disrupted. It is also important to ensure that full mobility is achieved at the upper aspect of nerve roots C5 and C6, which can be entrapped by the origins of the scalene muscles or other fibrous tissues at the apex of the scalene triangle. This aspect of the operation is not complete until each nerve root from C5 to T1 is completely free and mobile throughout its course in the operative field.

Figure 7

Brachial plexus neurolysis is continued with each nerve root sequentially identified. Exposure of the lower nerve roots (C8 and T1) is best achieved by medial displacement of the brachial plexus from the border of the middle scalene muscle. The origin of the T1 nerve root may be compressed by fibrous bands along the posterior neck of the first rib; relief of this source of nerve compression also requires adequate visualization of the proximal first rib to effect complete nerve root mobility. The attachment of the middle scalene muscle to the first rib is readily apparent after mobilization and medial retraction of the brachial plexus nerve roots. The muscle courses in an oblique manner to a wide osseous insertion; in some cases, the middle scalene may insert upon the first rib as far anteriorly as the scalene tubercle (the bony site of attachment of the anterior scalene muscle tendon) leaving little space for the neurovascular structures. The composition of the middle scalene muscle may also be firm and tendinous in this region, thereby serving as another potential source of nerve root compression and/or irritation; it is also important to note that when present, cervical ribs (or their soft tissue counterparts) are found within the same plane as the middle scalene muscle. Before detaching the middle scalene muscle from the first rib, the long thoracic nerve is identified where it passes through the middle scalene muscle and is thereafter protected from injury. The attachment of the middle scalene muscle to the first rib is initially divided using a cautery under direct vision, then detached along the lateral aspect of the rib using a periosteal elevator or curved Mayo scissors. After identifying the plane of separation between the middle and posterior scalene muscles as defined by the course of the long thoracic nerve, the middle scalene muscle anterior to the nerve is excised. It is important to note that the long thoracic nerve is often represented by two or three branches at this level rather than a single nerve as often described. With lateral displacement of the long thoracic nerve, the remaining portion of the middle scalene muscle is then detached from the upper surface of the first rib as far posterior as necessary to expose the neck of the rib and the T1 nerve root.

Figure 6

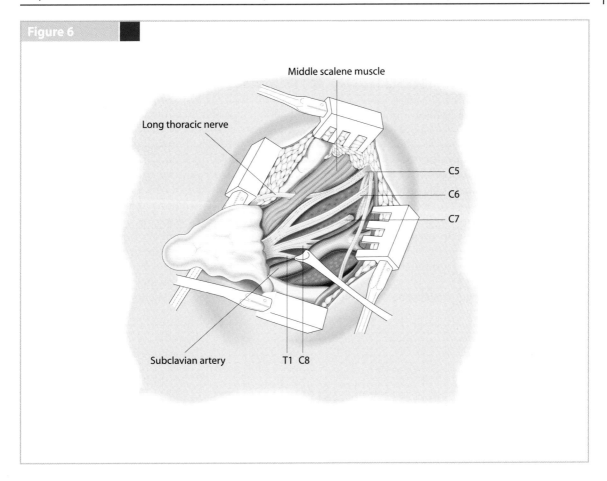

Middle scalene muscle

Long thoracic nerve

C5

C6

C7

Subclavian artery

T1 C8

Figure 7

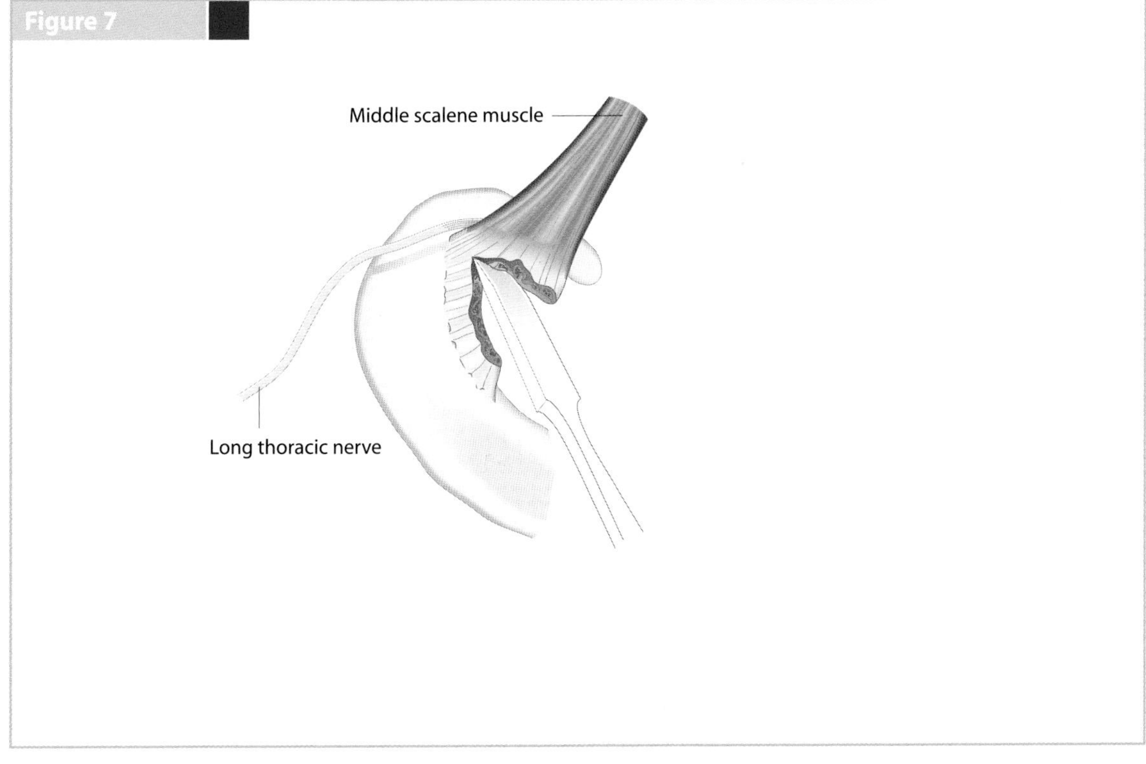

Figure 8

Resection of the first rib is readily accomplished given the extent of anatomic exposure achieved at this stage of supraclavicular thoracic outlet decompression. Using blunt dissection, the pleural membrane is separated from the inferior aspect of the first rib and the intercostal muscle attachments are divided with a periosteal elevator or cautery, such that the posterior and lateral aspects of the first rib are circumferentially exposed (**A**). Additional intercostal attachments are divided along the anterolateral aspect of the rib up to the level of the scalene tubercle. With the brachial plexus nerve roots well visualized and protected by gentle medial retraction, a small rib cutter is inserted around the posterior neck of the rib and applied (**B**). The rib is then displaced inferiorly to help expand visualization of the costoclavicular space, and the rib cutter is inserted around the anterior portion of the rib at the level of the scalene tubercle. The anterior rib is divided and any remaining muscular attachments to the rib are divided under traction, and the bone is removed from the operative field. The remaining posterior edge of the rib is remodeled to a smooth surface using a Kerrison bone rongeur, ensuring that there is no residual impingement on the T1 nerve root (**C**). The anterior edge of the rib is similarly remodeled to a smooth surface, but it is not necessary to remove the entire distal portion of the first rib (medial to the scalene tubercle) for patients with neurogenic or arterial thoracic outlet syndromes. Additional maneuvers to remove the remaining medial portion of the rib are necessary, however, in patients with venous TOS.

Figure 9

Subclavian artery reconstruction is indicated for any degree of aneurysmal degeneration or for persistent occlusive lesions of the arterial wall that are still evident after scalenectomy, particularly if the patient has had preoperative symptoms of digital thromboembolism. This is easily accomplished by direct excision of the diseased subclavian artery and interposition bypass grafting with end-to-end anastomoses, especially given the generous exposure of the proximal subclavian artery afforded by supraclavicular exploration. Because distal control of the subclavian or axillary artery is often inadequate through supraclavicular exposure alone, this may require a second (infraclavicular) incision placed over the deltopectoral groove to permit exposure of the axillary artery just underneath the pectoralis minor muscle, much the same as that used for axillofemoral bypass operations. In this situation the graft is easily passed through the subclavicular space afforded by removal of the first rib. Although prosthetic graft materials of either Dacron or externally supported polytetrafluoroethylene (PTFE) may be used effectively in the subclavian position, in young active patients where the arm will be subject to considerable motion and extended use, autologous arterial conduits may be preferred. In the latter case, subclavian artery reconstruction is performed with a size-matched segment of the external iliac artery, which is then replaced with a separate prosthetic graft.

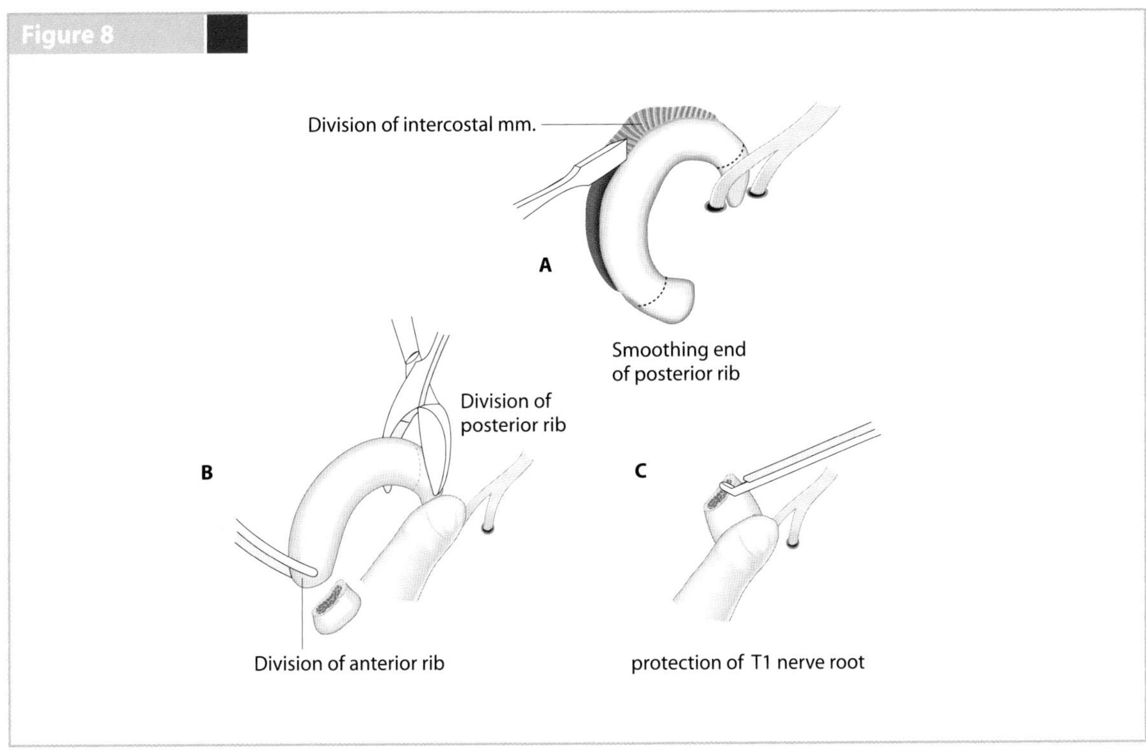

Figure 8

Figure 9

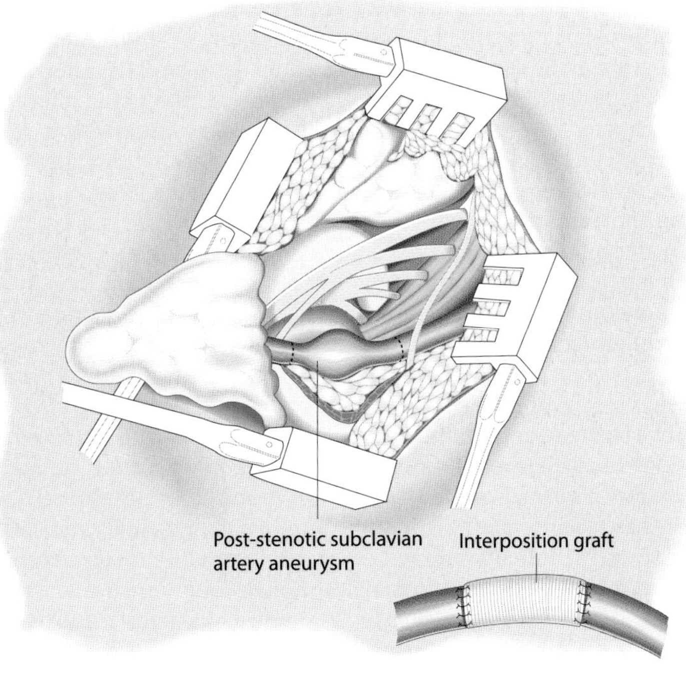

Post-stenotic subclavian
artery aneurysm

Interposition graft

Figure 10

Several additional considerations to the standard supraclavicular exploration are involved in thoracic outlet decompression for venous TOS (effort thrombosis syndrome). Although the initial stages of the operation are performed exactly as described for neurogenic TOS (including scalenectomy, brachial plexus neurolysis and partial resection of the first rib), attention is then specifically directed toward removal of the remaining medial portion of the first rib and correction of the venous problem, either by circumferential venolysis and/or venous reconstruction. It is important to note that complete resection of the medial first rib, where it contributes most to venous compression, cannot be performed through the supraclavicular approach alone. To accomplish this component of venous decompression an additional incision is made over the medial infraclavicular space, extending from the edge of the sternum. The sternal attachment of the first rib is identified by palpation and its anterior surface exposed using the cautery. With downward pressure applied to the remaining segment of the first rib through the supraclavicular incision to place its attachments to the clavicle under tension, the costoclavicular ligaments are divided under direct vision through the infraclavicular incision. Great care is taken during this dissection to prevent injury to the proximal subclavian vein, which would be exceptionally difficult to control in this area. Once this has been accomplished, the remaining portion of the first rib is removed by detaching it from the sternum, and the subclavian vein is exposed as far centrally as its junction with the jugular vein to form the innominate vein.

Figure 11

After paraclavicular decompression of the thoracic outlet with removal of the proximal first rib, the subclavian vein is visualized through the supraclavicular incision. The proximal subclavian vein is dissected free of surrounding scar tissue, from the supraclavicular space to its junction with the internal jugular vein, and into the upper mediastinum if necessary. Dense fibrosis encasing the vein is unusually encountered regardless of the timing of operation in relation to an effort thrombosis event, as a result of repeated compression, previous episodes of venous thrombosis and local inflammation. Despite the venographic appearance of persistent venous thrombosis, the subclavian vein itself is often patent without permanent obstructive changes, and for this reason, relief of the encasing scar tissue usually results in re-distention of the vein to a normal caliber. Furthermore, once the vein has been circumferentially exposed by external venolysis, it is often found to be soft, compressible and free of residual intraluminal obstruction or thrombus. The subclavian vein is therefore dissected out in its entirety before considering the need for other forms of venous reconstruction.

Direct venous reconstruction is required in situations where external venolysis is insufficient to ensure relief from venous obstruction. The subclavian vein is clamped and a longitudinal venotomy is created up the level of the internal jugular vein to permit visual inspection of the internal surface. If the luminal lining is intact with a smooth endothelialized surface, simple patch angioplasty using a segment of autologous saphenous vein may be sufficient; when this form of closure is used, the patch is constructed with a long tail that is attached along the side of the internal jugular vein, thereby helping to widen the jugular-subclavian junction (**A**). When the subclavian vein is opened and any degree of surface ulceration, residual thrombus or significant wall thickening is encountered, the affected subclavian vein is simply excised and replaced. The most common form of reconstruction in our practice is interposition grafting, using a panel graft constructed from autologous saphenous vein (**B**). Cryopreserved arterial homografts have also been used for this purpose, although long-term results with these conduits are unknown. As an alternative form of venous reconstruction when the damaged segment of subclavian vein is particularly long, the ipsilateral internal jugular vein may be divided high in the neck, with its cephalad end turned down to be connected with the distal subclavian or axillary vein.

Figure 10

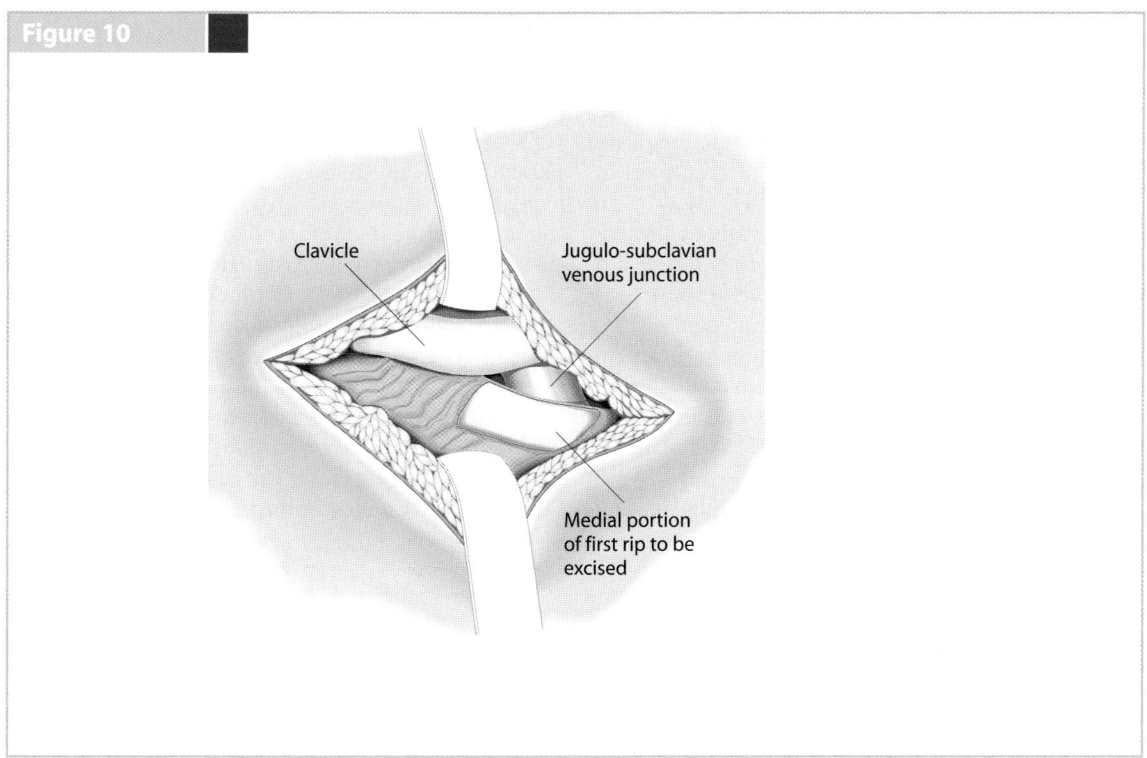

Figure 11

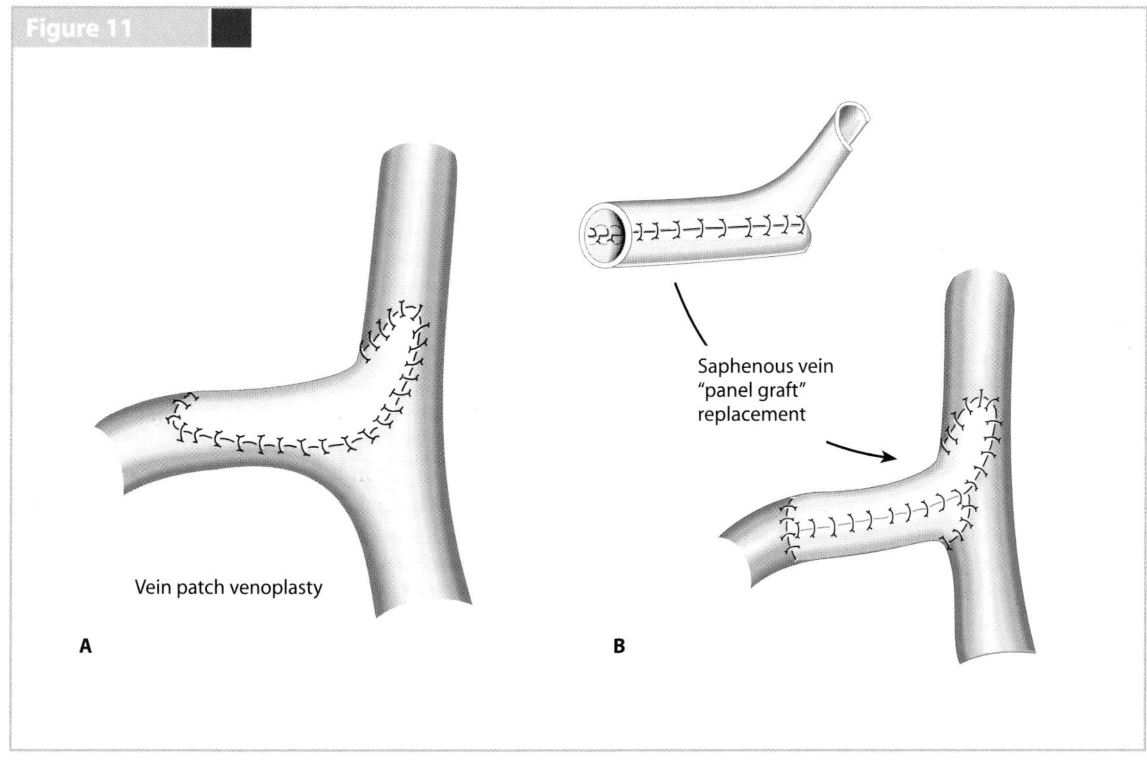

Figure 12

Patients with disabling neurogenic or arterial TOS may also present with symptoms characteristic of peripheral sympathetic overactivity, resulting in painful vasospasm, delayed healing of digital skin lesions, and at times even reflex sympathetic dystrophy. In these situations it may be preferable to include cervical sympathectomy with the primary procedure done for thoracic outlet decompression. Indeed, this adds little to the procedure itself and it may be of substantial benefit with respect to alleviating vasospastic complaints or in facilitating healing of digital lesions caused by atheroemboli or ischemic injury. Through the supraclavicular exposure, the cervical sympathetic chain is identified by palpation along the inner edge of the posterior first or second rib, where it will feel like a rubber band-like structure passing vertically over the neck of the bone. The sympathetic chain is elevated with a nerve hook and the lateral attachments (rami) to each ganglion are divided sharply. The sympathetic chain is mobilized distally to the level of the third rib, where metal clips are placed at the end of the chain prior to dividing it sharply. The chain is then elevated and mobilized proximally to the level of the stellate ganglion. In order to minimize the incidence of postoperative Horner's syndrome, metal clips are placed at the lower half of the stellate ganglion and the sympathetic chain is divided immediately below that level.

CONCLUSION

Postoperative pain medication is provided by patient-controlled intravenous analgesia until adequate control can be achieved by oral medications. Oral narcotics, muscle relaxants and non-steroidal anti-inflammatory agents are routinely prescribed for the first 3 weeks following surgery. The closed suction drain placed at the time of operation is removed within 2 days unless persistent lymphatic fluid is evident, in which case the patient is discharged and the drain is removed in the outpatient office when the leak has subsided. Patients are not specifically restricted with respect to use of the upper extremity, but are advised against excessive reaching overhead or heavy lifting. Resumption of physical therapy is encouraged as soon as feasible, usually upon discharge from the hospital. Although excessive activity in the first several weeks can result in muscle strain and spasm, with significant pain that is referred to the sternocleidomastoid, trapezius and other neck muscles, the majority of patients resume fairly regular activity within several weeks after operation. Cautious return to work is recommended by 6 weeks if possible, but heavy activity is restricted during the early stages to avoid excessive lifting or repetitive activities that may contribute to postoperative complaints. Patients with long-standing neurogenic TOS often display residual symptoms of dysesthesias, numbness, or other tolerable complaints that may not be eliminated by thoracic outlet decompression, and must be provided continuing support and reassurance during recovery and rehabilitation. Physical therapy is continued for as long as necessary to allow the patient to return to an optimal level of function, and patients are seen at twice-yearly intervals to assess the long-term results of operative intervention.

Patients with venous TOS undergo contrast venography 3–4 weeks after operation, both to assess the adequacy of venous decompression on the operative side and, if not previously determined, to determine if positional venous compression exists on the contralateral side. Any residual venous stenosis may be safely treated at this time by transluminal balloon angioplasty; although this was necessary in approximately one-third of patients early in our experience, with more uniform application of subclavian vein replacement the need for follow-up balloon angioplasty has been largely eliminated.

Minor degrees of diaphragmatic paralysis are not uncommon early after supraclavicular thoracic outlet decompression, usually resolving within several days to weeks. This is often unnoticed by the patient, but may result in shortness of breath with exertion. When phrenic neuropraxia requires nerve regrowth from the neck to the level of the diaphragm, this may take up to 10 months to resolve. It is therefore essential to ensure that any degree of phrenic nerve paresis has completely resolved prior to considering any form of operation for TOS on the contralateral side, using fluoroscopic examination to visualize diaphragmatic function and complete return of innervation.

In summary, supraclavicular exploration has become a widely utilized, versatile and effective approach in the treatment of thoracic outlet compression syndromes. It is applicable to virtually all forms of TOS, including neurogenic, arterial and venous,

Figure 12

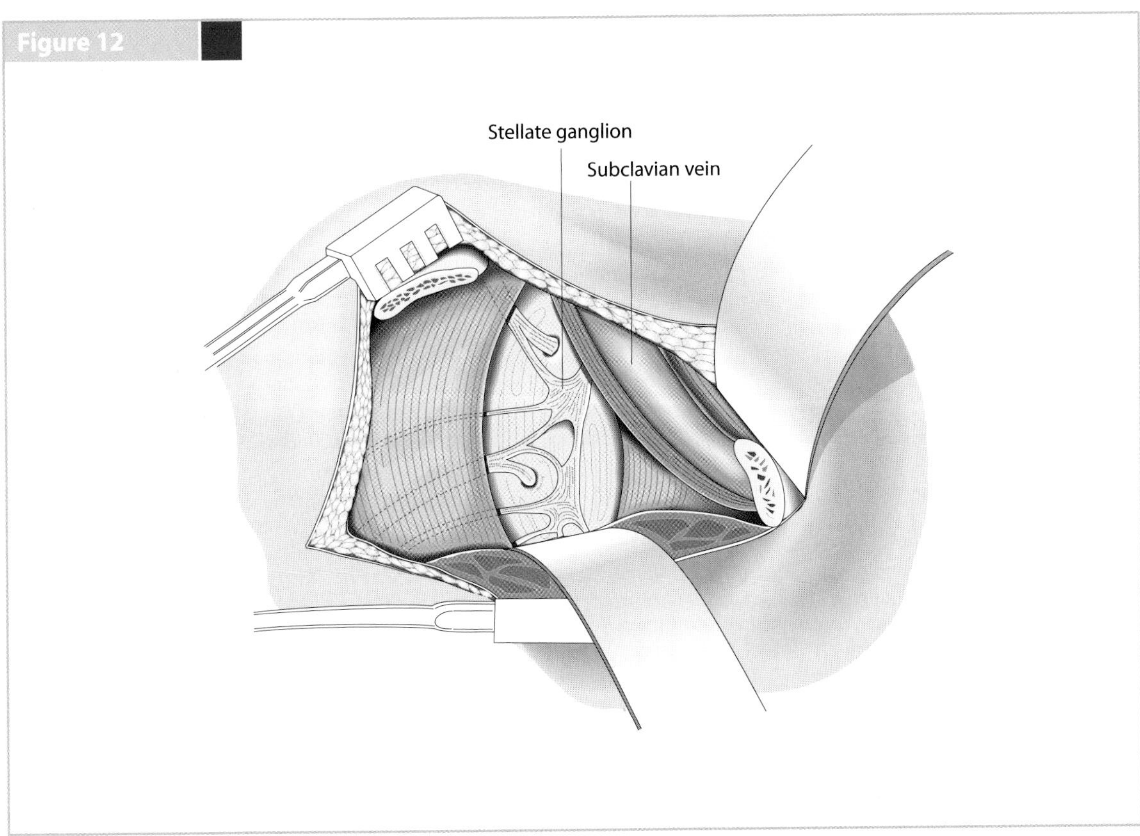

and permits a sufficient degree of operative flexibility to address individual variations. Although certain aspects of the surgical anatomy are quite familiar to most vascular surgeons, considerable attention must be given to the details of this procedure to avoid inadequate decompression, serious injury, or predictable causes of recurrent compression. Supraclavicular exploration and its variations provide an excellent approach to the entire spectrum of problems encountered in patients with TOS, and in many centers it has superseded the transaxillary approach previously popularized for these disorders. Because supraclavicular exploration for TOS involves a number of unique technical considerations and because it is typically applied to a difficult clinical problem outside the routine experience of most vascular surgeons, it should be undertaken only with appropriate training and interest in the comprehensive management of patients with TOS.

SELECTED BIBLIOGRAPHY

Azakie A, McElhinney DB, Thompson RW, Raven RB, Messina LM, Stoney RJ (1998) Surgical management of subclavian vein "effort" thrombosis secondary to thoracic outlet compression. J Vasc Surg 28:777–786

Hempel GK, Shutze WP, Anderson JF, Bukhari HI (1996) 770 consecutive supraclavicular first rib resections for thoracic outlet syndrome. Ann Vasc Surg 10:456–463

Machleder HI, Moll F, Verity MA (1986) The anterior scalene muscle in thoracic outlet compression syndrome: histochemical and morphometric studies. Arch Surg 121:1141–1144

Reilly LM, Stoney RJ (1988) Supraclavicular approach for thoracic outlet decompression. J Vasc Surg 8:329–334

Roos DB (1976) Congenital anomalies associated with thoracic outlet syndrome. Am J Surg 132:771–778

Sanders RJ (1991) Thoracic outlet syndrome: a common sequela of neck injuries. JB Lippincott, Philadelphia

Sanders RJ, Raymer S (1985) The supraclavicular approach to scalenectomy and first rib resection: description of technique. J Vasc Surg 2:751–756

Thompson RW, Petrinec D (1997) Surgical treatment of thoracic outlet compression syndromes. I. Diagnostic considerations and transaxillary first rib resection. Ann Vasc Surg 11:315–323

Thompson RW, Schneider PA, Nelken NA, Skioldebrand CG, Stoney RJ (1992) Circumferential venolysis and paraclavicular thoracic outlet decompression for "effort thrombosis" of the subclavian vein. J Vasc Surg 16:723–732

Thompson RW, Petrinec D, Toursarkissian B (1997) Surgical treatment of thoracic outlet compression syndromes. II. Supraclavicular exploration and vascular reconstruction. Ann Vasc Surg 11:442–451

10

CHAPTER 11

Digital Sympathectomy for Scleroderma

Nicholas J. Goddard

INTRODUCTION

Systemic sclerosis (scleroderma) is a widespread disease affecting the skin, gastrointestinal tract, heart, lungs and hands. Most patients with systemic sclerosis of the hand present with Raynaud's phenomenon (see below) and may have no progression beyond that. In more advanced cases, the ischemic changes may include fingertip pain, digital tip ischemia, ulceration and gangrene. Sclerodactyly, loss of fingertip pulp and joint contractures (especially those affecting the interphalangeal joints) are another form of presentation. There is often overlap between the two forms of presentation and both may be associated with painful cutaneous calcinosis.

Treatment of the hand is primarily aimed at reversing the ischemic changes, followed by excision of the calcinotic deposits. Finally, function is restored by improving the position of the affected digits, generally by fusion of the interphalangeal joints in a more favorable position.

RAYNAUD'S PHENOMENON AND DIGITAL ISCHEMIA

In 1865, Maurice Raynaud first described the characteristic color changes caused by paroxysmal blanching, cyanosis and secondary hyperemia of the digits that occur in Raynaud's phenomenon. The symptoms are intermittent and attacks are generally provoked by exposure to cold or the increased sympathetic output associated with emotional upset. Although Raynaud's phenomenon may never progress, it is commonly the initial presentation of systemic sclerosis, which may take many years to become apparent.

Two theories have been put forward to explain Raynaud's phenomenon. The first proposes that the exaggerated vasomotor signs are caused by an excessive sympathetic response to cold or stress. This theory explains the reported efficacy of treatment aimed at reducing sympathetic vasoconstrictor tone (i.e., alpha-agonists, cervical sympathectomy, digital sympathectomy). The second theory suggests that the sympathetic response is normal, but the arteries of the hand and digits are abnormal. Angiographic and histological studies, in patients with systemic sclerosis, have demonstrated multiple small areas of narrowing and occlusion of the ulnar artery at the wrist (up to 50% of cases), the superficial palmar arch (10%) and the main digital arteries. The radial artery and common digital arteries are less commonly involved. Paradoxically, ischemic change is most common in the index and middle fingers, with the thumb seldom affected.

Postmortem histological studies of digital arteries in patients with systemic sclerosis and Raynaud's phenomenon show that 80% have more than 75% luminal narrowing as a result of intimal hyperplasia and fibrosis. These findings are commonly associated with adventitial fibrosis and telangiectasia of the vasa vasorum of the adventitia, a relatively common observation at operation. This intimal thickening results in a permanent increase in the wall-to-lumen ratio and consequently a significant reduction in blood flow to the fingers (flow is proportional to the fourth power of the radius). Thus, even a minimal increase in the vasoconstrictive response to cold may produce further functional narrowing in an artery that is already partially occluded by structural changes.

NON-SURGICAL TREATMENT

The patient should be advised to avoid factors that provoke onset of symptoms and, most importantly, should stop smoking. The patient should avoid exposure to cold by wearing gloves or using warming devices to protect the fingers, and hats and scarves to protect the ears.

Drugs that reduce sympathetic activity and promote vasodilatation are beneficial in the control of Raynaud's phenomenon and healing digital ulcers.

- Nifedipine is a calcium channel blocker that induces vasodilatation.
- Prazosin has a direct effect on arterial smooth muscle relaxation, promoting vasodilatation.

In the author's unit, a synthetic prostacyclin infusion is used for critical ischemia and as a prelude to surgery.

SURGICAL TREATMENT

The early theories of Raynaud's phenomenon suggested that it was caused by an exaggerated sympathetic response. Surgical interruption of the sympathetic outflow by cervical sympathectomy was therefore used to treat Raynaud's phenomenon.

Although the short-term results were encouraging, the long-term results were poor in most patients. This is probably because many sympathetic nerve fibers bypass the cervicothoracic trunk and feed in distally, to provide additional contributions to the sympathetic nerve supply of the upper limb. More recently, thoracoscopic sympathectomy has been used.

The results of this procedure are awaited with interest, especially in view of its reported low morbidity and the ease with which the sympathetic chain can be identified.

Figure 1: Digital Anatomy

The poor results obtained with cervical sympathectomy led to attention being directed to the digital vessels. It was observed that additional sympathetic nerve fibers leave the median and ulnar nerves at the level of the wrist, to innervate the radial and ulnar arteries and superficial palmar arch. In addition, the common digital and main digital arteries receive direct input from the adjacent digital nerves. These observations led to the development of the technique of digital sympathectomy in 1980. When first described, the operation was performed at the level of the common digital and proper digital arteries. All neural connections between the digital nerve and artery were divided and the adventitia stripped from the main digital vessel. In contrast to cervical sympathectomy, this operation showed good results in Raynaud's disease after 10 years of follow-up. In systemic sclerosis, however, the results were not as impressive, except with regard to pain relief.

The operation has since been modified, with encouraging results being reported for systemic sclerosis. Modifications range from a simple extension of the operation to include the common digital artery as well as the main arteries, to complete adventitial stripping of the main radial and ulnar arteries at the wrist, the superficial palmar arch, and the common and main digital arteries of the fingers, with reversed interposition vein grafting for sites of total vessel occlusion.

Digital sympathectomy may improve blood flow in the digital arteries by interrupting the sympathetic vasoconstrictor supply to the digital arteries, and by removing the external constrictive cuff or periadventitial fibrosis from around the arteries. It has been suggested that the operation be renamed decompression arteriolysis or radical microarteriolysis.

Patients with disabling symptoms of Raynaud's phenomenon, fingertip pain and chronic digital ulceration refractory to medical management are most likely to benefit from surgery.

THE AUTHOR'S APPROACH

■ **Investigations.** The standard preoperative investigations include thermography and cold stress testing to quantify fingertip temperatures and to assess the rate of rewarming. Routine use of digital subtraction angiography has been largely abandoned, though it is still used for more difficult cases. The author has attempted to quantify blood flow using radionuclides, but this can be painful (xenon clearance involves an injection into the pulp) and the results are variable and unreliable.

Figure 1

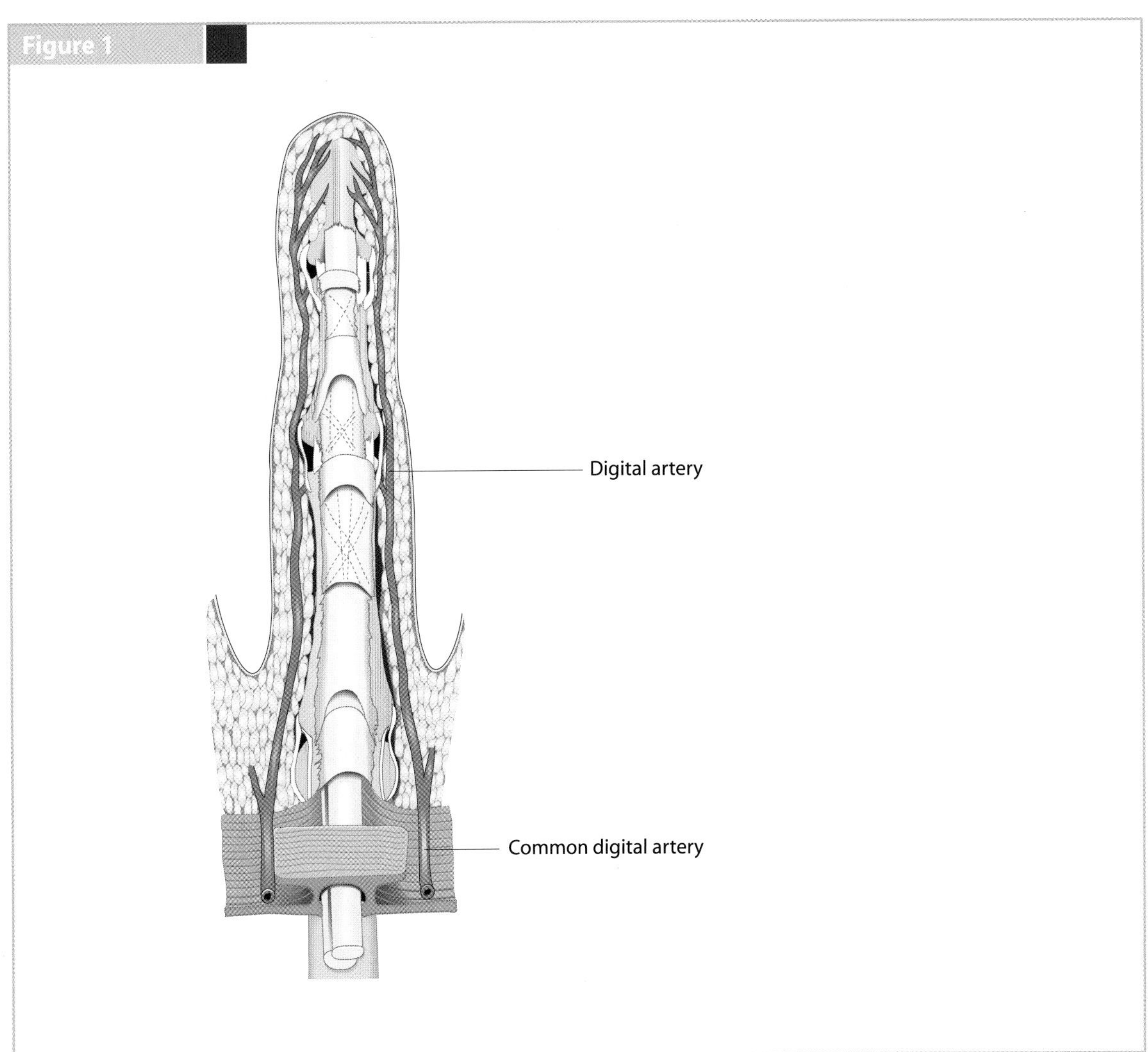

Figure 2: Technique

The technique used is essentially the same as that originally described by Flatt (1980) with some minor modifications. A relatively limited sympathectomy is performed, confined to the affected digits and occasionally to the main radial and ulnar arteries when indicated (Ballogh 2002). Results are comparable with those of more extensive operations (O'Brien et al. 1992).

The operation is performed with the patient under general or regional anesthesia. Many of these patients have lung and cardiac involvement and most have some esophageal reflux. Antacid or H_2-antagonist (omeprazole) is therefore given preoperatively to minimize the risk of aspiration. Intubation may also be hazardous because of jaw stiffness.

In common with all hand surgery a pneumatic tourniquet is essential; there have been no complications caused by the tourniquet. Some form of magnification, either binocular loupes or an operating microscope, is mandatory.

A Y-shaped palmar incision is used with the vertical limb situated between the two most severely affected fingers, generally the index and middle. Such an incision generally gives adequate access to the common digital artery, the bifurcation and the proper digital arteries to the level of the proximal interphalangeal joint. If necessary, the incision can be extended distally in a Brunner fashion (zigzag) to enhance exposure of the digital vessels. The subcutaneous tissues are generally abnormal with a striking degree of proliferative fibrous tissue in the palm, similar to that seen in Dupuytren's disease. This extends down on either side of the neurovascular bundles, making their exposure more difficult.

Figure 3: Adventitial Release of Digital Artery

The adventitia is easily identified by the vena comitans and is often inflamed and thickened. Removal of the adventitia is straightforward with a pair of fine watchmaker's forceps or micro-scissors. Following removal, the vessel takes on a different hue and appear slightly dull. Care should be taken around the small branches arising from the artery, not only to avoid damaging them, but also to ensure that the adventitia is adequately stripped and has not bunched up at the level of the branch causing a localized constriction. The adventitia is then divided to sever any remaining sympathetic nerve fibers that it may contain.

Figure 2

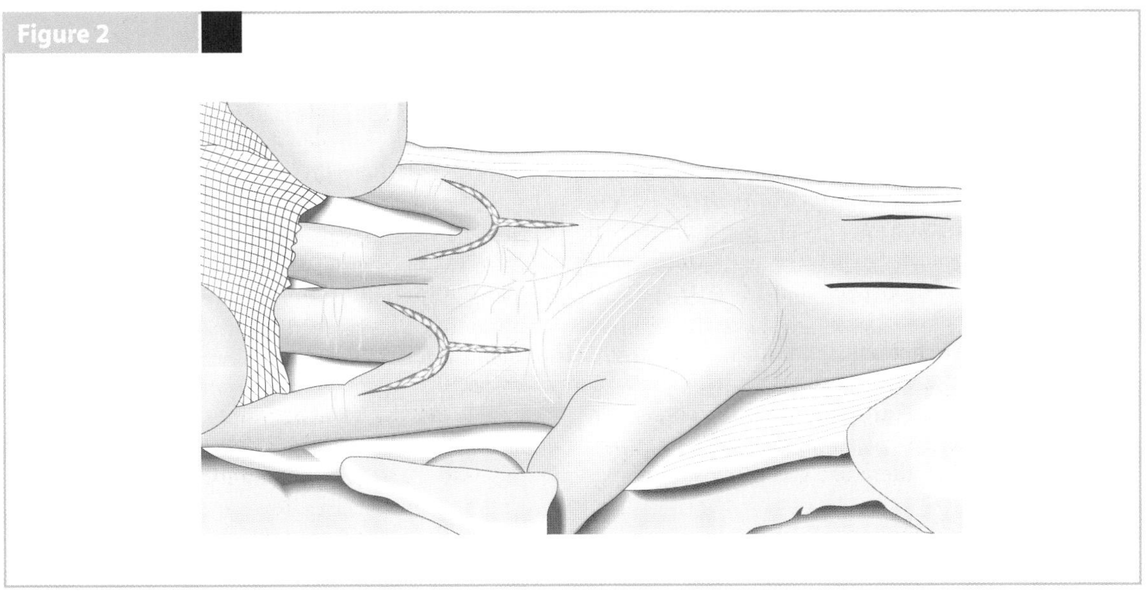

Figure 3

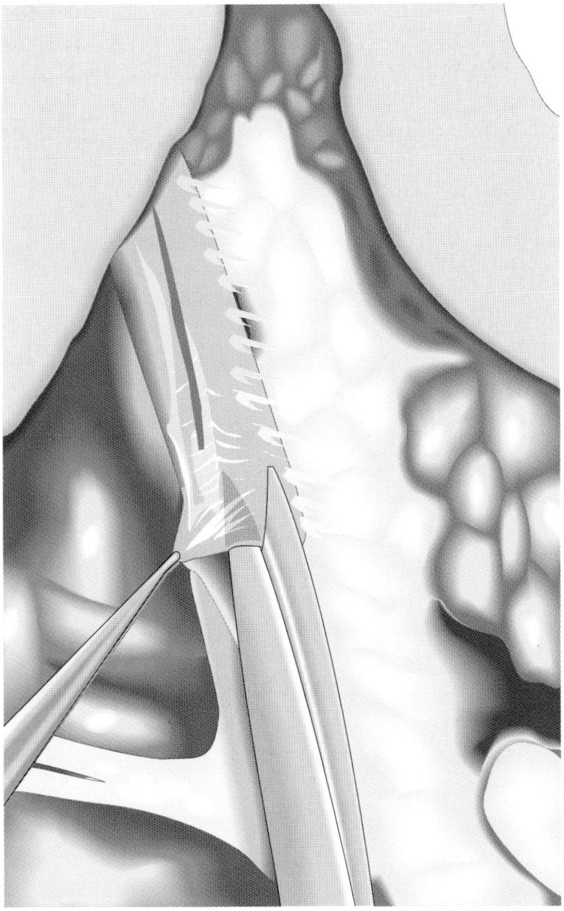

Figure 4: Completed Dissection of the Common Digital Vessels

The dissection is confined to the common digital vessel as it arises from the superficial palmar arch and this is traced distally to include the radial and ulnar proper digital arteries of the affected fingers to the level of the proximal interphalangeal joint. Wherever possible both vessels should be stripped, but if this is not possible, the dissection is restricted to the dominant vessel (i.e., that which faces the median axis of the hand). The author's unit, unlike others, does not use reversed vein grafts if there is an area of occlusion; occasionally, a small arteriotomy has been necessary to remove a large intra-arterial thrombus.

The tourniquet is released before closure and any bleeding points secured with bipolar diathermy. Attention should be paid to the viability of the skin flaps and to the time taken for the fingers to revascularize. The wound is closed with non-absorbable sutures to the skin only, and a light non-compressive dressing is applied. Postoperatively, the hand is kept warm and not elevated. The dressing is reduced the following day and the sutures removed at 10 days.

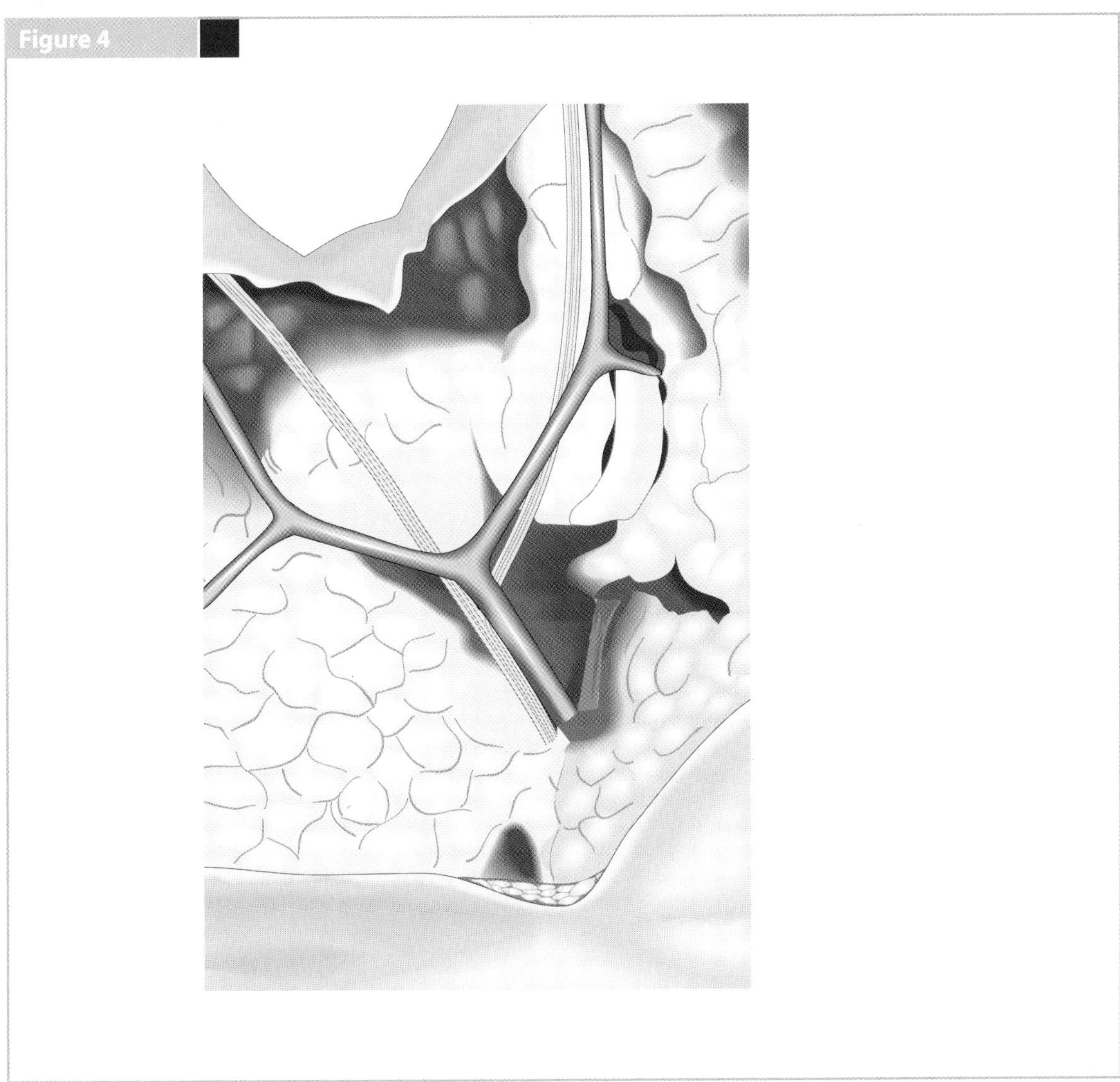

Figure 4

CONCLUSION

Over the past 14 years, the author's unit has carried out digital sympathectomies on over 200 patients with over 700 affected digits. The main experience has been of operating on the hand, predominantly the index and middle fingers. The thumb and ulnar two fingers are less commonly affected. The major indications for surgery have been for chronic ulceration refractory to conservative measures, unremitting fingertip pain, dramatically symptomatic Raynaud' s phenomenon and as a prelude to surgery for fusion of the proximal interphalangeal joints.

The procedure has achieved widespread patient satisfaction and has been shown to be effective for healing digital ulcers (after 25 years in one case), pain relief, cold intolerance and reducing the frequency, but not necessarily the severity, of symptoms of Raynaud's phenomenon. Results at 10 years are encouraging with no major complications and a low rate of recurrent ulceration (5% at 5 years). Similar results have been reported from other centers.

REFERENCES

Balogh B, Mayer W, Vesely M, Mayer S, Partsch H, Piza-Katzer H (2002) Adventitial stripping of the radial and ulnar arteries in Raynaud's disease. J Hand Surg (Am) 2002 Nov;27(6):1073-80

Bogoch ER, Gross DK (2005) Surgery of the hand in patients with systemic sclerosis: outcomes and considerations. J Rheumatol. 2005 Apr; 32(4):642-8

Egloff DV, Mifsud RF, Verdan D (1983) Superselective digital sympathectomy in Raynaud's phenomenon. Hand 15:110–114

Flatt A (1980) Digital artery sympathectomy. J Hand Surg [Am]. 5(6):550–556

Jones NF, Imbriglia JE, Steen VD, Medsger TA (1987) Surgery for scleroderma of the hand. J Hand Surg (Am) May; 12(3):391-400.

Melone CP, Beldner S, Polatsch DB, Thomas AD (2004) Digital sympathectomy for Raynaud's syndrome in limited systemic sclerosis (crest syndrome). Podium presentation American Society of Surgery of the Hand, Sept 2004

O'Brien BM, Kumar PA, Mellow CO, Oliver TV (1992) Radical microarteriolysis in the treatment of vasospastic disorders of the hand. J Hand Surg 17B:447—452

Ruch DS, Holden M, Smith BP, Smith TL, Koman LA (2002) Periarterial sympathectomy in scleroderma patients: intermediate-term follow-up. J Hand Surg [Am]. 2002 Mar; 27(2):258-64.

Stratton R, Howell K, Goddard NJ, Black C (1997) Digital sympathectomy for ischaemia in scleroderma. Br J Rheumatol 36:1338–1339

Wilgis EFS (1981) Evaluation and treatment of chronic digital ischaemia. Ann Surg 193:693–696

CHAPTER 12

Thoracoscopic Cervical Sympathectomy

Alun H. Davies

INTRODUCTION

Hyperhidrosis is a disabling condition, often affecting the young, with profound effects on their employment, social lifestyle and quality of life. Excessive sweating has been estimated to affect between 0.6% and 1% of the population (Adar et al. 1977). At present, non-surgical management options give unpredictable results. Laparoscopic cervical sympathectomy is a proven alternative, without the significant morbidity associated with traditional open surgical techniques.

Patient selection includes those in whom sweating is severe enough to interfere significantly with their occupation or enjoyment of life. Quantification and descriptive qualitation of this disease is difficult. Several scales include the use of a perspirator, blot test or hyperhidrosis scoring system, combining values for dampness, quality of life and blot test in three grades (Krasna et al. 1998).

The approaches to the sympathetic chain have been described as supra clavicular, axillary or posterior using open techniques. However, the advent of endoscopic surgery has largely superseded these procedures.

Patients require preoperative chest X-ray, thyroid function tests and examination to exclude a systemic disease causing excessive sweating. Those with more generalized hyperhidrosis attributable to another cause and those with pleural adhesions should be excluded.

SYMPATHETIC NERVOUS SYSTEM

Each of the 31 pairs of spinal nerves are formed within the intervertebral foramen by the union of the anterior and posterior roots. The nerve divides quickly into an anterior and posterior ramus, contributing to the great nerve plexuses and body wall innervation. Preganglionic sympathetic fibers leave the lateral column of the spinal cord and pass in all the thoracic and upper two lumbar spinal nerves to the sympathetic chain. These myelinated fibers (white rami communicans) synapse in the chain.

Unmyelinated postganglionic sympathetic fibers to the arm leave the chain to pass with the second and third thoracic nerves, only leaving the nerve at the distal target. The fibers are vasoconstrictor, pilomotor and sudomotor.

The cervical part of the sympathetic trunk receives sympathetic fibers from the first thoracic nerve; it lies within the deep fascia between the carotid sheath and the prevertebral layer of deep fascia. The superior cervical ganglion lies opposite the second and third cervical transverse processes and behind the angle of the mandible. The middle cervical ganglion lies at the level of the cricoid cartilage and the inferior ganglion opposite the seventh cervical vertebra. The inferior ganglion frequently combines with the first thoracic ganglion to form the stellate ganglion on the neck of the first rib.

Figure 1: Operation

Both sides of the chest can be operated on under the same anesthetic. The procedure is performed with the patient under general anesthesia using one lung ventilation by means of a double lumen endobronchial tube. The patient is placed supine with both arms abducted to 60° and supported on arm boards. Incisions are planned for the fourth intercostal space midaxillary line and second intercostal space midclavicular line.

Blunt dissection is used to introduce a size 10-mm thoracoscope through the formed skin incision. A 5-mm cannula is placed under direct vision through the second intercostal space in the midclavicular line. An insulated monopolar diathermy electrode is introduced though this port.

Figure 1 shows an intubated patient, skin marks and the hand of the surgeon with thoracoscope.

Figure 2

The thoracoscope provides an excellent view of the sympathetic chain. The second rib is the highest rib visible. The sympathetic chain may be identified by following the ribs medially until it appears in view overlying the neck of the ribs lying deep to the pleura. Gentle inspection with the diathermy probe confirms its soft consistency. In operations on the right side of the chest, the superior vena cava, azygos vein and vagus nerve can be identified. On the left side the subclavian artery and vagus nerve can be seen medially.

The pleura overlying the sympathetic chain is identified and excised using the diathermy probe.

The second and third thoracic ganglia and intervening trunk are resected. The first thoracic ganglia is not excised as preganglionic sympathetic fibers supplying the upper limb originate from T1 in only 10% of people. Removal of this ganglion results in a Horner's syndrome.

In the resection of the ganglia the diathermy current is applied laterally for 2 cm along the neck of the second and third ribs in order to ablate the nerve of Kuntz (1927). Alternative methods using a single thoracoscope inserted on the fourth intercostal space in the midaxillary line, with a resectoscope with a single side channel for a diathermy hook, have been described.

The diathermy probe and cannula are removed under direct vision and the lung reinflated. If there is no residual pneumothorax the thoracoscope and cannula are removed and the wounds sutured. A chest drain is not necessary.

A postoperative chest X-ray should be performed to confirm lung inflation.

Figure 1

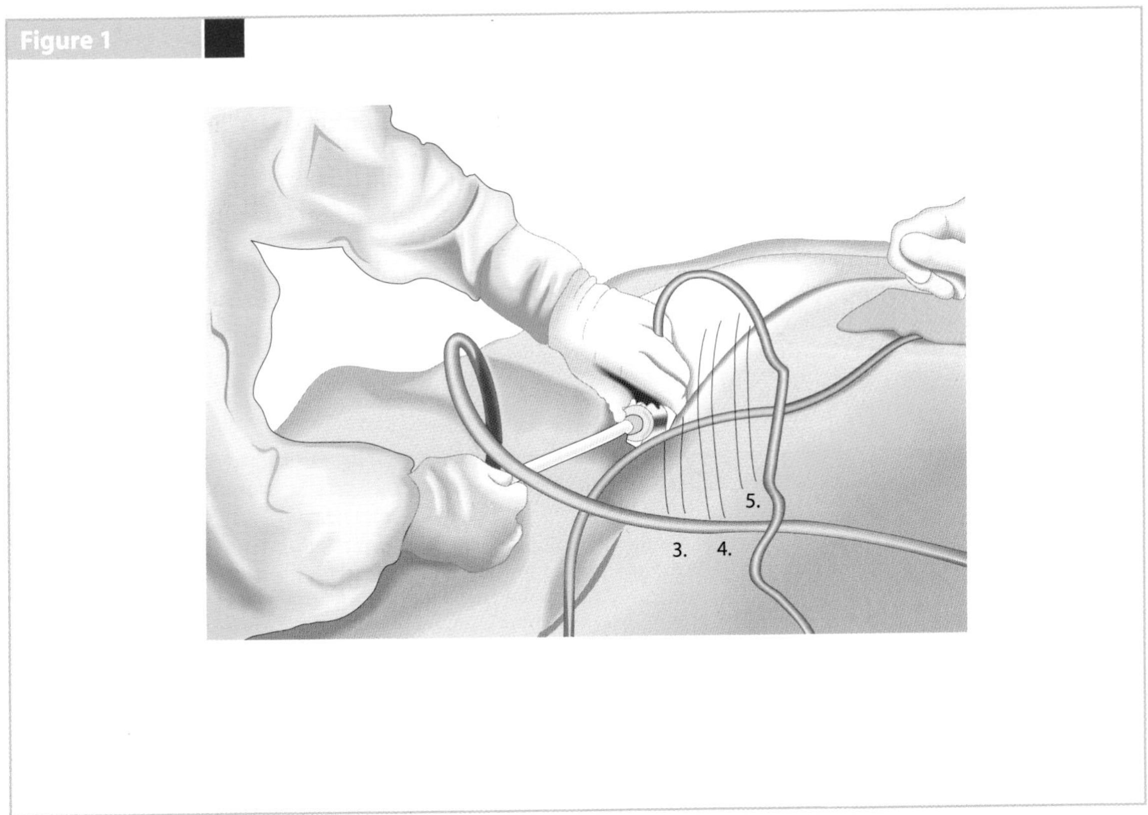

Figure 2

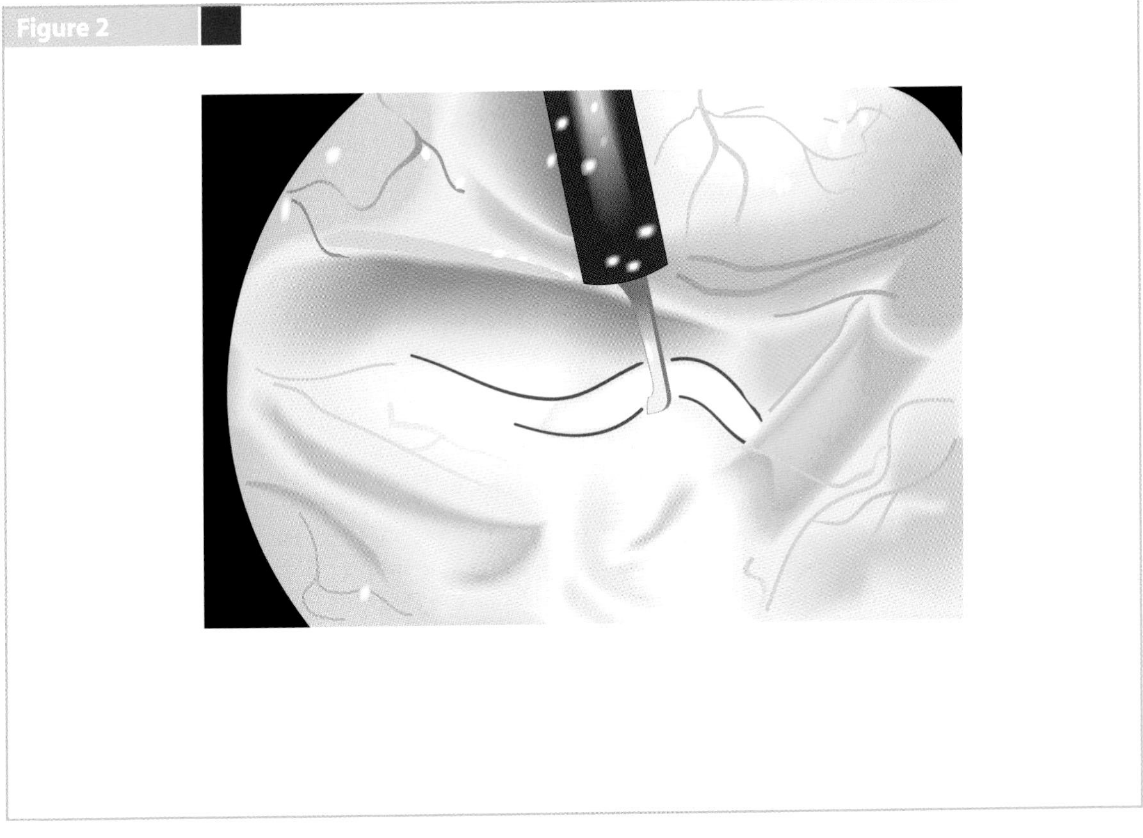

CONCLUSION

Laparoscopic cervical sympathectomy has become a well established technique. A review of the literature describing cervical sympathectomy has reported success rates of over 90% (Gordon et al. 1994). However, complications do occur and it is important that these are explained to the patient whilst obtaining written informed consent prior to the procedure.

Horner's syndrome has been variously reported to occur in 0.01–3% of cases (Gordon et al. 1994). Using a low diathermy current and dissection only below the second rib may help to avoid this complication. Compensatory hyperhidrosis affecting the axilla, face or body and gustatory sweating may be seen after both open or thoracoscopic surgery, and occurs in up to 50% of patients (Rennie 1996). A small pneumothorax may persist for 24 h postoperatively and pleuritic chest pain is common.

REFERENCES

Adar R, Kurchin A, Zweig A, Moses M (1977) Palmar hyperhidrosis and its surgical treatment: a report of 100 cases. Ann Surg 186:34–41

Gordon A, Zechmeister K, Collin J (1994) The role of sympathectomy in current surgical practice. Eur J Vasc Surg 8:129–137

Krasna MJ, Demmy TL, McKenna RJ, Mack MJ (1998) Thoracoscopic sympathectomy: the US experience. Eur J Surg 580:19–21

Kuntz A (1927) Distribution of the sympathetic rami to the brachial plexus: its relation to sympathectomy affecting the upper extremity. Arch Surg 113:264

Rennie J (1996) Compensatory sweating: an avoidable complication of thoracoscopic sympathectomy? Minim Invasive Ther Allied Technol 5:101

CHAPTER 13

Lumbar Sympathectomy

John Lumley

INTRODUCTION

Denervation of the sympathetic vascular supply of the foot is achieved by excision of the lowest (4th lumbar) ganglion of the thoracolumbar sympathetic chain. The procedure is effective in the treatment of vasospastic disorders, such as chilblains, and may help the vasculitic manifestations of collagen diseases, such as scleroderma; it can be of value in frostbite. Its effect is primarily on the cutaneous blood supply, and although it helps vasculitic ulcers, its effect on the ulceration and rest pain of severe ischemia is less predictable. Nevertheless, a number of vascular units undertake phenol injection of the lumbar sympathetic chain, under radiological control, when other measures are not available.

The procedure is equally effective in stopping foot sweating, as cervical sympathectomy is in the hand, but this problem is usually less troublesome, and bilateral lumbar sympathetic denervation can interfere with ejaculation; the risk of producing retrograde ejaculation must always be considered in male patients. Denervation of the upper and lower limbs can also increase trunk sweating to a troublesome level.

Sympathectomy does not influence muscle blood flow and theoretically could divert the muscle blood supply to the skin. It is therefore not effective in the treatment of claudication. It does have a marked initial effect on the blood flow after lower limb reconstruction; this effect, however, reduces within a few hours, and long-term results are not available to support routine use in these procedures.

Diabetic patients have usually undergone an autosympathectomy by the time they develop lower limb vascular problems; the procedure is thus of little value.

The operation of lumbar sympathectomy is undertaken with the patient under general anesthesia, with tracheal intubation, to allow relaxation of the anterior abdominal wall musculature. The patient is placed supine, with their arms strapped across the chest. A 20% raise of the ipsilateral pelvis with a sandbag improves access; in bilateral procedures, this position is achieved by tilting the operating table to each side in turn.

Figure 1

Skin preparation extends from the nipples to the pubis and to the posterior axillary line bilaterally, or across the midline in unilateral procedures. A double layer of rectangular towels is held in position by a Steridrape around the prepared area (Fig. 1). The abdominal wall incision is the same on both sides. The skin is incised along the middle third of a line joining the tip of the 12th rib to the umbilicus; it is extended through the fat and layers of superficial fascia to the external oblique muscle, exposure including the lateral aspect of the rectus sheath.

The three abdominal wall muscles are split in the line of their fibers, centered over the mid-incision. This gridiron approach provides sufficient exposure of the sympathetic chain, without the need to divide any muscle fibers. Inserting and opening the points of a pair of scissors starts the separation of the muscle fibers; it is extended digitally or by pulling on a pair of retractors. The split may extend into the edge of the rectus sheath, and should aim to preserve the nerves supplying the abdominal wall.

The transversalis fascia beneath the abdominal wall muscles, and overlying the extraperitoneal fat and peritoneum, is thinnest posteriorly. Digital pressure is applied at this site to enter the extraperitoneal space, rather than more anteriorly, where the peritoneum may be torn, the peritoneal contents subsequently interfering with the operative exposure. Once the extraperitoneal space has been entered, the peritoneum and ureter are lifted forward, the hand passing around the posterior abdominal wall. The lateral edge of the psoas muscle is reached, and the manual dissection advances anterior to psoas to the vertebral bodies. The fourth or fifth vertebral body is first felt and, by palpating distally, the lower medial border of the psoas and the promontory of the sacrum are useful in identifying the body of the fifth lumbar vertebra, which is where the target ganglion is situated. At this stage the exposure is helped by the insertion of two deep abdominal retractors; subsequent dissection differs on the two sides.

Figure 2

On the right side, the first deep square retractor is used to expose the inferior vena cava. The blade is placed under the peritoneum and the right ureter, and the end is passed medially onto the fifth lumbar vertebral body. The second retractor is placed on the cranial side of the wound, at right angles to the first, and is used to retract the kidney and perinephric fat cranially; the two retractors lie against each other and this helps exposure.

Medial retraction on the first retractor exposes the inferior vena cava; this is gently pulled to the opposite side, to expose the fat filled angle, between the cava and vertebra, containing the sympathetic chain. The chain is first palpated by rolling it against the vertebra, a nerve hook is then used to gently lift it, and it is freed from adherent fat and lymphatic tissue with a pair of scissors.

The sympathetic chain expands into the fourth lumbar ganglion. The rami communicantes, and a 2.5-cm length of the chain containing the ganglion, are excised, thus denervating the foot. A transverse diathermy cut is made across the side of the vertebra, taking care not to damage the cava; this removes any additional descending autonomic fibers.

Figure 2 shows the two retractors that have been inserted; the one on the left of the picture is retracting the kidney and perinephric fat. The retractor in the upper part of the picture is retracting the peritoneum and the ureter and will later be inserted deeper to retract the inferior vena cava from the operating field. The plane between the inferior vena cava and the psoas muscle is being gently dissected to separate lymphatic and fatty tissue from the underlying sympathetic chain.

Figure 1

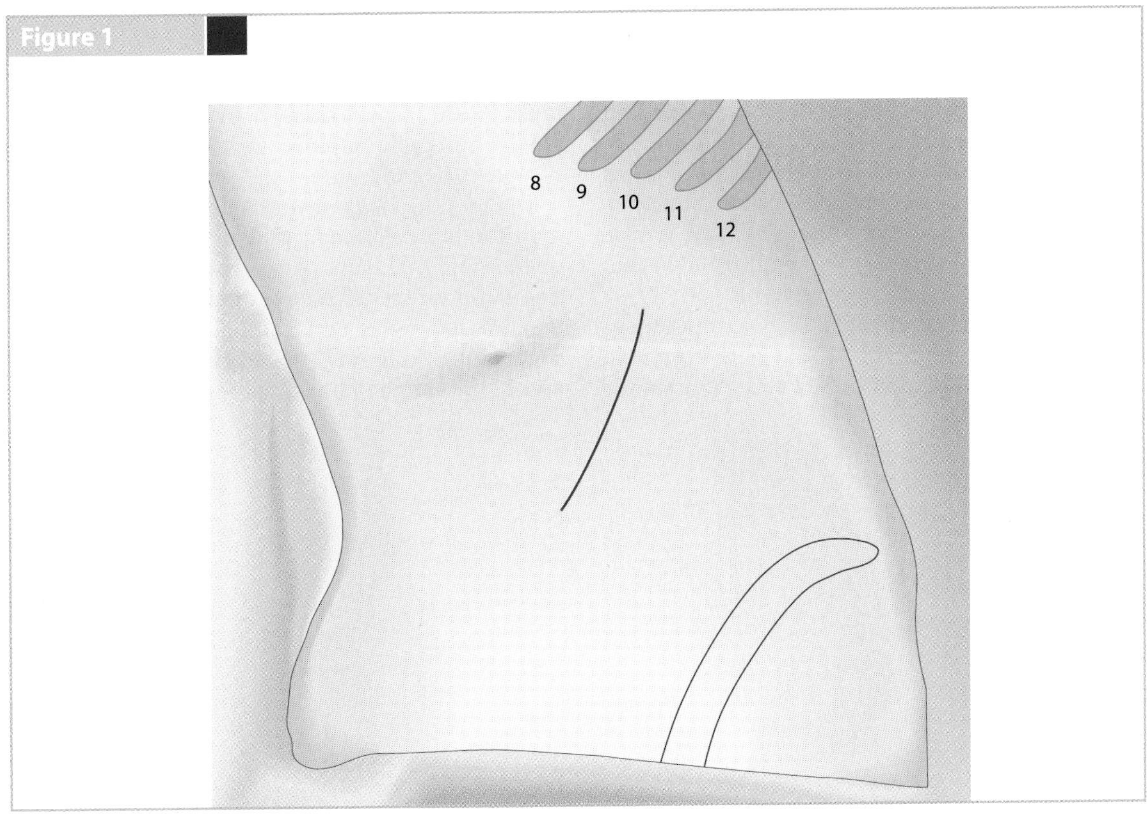

Figure 2

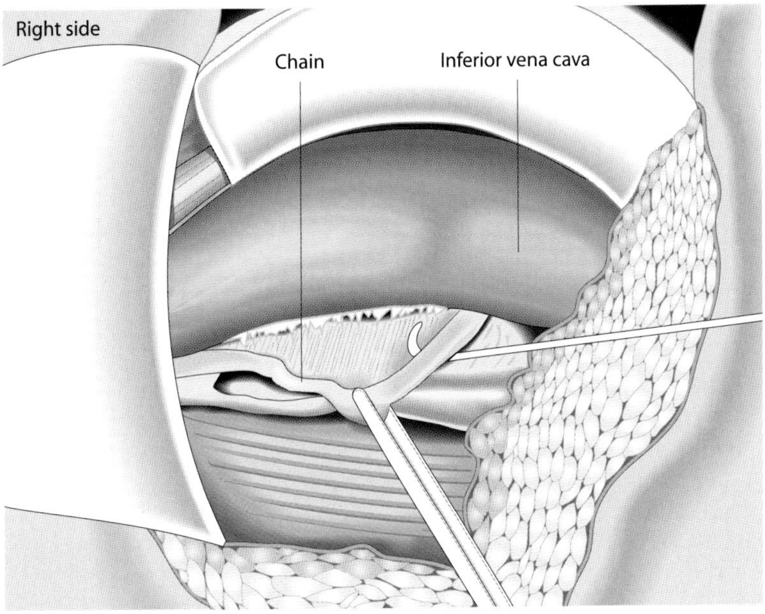

Right side
Chain
Inferior vena cava

Figure 3

Left lumbar sympathectomy follows the same steps described for the right. The first retractor, in this case, pulls the aorta and left common iliac artery medially. The chain may not be as distinct on the left, and if this is so on either side, particular care is taken to diathermy across the vertebral body from the midline to the medial fibers of the psoas muscle.

Hemostasis is essential in the retroperitoneal space; lumbar or other vessels may have been damaged, and must be diathermied. The abdominal wall muscles are reapproximated with a few lightly applied absorbable sutures; facial and skin closure complete the procedure.

In Fig. 3 the sympathetic chain and its rami communicantes have been identified; the latter have been divided and the chains being raised on a nerve hook. The chain on the left side is often less discrete than that on the right, and additional fibers must be sought and diathermy used to clear the anterior aspect of the vertebral body, as previously described.

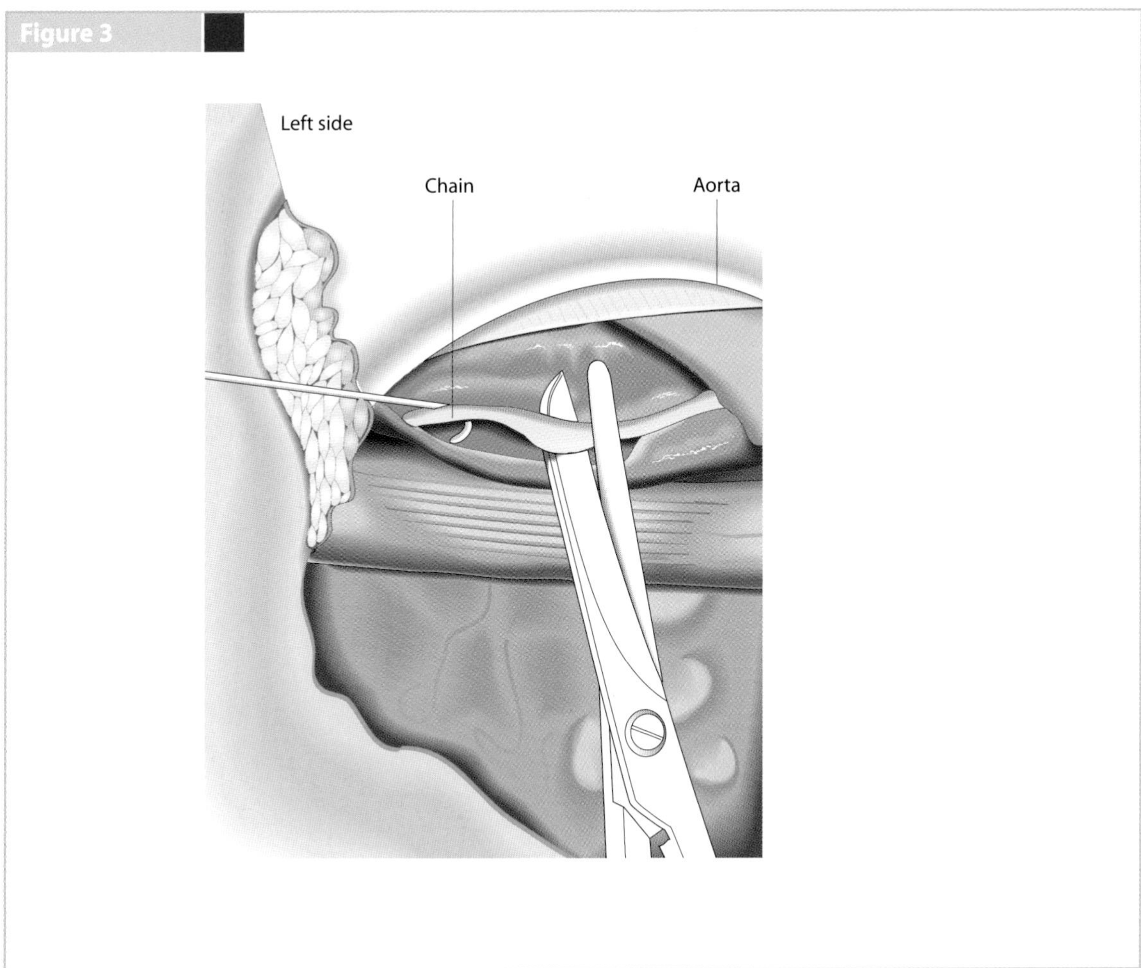
Figure 3
Left side
Chain
Aorta

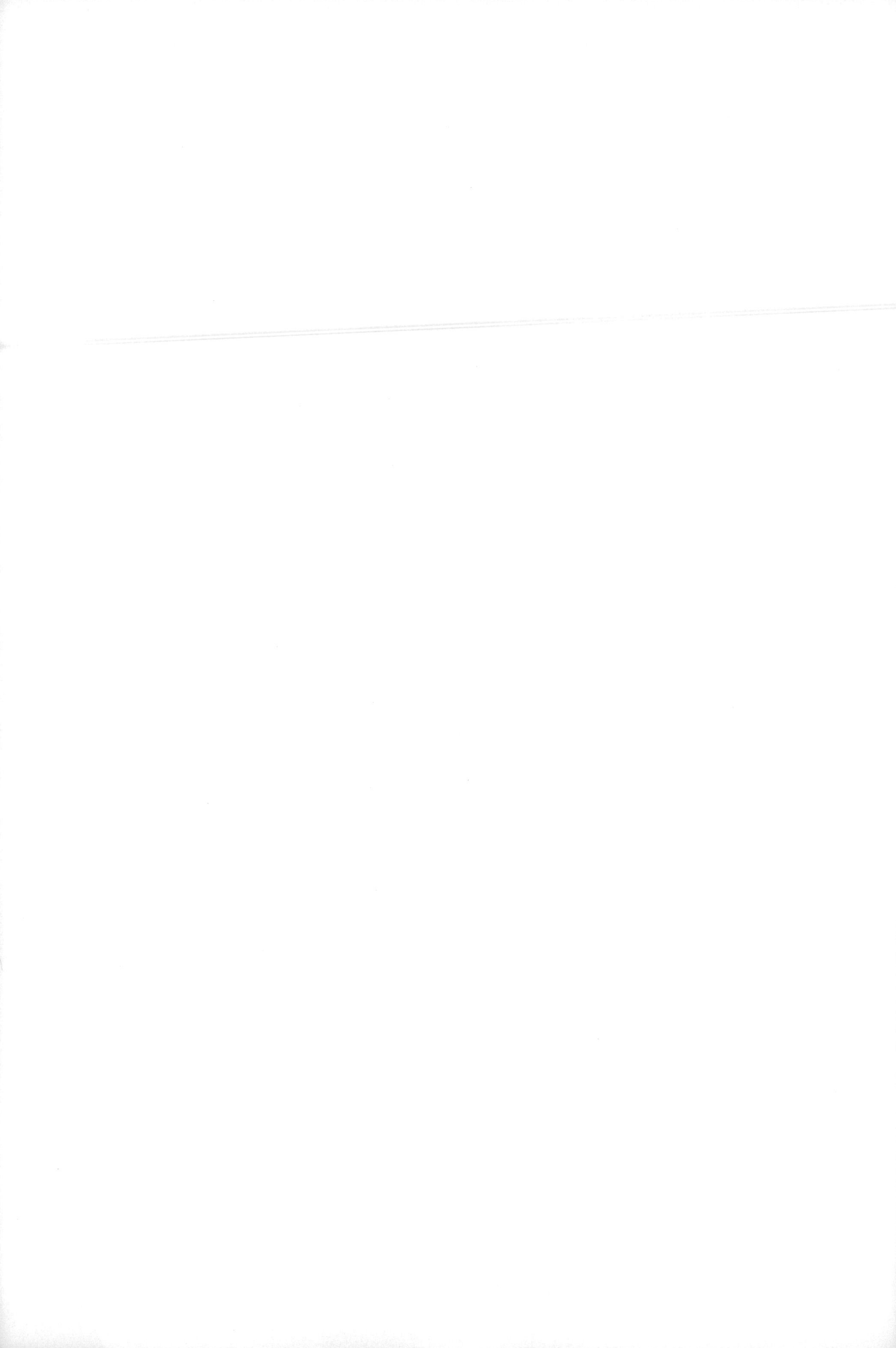

Part III Thoracic Aneurysms

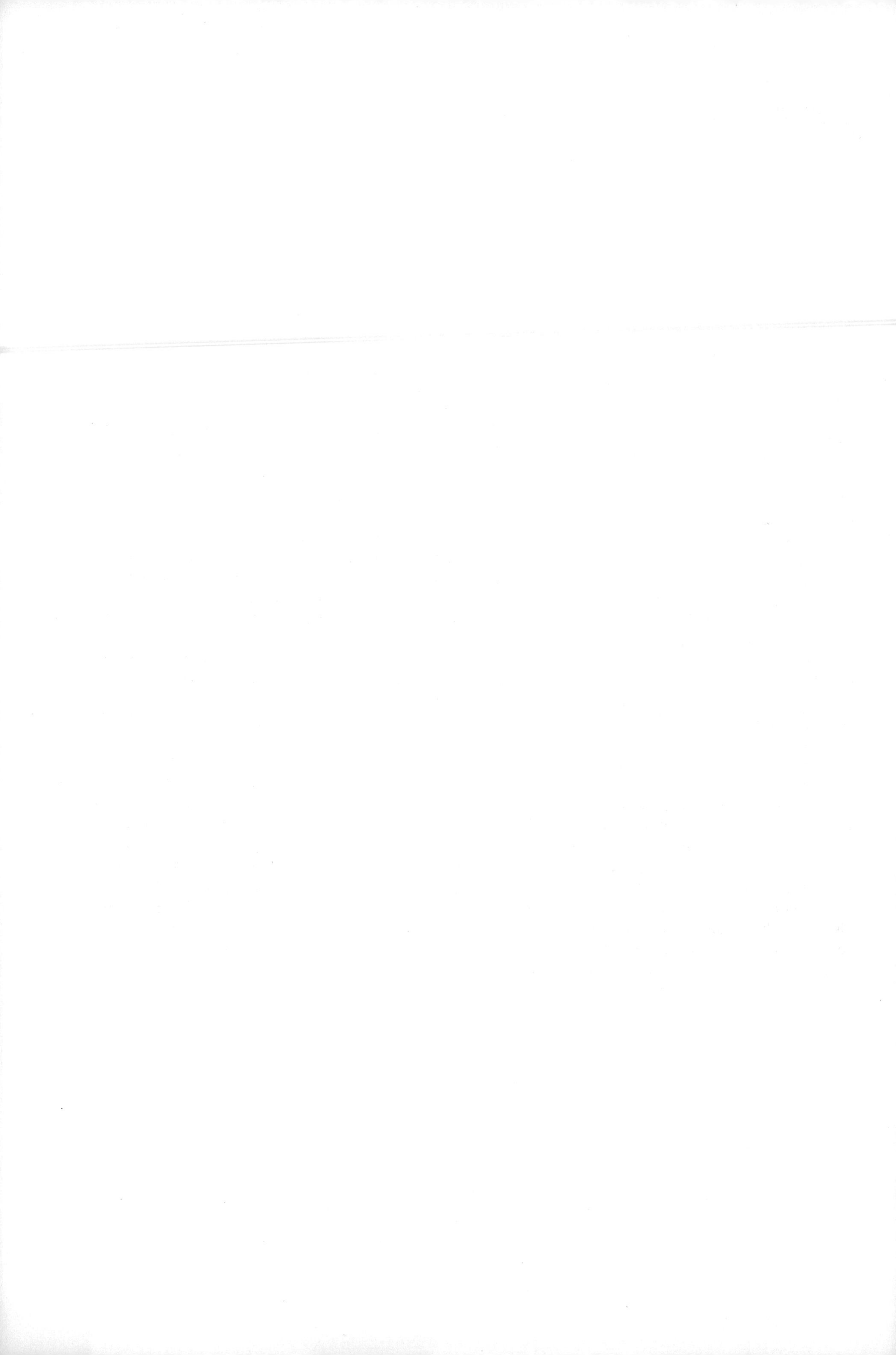

CHAPTER 14

Repair of Thoracoabdominal Aortic Aneurysms

Hazim J. Safi, Anthony L. Estrera

INTRODUCTION

In the United States as the aging population grows the incidence of thoracoabdominal aortic aneurysms (TAA) has gradually increased. The mean age of TAA patients is between 59 and 69 years with a male predominance, although the incidence of TAA in women has grown in recent years. Left untreated, the survival rate for patients with thoracic aortic aneurysms is dismal, estimated to be between 13% and 39% at 5 years. The most common cause of death in the untreated aneurysm patient is aortic rupture, the probability of which is between 75% and 80%. Moreover, patients who survive rupture to operation sustain significant morbidity, prolonged hospital course and, ultimately, a poor quality of life.

The decision to intervene surgically is generally based on the size of the aneurysm, the rate of aneurysm growth and patient symptoms. Aneurysm symptoms may include back pain, although it is difficult to differentiate between musculoskeletal problems and acute aneurysm expansion or rupture. Pressure on adjacent organs such as the recurrent laryngeal or vagus nerves can produce vocal cord paralysis or hoarseness; on the pulmonary artery, a fistula or bleeding leading to pulmonary hypertension and edema; on the esophagus, dysphagia; and on the tracheobronchial tree, dyspnea. Because about 5% of thoracoabdominal aortic aneurysm patients also have atherosclerotic occlusive disease of the visceral and renal arteries, there may be frank intestinal angina or renovascular hypertension. A new outbreak of pain in a patient with detected aneurysm is highly significant and may indicate rapid expansion, leakage, or impending rupture.

The diagnostic modalities for TAA characterization include computed tomography (CT), magnetic resonance angiography (MRA), contrast aortography, and transesophageal echocardiography (TEE). Computed tomography remains the first choice for initial screening and follow-up. Aortography is used selectively, for example, in cases of pseudoaneurysm, reoperative aortic surgery or renovascular hypertension. TEE is limited to the descending thoracic aorta, but may identify significant atheromatous plaquing as well as acute or chronic dissection.

Since 1991, for all patients undergoing elective repair of either descending thoracic or TAA aneurysms, we have utilized the combined adjuncts of distal aortic perfusion and cerebrospinal fluid (CSF) drainage. We believe that this combination provides significant spinal cord protection. Cross-clamping of the descending thoracic aorta results in both a decreased distal mean arterial pressure and increased cerebrospinal fluid pressure, which may lead to a significant reduction in spinal cord perfusion pressure. By draining the excess cerebrospinal fluid, CSF pressure is reduced, augmenting perfusion to the spinal cord. At the same time, distal aortic perfusion increases the distal aortic pressure and increases perfusion pressure to the spinal cord.

Figure 1

The patient is intubated using a left-sided double lumen endotracheal tube. Hemodynamics are monitored using an arterial blood pressure line (placed in the right radial artery) and a pulmonary artery catheter. Transesophageal echocardiography monitors cardiac function and aortic pathology. Spinal cord protection is imperative, and critical to our strategy are the adjuncts CSF drainage and distal aortic perfusion. A CSF catheter placed in the 3rd or 4th lumbar space provides CSF drainage and monitoring of CSF pressure. The CSF pressure is maintained at less than 10 mmHg throughout the procedure. In addition, electrodes attached to the scalp for electroencephalograms (EEG) and along the spinal cord for measurement of somatosensory evoked potential (SSEP) assess brain function and spinal cord status throughout the case. After insertion of the CSF drain and anesthetic preparation, the patient is positioned in the right lateral decubitus position with the hip flexed 45° for accessibility of the left and right groins. The chest, abdomen, and groins are sterilely prepared. Figure 1 shows the anesthetic preparation, cerebrospinal fluid catheter insertion, and patient positions.

Figure 2

The incision is tailored to complement the extent of the aneurysm. A modified thoracoabdominal incision is used for aneurysms that extend only to above the celiac axis (Safi 1999). A full thoracoabdominal incision begins inferiorly above the symphysis pubis, goes midline to the umbilicus, curves into the costal cartilage and the bed of the 6th rib, and is then extended between the scapula and the vertebral column.

The skin and subcutaneous tissues, and the latissimus and serratus muscles, are divided and the sixth rib identified. The sixth rib is removed for all cases except extent IV TAA (from the diaphragm to the aortic bifurcation). The resected rib space allows intraoperative identification of the dimension of the aneurysm, i.e., classification and the intercostal artery location. The left lung is collapsed. A self-retaining retractor fully exposes the aneurysm. Taking care to avoid injury to the phrenic nerve, the aortic hiatus and the crus of the diaphragm are cut for passage of the aortic graft. In dividing the diaphragm, only a small part of the muscular portion is divided. We have found that preserving the diaphragm lowers the incidence of pulmonary complications and shortens the length of stay.

For abdominal exposure, a plane in the retroperitoneal space is developed and the viscera rotated medially. Care is taken to avoid injuring the spleen. The renal artery is identified and the kidney exposed for insertion of a temperature probe if renal cooling is required.

The pump circuit for distal aortic perfusion involves a BioMedicus centrifugal pump (Minneapolis, MN) with an in-line heat exchanger and reservoir attached to perfusion tubing that can also be used for active visceral perfusion. After complete exposure, the pericardium is opened posterior to the phrenic nerve to expose the left atrium for distal aortic perfusion outflow. The left atrium can be cannulated via the left inferior pulmonary vein or the left atrial appendage. We prefer opening the pericardium at the level of the pulmonary veins for easier identification and to confirm accurate placement of the cannula. Opening the pericardium also prevents postoperative pericardial tamponade in the case of cannulation site leakage.

Distal aortic perfusion inflow is established by cannulating the left common femoral artery. If the left common femoral artery is severely calcified and cannot be cannulated, we use the descending thoracic aorta [for descending thoracic aneurysms or (extent I) TAA] or the infrarenal aorta [TAA (extents II, III, IV or V)]. Prior to initiation of distal aortic perfusion, the patient is systemically anticoagulated with sodium heparin at a dose of 1 mg/kg body weight.

Figure 2 shows the initial skin incision. This is deepened through the superficial muscles, enabling the ribs to be counted under the scapula.

Figure 1

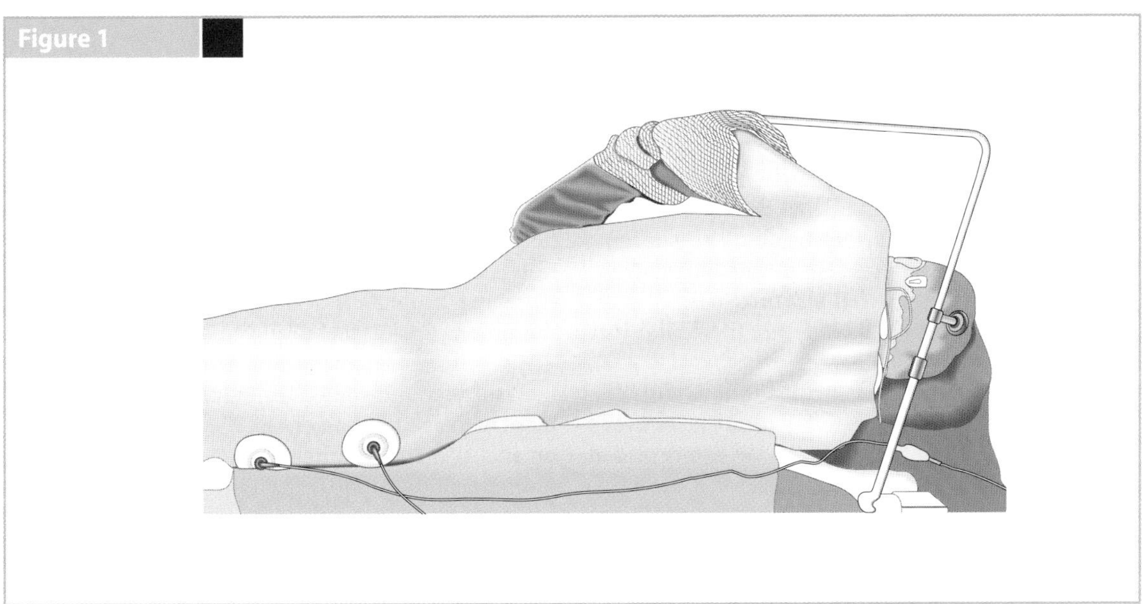

Figure 2

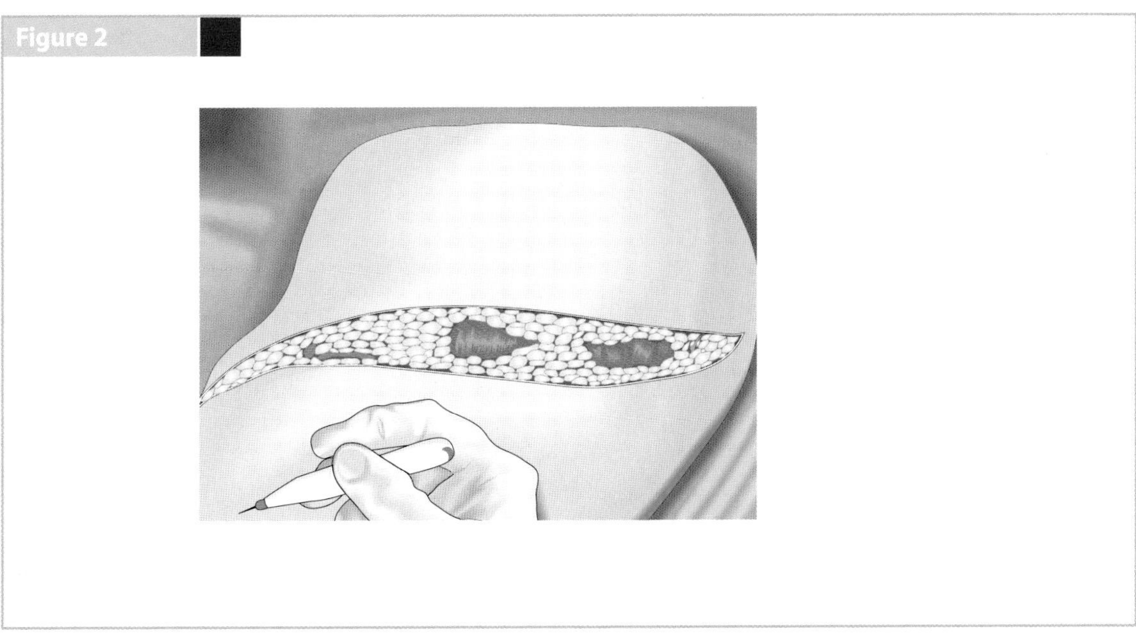

Figures 3, 4

The deflated lung is retracted medially, exposing the distal aortic arch and descending thoracic aorta. Dissection begins in the aortopulmonary window on the surface of the aorta and is carried proximally to the level of the subclavian artery origin. The supreme intercostal vein is often present on the aorta at this level and is divided. The *ligamentum arteriosum* is identified and transected, taking care to avoid injury to the recurrent laryngeal nerve.

We use sequential clamping, beginning with dissection of the descending thoracic aorta between clamps applied distal to the subclavian artery and at the level of the 6th intercostal space. We use large clamps applied to heavy silk suture placed into the walls of the aneurysm for retraction and visualization. In general, we prefer to clamp distal to the subclavian artery origin since the subclavian artery and branches (e.g., left internal mammary artery, thyrocervical trunk, or thoracodorsal artery) may provide collateral circulation to the spinal cord. If the aneurysm involves the origin of the left subclavian artery, we clamp proximal to this point or, less commonly, utilize profound hypothermic circulatory arrest for the arch replacement.

The aorta is inspected from the inside and the neck of the aneurysm identified. Complete transection is performed with separation of the native aorta from the esophagus. Complete transection rather than the inclusion technique has decreased the incidence of aorto-esophageal fistula.

We prefer a woven Dacron graft for aortic replacement with graft diameter and length determined upon aneurysm inspection. We suture the graft in end-to-end fashion to the descending thoracic aorta, using a running 3-0 or 2-0 monofilament polypropylene suture. The anastomosis is checked for bleeding and reinforced with 3-0 pledgeted sutures, if necessary.

Figure 3 shows: opening the dissecting aneurysm. Figure 4 shows: trimmed dissection walls and start of the proximal anastomosis.

Figure 3

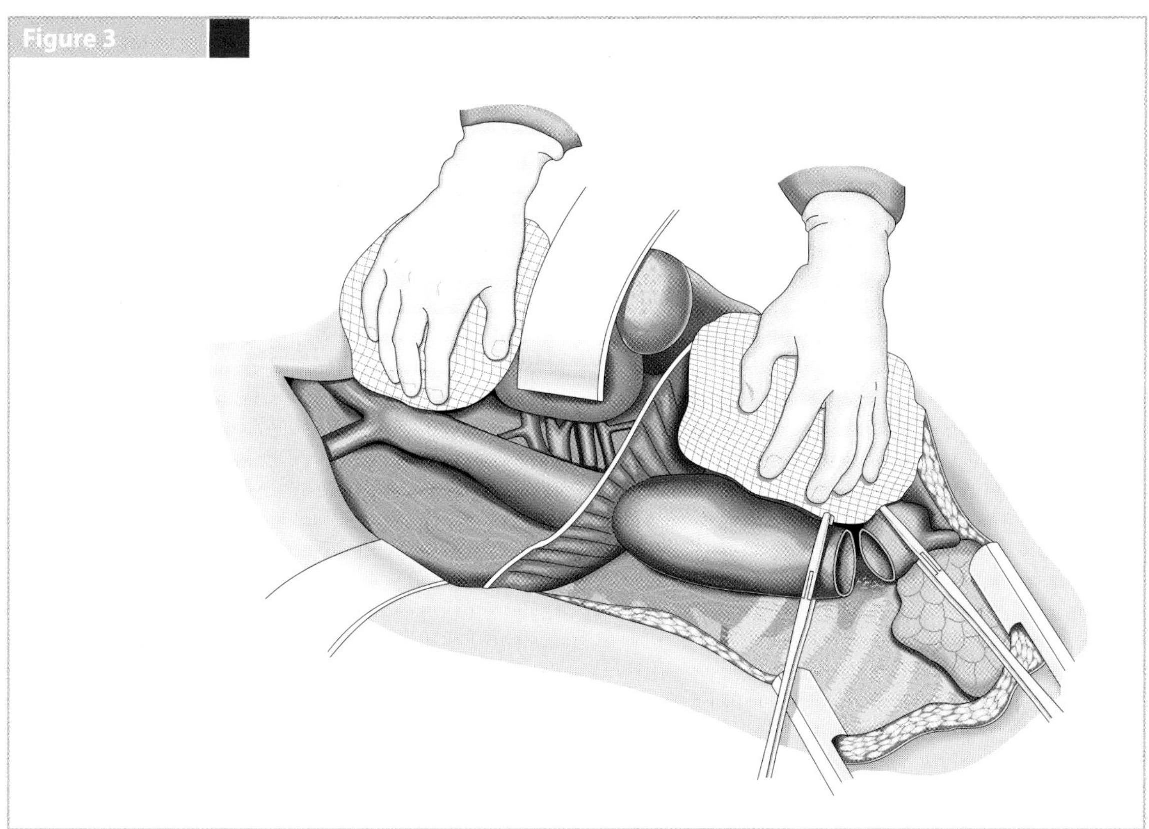

Figure 4

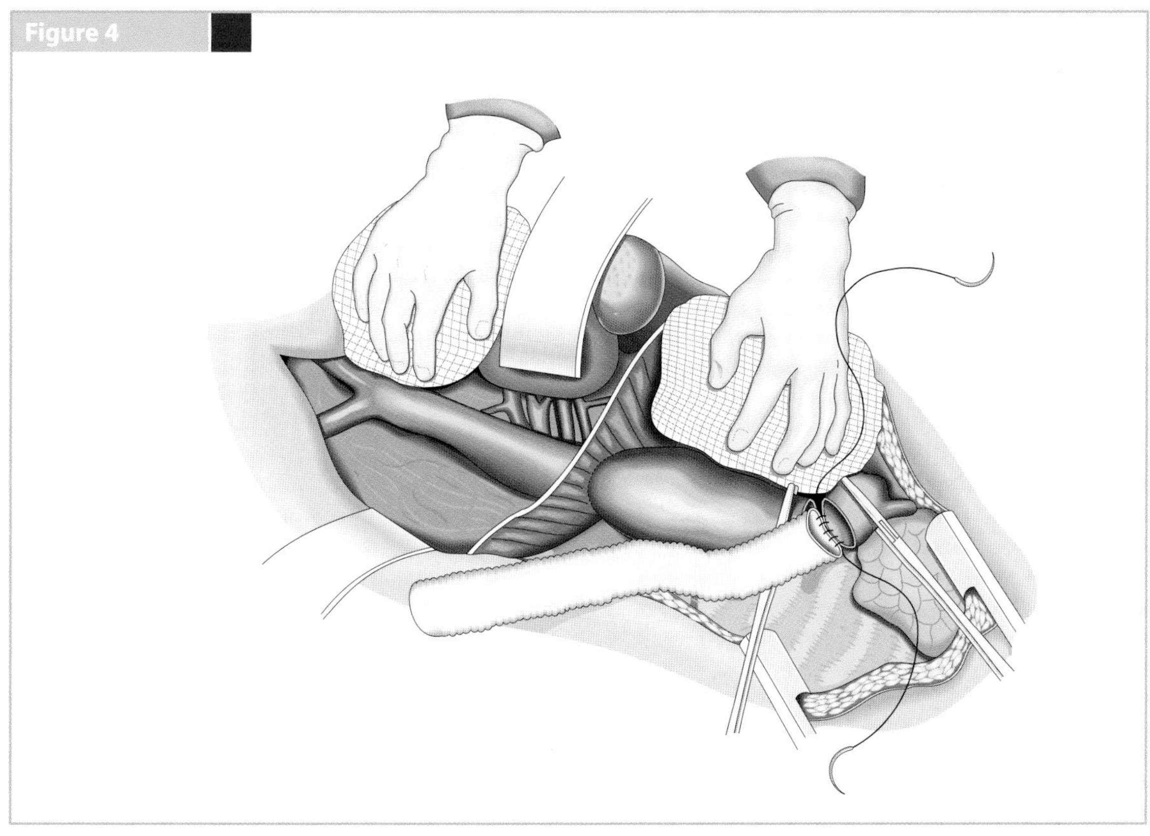

Figure 5: Intercostals

After completion of the proximal anastomosis, the separate aortic clamp is placed distally on the aorta above the celiac axis. The mid-descending thoracic aortic clamp is removed, and the distal descending thoracic aorta is opening longitudinally to the level of the diaphragm (T12). The intercostal arteries are inspected. Because we have found that intercostal artery reattachment enhances spinal cord protection, we reattach those that are patent between thoracic level eight (T8) to thoracic level twelve (T12). The determination of the intercostal artery patency is subjective, but generally arteries with high or low flow emanating from the orifice with dark or bright red blood are identified as patent. Patent arteries are then occluded temporarily with balloon catheters to decrease blood loss during reattachment.

The Dacron graft is stretched and a hole is cut in the graft to accommodate the intercostal arteries to be reattached as a patch island. This anastomosis is performed using either 2-0 or 3-0 polypropylene sutures. After completion of the intercostal artery reattachment, the proximal aortic clamp is released and placed distally onto the aortic graft beyond the level of the intercostal arteries. This re-establishes pulsatile flow to the intercostal arteries.

Figure 5 shows: matching of intercostal graft opening to aortic intercostal island prior to anastomosis.

Figure 6: Visceral arteries

14

After completion of the intercostal artery reattachment, attention is turned to the abdominal segment of the aorta. Distal aortic perfusion is briefly discontinued while the clamp is removed from the aorta at the level of the celiac axis, and placed onto the infrarenal aorta. Distal aortic perfusion is restarted. Figure 6 shows active visceral perfusion.

The abdominal aorta is opened longitudinally and the visceral vessels are inspected. The celiac, superior mesenteric, and renal arteries are perfused using #9 Pruitt catheters (Cryolife, St. Petersburg, FL). The amount of cold perfusate (blood at 4°C) delivered to the viscera depends on proximal aortic pressure and is maintained at between 300 and 600 ml/min. Renal temperature is directly monitored and kept at approximately 20°C. Since cold visceral perfusion can cause hypothermia, core body temperature is kept between 33 and 34°C by warming the lower circulation, i.e., lower extremities. If we cannot clamp the infrarenal abdominal aorta because of problems such as aortic calcification or an overly large aorta, distal circulatory warming cannot be performed and cold visceral perfusion is avoided, to prevent core body cooling that could result in cardiac dysrhythmias.

Figure 5

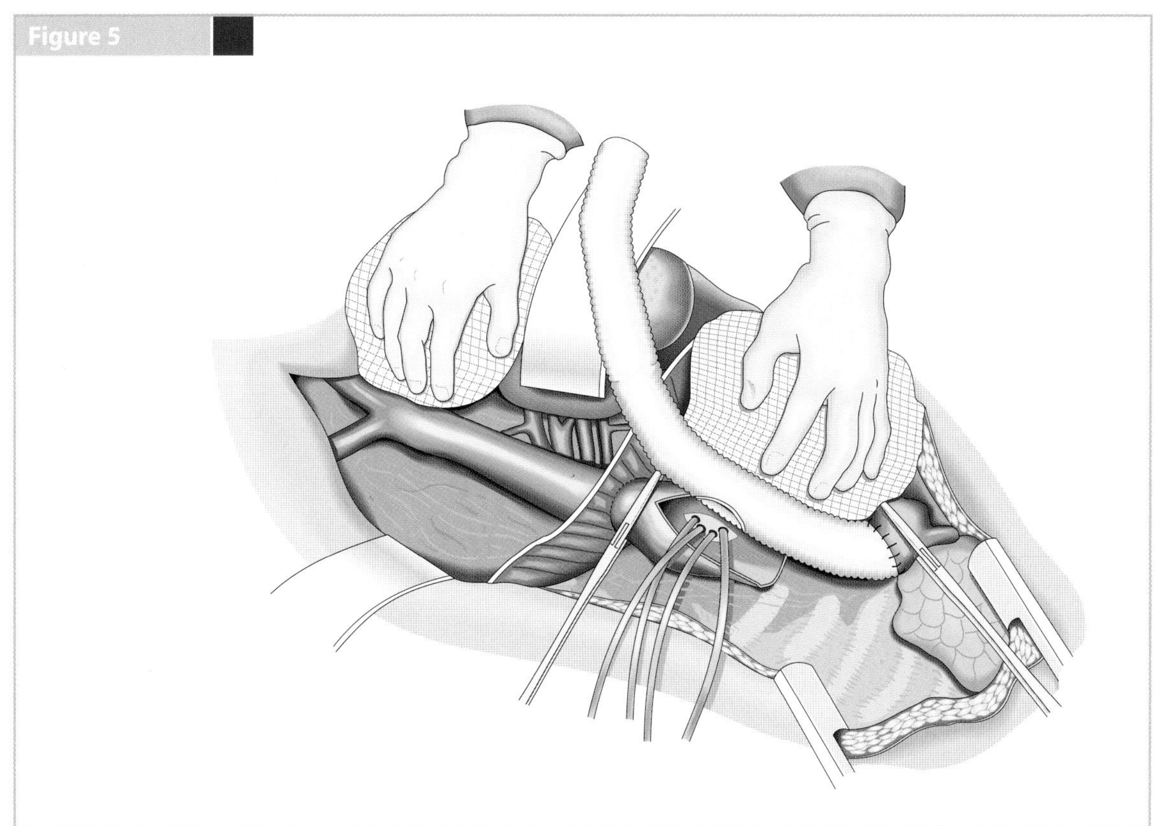

Figure 6

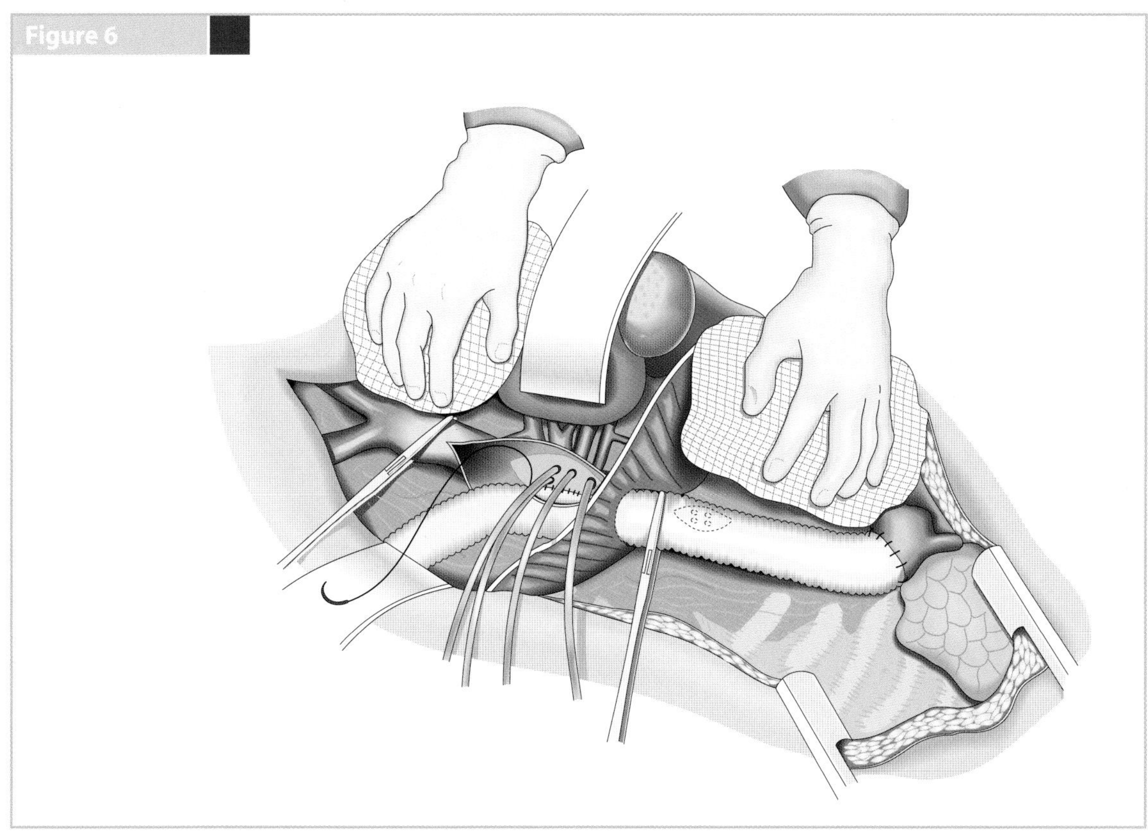

Figures 7, 8

After perfusing the viscera, the Dacron graft is tunneled through the aortic hiatus through the diaphragm. An elliptical cut is made in the graft opposite the celiac, superior mesenteric, and renal arteries for a visceral patch, using either 2-0 or 3-0 polypropylene sutures. Sometimes the left and right renal arteries are far apart, requiring separate interposition grafts for reattachment. Prior to completion of this anastomosis, the Pruitt catheters are removed. The proximal aortic clamp, distal to the intercostal artery reattachment, is then removed from the aortic graft and placed onto the graft distal to the visceral artery reattachment. This re-establishes pulsatile blood flow to the viscera. Figure 7 shows visceral perfusion and Fig. 8 shows the start of the graft.

Figure 7

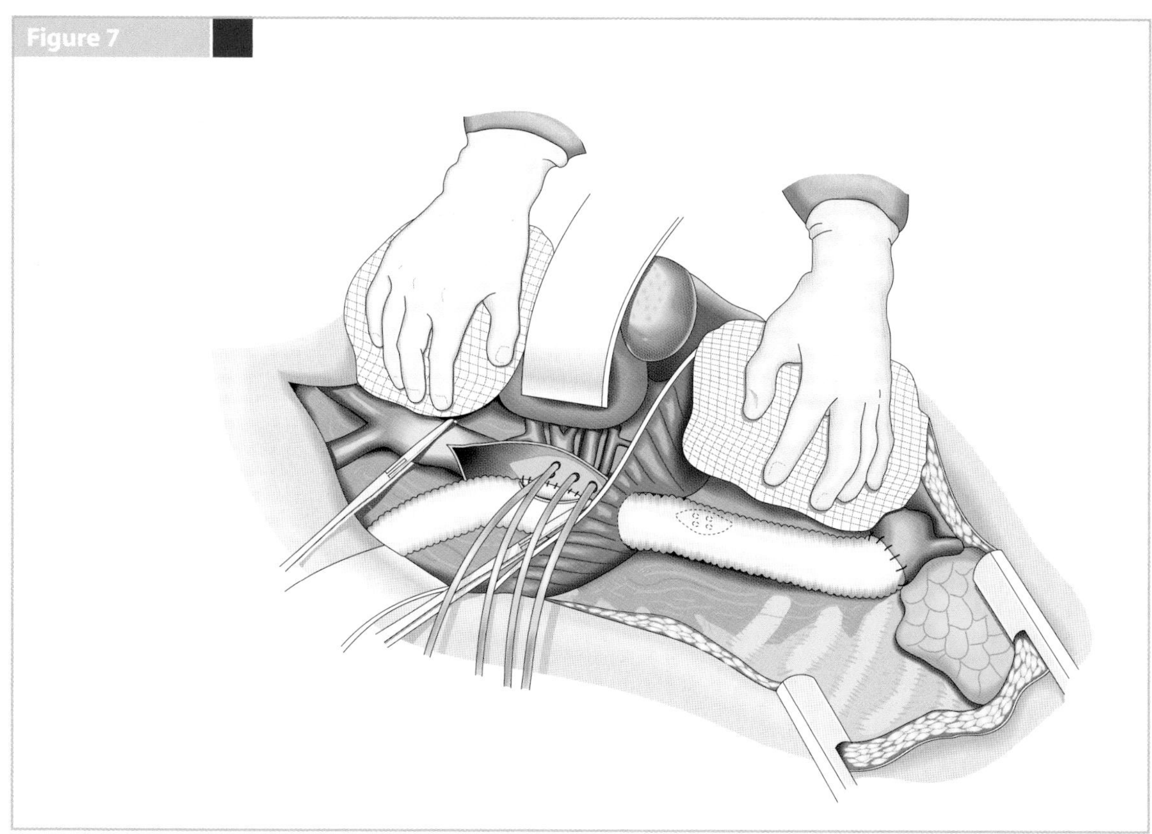

Figure 8

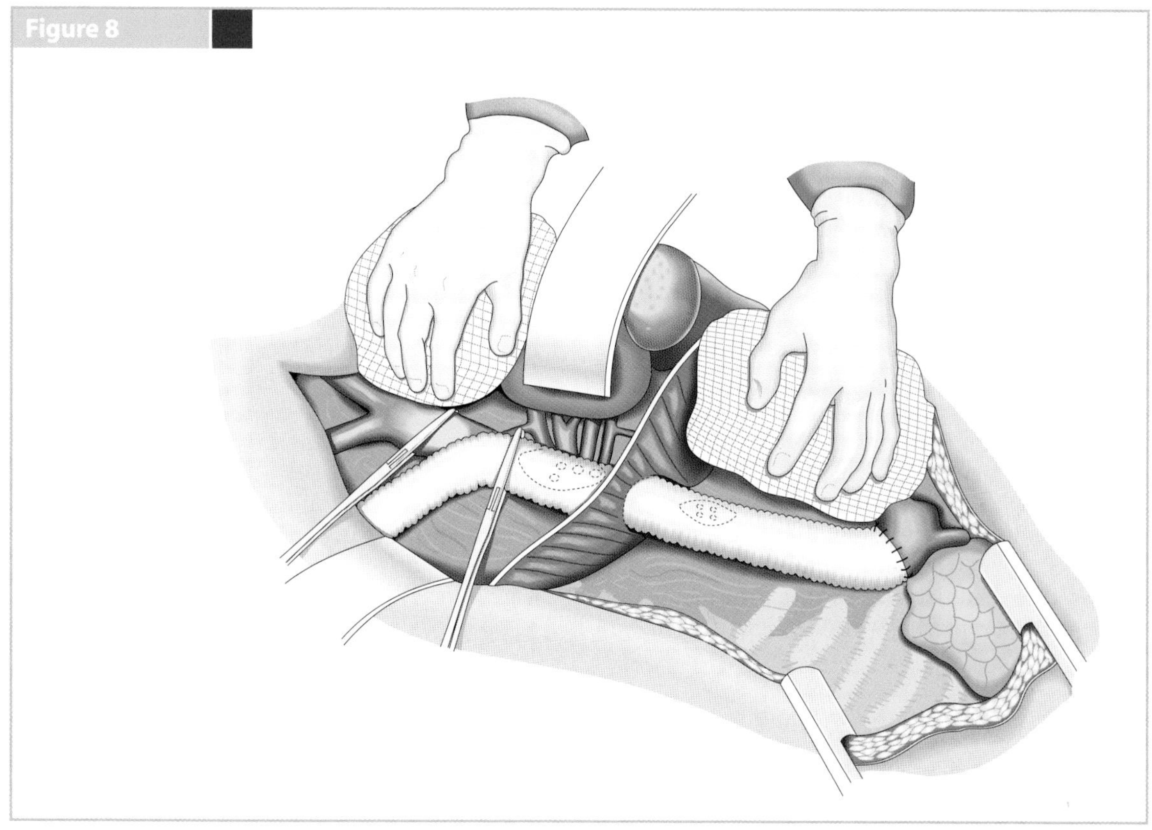

Figure 9

The infrarenal aorta is opened and inspected from the inside to identify a neck. The distal aorta is then prepared, and the anastomosis performed using either 2-0 or 3-0 polypropylene sutures. Prior to completion of the distal anastomosis, the graft is flushed proximally and the aorta distally. We wean the patient from partial bypass once the rectal temperature reaches 37°C. Protamine is administered and the atrial and femoral cannulae are removed. Figure 9 shows the start of iliac anastomosis.

Figure 10

Once hemostasis is achieved, three tubes are placed in the chest for pleural cavity drainage. The pericostal space is approximated using braided absorbable sutures, and the muscular fascia of the chest closed using monofilament absorbable sutures. The diaphragm and abdominal walls are closed in multiple layers with heavy polypropylene sutures, and the skin is approximated with staples.

Postoperatively, with the patient in a supine position, a single endotracheal tube is exchanged for the bifurcated endotracheal tube. If the vocal cords are swollen, the bifurcation tube is kept in place postoperatively. The length of stay in the intensive care unit is about 3 or 4 days. We try to wake the patient as quickly as possible to check neurological status. Even after the patient recovers from anesthesia and is moving all extremities, we still have to be on the alert for delayed paraplegia. Warning signs for delayed paraplegia are unstable blood pressure, hypoxia after extubation or CSF pressure above 10 mmHg. Cerebrospinal fluid drainage is discontinued on the third postoperative day, and the patient is discharged to the regular floor. If the patient develops delayed paraplegia, the CSF drainage catheter has to be reinserted and drained for 3 days. Usually, the patient will recover if CSF drainage is restored within the first 2 or 3 h of insult. Once the patient is up and about, tolerating a regular diet, afebrile and has return of normal bowel function, they are discharged, usually in a period of 10–12 days following surgery. Following TAA repair we recommend biannual follow-up with CT scan for the 1st year postoperatively with subsequent yearly CT scan as long as the repair and native aorta remains stable.

Figure 10 shows completed graft.

Figure 9

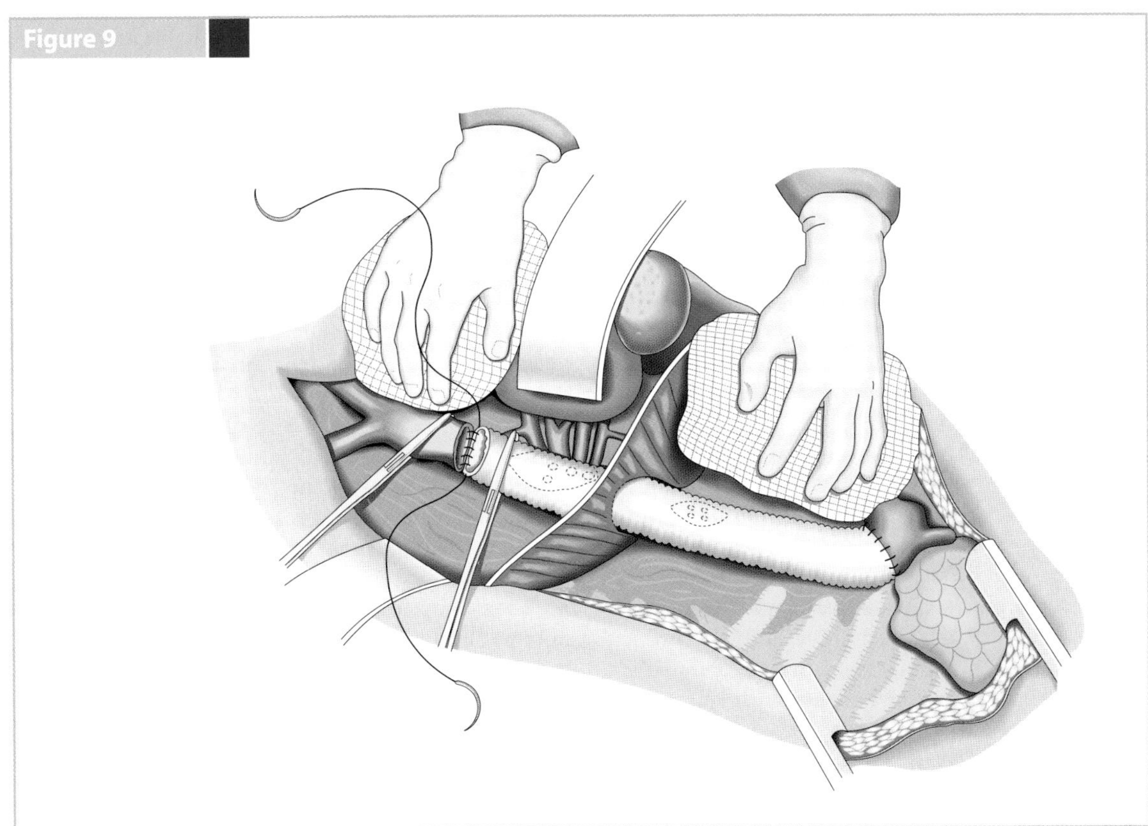

Figure 10

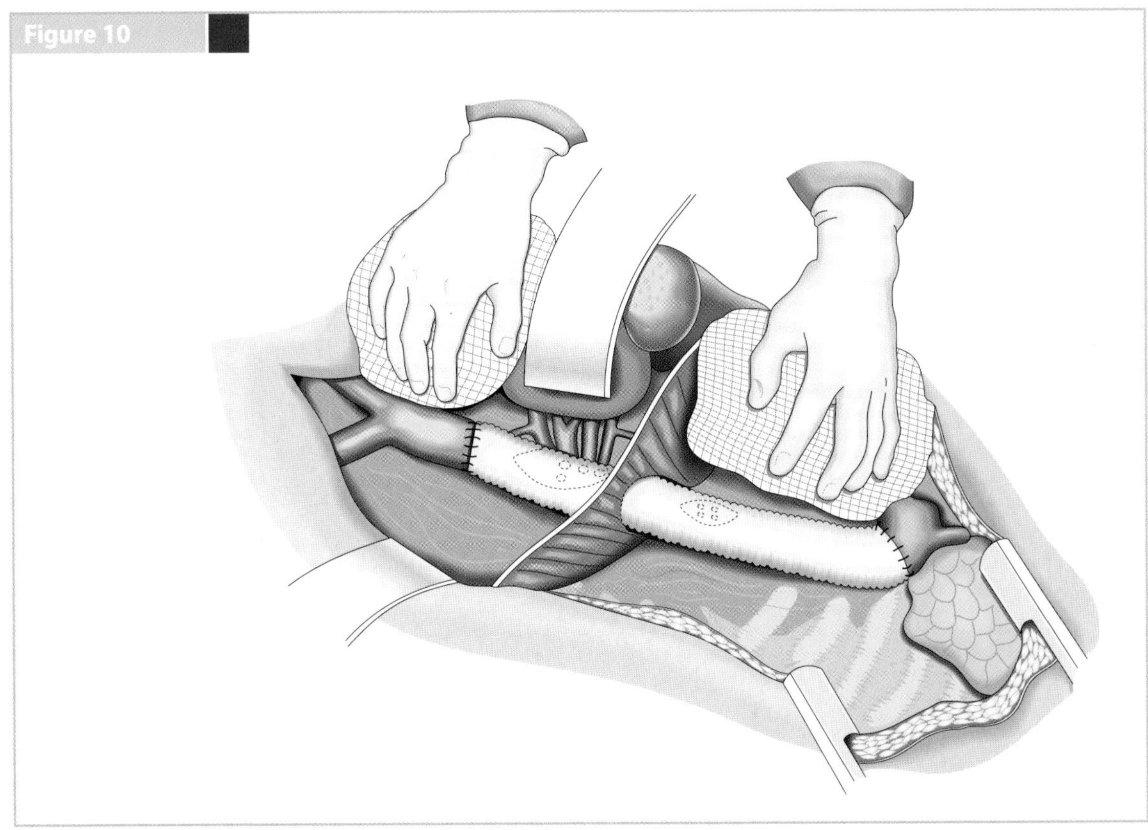

CONCLUSION

Untreated, TAA is associated with poor long-term survival. Aneurysm size and growth rate, and patient age, medical history and symptoms must be carefully weighed when considering surgical intervention, but elective surgery for TAA improves long-term survival (Safi et al. 1997). A thorough preoperative assessment should include cardiac, renal, neurologic and pulmonary evaluations. Aneurysm size of more than 5.0 cm, and a rate of expansion of greater than 0.5 cm/6 months, as well as the presence of symptoms are all indications for surgical intervention.

Historically, TAA repair involved replacement of the diseased aortic segment with a graft using the simple cross-clamp technique. For non-emergent cases, this approach was associated with a rate of neurologic deficit (paraplegia or paraparesis) of up to 30% and a mortality rate of 20–25% (Svensson et al. 1992). With modern techniques and the surgical adjuncts of cerebrospinal fluid drainage and distal aortic perfusion, we have seen improvements in morbidity and mortality (Estrera et al. 2001). Distal aortic perfusion (partial left heart bypass) provides cardiac unloading and increases ischemic tolerance to the spinal cord, viscera and kidneys (Safi et al. 1996). Cerebrospinal fluid drainage may alleviate the "compartment syndrome" caused by aortic cross-clamping and reperfusion injury. Reimplantation of intercostal arteries, which became feasible with the introduction of perfusion adjuncts, has also improved results dramatically (Safi et al. 1998). While complications following TAA surgery remain a threat, our current short-term mortality for TAA surgery is 5–10%. The overall incidence of neurologic deficit is 3.3% and for the most extensive (type II) TAA has fallen below 7%.

Because diseases of the thoracoabdominal aorta require multiple organ protection, it is our philosophy that treatment must rely on a multifaceted approach. Our current system involves a multidisciplinary team that includes anesthesia, perfusion technology, nursing, physical therapy, critical care (renal, pulmonary, cardiology, neurology) and surgery. Each of these components must be able to optimally communicate and cooperate in order to care for these often critically ill patients and to obtain the best results.

REFERENCES

Estrera AL, Miller CC 3rd, Huynh TT, Porat E, Safi HJ (2001) Neurologic outcome after thoracic and thoracoabdominal aortic aneurysm repair. Ann Thorac Surg 72:1225–1230; discussion 1230–1231

Safi HJ (1999) How I do it: thoracoabdominal aortic aneurysm graft replacement. Cardiovasc Surg 7:607–613

Safi HJ, Harlin SA, Miller CC et al. (1996) Predictive factors for acute renal failure in thoracic and thoracoabdominal aortic aneurysm surgery [published erratum appears in J Vasc Surg 1997 25(1):93]. J Vasc Surg 24:338–344; discussion 344–345

Safi HJ, Miller CC 3rd, Iliopoulos DC, Griffiths G (1997) Long-term results following thoracoabdominal aortic aneurysm repair. In: Branchereau A, Jacobs MJHM (eds) European Vascular Course: long-term results of arterial interventions. Futura Publishing, NY

Safi H, Miller CI, Carr C, Illiopoulos D, Dorsay D, Baldwin J (1998) The importance of intercostal artery reattachment during thoracoabdominal aortic aneurysm repair. J Vasc Surg 27:58–68

Svensson LG, Crawford ES, Hess KR, Coselli JS, Safi HJ (1992) Experience with 1509 patients undergoing thoracoabdominal aortic operations. J Vasc Surg 17:357–368; discussion 386–370

Part IV Abdominal Aorta and its Branches

CHAPTER 15

Transabdominal Replacement of Abdominal Aortic Aneurysms

Michael S. Conners III, John W. York, Samuel R. Money

INTRODUCTION

Aneurysmal disease of the abdominal aorta was responsible for approximately 16,000 (0.7%) deaths in the United States in 1999. It was the 11th leading cause of death during the same time period for the age range of 65–79 years (National Vital Statistics Reports 2001). The overall incidence is increasing and this is unrelated to the general aging of the population (Cronenwett et al. 2000; Hollier et al. 1992). Males have a four to six times higher prevalence than females and Caucasians are affected more often than other races. Population-based studies vary but generally agree that the overall prevalence in patients >55 years of age is roughly 6.0% in males and 1.5% in females (Pleumeekers et al. 1995; Singh et al. 2001). Differences in the criteria used to define aneurysms may account for the disparity of various reports. Currently, accepted standards classify an abdominal aorta as aneurysmal if an isolated segment of the infrarenal aorta is ≥3.0 cm in diameter or if the diameter of the infrarenal aorta is 1.5× the diameter of the suprarenal aorta (Cronenwett et al. 2000). Aneurysm size is the most important prognostic factor in determining the risk of aneurysm rupture.

Degenerative AAA aneurysms are the result of a multifactorial process, and leading theories focus on either abnormal synthesis or deficiencies in arterial wall elastin (and/or collagen) as well as an overabundance of degradation enzymes (Cronenwett et al. 2000). A core genetic or familial component is responsible for 15% of AAAs and these may rupture at a smaller size (Cronenwett et al. 2000).

The most significant independent risk factor is age (Pleumeekers et al. 1995; Singh et al. 2001).

A second factor associated with the development of an AAA is cigarette smoking, this being the duration rather than the quantity of cigarettes smoked (Singh et al. 2001). Other contributing factors are hypertension and hypercholesterolemia (Pleumeekers et al. 1995; Singh et al. 2001). Historically, atherosclerosis was considered the cause of AAAs but this is only one of many contribution factors.

The purpose of elective AAA repair is to avoid aneurysm rupture and the accompanying high mortality rate. Death rates associated with a ruptured aneurysm are difficult to estimate because many individuals expire in the field. However, mortality rates as high as 50% are experienced in patients who survive long enough to arrive at the hospital. This is in contrast to a mortality rate of <5% for elective aneurysm repair (Hollier et al. 1992).

Predicting which aneurysm will rupture is impossible, but aneurysms ≥5.5 cm size and/or expansion ≥0.5 cm/year are high risk. In addition, the risk of rupture increases with increasing aneurysm size (Guirguis et al. 1991). Aneurysms <5 cm can rupture but the incidence is ≤1%/year and the potential risk associated with surgical repair exceeds the expected benefit. As the size of the aneurysm surpasses 5 cm the risk of rupture per year starts to outweigh the risk associated with an elective repair in most patients.

Each aneurysm is unique in the timing and rate of growth, but generally accepted rates of growth are 0.3–0.5 cm/year (Guirguis et al. 1991); greater than this carries a high risk of rupture.

As approximately 90% of abdominal aortic aneurysms occur in the infrarenal aorta, the following pages examine the steps involved in *elective* repair (± associated iliac aneurysms) of aneurysms at this site. Notations are made for deviations from this practice (i.e., when repairing a ruptured aneurysm).

Figure 1: Patient Positioning and Skin

Transabdominal aortic aneurysm repair is a major operative procedure that requires a general anesthetic and not infrequently invasive cardiac monitoring. Proper patient positioning is paramount in avoiding inadequate operative exposure. The author's choice is to have the patient supine on the operative table with the arms secured in the adducted position. This leaves ample room for placement of a table mounted self-retaining retractor. In contrast, when managing a ruptured aneurysm, patients will routinely have their arms abducted to 90°. This allows the anesthesiologist the opportunity to obtain arterial and venous access while simultaneous preparation for the laparotomy is under way. In either case, a sterile preparation extending from the patient's nipple-line to the mid-thighs must be arranged in the event that access to the femoral vessels is desired.

Once the operating field has been sterilely prepped and draped a midline incision is carried from the xiphoid process to the pubic symphysis. This allows adequate exposure of the entire abdominal aorta as well as the iliac arteries. If further distal control is warranted a counterincision in the groin can be used to expose the femoral artery. On occasion, in thin patients, the use of a more limited laparotomy may be acceptable when dealing with aneurysms of limited size and complexity.

Figure 2: Aneurysm Exposure

Upon entering the peritoneal cavity, a thorough manual inspection of all abdominal contents proceeds in a systematic fashion. Occasionally other pathology is encountered but the temptation to intervene must be resisted when planning to place a synthetic conduit in the aorta.

15

Adequate exposure of the aorta is essential in achieving a safe and proficient aneurysm repair. The initial step of exposure involves retraction of the transverse colon and greater omentum superiorly. This exposes the small intestine from the distal duodenum to the ileocecal junction. Lateral retraction of the small bowel to the right permits identification of the root of the mesentery and the ligament of Treitz. Subsequent placement of the sigmoid colon into the left pelvis clearly exposes the retroperitoneum overlying the aneurysm. In this situation the author prefers a self-retaining device that is capable of maintaining retraction in various directions by the addition of individual retractors (Omni retractor).

Dissection begins with careful separation of the duodenum from the neighboring soft tissue overlying the aorta. Meticulous care in avoiding a duodenal injury at this early step can prevent a disaster. Once the duodenum is freely mobilized, incising the retroperitoneum anterior to the aorta allows exposure of the anterior aortic wall. Extending the retroperitoneal incision cephalad toward the proximal neck of the aneurysm will permit identification of the left renal vein. Frequently the vein is stretched across the neck of the aneurysm so careful dissection is paramount in avoiding a serious venous injury. Occasionally, division of the left renal vein is required to expose the proximal infrarenal aorta. Very occasionally the left renal vein may be in a retroaortic position, so preoperative knowledge of the patient's anatomy is helpful in avoiding a catastrophic venous injury when placing a proximal aortic clamp.

Distal exposure of the aneurysm is accomplished by extending the retroperitoneal incision down the right anterior surface of the aneurysm. The inferior mesenteric artery (IMA) is frequently located on the left anterior surface of the aneurysm; therefore care should be taken to avoid an injury to the IMA upon opening the aneurysm sac. Depending on the distal extent of the aneurysm, the retroperitoneal incision may need to be advanced down the iliac vessels. Autonomic nerves responsible for sexual function in the male are routinely located overlying the left common iliac artery, so avoidance of this area is recommended. If the aneurysm extends down the left common iliac artery, some advocate a second retroperitoneal incision lateral to the sigmoid mesocolon to allow access of the left iliac bifurcation.

Figure 1

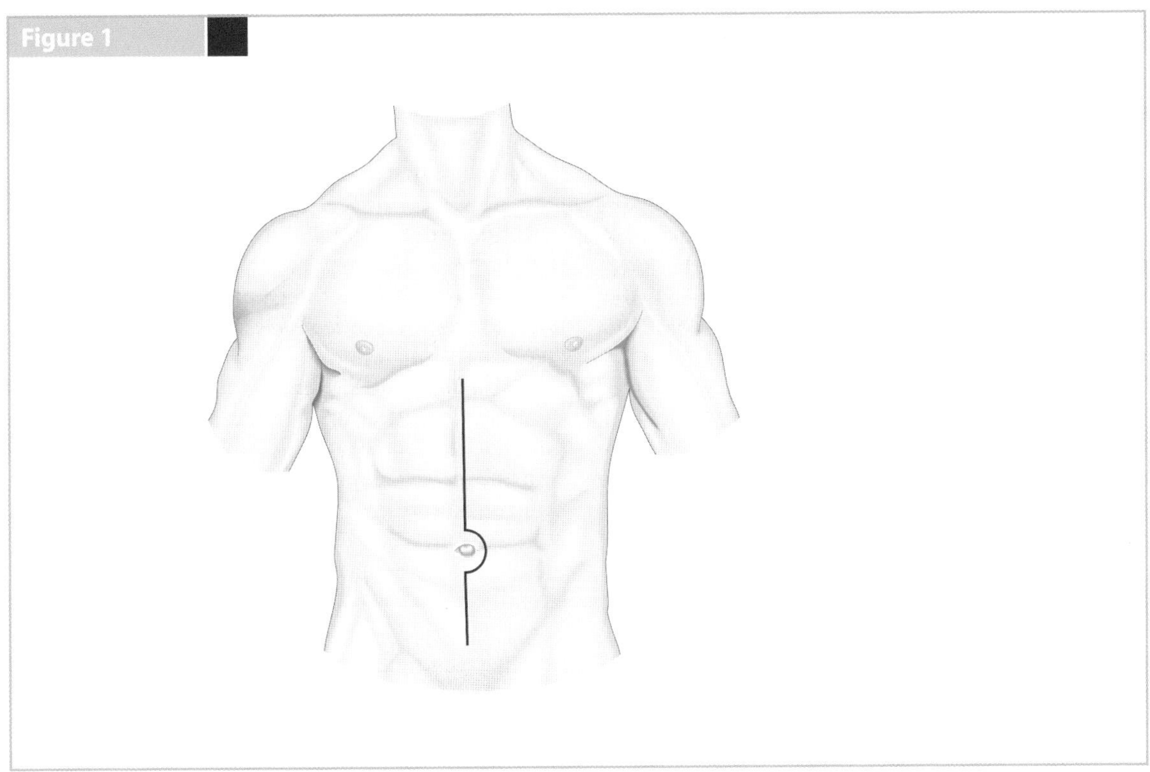

Figure 2

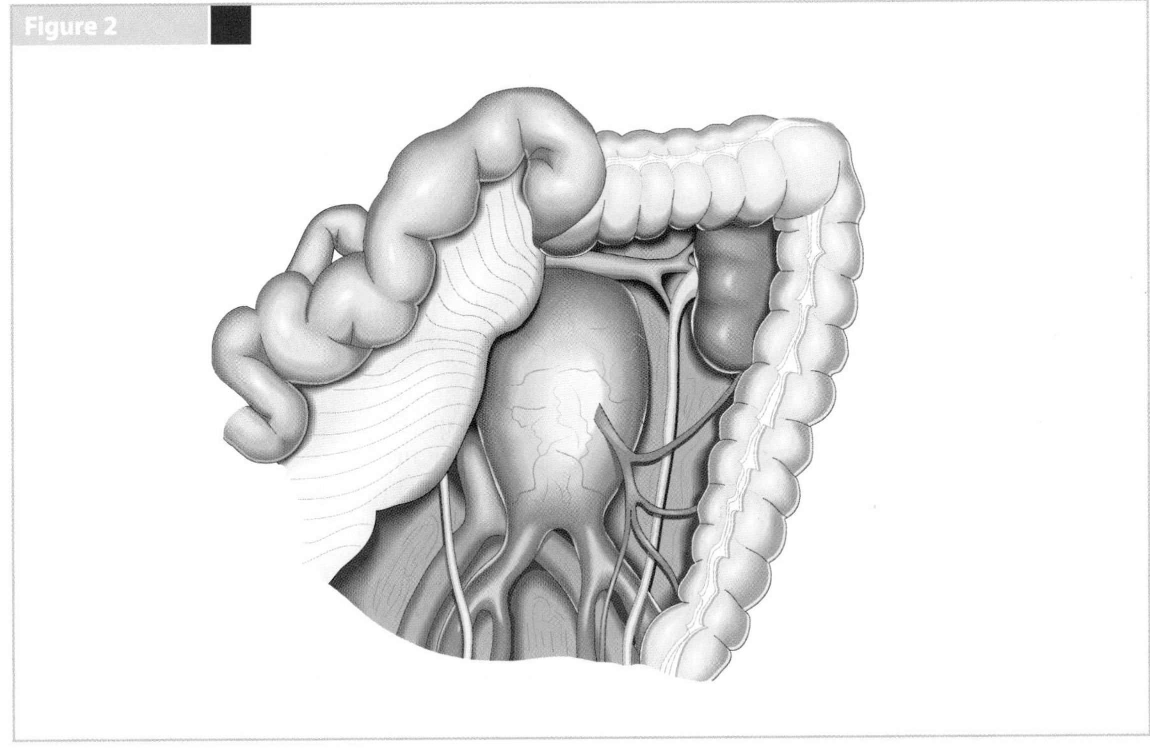

Figure 3: Proximal Control

Once the retroperitoneum overlying the aorta is completely opened, attention is directed at gaining proximal control. At the proximal aneurysm neck the left renal vein is mobilized cephalad allowing clear exposure of the proximal infrarenal aorta. In certain situations the proximal aspect of the aneurysm may necessitate division of the left renal vein, so important anatomic considerations must be kept in mind. Three important venous branches (adrenal, lumbar and gonadal) serve as the sole drainage of the kidney in the event the left renal vein is divided. Transection of the vein must be on the caval side of these branches to allow adequate venous outflow of the left kidney. After proper mobilization (or division) of the left renal vein, dissection of the proximal aorta is limited to the soft tissue intimately associated with the neck of the aneurysm ("slotting the aorta"). Avoiding haphazard dissection helps eliminate inadvertent injury to lumbar arteries that exit the posterior aorta. Circumferential dissection of the aorta is rarely needed and only risks injury to the posteriorly located lumbar vessels. On occasion large lymphatic channels are found coursing over the aneurysm neck. Ligation of these channels helps prevent postoperative lymphatic leakage.

Identification of the renal arteries at this point permits decisions regarding placement of the aortic clamp. A non-aneurysmal infrarenal aortic length of approximately 1 cm is needed to avoid placing a suprarenal aortic clamp. This distance allows adequate room for placement of an infrarenal aortic clamp and leaves enough aortic cuff length to complete the proximal anastomosis.

The exception to gaining proximal control in the above-described manner is in the management of a ruptured aneurysm. In this situation immediate proximal control is gained after opening the peritoneal cavity. Manual palpation at the level of the diaphragmatic hiatus allows identification of the supraceliac aorta and the opportunity to gain aortic control at this level. When removing the supraceliac control careful attention and slow release helps prevent sudden drops in system blood pressure. Frequently the hematoma has done the dissection itself and proximal control is relatively easy. However, sometimes infrarenal proximal control is difficult.

Figure 4: Distal Control

The exact position of distal control will vary depending on the extent of the aneurysm. If the aneurysm is limited to the aorta, control at the proximal common iliac arteries will usually suffice. Careful dissection and thorough understanding of the anatomic relationships between the iliac arteries and veins is important in preventing a serious venous injury. Venous bleeding within the pelvis can be profuse, difficult to control and not infrequently culminates in a fatal situation. As with the proximal aorta, circumferential dissection of the common iliac arteries is not routinely required and exposes the underlying veins to potential injury. Another important anatomic relationship that requires strict attention is that of the ureters. Prior to descending into the pelvis the ureters cross the distal common iliac arteries bilaterally. In an effort to avoid injury of their tenuous vascular supply, manipulation of the ureters should be kept to a minimum and done with caution.

When aneurysmal disease involves the common iliac arteries, distal control is typically gained beyond the iliac bifurcation. This rather common scenario requires dissection of both the proximal internal and external iliac arteries. In this situation the distal anastomosis is usually constructed at the level of the iliac bifurcation. For reasons discussed above, dissection over the left common iliac artery is avoided when feasible. However, if control of the left common iliac bifurcation is anticipated preoperatively, appropriate counseling concerning the risk of postoperative sexual dysfunction in the male is important.

In the unfortunate circumstance of internal iliac aneurysmal disease, distal control can be difficult to obtain. Intraluminal balloon occlusion techniques are helpful and permit either intraluminal oversewing or revascularization of pelvic blood flow. Reestablishment of pelvic blood flow is accomplished by creating a side limb off the iliac limb of the bifurcated aortic graft.

Regardless of the level of distal control, an overemphasis needs to be placed on the avoidance of a venous injury. These potentially lethal insults can lead to total vascular collapse rather rapidly.

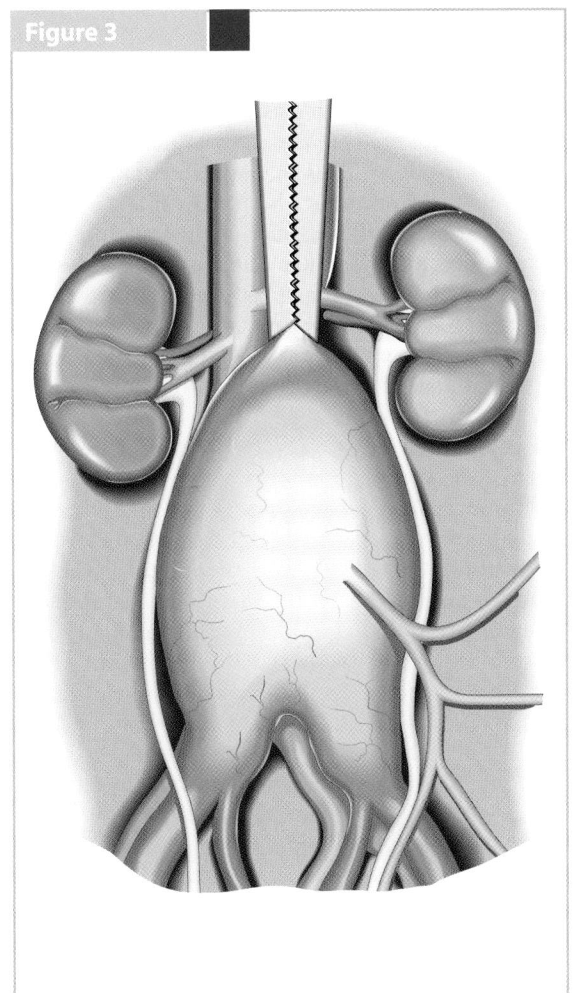
Figure 3

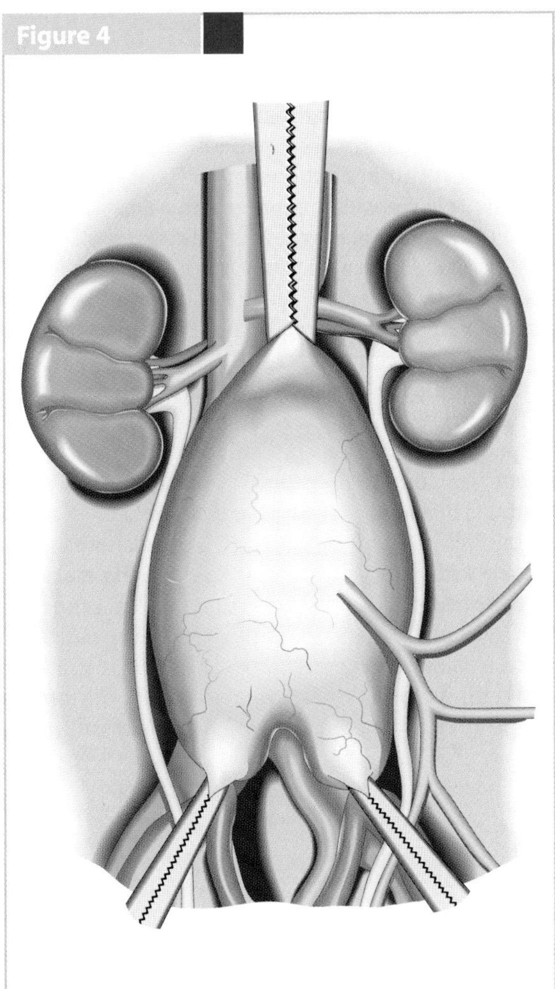
Figure 4

Figure 5: Opening Aneurysm

Once appropriate proximal and distal control has been established, the patient is systemically heparinized. Roughly 5000–7000 IU of heparin is given intravenously as a bolus. After allowing sufficient time for circulation, the distal clamps are placed first to avoid potential embolization as a result of clamping the proximal aorta. The specific type of clamp used both proximally and distally is down to the surgeon's preference; however, certain anatomic restraints dictate this choice, especially in the pelvis. Before making the aortotomy the aneurysm should be palpated to verify the absence of a pulse. If the aneurysm continues to have a pulse the proximal clamp is inadequate and must be reapplied.

Initially the anterior surface of the aneurysm is scored with the electrocautery; then using a scalpel and the heavy Mayo scissors the aneurysm is opened along its anterior surface. Similar to the retroperitoneal incision, cheating slightly to the right will help avoid injury to the IMA. Extension of the aortotomy to the proximalmost aspect of the aneurysm is accomplished with heavy scissors. At this point partial transection of the proximal aorta results in a T-shaped aortotomy. This maneuver opens the aneurysm in such a way that the proximal aortic cuff is clearly exposed. When extending the aortotomy posteriorly care must be taken in achieving a plane perpendicular to the spine. This prevents inadvertent shortening of the posterior aspect of the aortic cuff (at least 1 cm proximal aortic cuff is desired). A similar technique is utilized when extending the aortotomy distally. If iliac aneurysms are present the aortotomy is carried to the iliac bifurcation.

Once the aneurysm is completely opened, the mural thrombus is removed from the aneurysm sac. Backbleeding from the IMA and lumbar vessels may be profuse. A small non-crushing vascular clamp is used to control the IMA temporally. The decision whether or not to reimplant the IMA is made after reestablishing blood flow to the pelvis. Bleeding lumbar vessels are oversewn with 2.0-silk suture.

Figure 5

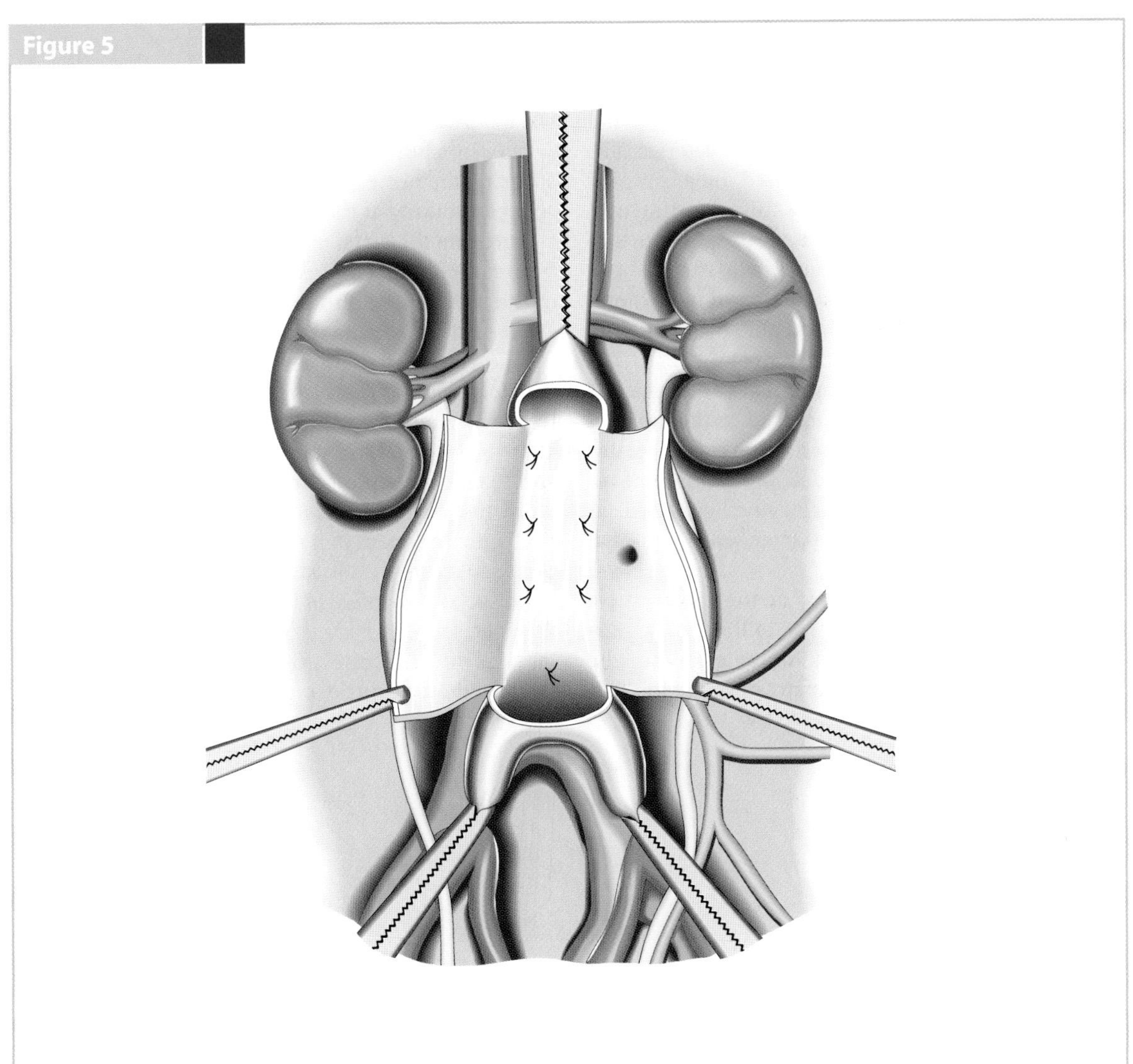

Figure 6: Placement of the Graft

Graft size is determined by estimating the diameter of the proximal aortic cuff and the iliac arteries. The proximal anastomosis is completed in a running fashion using 3-0 polypropylene suture. Starting with the initial knot posteriorly, the surgeon is able to easily sew up each side of the anastomosis. Suture bites should be approximately 1 mm apart and care should be taken not to place all bites an equal distance from the edge. This would create an environment susceptible to disruption. Once the proximal anastomosis is complete, the aortic clamp is moved to the graft allowing inspection for hemostasis across the anastomosis. If extra sutures are needed, the addition of felt pledgets can lend support to achieving hemostasis as well as help prevent the sutures from tearing though the degenerated aorta.

Depending on the anatomy of the aneurysm a tube or bifurcated graft may be utilized. If a tube graft is employed the distal end of the graft must be shortened. This prevents the graft from bulging forward once the repair is complete. If a bifurcated graft is chosen, shortening of the proximal end prior to suturing the proximal anastomosis will prevent subsequent kinking at the level of the aortic bifurcation.

Suturing the distal end of a tube graft to the aortic bifurcation is approached in a method similar to that of the proximal anastomosis. If the distal anastomosis is planned for the iliac bifurcation, 4-0 polypropylene suture is used. Prior to completing the last anastomosis, the graft is flushed retrograde then antegrade by releasing the individual clamps in a controlled manner. Lastly, all anastomosis sites are inspected for meticulous hemostasis.

Perfusion to the sigmoid colon is evaluated prior to closing the aneurysm sac. If the colon appears well perfused a simple silk suture is placed in the aneurysm sac at the orifice of the IMA. Reimplantation of the IMA into the side of the aortic graft is recommended if the slightest doubt exists regarding adequate colonic perfusion.

Figure 6

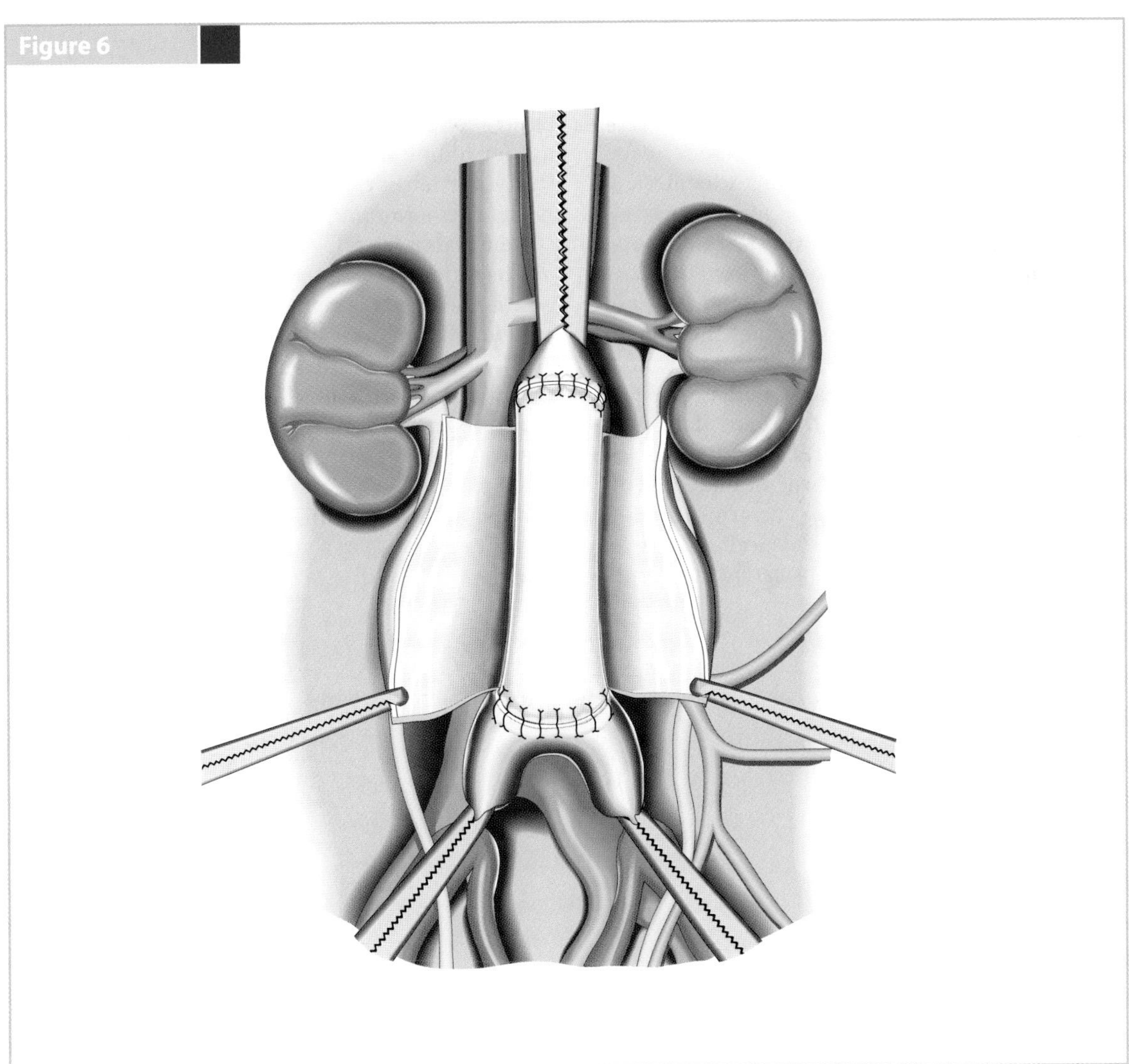

Figure 7: Closure of the Aneurysm Sac

After complete hemostasis is achieved, the aneurysm sac is closed over the graft. The idea here is to avoid the devastating complication of an aortoenteric fistula. An aortoenteric fistula necessitates removal of the graft and a subsequent revascularization procedure. When closing the aneurysm sac, the native aortic wall or the overlying retroperitoneum must cover all areas of the graft. Starting at the proximal aspect of the open aorta, a running suture, of the surgeon's choice, is used to reapproximate the aortic wall over the synthetic graft. The region of the proximal anastomosis deserves particular attention, due to the fact that the duodenum will ultimately lie over this area. If covering a simple tube graft the native aortic wall usually conceals the graft completely. However, if a bifurcated graft is carried to the iliac bifurcation, the additional use of the retroperitoneum for hiding the iliac limbs is frequently needed. Lastly, the retroperitoneum is closed over the aneurysm sac in a running fashion.

Removal of the self-retaining retractor and return of the abdominal contents to their usual anatomic position allows a last inspection of all viscera. The anterior abdominal wall can be closed in a multitude of ways (running, interrupted, running with additional interrupted), all of which are adequate when done properly. Despite which method of closure is chosen, secure approximation of the fascia is of utmost importance. Closure is concluded with approximation of the epidermis using either a subcuticular stitch (our choice) or a stapling device.

Figure 7

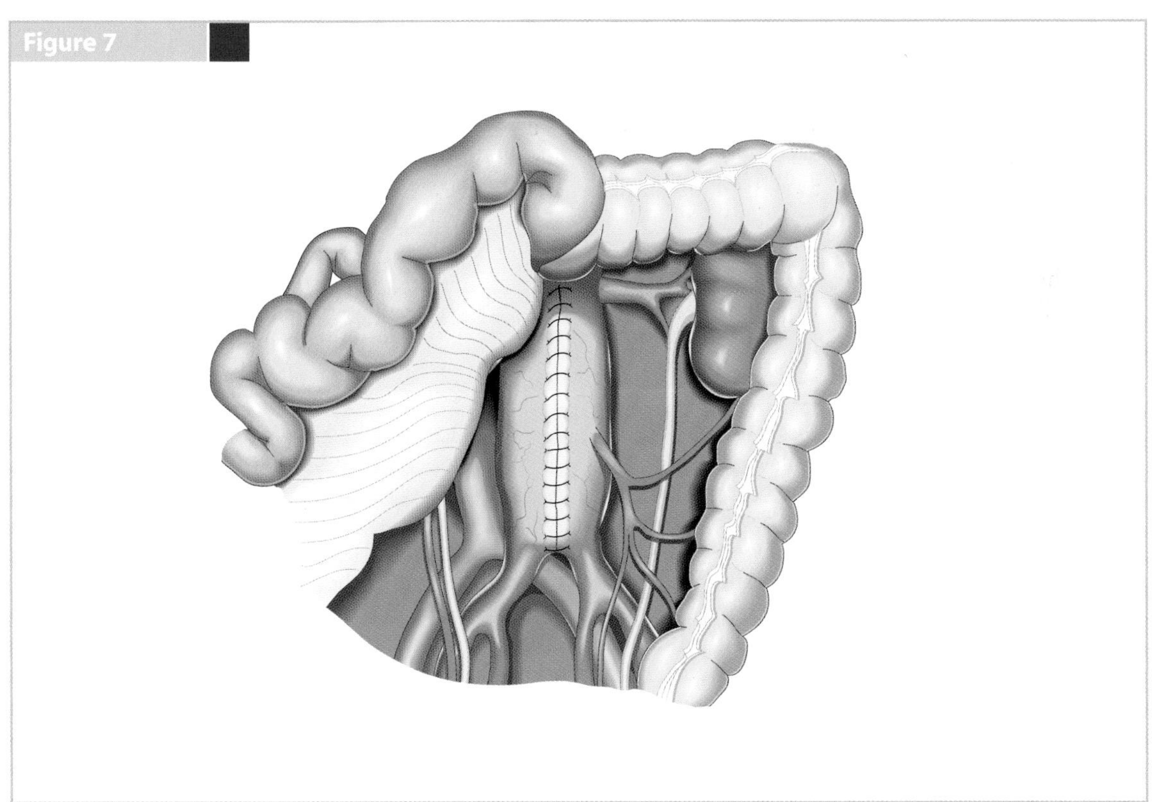

CONCLUSION

Elective abdominal aortic aneurysm repair can be rewarding to both the patient and physician. Keys to success begin with proper preoperative patient evaluation. Aneurysm patients are frequently victims of diffuse vascular disease. This may be in the form of other aneurysms (femoral, popliteal) or occlusive disease (coronary, carotid or infrainguinal). Preoperative identification of these comorbid conditions is important and may alter decisions regarding the timing and method of aneurysm treatment. Proper explanation of the inherent risk associated with AAA repair is another preoperative must as well as a physician obligation.

Knowledge of the natural history of aneurysmal disease is mandatory. Continual growth and subsequent rupture is the norm but predicting the rate of growth and the timing of rupture are impossible. For this reason, patient education and the institution of a structured follow-up program are essential to the success of abdominal aortic aneurysm management. The imaging modalities utilized for follow-up are dependent on physician preference and the risks (contrast-enhanced computed-tomography scan) and limitations (abdominal ultrasonography) of each must be recognized.

The timing of treatment or the question of "when to repair an aneurysm" is generally dictated by the aneurysm size, growth rate or the presence of symptoms and the patient's overall physical status. All symptomatic aneurysms are repaired regardless of size but the converse holds true only for stable asymptomatic aneurysms 5 cm in size. As fusiform aneurysms of the infrarenal aorta exceed ≥5 cm in diameter or approach a growth rate of 1 cm/year, the risk of rupture starts to outweigh the accepted risk associated with elective surgical repair in "healthy" individuals. At this point appropriate patient counseling regarding the mortality rate associated with aneurysm rupture is warranted. Like symptomatic aneurysms, saccular and inflammatory aneurysms are repaired more liberally.

A through understanding of the principles described in this chapter is essential to the success of a transabdominal aortic aneurysm repair. Transabdominal aortic aneurysm repair is a major vascular procedure with significant potential to turn fatal in a matter of moments. Small errors in detail can offer significant consequences. As with all surgical procedures, meticulous attention to detail is paramount in avoiding a disaster.

REFERENCES

Cronenwett JL et al. (2000) Abdominal aortic and iliac aneurysms. In: Rutherford RB (ed) Vascular surgery. WB Saunders, Philadelphia, pp 1246–1280

Guirguis EM et al. (1991) The natural history of abdominal aortic aneurysms. Am J Surg 162:481–483

Hollier LH et al. (1992) Recommended indications for operative treatment of abdominal aortic aneurysms. J Vasc Surg 15(6):1046–1053

National Vital Statistics Reports (2001) Deaths: preliminary data for 1999. Vol 49(3):1–49

Pleumeekers HJCM et al. (1995) Aneurysms of the abdominal aorta in older adults. Am J Epidemiol 142:1291–1299

Singh K et al. (2001) Prevalence of and risk factors for abdominal aortic aneurysms in a population-based study. Am J Epidemiol 154:236–244

CHAPTER 16

Retroperitoneal Replacement of Abdominal Aortic Aneurysm

Patrick J. Geraghty, Gregorio A. Sicard

INTRODUCTION

Infrarenal abdominal aortic aneurysm (AAA) disease is a significant cause of mortality in the United States, accounting for over 15,000 deaths annually (Minino et al. 2002). Following FDA approval of commercial stent-graft systems for aortic repair in 1999, a significant proportion of infrarenal AAAs have been repaired using stent-grafts. Despite the popularity of endoluminal repair, traditional open repair remains the gold standard against which all other approaches must be compared.

Indications for repair are based on maximal aneurysm diameter, the presence of abdominal/back discomfort, thrombosis, distal embolization, and rupture. With regards to aneurysm diameter as a criterion for repair, patients had historically been offered repair when the maximal transverse diameter reached 5.0 cm. However, two recent multicenter, randomized trials, the UK Small Aneurysm Trial and the ADAM Trial, compared open surgical repair to watchful waiting for asymptomatic AAAs with diameters from 4.0 to 5.5 cm (Lederle et al. 2002; The UK Small Aneurysm Trial Participants 1998). No survival benefit was seen in patients who underwent repair of AAAs that were less than 5.5 cm in diameter.

When appropriate selection criteria for offering repair are present, attempts must be made to stratify the patient's cardiac risk. If indicated, cardiac catheterization and coronary revascularization should be pursued prior to elective AAA repair. The preoperative history and physical examination should also search for concomitant disease processes that may alter surgical planning, such as chronic mesenteric angina, renovascular hypertension, and aortoiliac occlusive disease.

Centers of excellence have demonstrated operative mortality rates less than 3% (Cambria et al. 1992; Sicard et al. 1995). As mortality rates correlate with both the surgeon's experience and institutional volume, state and nationwide outcomes for elective open AAA repair are slightly poorer than those reported from high-volume institutions (Dardik et al. 1999; Katz et al. 1994; Richardson and Main 1991).

We preferentially employ the retroperitoneal approach for open repair of infrarenal AAAs. Studies have demonstrated that this approach may diminish the duration of postoperative ileus and the length of stay in the intensive care unit (Sicard et al. 1995). The left renal and left iliac vessels are readily visualized in the course of the approach. Proximal extension may be performed with minimal difficulty, should the need for suprarenal or supraceliac aortic exposure arise. Inflammatory aneurysms and aneurysms with crossed/fused renal ectopia are more easily approached via the retroperitoneal route. Intraperitoneal adhesions and stomas from previous transperitoneal operations are avoided, and in massively obese patients anterior displacement of the pannus may facilitate an otherwise difficult operation.

Several instances exist where conventional transperitoneal exposure may be the more suitable choice. The presence of a left-sided inferior vena cava dictates against the use of the retroperitoneal approach. Likewise, concomitant right renal artery revascularization at the time of aneurysm repair may be more easily approached via a midline incision.

Figure 1A, B

The patient is positioned supine for the induction of anesthesia and placement of central venous and arterial monitoring catheters. The beanbag used to maintain positioning should be positioned beneath the patient prior to induction. Following induction, line placement, and urinary catheter placement, the patient is lifted and rolled into the right lateral decubitus position. The shoulders are positioned at an angle of 60 degrees from the bed, and the hips are positioned at approximately 45 degrees. The greater lateral relaxation of the hips affords easier exposure to the femoral vessels. Appropriate axillary protection is maintained by the anesthesiologist to avoid brachial plexus neuropathy. The left arm is placed in a padded sled, and the lower extremities are padded to prevent compression over the peroneal nerve and bony prominences.

Next, the beanbag is aspirated to maintain the desired position. Note that the posterior edge of the beanbag should not be higher than the spinal column, and that the anterior edge must accommodate access to the right groin, as well as extension of the incision to the midline. The kidney rest is raised, and the table flexed. Addition of reverse Trendelenburg tilt is also required to ensure that the patient's head is not kept in a severely dependent position throughout the procedure, as significant facial edema will result. The patient is then prepped from the nipples to the distal thighs. Retention of sterile towels is facilitated by use of an occlusive surgical drape.

Orientation of the incision depends upon the anticipated level of proximal exposure that will be required. *Line A* indicates the incision used for iliac exposure. *Lines B* and *C* indicate the incisions used for infrarenal aortic and aortoiliac exposure, respectively. The lateral termini of the incisions in Lines B and C are at the 12th rib tip, or between the 11th and 12th rib tips. (Figures 1–8 are taken from Sicard and Reilly 1994: Left retroperitoneal approach to the aorta and its branches: part I. *Ann Vasc Surg* 8(2):212–219.)

Figure 1A

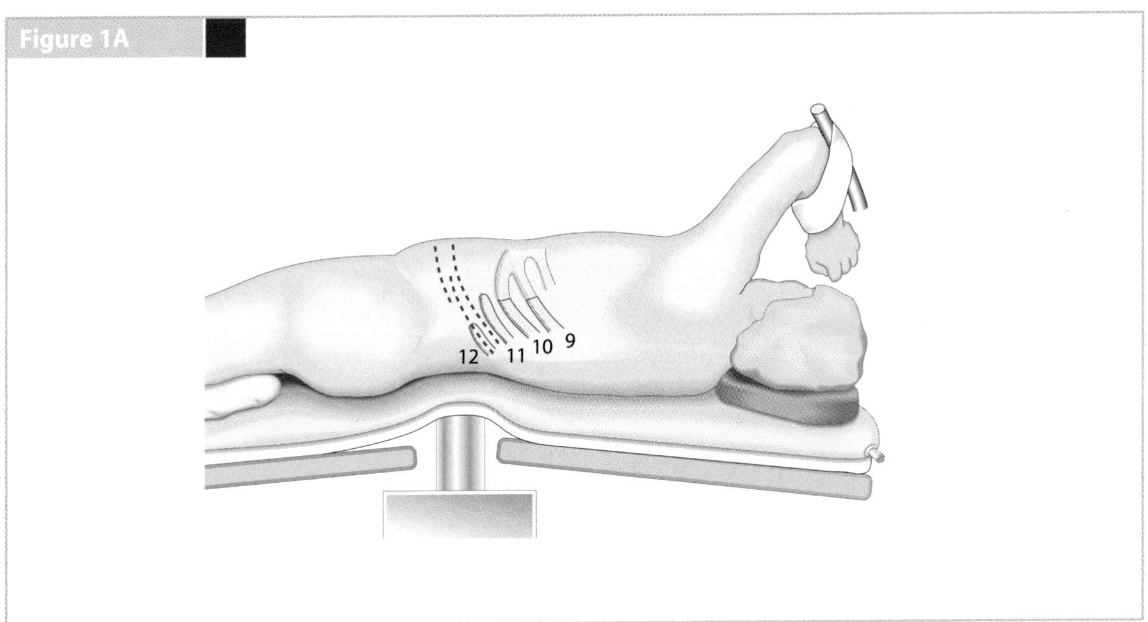

Figure 1B

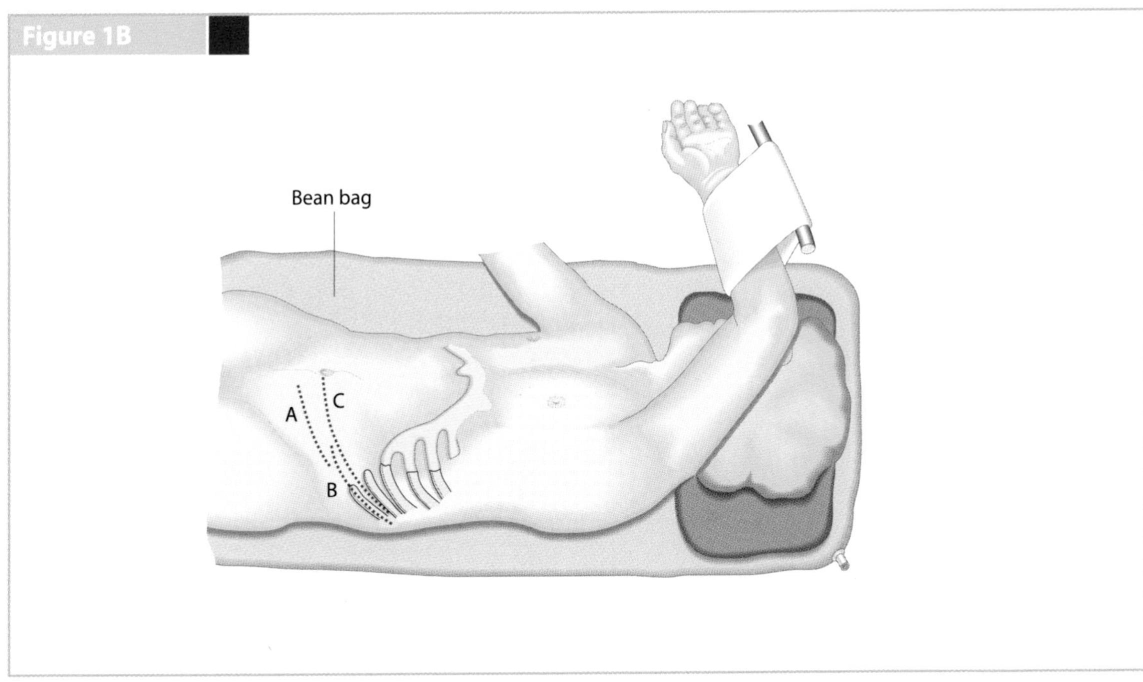

Figure 2A, B

The approach is altered when juxtarenal and suprarenal aortic crossclamping is anticipated, and may also vary depending on the patient's body habitus. *Line D*, with extension to the 11th rib, provides adequate exposure of the juxtarenal aorta. Extension to the 10th or 9th rib spaces, shown by *Lines E* and *F*, is used when supramesenteric or supraceliac control is anticipated, as in the case of type IV thoracoabdominal aneurysms. Repair of type III thoracoabdominal aneurysms is performed by extending the abdominal incision across the costal margin to the 6th rib shown by *Line G*.

Figure 2A

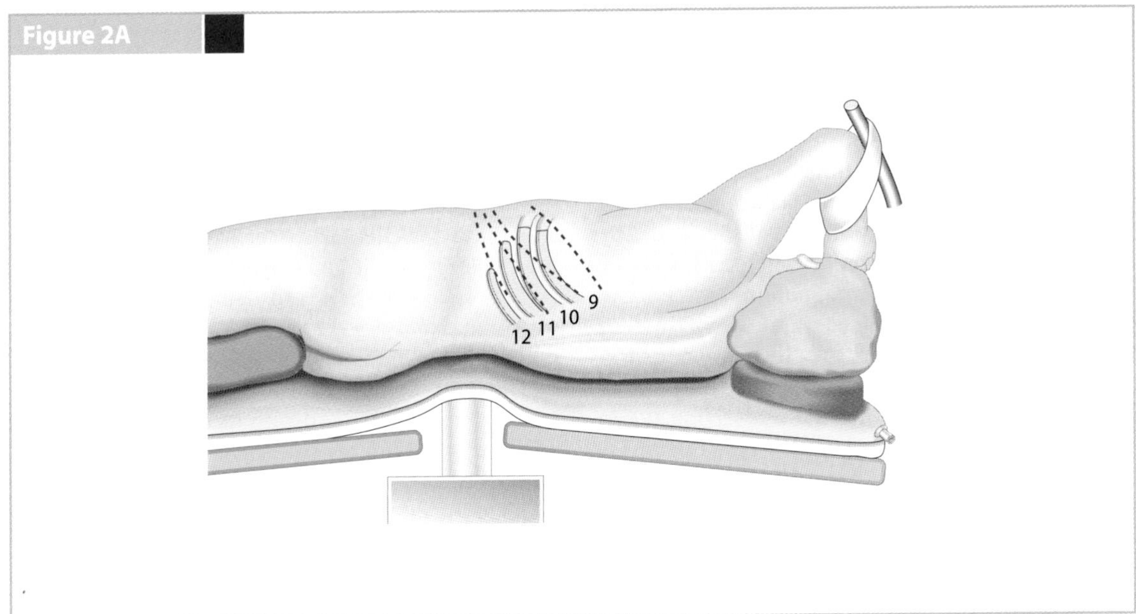

Figure 2B

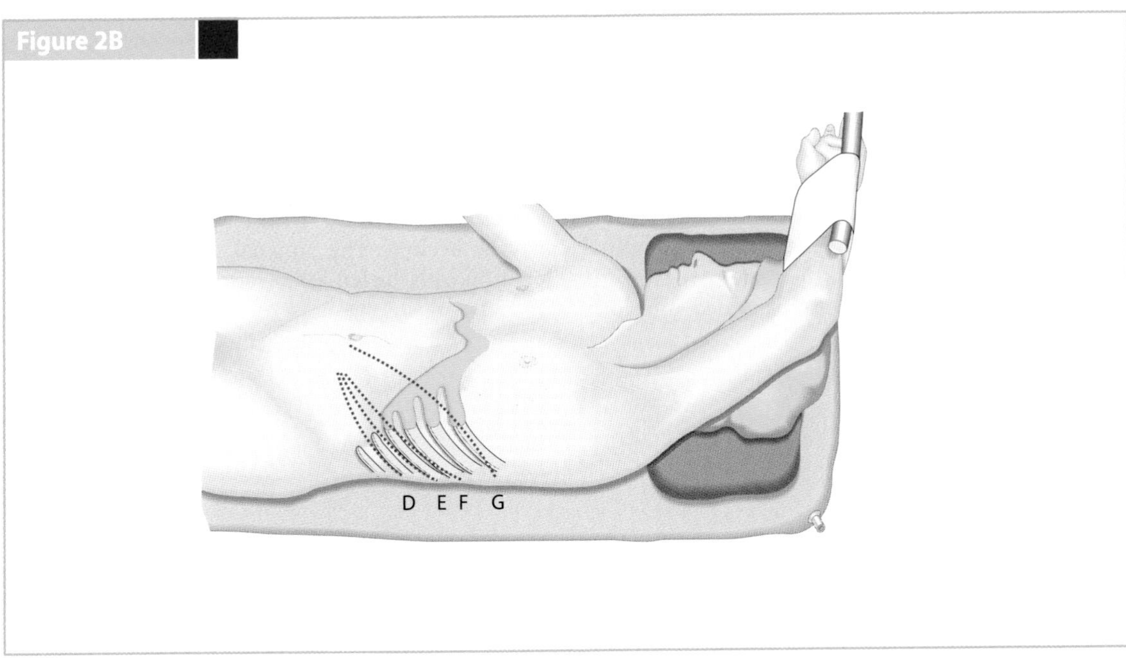

Figure 3

The subcutaneous tissue is divided with cautery. The lateral aspect of the anterior rectus sheath is incised, and the lateral half of the left rectus abdominis muscle is divided, defining the decussation at the lateral border of the rectus sheath. If the inferior epigastric vessels are encountered, they are ligated with silk ties prior to division. The external oblique fibers are divided along the remaining length of the incision, extending several centimeters over the rib. The fibrous decussation at the lateral aspect of the rectus sheath is sharply incised, exposing the underlying peritoneum.

The peritoneum is gently reflected off the overlying muscles, and the incision is extended 8–10 cm laterally. At this point, the musculotendinous wound edges are grasped with Kocher clamps, and the surgeon's finger is used to sweep the underlying peritoneum free of the musculature beneath the intended line of incision. The peritoneum should be reflected for 6–8 cm superior to the obliquely oriented incision, which facilitates later retractor placement. Inferiorly, the peritoneum is freed to the level of the inguinal region. The overlying inferior oblique and transversus abdominis muscles are elevated on the surgeon's fingers and divided. The exposed rib tip is resected in subperiosteal fashion.

At the level of the mid-axillary line, the fingers bluntly dissecting the peritoneum off the abdominal wall will be felt to drop into the fatty tissues of the retroperitoneum. This plane is extended inferiorly into the pelvis until the left iliac pulsation can be palpated. The assistant can then retract the peritoneal sac medially. At the lateral aspect of the incision, the exposed rib tip is resected, taking care to avoid entry into the pleural space. A sternal retractor is then secured to the muscular layers of the incision with large silk sutures and deployed. An Omni retractor is also utilized to provide stable visualization of the surgical field.

The left ureter is identified at the base of the retracted peritoneum, and with its accompanying vascular pedicle is loosely encircled with a Silastic vessel loop. The ureteral pedicle is then dissected proximally to the inferior pole of the left kidney, and inferiorly to the level of the iliac artery. Careful sharp dissection may be required to separate an adherent ureter from an aneurysmal left common iliac artery.

For routine infrarenal AAA repair, the left kidney is left in situ in its retroperitoneal location. To identify the plane between the left colon and Gerota's fascia, the left gonadal vein is located along the lateral aspect of the peritoneal sac and traced proximally to its junction with the left renal vein. The overlying fatty tissues are carefully thinned and the edge of the peritoneal sac is left inviolate and reflected medially. A large pedicle of excess fatty tissue is often noted anterior to the true Gerota's fascia, and may be excised. The gonadal vein is ligated at its junction with the left renal vein and divided.

Figure 3

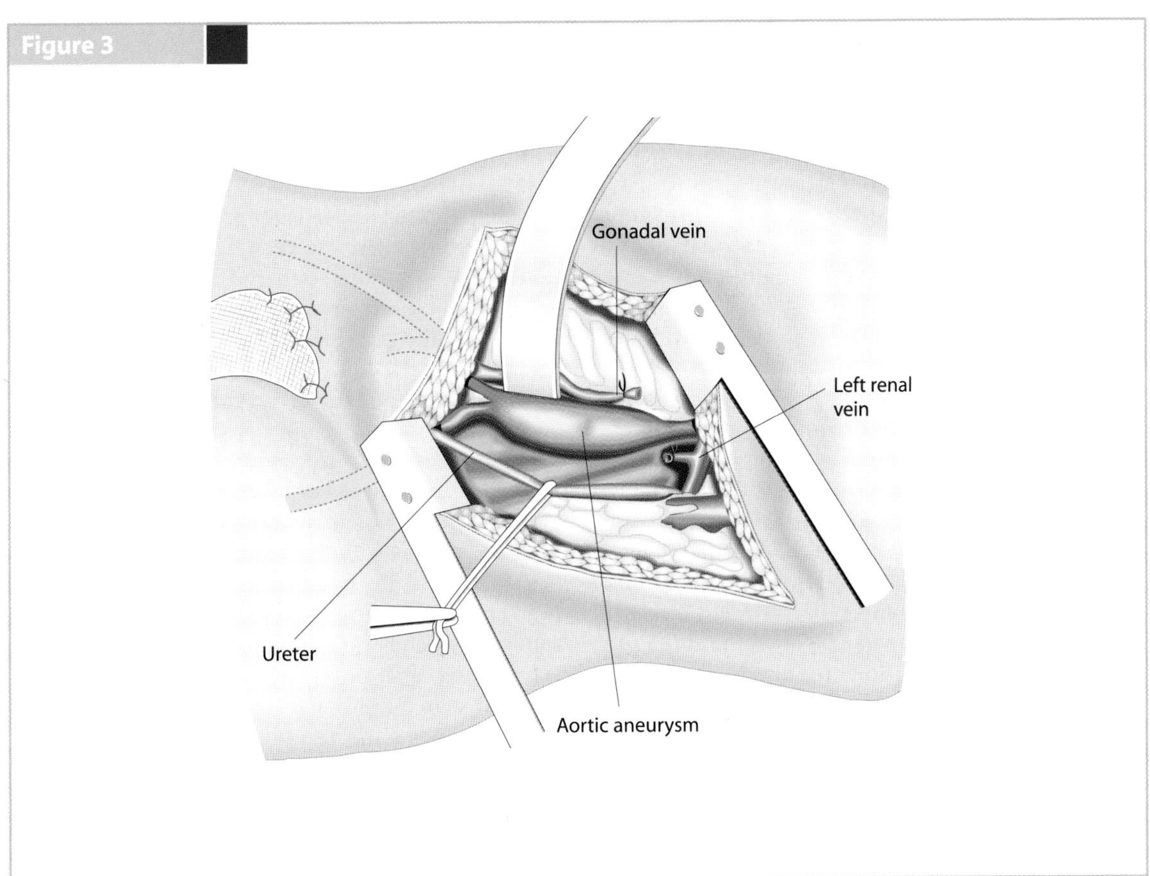

Figure 4A, B

The inferior edge of the left renal vein is sharply dissected free. The pulsatile aneurysm neck is felt directly inferior to the vein. The surgeon's finger is used to bluntly dissect space for clamp placement anterior and posterior to the aorta, at the level of or just inferior to the renal vein. The posterior dissection should proceed in the clear space between lumbar artery branches. No attempt is made to fully encircle the aortic neck, as this blind maneuver may lead to significant caval injury

Distal control of the left common, external, and internal iliac arteries is readily obtained. The parasympathetic neural fibers crossing the proximal left common iliac artery are preserved. Elevation of the areolar tissue and superior rectal vascular pedicle from the aortic bifurcation allows visualization of the proximal right common iliac artery. Control of the right iliac artery may also be obtained at the time of aneurysm sac entry using Pruitt balloon occlusion catheters. If extension of the graft limbs to one or both femoral arteries is required, exposure of the femoral vessels should be obtained at this time.

After systemic heparinization, proximal and distal clamps are applied and the aneurysm sac is entered along its left lateral surface. A Weitlaner retractor or silk stay sutures can be used to maintain exposure of the sac. Mural thrombus is manually evacuated, taking care not to displace any clot into the proximal iliac vessels or inferior mesenteric artery. Proximally, the longitudinal incision is extended anteriorly and posteriorly to facilitate visualization of the aneurysm neck. Backbleeding from paired lumbar arteries and the inferior mesenteric artery is controlled with silk sutures from inside the aneurysm sac (Fig. 4A). If the aneurysm shell is heavily calcified, limited endarterectomy of the sac may facilitate suturing of these vessels.

The graft is brought onto the field. If using a bifurcated graft, the proximal trunk must be shortened to ensure that the graft bifurcation remains proximal to the native aortic bifurcation. The proximal anastomosis is performed using running 2-0 or 3-0 Prolene suture. Use of a continuous reinforcing strip of Teflon felt pledget is recommended when the surgeon is faced with a thinned or heavily diseased aortic wall at the anastomotic site. After completion of the proximal anastomosis, the proximal clamp is briefly released to clear the graft of any debris. The graft is then clamped several centimeters distal to the anastomosis, which is carefully inspected for hemostasis. Hemostasis can be addressed using mattressed, doubly pledgeted 3-0 Prolene sutures. The distal graft is flushed with heparinized saline.

The distal anastomoses are then created in the desired configuration. Figure 4B demonstrates a tube graft repair. Prior to anastomosis completion, the native vessels and graft are allowed to flush out via the incomplete suture line. The lumen is irrigated with heparinized saline and the suture line is completed. Gradual restoration of lower extremity flow, accompanied by administration of intravenous fluids, will avoid precipitous changes in blood pressure.

Figure 4A

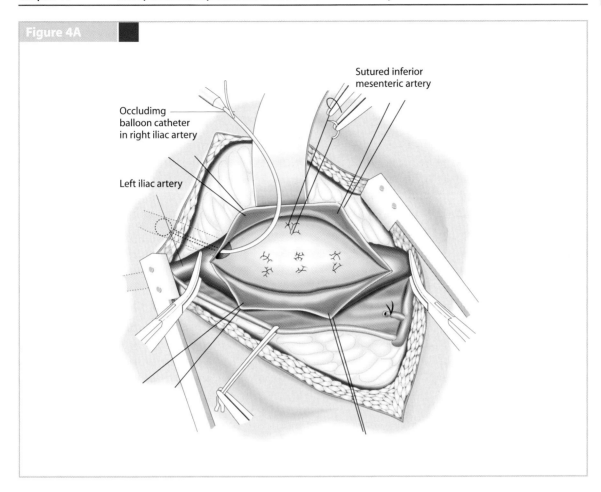

Sutured inferior mesenteric artery

Occludimg balloon catheter in right iliac artery

Left iliac artery

Figure 4B

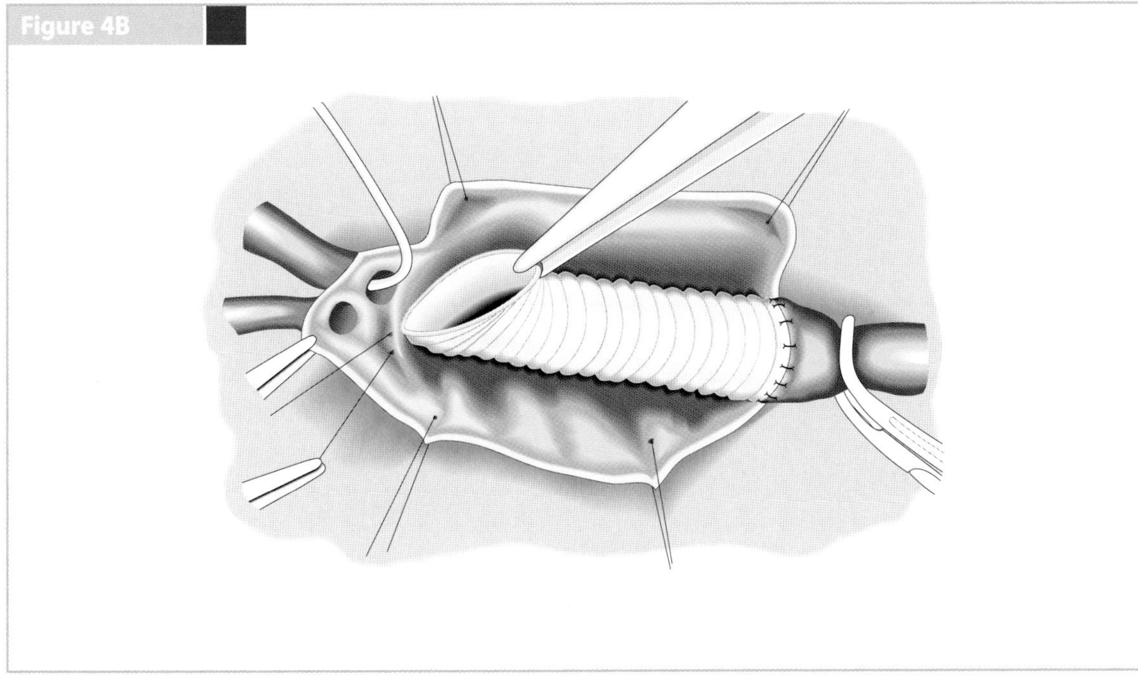

Figure 5A, B

In the presence of iliac occlusive or aneurysmal disease, aortic reconstruction is performed with a bifurcated graft. For purely occlusive disease, an end-to-side proximal anastomosis may be created (Fig. 5A), whereas for aneurysmal disease, an end-to-end proximal anastomosis (Fig. 5B) is chosen to exclude the aneurysm sac. The limbs of the graft are tunneled to the groin incisions along the course of the native iliac vessels, and positioned posterior to the overlying ureters.

Figure 5A

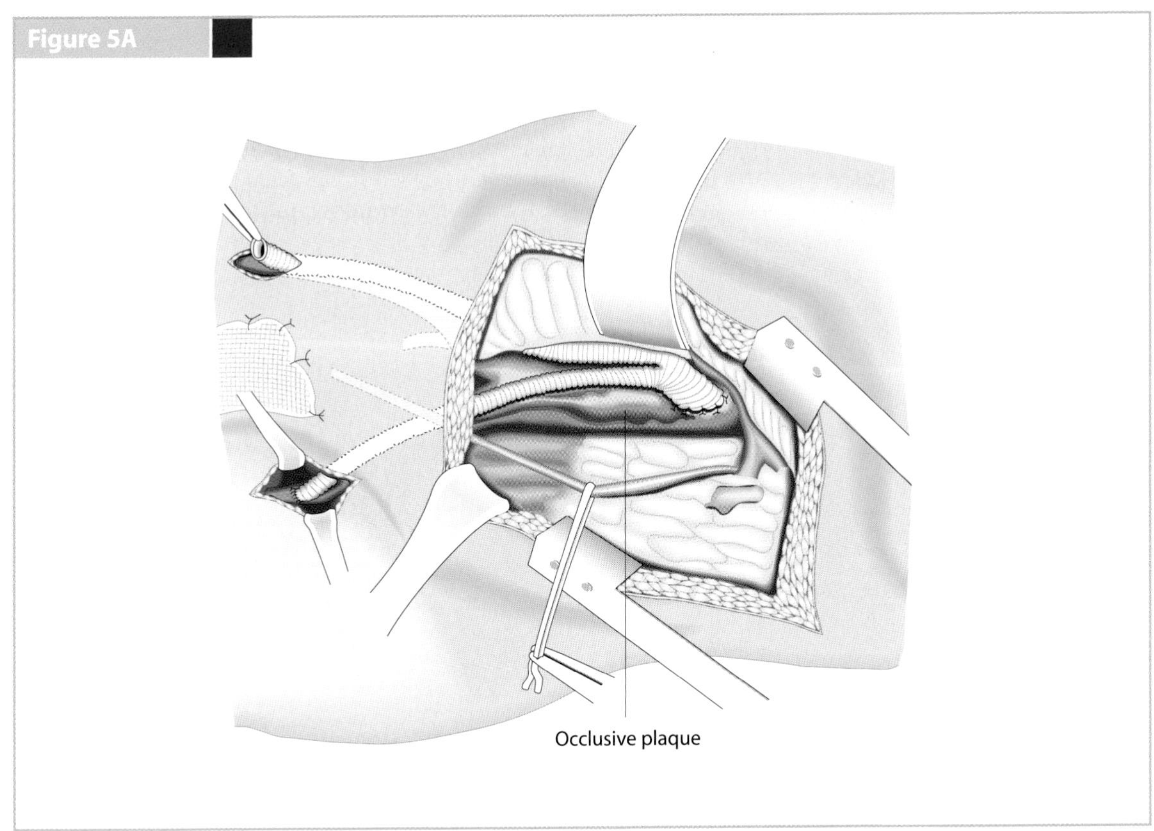

Figure 5B

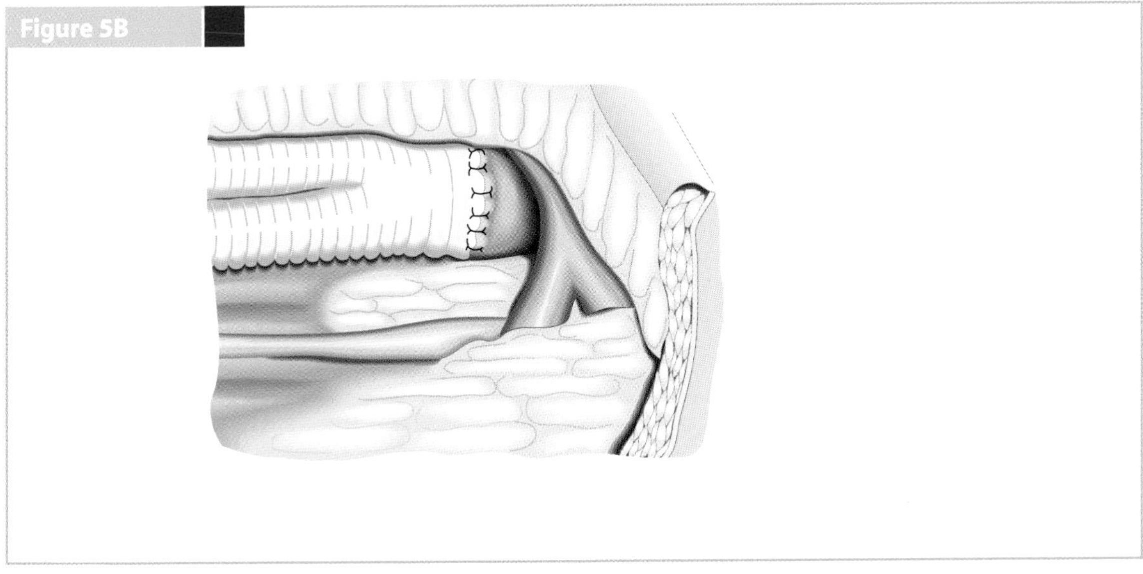

Figure 6

For repairs extending above the renal arteries, the diaphragmatic crura are opened proximally along the left posterolateral aspect of the aorta (Fig. 6A). If needed, the diaphragm may be incised circumferentially to improve exposure, leaving a 2-cm rim attached to the chest wall to facilitate later closure. The kidney may be left in the renal fossa, or rotated anteriorly with the peritoneum (Fig. 6B).

Figure 6A

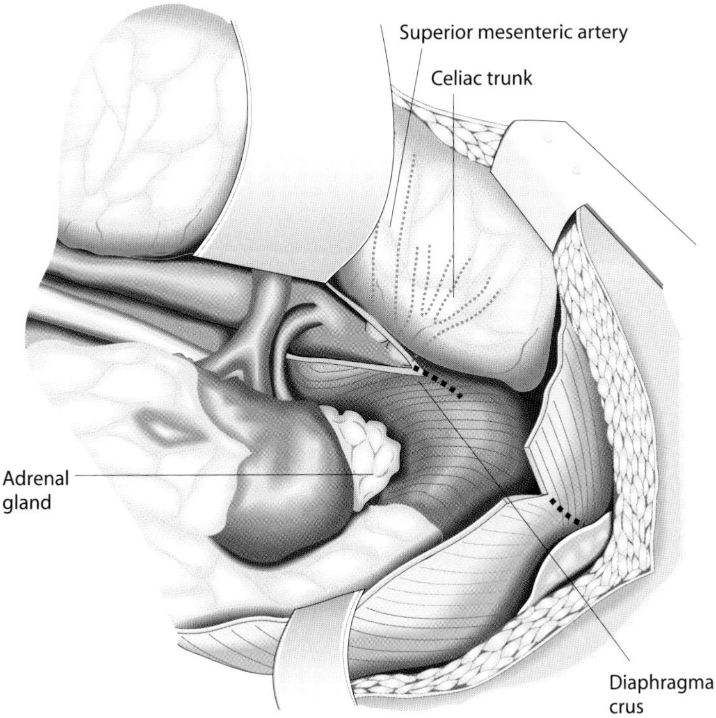

Superior mesenteric artery
Celiac trunk
Adrenal gland
Diaphragma crus

Figure 6B

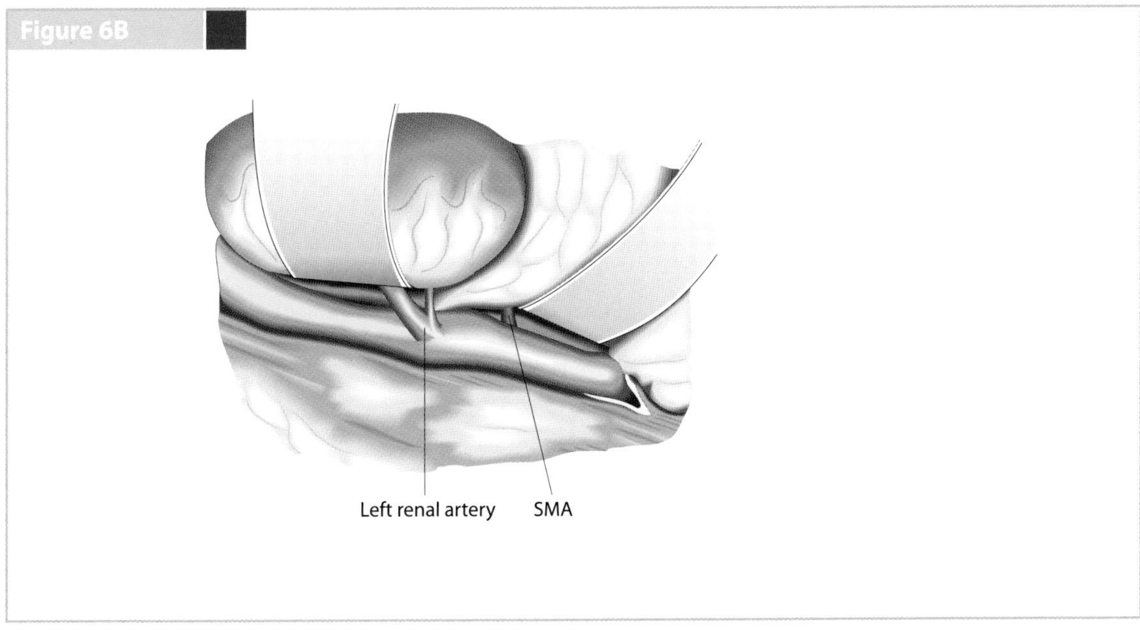

Figure 7

As shown in Fig. 7A, B, the repair can be performed with the kidney up or down. The proximal clamp may be placed between the renal arteries and SMA if an adequate length of nondiseased aorta is present. If not, a supraceliac crossclamp (Fig. 7C) is used.

Figure 7A

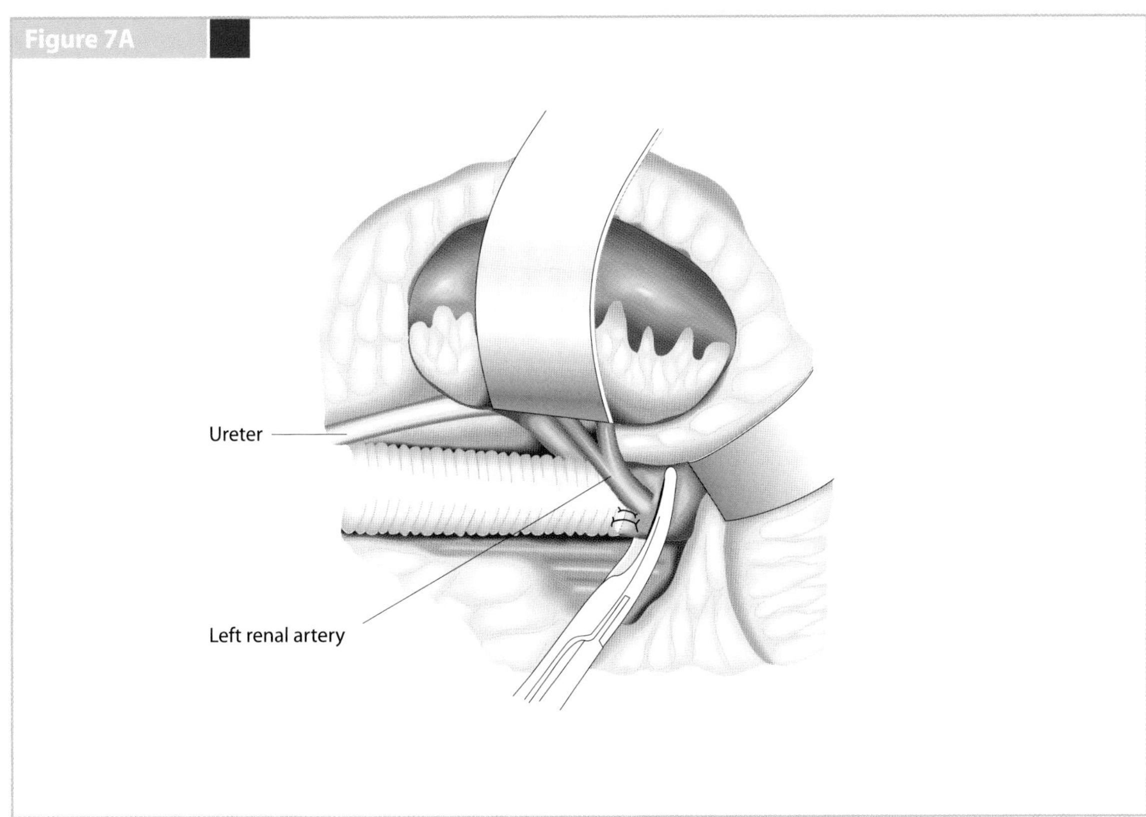

Figure 7B

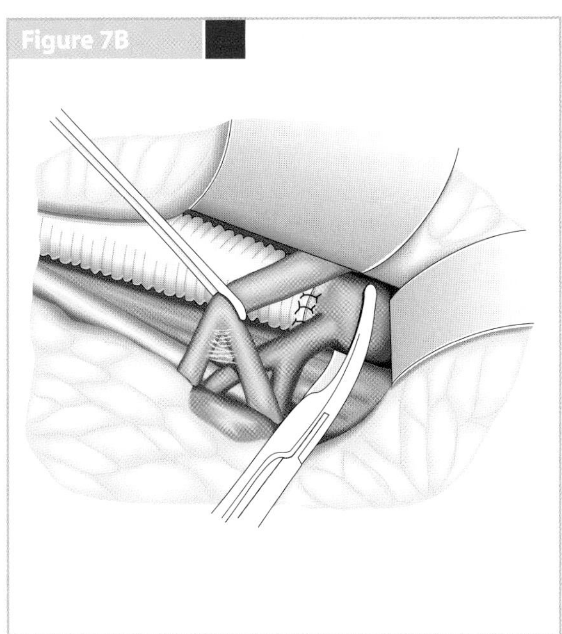

Figure 7C

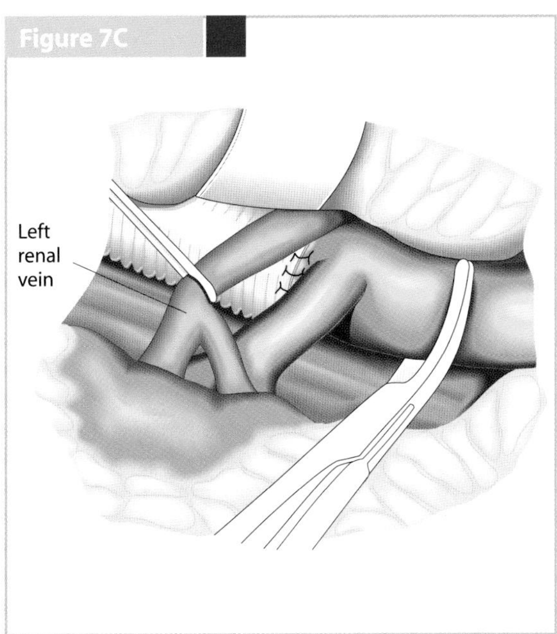

Figure 8

For aneurysmal disease extending proximal to the renal artery orifices, a beveled graft configuration is often used at the proximal anastomosis. The aorta is opened posterior to the left renal artery. An anterior patch that includes the orifices of the visceral vessels and right renal artery is fashioned. The renal vessels are perfused with cold heparinized saline solution via balloon irrigation catheters while the anastomosis is constructed. The left renal artery may be resected from the aorta as a Carrel patch, perfused during completion of the proximal anastomosis (Fig. 8A), and later reimplanted on the lateral aspect of the new graft (Fig. 8B).

After restoration of pelvic and lower extremity flow, the inferior mesenteric artery and left colonic perfusion are assessed. If needed, a small window may be created in the peritoneum to allow direct visualization of the left and sigmoid colon, and later closed with absorbable suture. In the setting of inadequate colonic perfusion, the IMA orifice is excised from the aneurysm sac as a Carrel patch, and reimplanted on the adjacent graft using a side-biting clamp. Adequate pedal, renal, and visceral flow is confirmed prior to preparing for closure.

After hemostasis has been obtained, the field is irrigated and the retractors removed. The aneurysm shell is allowed to collapse over the graft. No closure of the redundant aneurysm sac is required. The peritoneum and its contents are returned to their native position. The table is returned to the neutral position, facilitating a tension-free closure.

The abdominal wall is closed in two layers using heavy looped PDS suture. The deep layer is composed of the posterior rectus sheath, transversus abdominis and inferior oblique muscles. The superficial layer is composed of the anterior rectus sheath and external oblique muscle. The skin is approximated with staples and an occlusive dressing is placed. Closure of groin incisions is performed with several layers of running absorbable suture.

Figure 8A

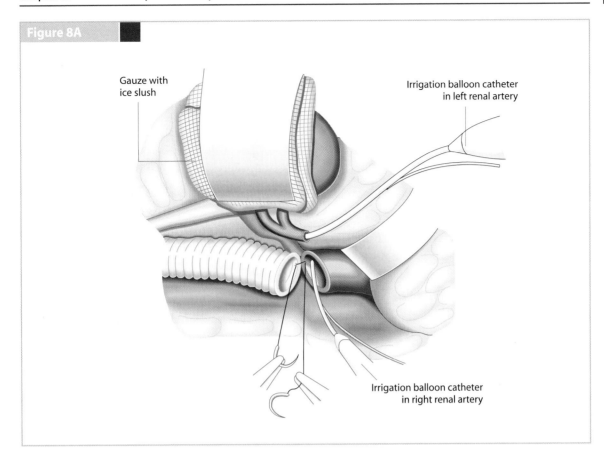

Gauze with ice slush

Irrigation balloon catheter in left renal artery

Irrigation balloon catheter in right renal artery

Figure 8B

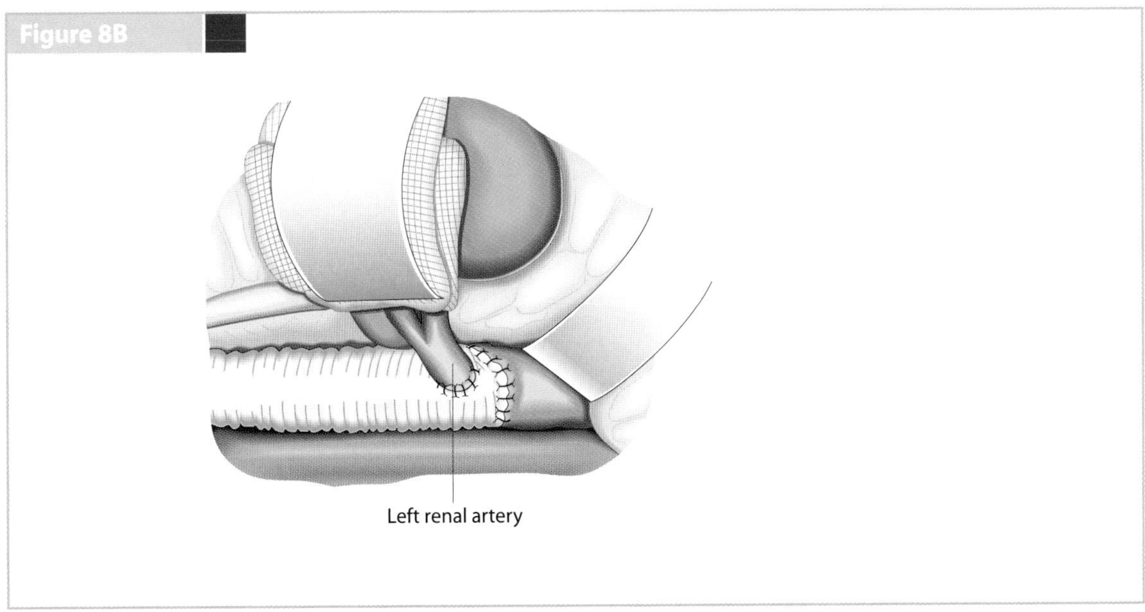

CONCLUSION

Long-term survival following successful AAA repair is largely dependent on the progression of coronary atherosclerosis. Continued follow-up is essential to detect possible late complications of open repair, including graft infection and anastomotic pseudoaneurysm formation. It has been our practice to perform computed tomography of the chest, abdomen, and pelvis 5 years after infrarenal AAA repair, to assess for development of new aneurysms in the proximal or distal vasculature.

REFERENCES

Cambria RP et al. (1992) The impact of selective use of dipyridamole-thallium scans and surgical factors on the current morbidity of aortic surgery. J Vasc Surg 15(1):43–50; discussion 51

Dardik A et al. (1999) Results of elective abdominal aortic aneurysm repair in the 1990s: A population-based analysis of 2335 cases. J Vasc Surg 30(6):985–995

Katz DJ, Stanley JC, Zelenock GB (1994) Operative mortality rates for intact and ruptured abdominal aortic aneurysms in Michigan: an eleven-year statewide experience. J Vasc Surg 19(5):804–815; discussion 816–817

Lederle FA et al. (2002) Immediate repair compared with surveillance of small abdominal aortic aneurysms. N Engl J Med 346(19):1437–1444

Minino AM et al. (2002) Deaths: final data for 2000. National Center for Health Statistics. National Vital Statistics Reports 50(6)

Richardson JD, Main KA (1991) Repair of abdominal aortic aneurysms. A statewide experience. Arch Surg 126(5):614–616

Sicard GA, Reilly JM (1994) Left retroperitoneal approach to the aorta and its branches: part I. Ann Vasc Surg 8(2):212–219

Sicard GA et al. (1995) Transabdominal versus retroperitoneal incision for abdominal aortic surgery: report of a prospective randomized trial. J Vasc Surg 21(2):174–181; discussion 181–183

The UK Small Aneurysm Trial Participants (1998) Mortality results for randomised controlled trial of early elective surgery or ultrasonographic surveillance for small abdominal aortic aneurysms. Lancet 352(9141):1649–1655

CHAPTER 17

Endovascular Treatment of Abdominal Aortic Aneurysms

Alan B. Lumsden, Eric K. Peden, Ruth L. Bush, Peter H. Lin, Lyssa N. Ochoa, Jonathon C. Nelson

INTRODUCTION

Aneurysmal disease of the aorta affects 5% of the adult population in the United States and abdominal aortic aneurysms (AAA) are responsible for approximately 20,000 deaths per year, making it the 10th most common cause of death in males over age of 60 (Prisant and Mondy 2004; Scott et al. 1991; Spurgeon 2004). The majority of aneurysms are asymptomatic, most being diagnosed incidentally during physical examination or when undergoing abdominal imaging for an unrelated cause. Early diagnosis and treatment will dramatically improve the outcome of this lethal disease, since the mortality of an elective operation is approximately 2% (Blum et al. 1996).

The detection of a pulsatile abdominal mass and demonstration of an AAA by CT scan or ultrasound of an AAA >5.5 cm in diameter is an indication for surgery. AAA grow on average 0.4 cm per year. The annual rupture rate of a 5.5-cm AAA is 3–4%; however, the rupture rate increases exponentially with increasing diameter such that a 7.0-cm AAA has a 19%/year rupture rate (Brown and Powell 1999; Boyle et al. 2003).

The first widely read description of a prosthetic endovascular graft for repair of an AAA was by Parodi et al. in 1991. Since then, many studies have demonstrated the technical feasibility and effectiveness of AAA exclusion from the systemic circulation (Bush et al. 2003; May et al. 1998). Currently, approximately 40–50% of infrarenal AAA can be treated with endovascular stent-grafts. However, various anatomical features of AAA exclude many patients from endoluminal repair or lead to technical difficulties in stent-graft delivery. Anatomical limitations for the applicability of stent-grafts include a short or wide neck, severe neck angulation, and tortuous or stenotic access arteries. The criteria for candidate selection are in evolution as are the development of improved grafts and delivery systems. It is likely as experience with stent-grafts and endoluminal techniques increases, more patients with infrarenal AAA will be treatable in this manner. Furthermore, a smaller diameter, more flexible delivery system potentially could address several of the anatomical restrictions of stent-graft implantation.

There are currently two approaches to repair of AAA: either open via a transabdominal or retroperitoneal approach, or using an endovascular graft. The use of endovascular stent grafting has moved from the initial phase of overhyped exuberance to one of more objective evaluation of its limitations, troubleshooting of long term aneurysm remodeling effects, and management of endoleaks. Proper selection of patients with AAA for endovascular stent-grafting (ESG) is essential for successful outcome. Some of the more important current characteristics include: proximal AAA neck diameter <26 mm (32 mm for Zenith); proximal AAA neck length >15 mm; neck angulation <60 degrees; absence of thrombus in the neck of the AAA; iliac artery >5 mm with minimal calcification, stenosis, and tortuosity; and finally adequate visceral blood supply (the SMA and at least one internal iliac artery should remain patent).

Preoperative imaging consists of a spiral CT scan with IV and no PO contrast. CT accurately characterizes the AAA, demonstrates additional abnormalities (venous anomalies, horseshoe kidney, iliac aneurysms, gallstones, etc.) and reliably excludes patients from ESG. Angiography is being performed less frequently but, if performed, should employ a calibrated pigtail catheter to permit accurate length and diameter measurement.

Figures 1

There are presently four Food and Drug Administration (FDA)-approved systems: (1) the AneuRx (Medtronic Inc.) (Fig. 1), which is a fully supported graft with a nitinol exoskeleton that incorporates proximal aortic and iliac extender cuffs if needed (Zarins 2003); (2) the Excluder (WL Gore) (Fig. 9), which is a PTFE graft with a nitinol exoskeleton and proximal barbs to prevent distal migration (the Excluder also has extenders available) (Matsumura et al. 2001, 2003); (3) the Zenith (Cook Inc.) (Greenberg 2003); and (4) the Powerlink (Endologix) which is a unibody bifurcated system made of ePTFE supported by an endoskeleton constructed using a single wire of Cobalt Chromium (Figure 20). The type of system used depends on the personal expertise of the implanting physician. However, the diameter of the endograft must be oversized by at least 10% when compared to the aortic neck diameter. The Ancure device, which was a unibody bifurcated graft and was one of the first two approved, has subsequently been removed from the market (Moore et al. 2003).

The AneuRx endograft, by Medtronic Co. (Fig. 1), is a bifurcated modular device. The first generation AneuRx was made in 1994 and consisted of a stiff body design incorporating a thin polyester luminal fabric externally supported by a self-expanding Nitinol skeleton. The fabric and exoskeleton are bonded by more than 2000 hand tied sutures. The current generation AneuRx aortic endograft has an increased number of 1-cm Nitinol rings resulting in increased flexibility and fewer deployment and long-term complications. The main body of the endograft consists of a 3-cm aortic segment with an ipsilateral iliac limb of variable length. The contralateral portion of the main or bifurcated segment contains a gate into which the contralateral iliac limb must be inserted and deployed. The deficiencies relate to the lack of conformability and increased tendency for module separation.

In order to use this device the femoral arteries are exposed and introducer sheaths (8F) are placed. Systemic heparin is given. Guidewires (0.035“×180-cm stiff wire, ipsilateral and 180-cm Bentsen wire, contralateral) are placed.

A pigtail catheter is then placed in the suprarenal aorta through the ipsilateral common femoral artery and a straight angiographic catheter should be placed in the suprarenal aorta through the contralateral common femoral artery. An angiogram is performed through the pigtail catheter, and the positions of the renal arteries, aortic bifurcation and internal iliac arteries are noted and marked on the screen. Measurements are checked and the appropriate sized device selected.

Figures 2A, B, 3, 4

The ipsilateral guidewire is exchanged for an Amplatz Super Stiff 0.035“ wire well into the descending thoracic aorta. Via a transverse arteriotomy in the common femoral artery, the main delivery catheter is placed either "bare-back" or through a previously placed 22F sheath into the artery and is advanced over the wire into the suprarenal position. Although the blunt tip on the original AneuRx device necessitated use of a sheath, the current iteration has a nicely tapered tip (Fig. 2A) and consequently a sheathless technique can be performed. It is our preference to use a sheath if the host arteries are large enough as it facilitates device exchange and contrast injection. The device is rotated aligning the contralateral gate in the desired direction (Fig. 2B). In the most recent device there are three markers at the leading edge and a more proximal marker which can be used to orient the device. With intermittent contrast injection, very accurate positioning of the device at the level of the renal arteries is possible (Fig. 3). Positioning the gate anteriorly, or even crossing the limbs, may be beneficial depending on the configuration of the aneurysm to facilitate cannulation of the gate.

With the main body oriented properly, the graft is deployed by turning the handle, which slowly retracts the outer constraining sheath. Typically three to five revolutions are necessary before the graft begins to deploy. Once two to three stent rings are deployed, the device is retraced down to an approximate infrarenal position. Contrast injections through the remaining flush catheter are used to permit very accurate graft placement. The device is then deployed by continuing to rotate the handle. A variety of techniques are used to complete main body deployment. It is our practice to stop the deployment once the gate has been completely deployed (Fig. 4). A sheath through the contralateral groin will be used to buttress the main body during completion and runner withdrawal.

Figure 1

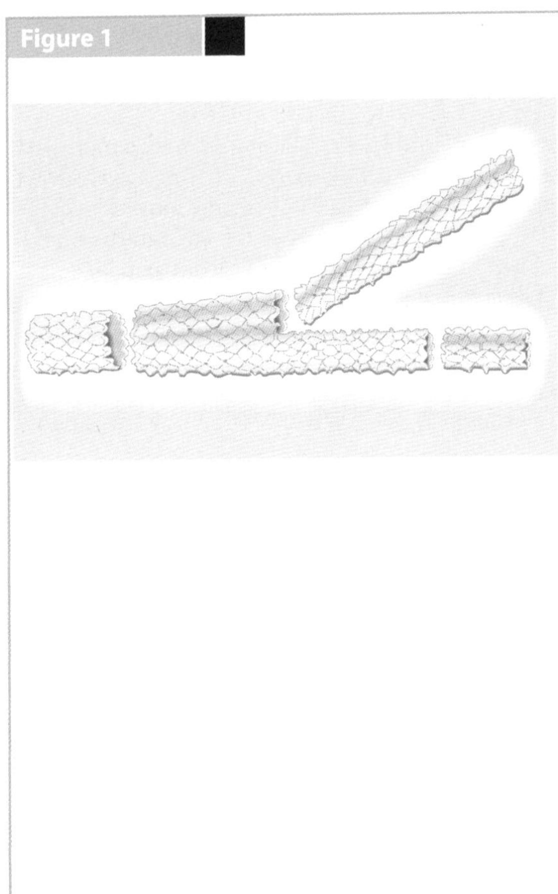

Figure 2A

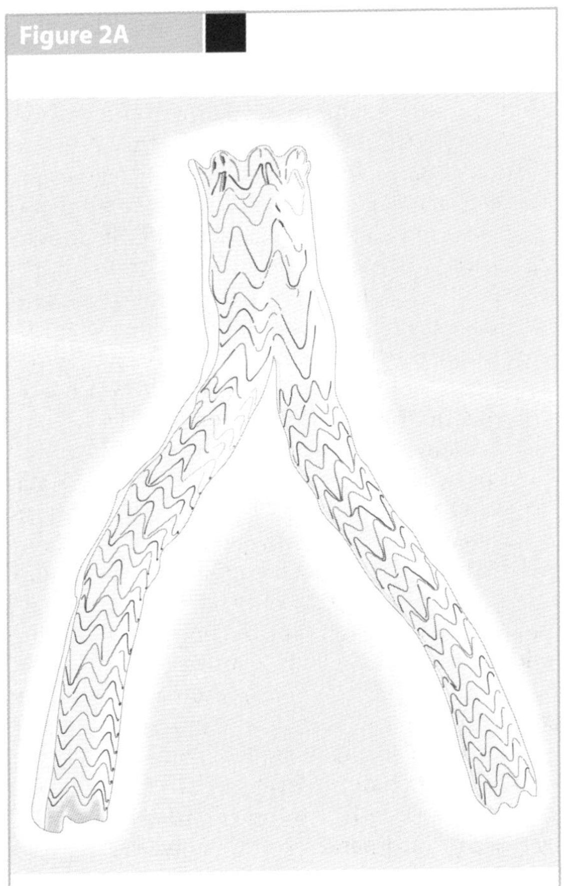

Figure 2B

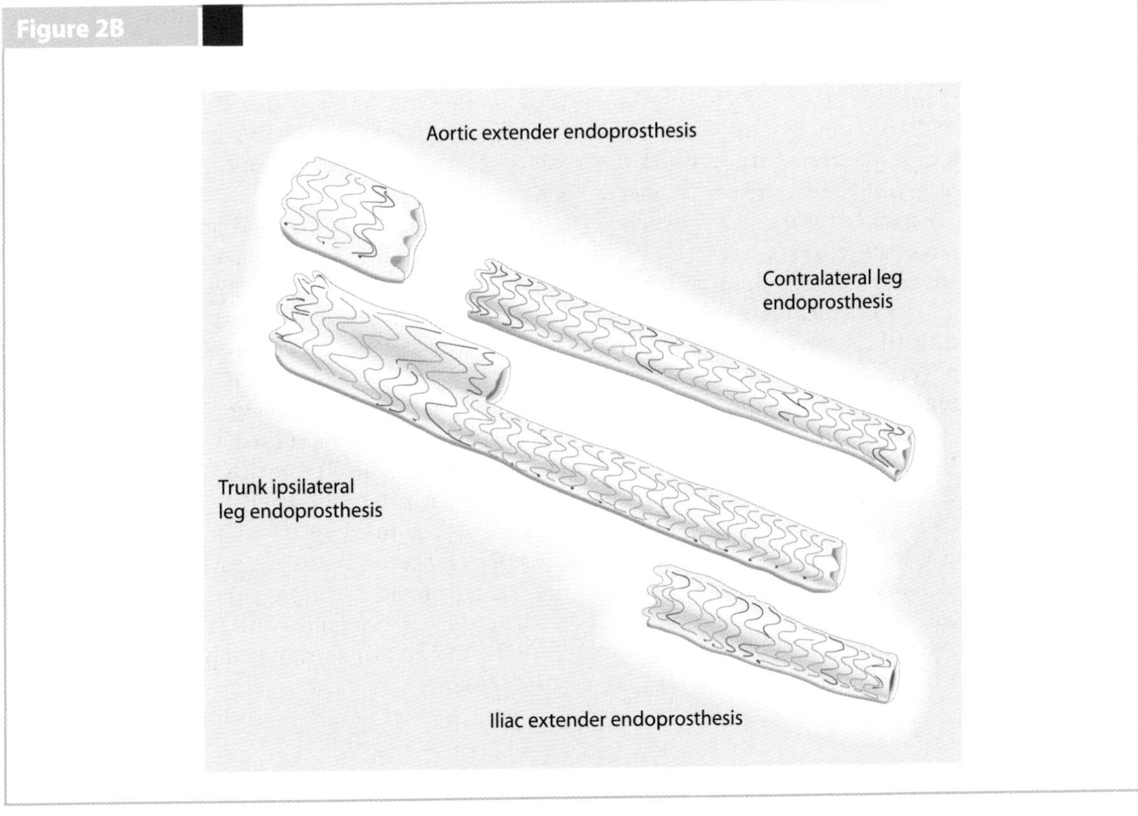

Figures 3, 4

Figure 3

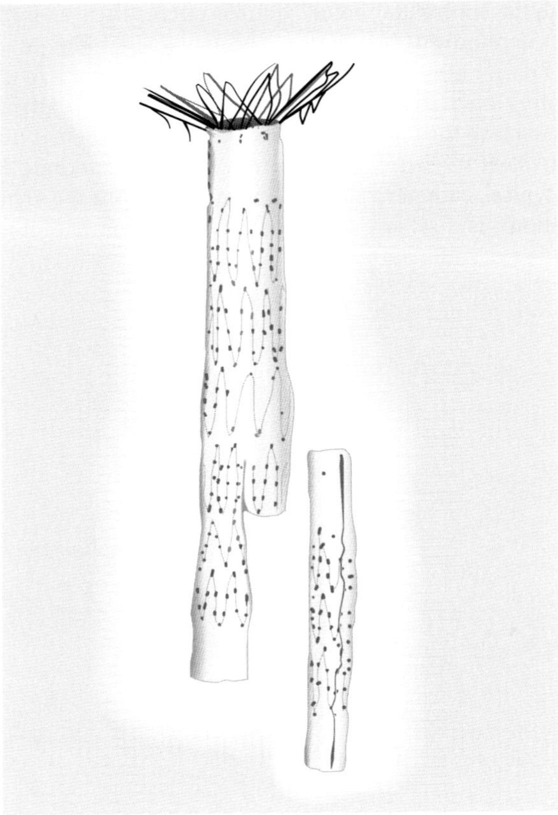

Figure 4

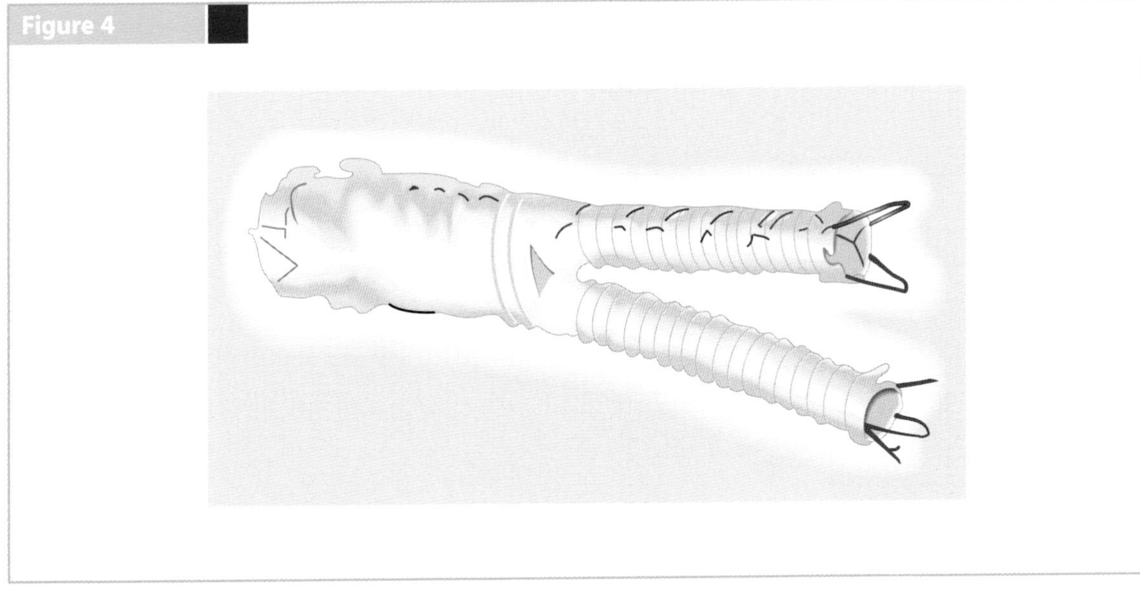

Figure 5A, B

An angled glide wire is placed through the contralateral straight catheter and the catheter is removed. A Bernstein catheter is advanced over the wire into the aneurysm sac and placed immediately below the contralateral gate, the wire is withdrawn into the aneurysm sac and the catheter is used to steer the wire to cannulate the gate (Fig. 5). Our typical catheter selection for difficult gate cannulations is first a Bernstein catheter followed by a Cobra 2 catheter, renal double curve, then a multipurpose catheter. Very occasionally, inability to cannulate the gate from below requires use of a reversed curve catheter to go over the bifurcation advancing a wire down into the aneurysm sac where it is snared and retracted into the groin. An alternate approach is to pass long (260 cm) wire from the arm down through the gate into the aneurysm where it is again snared.

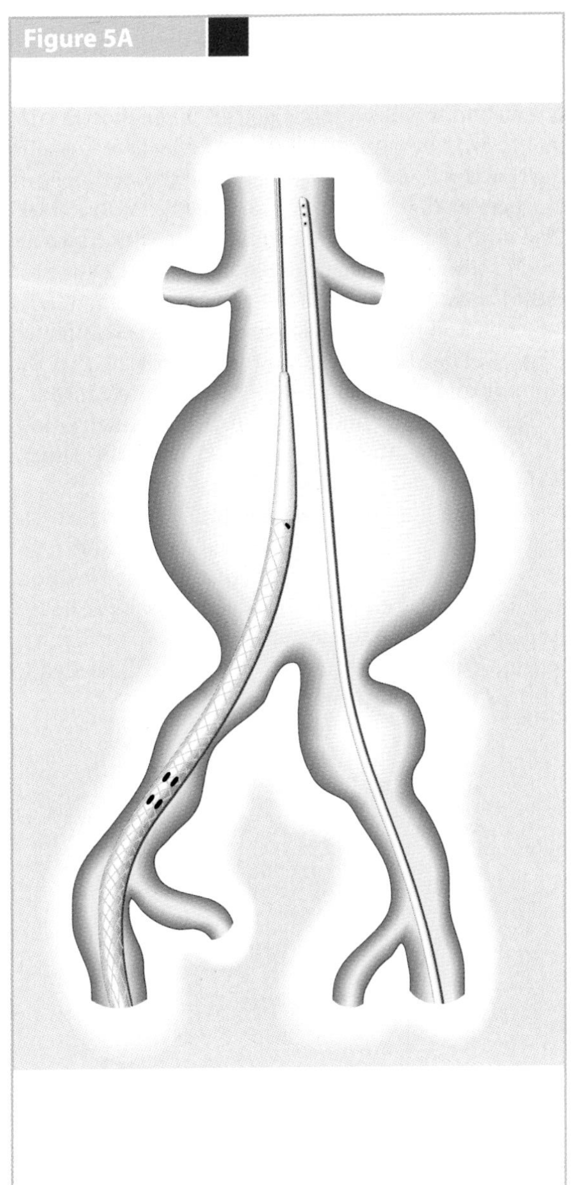
Figure 5A

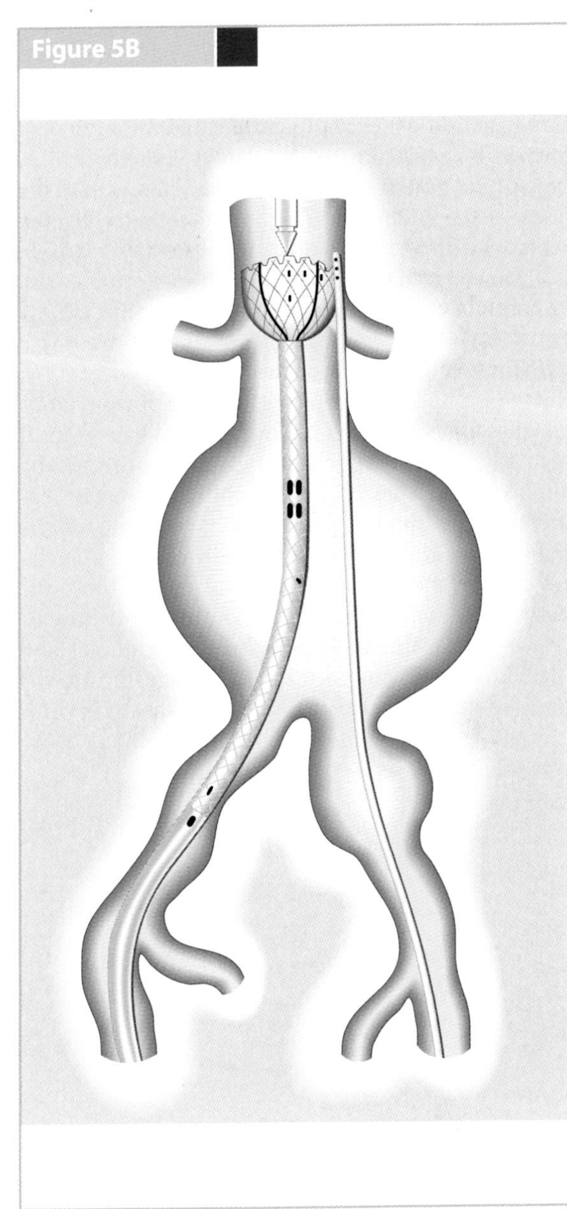
Figure 5B

Figures 6, 7A, B, 8A, B

Confirmation of successful gate cannulation is performed by replacing the Bernstein catheter with a pigtail and rotating the pigtail catheter within the body of the endograft. The pigtail catheter is then replaced with a 0.035" Amplatz Super Stiff wire which is advanced into the descending thoracic aorta. The 8F contralateral sheath is then replaced with a 16F/35-cm sheath delivered carefully under fluoroscopic guidance into the gate of the bifurcated device. At this point the dilator is retracted approximately 2 inches and the sheath is slowly pulled back until it just exits the gate. Gentle forward pressure can be applied to the sheath to buttress the bifurcated segment as the runners and delivery catheter of the main device are removed. After fully readvancing the 16F dilator, the 16F sheath is advanced well into the body of the main device in preparation for contralateral limb placement. The deployment catheter and iliac limb are advanced through the sheath into the body of the bifurcated segment. The sheath is withdrawn and the iliac limb is placed in position for deployment. The contralateral limb is deployed, ensuring maximal overlap by aligning the radiopaque markers at the top of the gate and the contralateral iliac limb (Fig. 6). The sheath must be withdrawn allowing clearance for safe deployment as was done for the bifurcated segment. The deployment handle is attached and the iliac limb deployment is completed (Fig. 7). The disconnect button is pressed and the runners and nose cone are retracted slowly into the delivery catheter under fluoroscopic visualization. The delivery catheter is removed from the sheath while maintaining guidewire access.

A completion angiogram is finally performed using a pigtail catheter (Fig. 8). Patency of the renal and hypogastric arteries, adequate graft position, and the presence or absence of endoleaks is noted. Angioplasty and the placement of aortic or iliac extension cuffs should then be performed if needed to address type I or type III endoleaks.

Figure 6

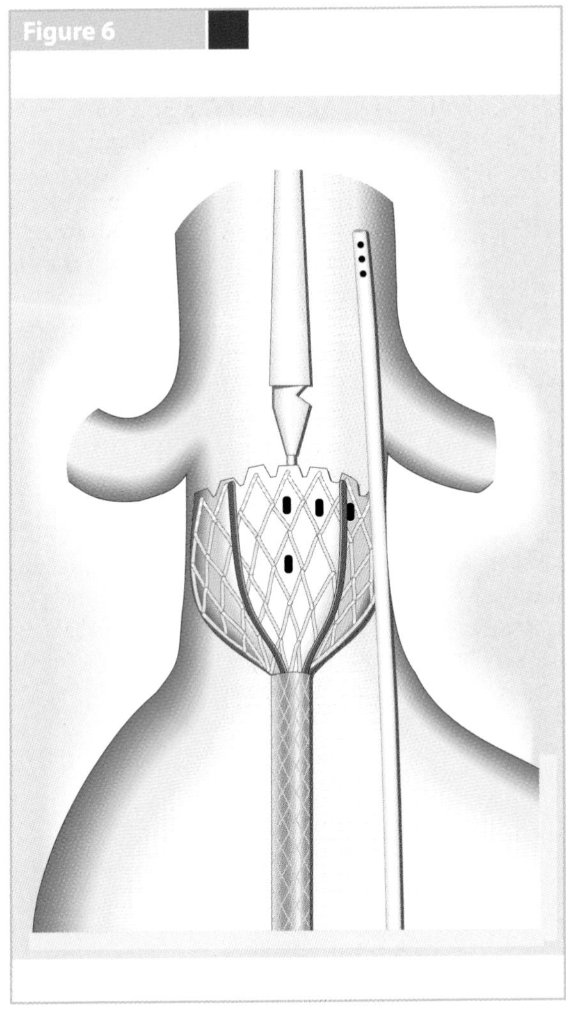

Figure 7A

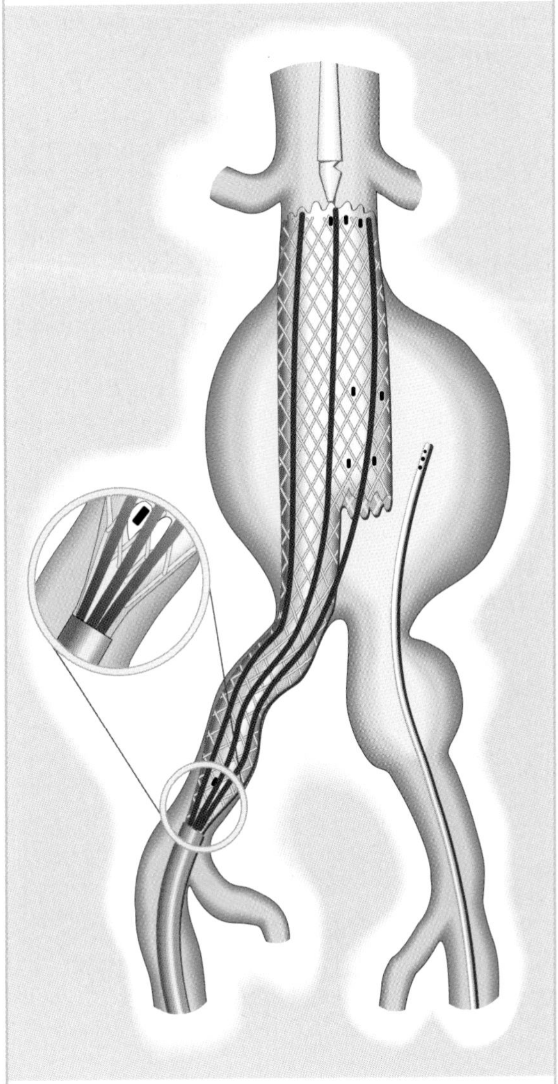

Figure 7B

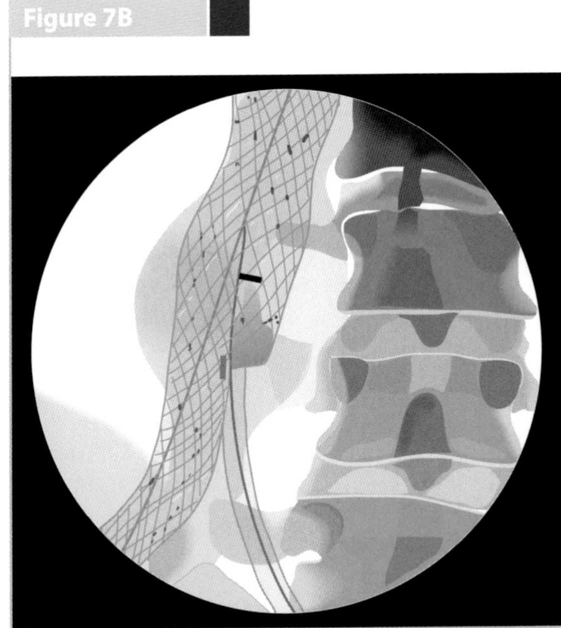

Figure 8A, B

Figure 8A

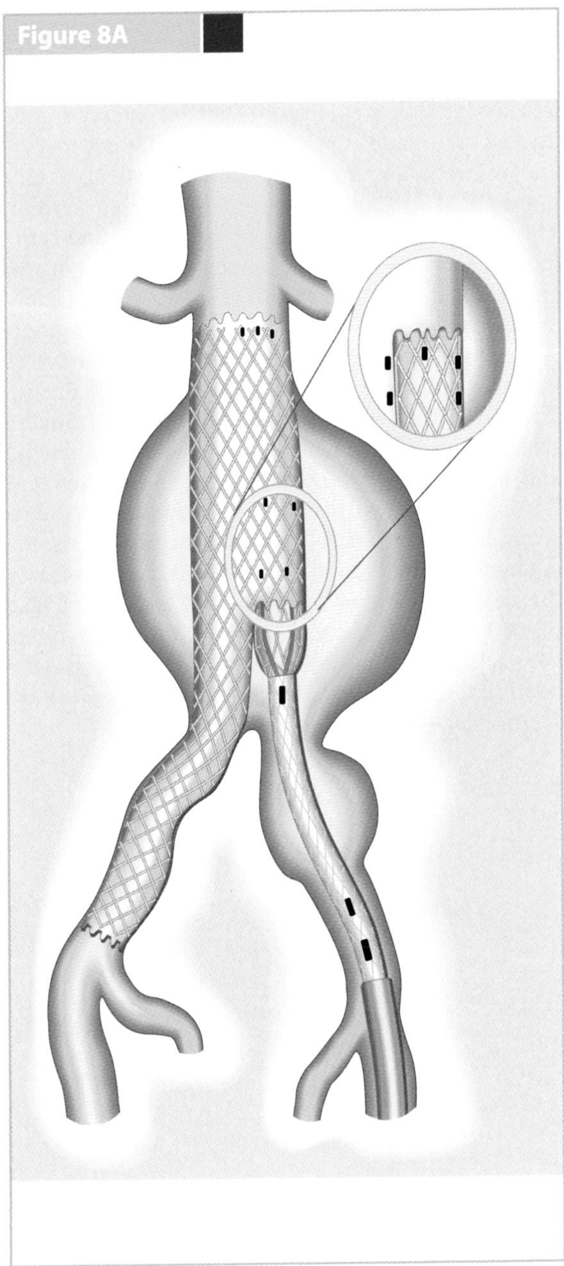

Figure 8B

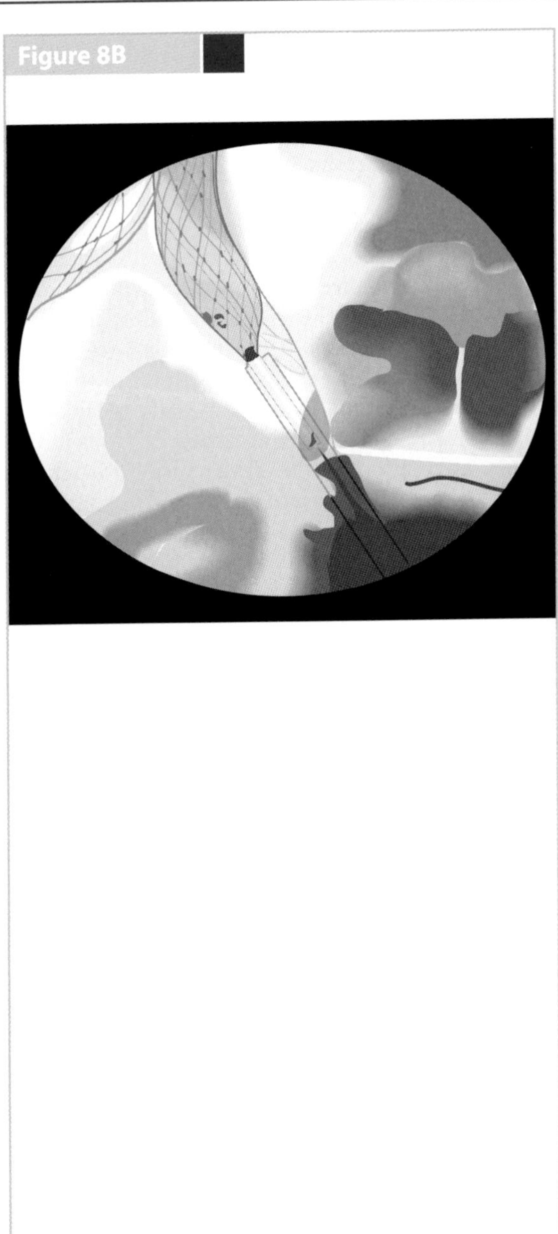

Figure 9A, B: The Excluder

The third device approved for use in the United States was the Gore Excluder. The Gore endoprosthesis is a modular system manufactured with an expanded polytetrafluoroethylene (ePTFE) prosthesis and is externally supported by a self-expanding nitinol stent structure (Fig. 9). Angled nitinol wire barbs are located at the proximal end of the main device (trunk-ipsilateral leg component) to provide additional anchoring support against the aortic wall. A radiopaque ring marks the contralateral leg opening. Radiopaque markers are present to facilitate proper orientation of the device prior to deployment. The contralateral prosthesis is also composed of a tapered ePTFE tube and a nitinol exoskeleton. The proximal end fits into the contralateral leg hole in the main device. Both components of the device have an attached sleeve (see Fig. 9) made of ePTFE that is sewn closed around the prostheses and functions to constrain them during positioning.

Aortic and iliac extenders are available and are designed to add additional length and/or to provide enhanced sealing. The aortic extenders allow for 1.5 cm of proximal extension. The iliac extenders give up to 4 cm of additional length to either the ipsilateral or contralateral leg components. Both accessory items are of similar composition as the main system. The Excluder has the smallest profile (18F) and is the most flexible. Therefore it is the graft of choice in patients with tortuous or small iliac vessels.

The self-expanding components of the Gore endoprosthesis come preloaded on delivery catheters that are similar for all modular components (Fig. 9). The outer shaft is reinforced with braided stainless steel and has two inner tubes, one for the guidewire and one for the deployment line. The deployment line is attached to the ePTFE sleeve that is sewn around the prosthesis. To release the prosthesis, the deployment line is pulled which effectively releases the sleeve and allows for device self-expansion. The trunk-ipsilateral leg component and aortic extenders are packaged within 18F delivery catheters while the contralateral leg component and iliac extenders are set on 12F delivery catheters.

Figure 9A

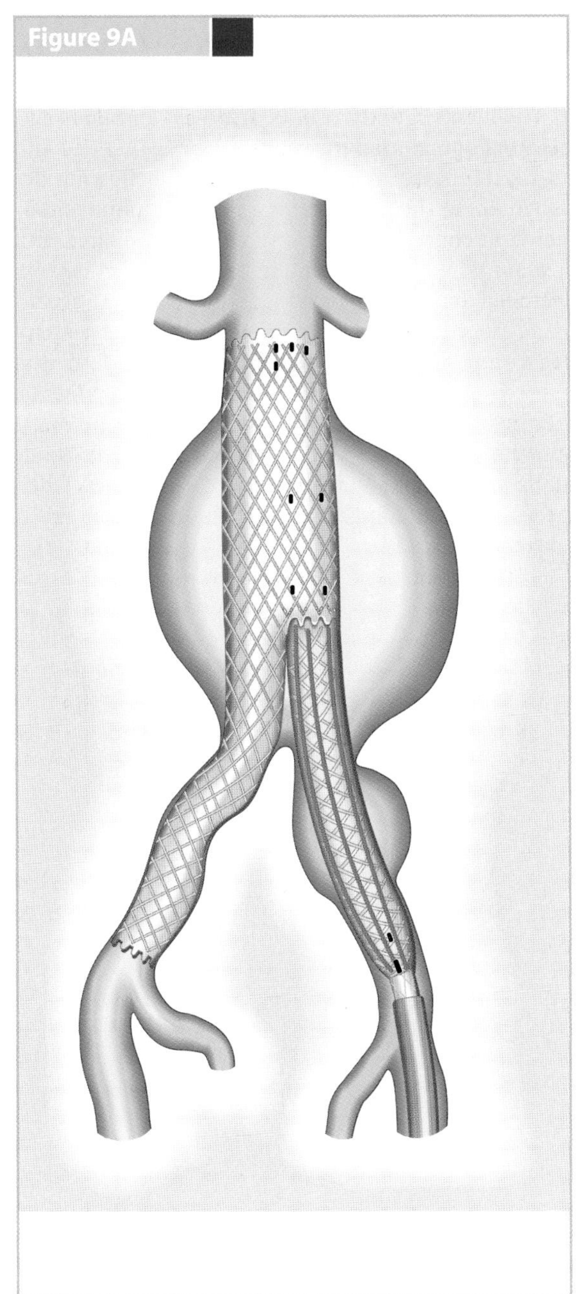

Figure 9B

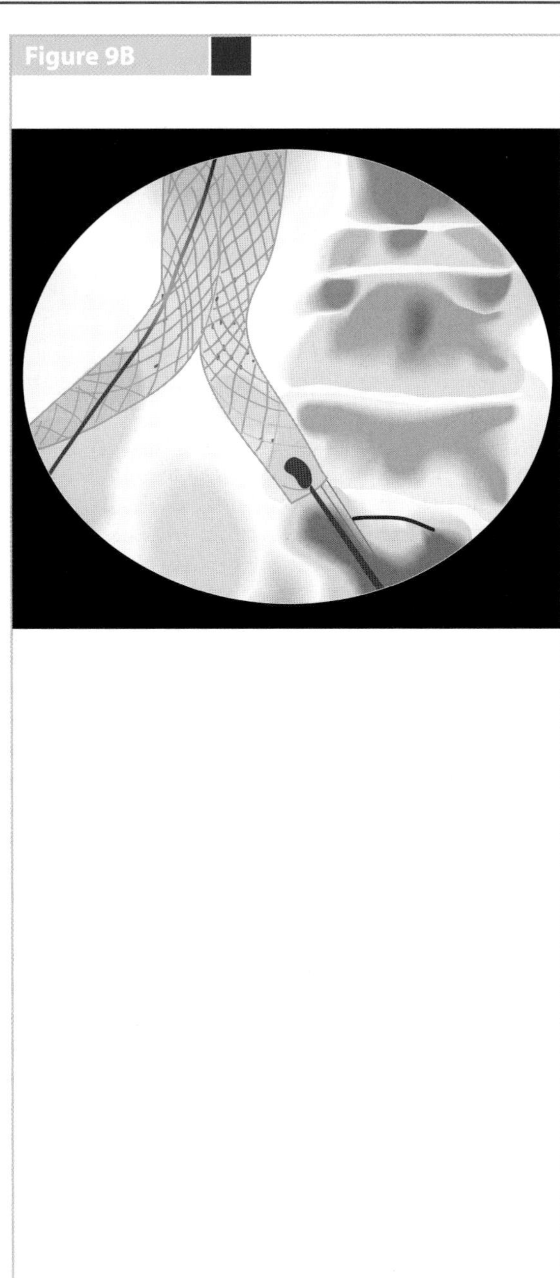

Figures 10–12

The common femoral arteries are again used as access sites and exposed via bilateral surgical cutdowns. Using an angiographic catheter with calibrated radiopaque markings (Cook Inc., Bloomington, IN, USA), an arteriogram is performed to verify AAA dimensions and determine future positioning of the device. Fluoroscopic guidance (OEC 9600, OEC Medical Systems, Inc., Thousand Oaks, CA, USA) is used for placement of the endoprosthesis throughout the entire procedure. Figure 10A–D demonstrates the process of deploying the Excluder. The radiopaque markers at the top of the graft are aligned with the renal arteries. The long marker depicting the contralateral limb is aligned either with the contralateral iliac artery or in some cases deliberately crossed to take up length to improve ease of cannulation. The main body is then deployed and an occlusion balloon is used to secure the proximal end and to fix the barbs into the aortic wall. Following deployment of the main trunk-ipsilateral limb component, the contralateral leg opening is cannulated with a glide wire in a retrograde fashion and then exchanged for an Amplatz super stiff wire. A 12F sheath is advanced through the gate and the contralateral leg component is inserted and positioned so that there is 3.0 cm of overlap between the components. The overlap zone, aortic bifurcation and the distal attachment sites are all angioplastied (Fig. 11). Additional procedures and extenders are utilized when necessary, and finally a completion angiogram is obtained (Fig. 12).

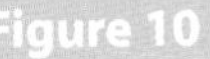
Figure 10

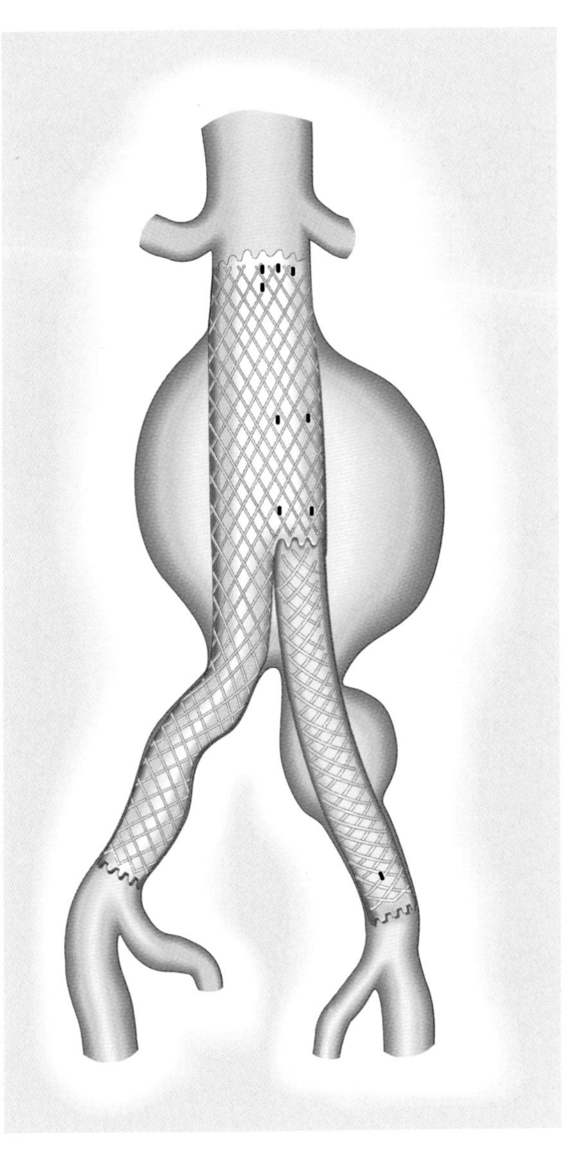

Figure 11A–C

Figure 11A

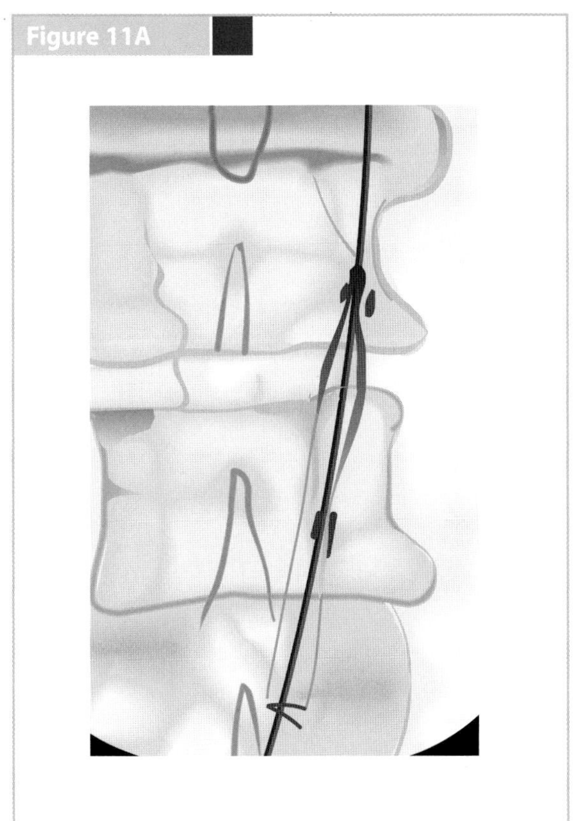

Figure 11B

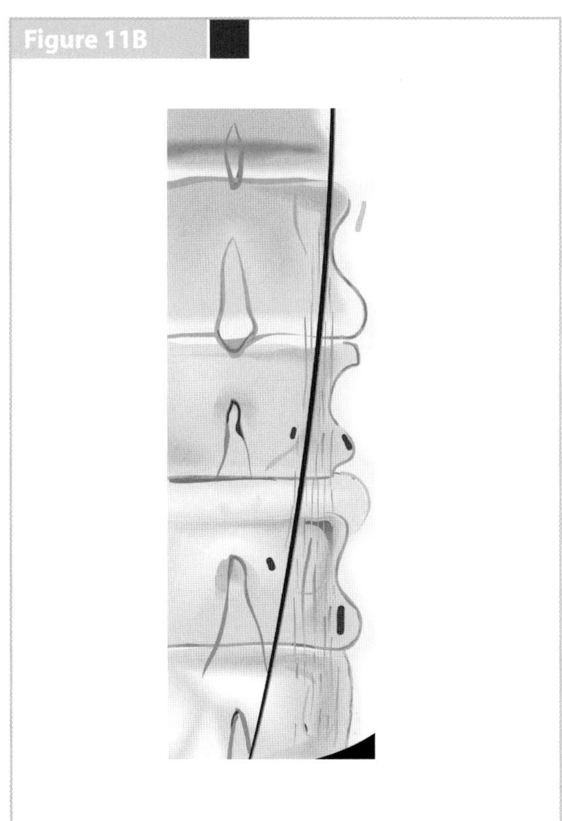

Figure 11C

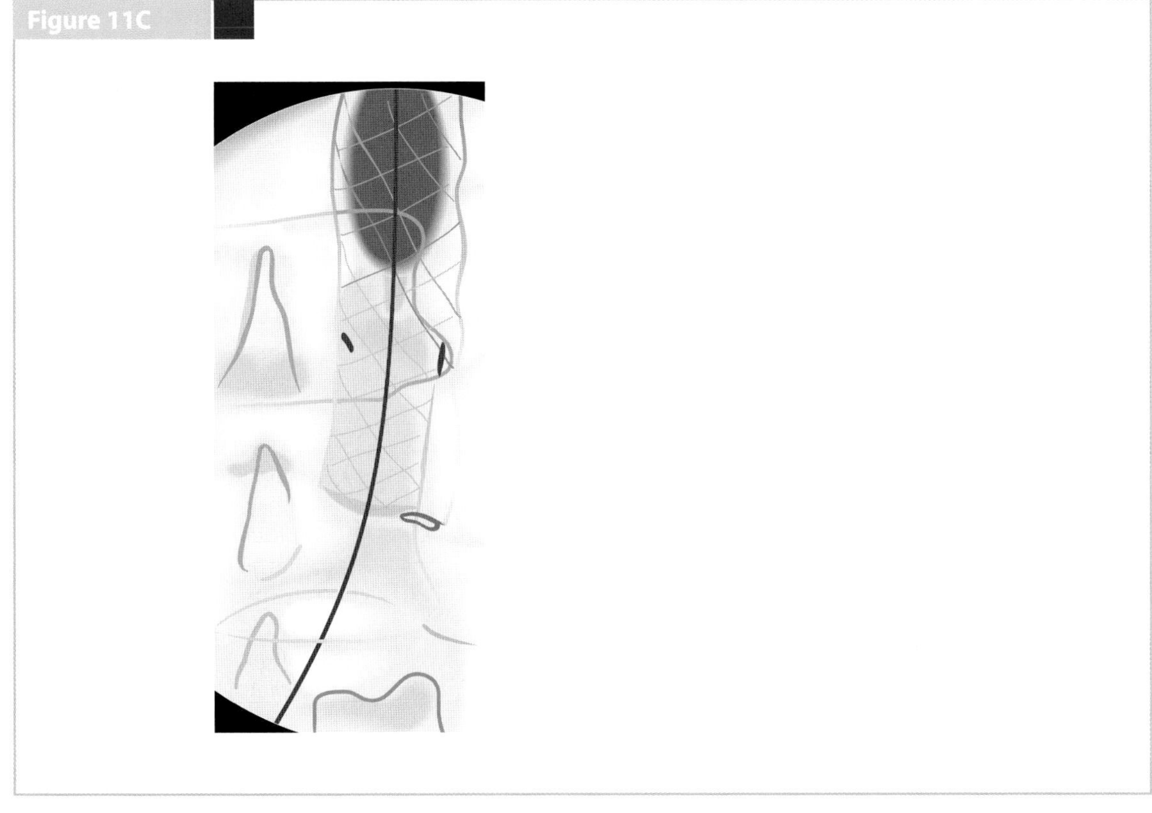

Figure 12A–C

Figure 12A

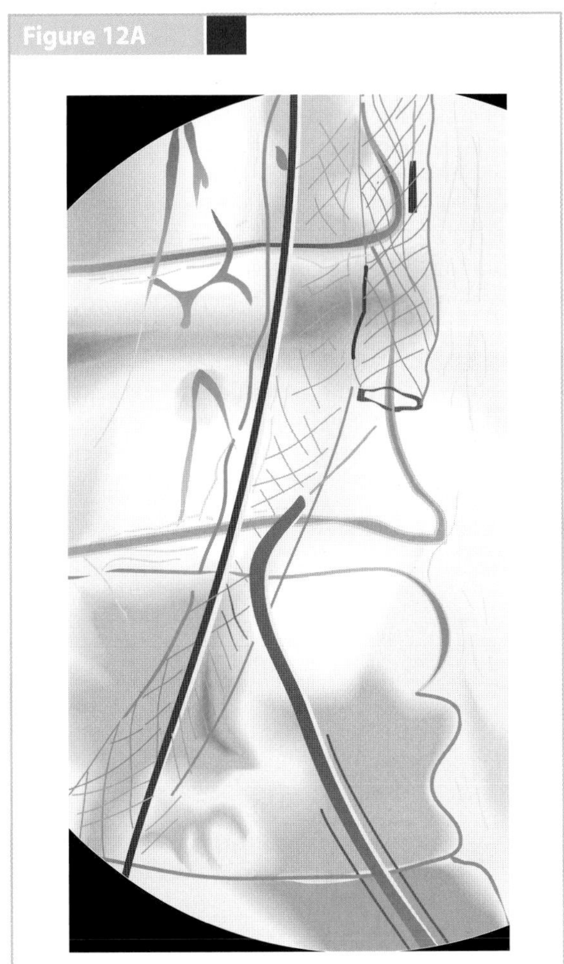

Figure 12B

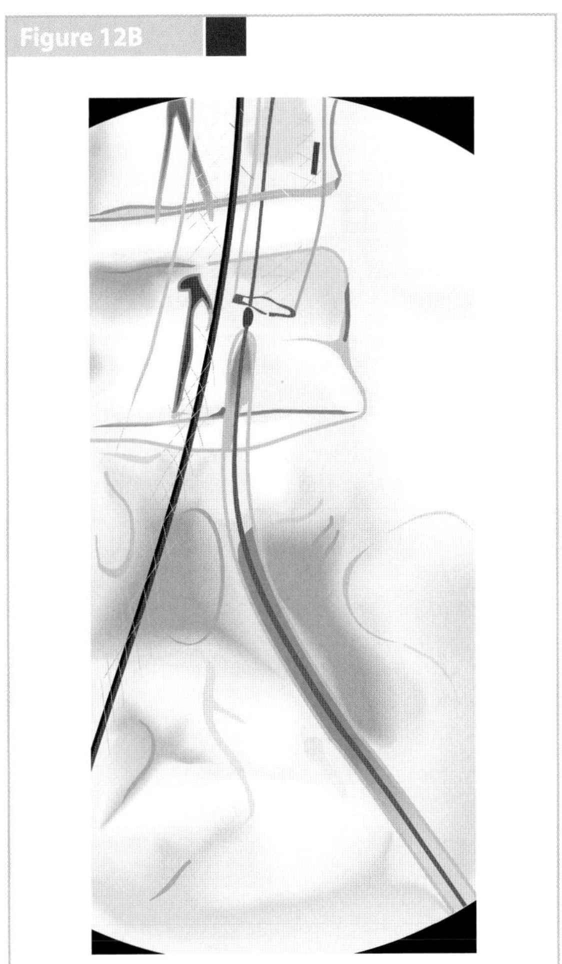

Figure 12C

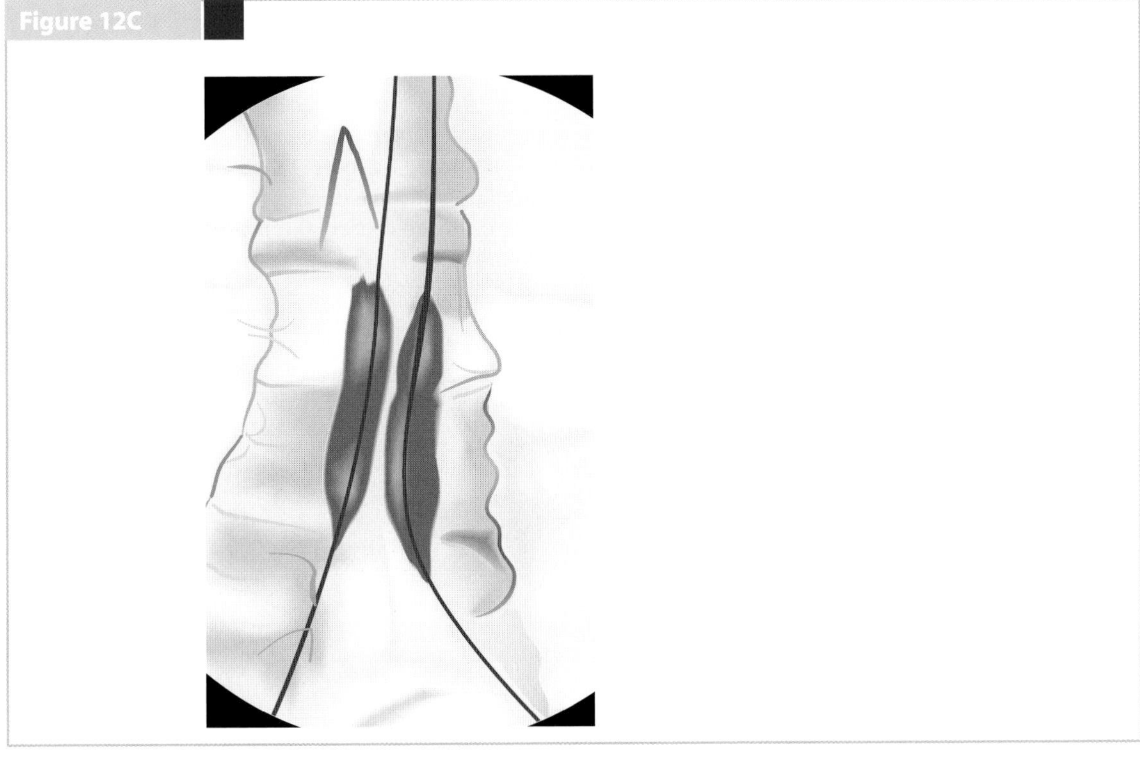

Figure 13: The Zenith AAA Endovascular Graft

This is another bifurcated modular system. It is composed of stainless steel Z stents and woven polyester graft material. However, it differs from the other two devices in that it is a three-component system. The aortic section consists of a main body with attached short contralateral iliac limb and an attached longer ipsilateral iliac limb. Separate contralateral and ipsilateral iliac legs are docked into the main body aortounilateral iliac graft. Another difference from the two devices described here is the suprarenal bare stent extensions and hooks designed to securely anchor the device into a disease free supra-aortic segment. This was also the first device to incorporate flaring of the iliac limbs to accommodate large iliac arteries. Additional unique features of this device include:

1. Ability to perform angiography through the dilator
2. Controlled release of the device after partial deployment using trigger wire which controls deployment of the suprarenal stent

In patients with a severely diseased iliac artery or an occluded common iliac artery, it is not possible to place a bifurcated graft. The Ancure aortoiliac system was the first to be approved by the FDA for this purpose. However, this device is no longer available. Currently the only commercially available AUI device is from Cooke. However, there are several techniques which permit conversion of a bifurcated graft into an aortounilateral iliac graft. Bifurcated devices can be converted using an aortic extender cuff to exclude the contralateral limb. Another technique is to use a second main body device in which the contralateral limb is rotated 180 degrees from the first device.

Figures 14–20: Zenith Deployment

The delivery system has been advanced, placing the gold radiopaque marker below the renal arteries (Fig. 14). The contralateral limb has been oriented to the contralateral iliac artery. While stabilizing the grey shaft (positioner), the sheath is withdrawn deploying the first two Z stents. After checking that the device is appropriately oriented, the contralateral limb is fully deployed by retracting the sheath.

The contralateral limb is cannulated with a guidewire and its position inside the graft confirmed (Fig. 15).

Prior to deploying the suprarenal stents, an angiogram is performed through the main body delivery system (15 cc/s @1200 psi. The proximal markers are deployed 2 mm below the lowest renal artery. The suprarenal stent is then deployed.

The contralateral wire is then advanced up into the descending thoracic aorta. The contralateral internal iliac artery is then localized with angiography, the contralateral limb advanced into the contralateral main body limb and deployed (Fig. 16).

The ipsilateral main body limb is then fully deployed. After localizing the ipsilateral internal iliac artery, the ipsilateral iliac limb is advanced into position and deployed (Figs. 17, 18).

A moulding balloon is then advanced into the suprarenal stent and dilated (Fig. 19). This is used to dilate both the proximal attachment system and the endograft below the renal arteries. Both iliac limb overlaps are also dilated as is the distal landing zone (Fig. 20).

Figure 13

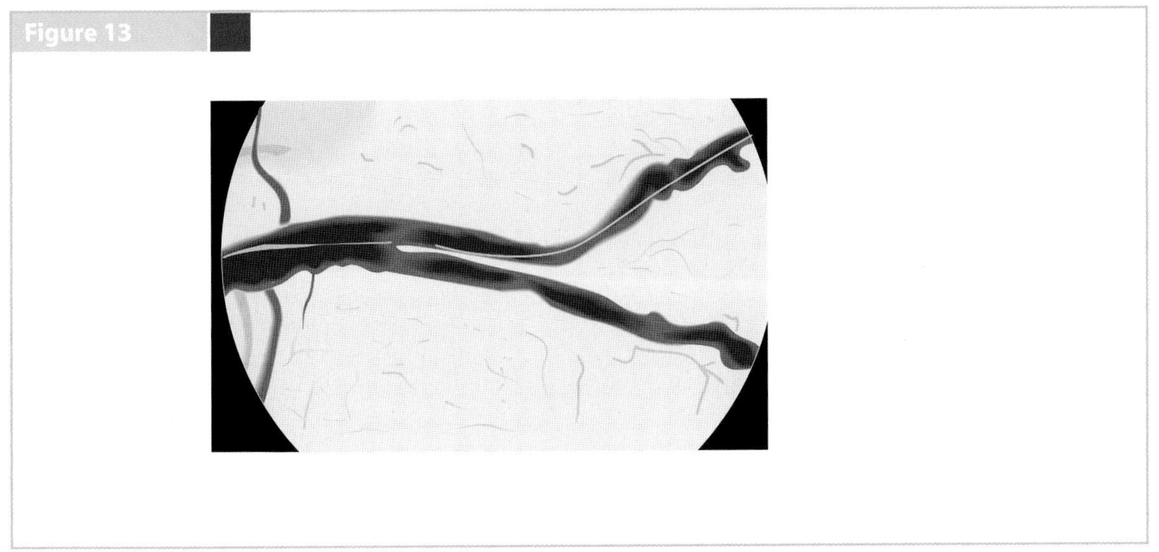

Figure 14A

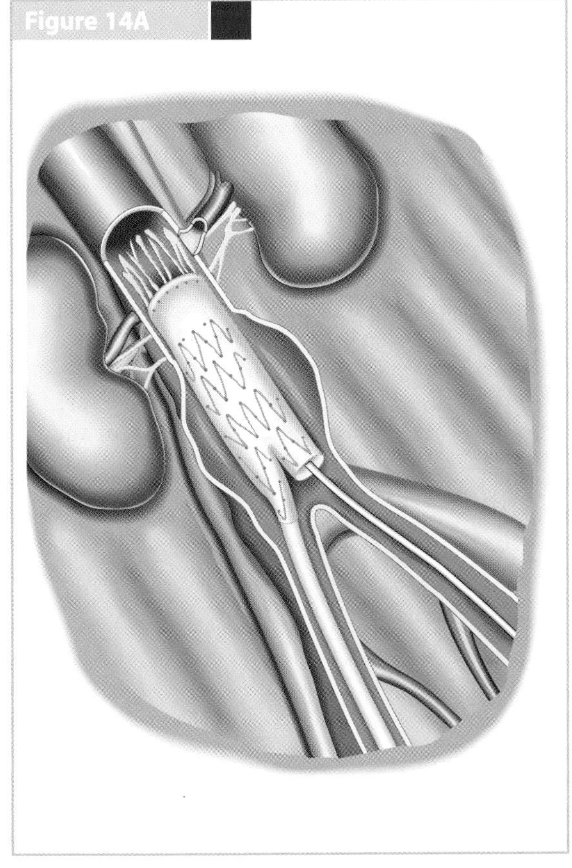

Figure 14B

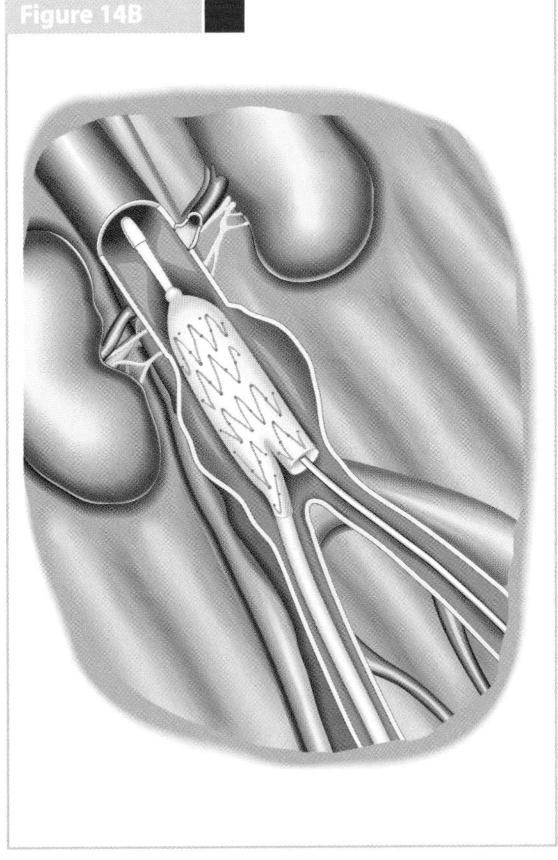

Figure 15–18

Figure 15

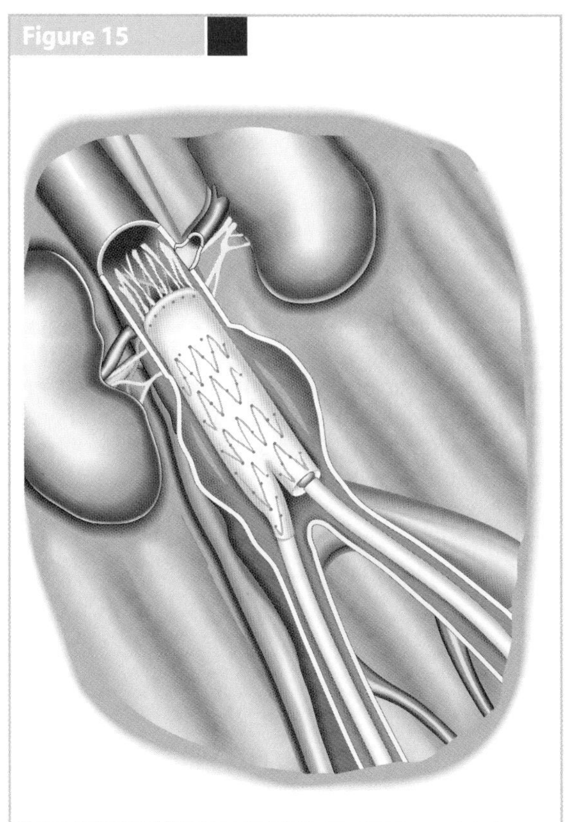

Figure 16

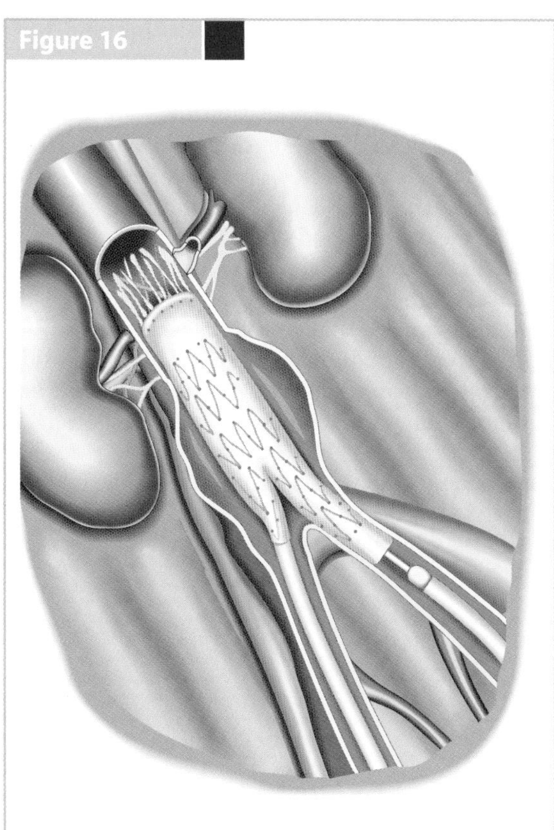

Figure 17

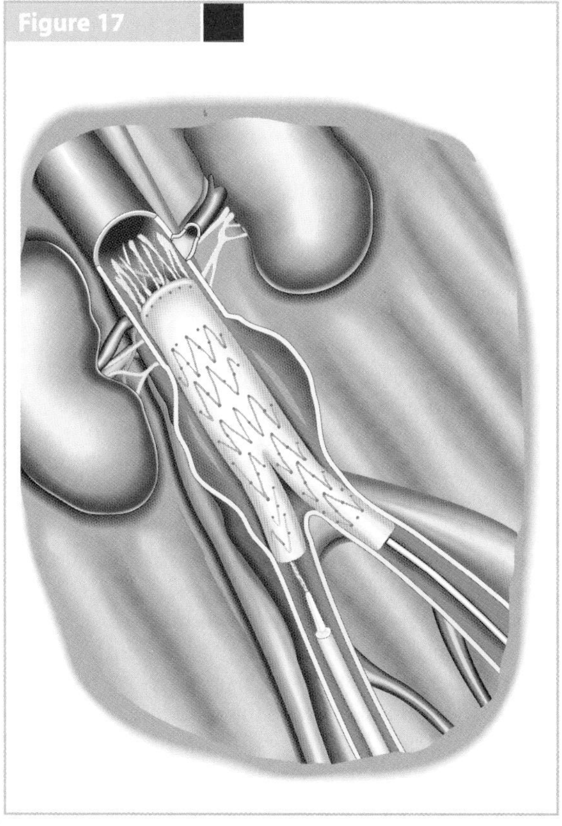

Figure 18

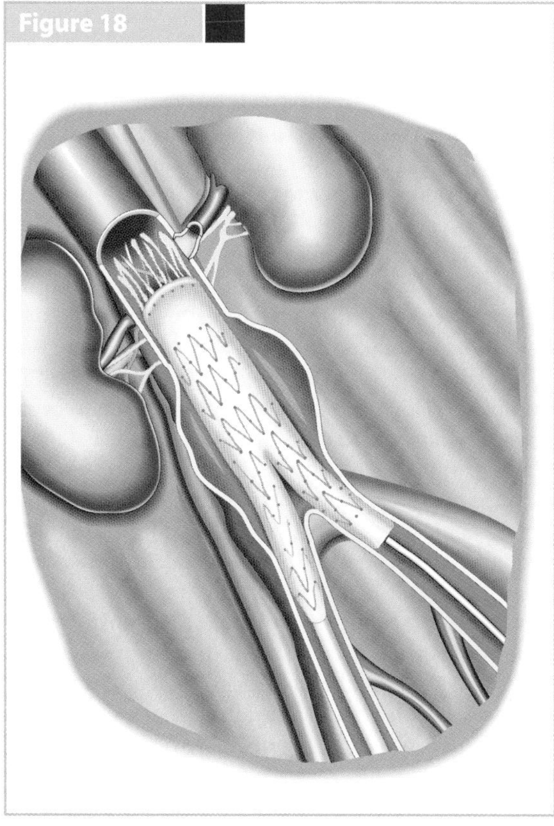

Figure 19, 20: Powerlink Deployment Sequence

Access is initially achieved with a cutdown on the ipsilateral side and a 9 French percutaneous access on the contralateral side. A snare catheter (EnSnare) is advanced up the ipsilateral side and a 180 cm guide wire up the contralateral side. The wire is snared and pulled out the ipsilateral side, achieving a transfemoral access with the 180 guide wire.

A dual lumen catheter (Endologix) is then advanced from the contralateral to the ipsilateral side. A stiff wire is passed through the proximal skive and advanced into the thoracic aorta. The Powerlink catheter is prepped and loaded on the stiff wire. The contralateral limb wire is removed from the housing and passed through the other lumen from the ipsilateral to the contralateral side. The dual lumen catheter is removed.

The device is then advanced into the aorta above the aortic bifurcation. The outer sheath on the Powerlink catheter is retracted to expose the iliac limbs. The Powerlink device is pulled down to the aortic bifurcation. The main body of the Powerlink is deployed by advancing the pusher-rod on the deployment catheter, unsheathing the main body from bottom to top. Pulling on the red hub of the deployment catheter, the front stop and front sheath are then retracted down through the main body. The ipsilateral iliac limb is deployed and the front sheath and outer sheath are mated up. The Powerlink catheter is then removed through the ipsilateral femoral artery. A 14–18F access sheath is inserted into the ipsilateral femoral artery. The contralateral limb wire is then pulled to deploy the contralateral limb.

ADJUNCTIVE PROCEDURES

Due to severe iliac disease (occlusive or tortuosity), occasionally it is not possible to deliver a stent graft from the femoral approach. In this case it is reasonable to make a retroperitoneal incision in the appropriate lower quadrant and expose the common iliac artery. This is performed by making an oblique "transplant" type incision, dividing the abdominal wall muscles and reflecting the peritoneum medially. Care has to be taken to avoid the ureter. The common iliac artery is isolated in an area which permits clamping. A longitudinal arteriotomy is made in the artery and an end-to-side anastomosis is created using a 10-mm Dacron graft (PTFE is to be avoided because of needle hole bleeding and difficulty in securing hemostasis with a tape and collar around the endograft delivery system). The conduit is then tunneled down to the groin incision anterior to the artery. It should not simply be pulled out through the abdominal incision as the angle the graft makes with the native artery makes it difficult to negotiate with a stiff device. After the endograft has been implanted, the option is to either divide and oversew the graft, or if the patient has severe occlusive disease use the graft as a iliofemoral bypass.

When the iliac artery is larger than can be safely treated with the endografts, the bell bottom technique can be employed. In this approach, an aortic extender cuff is used to flare out the distal end of the iliac limbs in order to create a seal. As manufacturers increase the inventory of graft sizes, it is likely that this technique will be used less as flared endografts become increasingly available.

■ **Outcome.** Primary technical success is defined by our institution as successful endograft deployment with no evidence of proximal or distal attachment site endoleak on completion arteriography. We do not consider a retrograde branch vessel filling of the aneurysm sac a technical failure as no immediate intervention is performed and the majority of these endoleaks thrombose spontaneously within a few months. No leakage between modular components has been observed in our patients. CT scanning at 1-, 6-, and 12-month follow-up visits assesses complete exclusion of the AAA from the systemic circulation. A CT scan is performed at 3 months if an endoleak is present and more frequent surveillance imaging will be performed as clinically indicated.

Figure 19

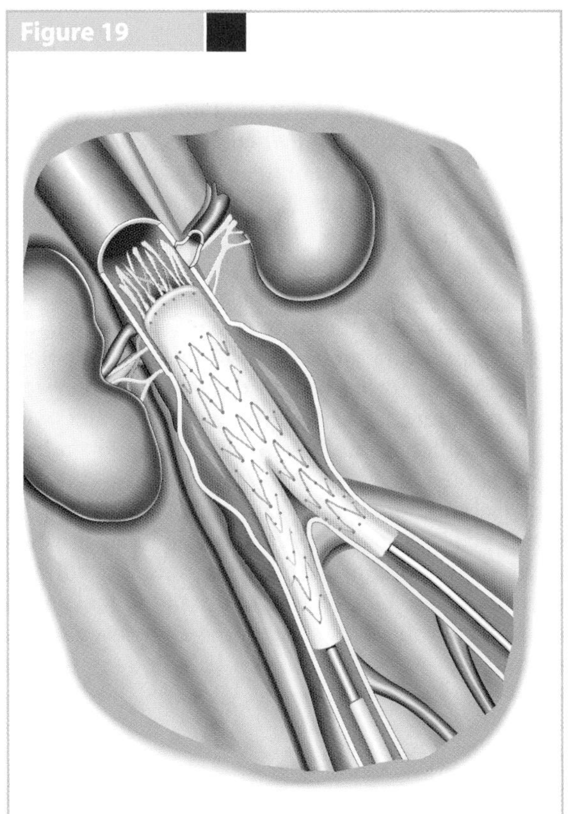

Figure 20

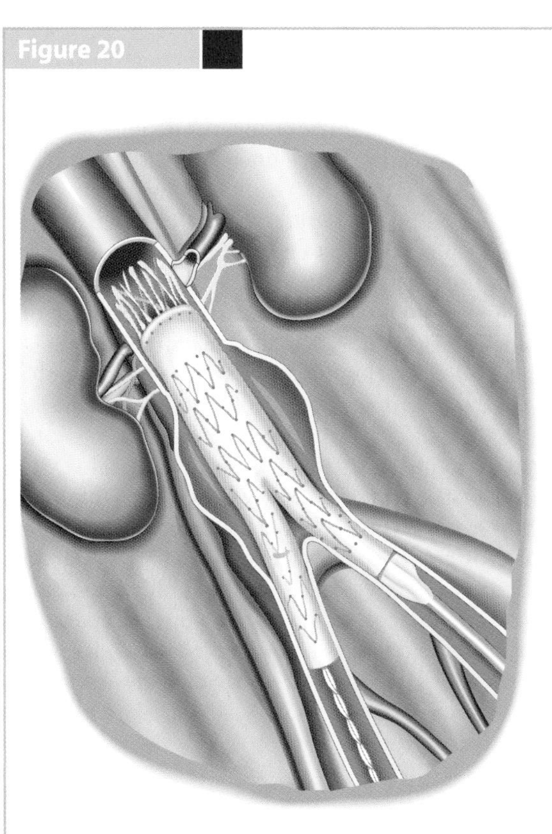

CONCLUSION

We have reviewed three systems in detail: the AneuRx (Medtronic Inc.), Excluder (WL Gore), and Zenith (Cooke Co.). The AneuRx is the most widely used device in the United States. It has been improved upon with the current generation of stents having increased flexibility and fewer deployment and long term complications. This is primarily due to the increased number of 1-cm nitinol rings. The biggest deficiencies of this device remain the increased tendency for module separation and the lack of conformability. The Excluder's modular system renders it the most flexible of all. As stated, it is therefore the graft of choice for patients with tortuous or small iliac vessels. Furthermore, the extenders allow for greater customization to accommodate the patient's anatomy. However, the multipiece system allows for the possibility of component separation. The Ancure system is no longer available. Its transmural hooks theoretically provided the maximum fixation and therefore minimized migration. Also, its one piece design prevented component separation. However, the large sheath diameter and a poor deployment system rendered it a more difficult system to use for implantation.

Aortic endograft technology is undergoing rapid evolution. During the time of writing, one device was removed from the US mark (Kibbe and Matsumura 2003; Matsumura and Chaikof 1999) and two new devices were approved. Many challenges remain with both stent and fabric technology. New devices will have a smaller profile, be more flexible and have better fixation systems. Long term follow-up is essential and techniques for endoleak management will be developed (Lin et al. 2003). It is certain that with new technology and improved devices a larger portion of patients undergoing treatment for abdominal aortic aneurysms will be candidates for endovascular repair.

REFERENCES

Blum U, Langer M, Spillner G, Mialhe C, Beyersdorf F, Buitrago-Tellez C, et al. (1996) Abdominal aortic aneurysms: preliminary technical and clinical results with transfemoral placement of endovascular self-expanding stent-grafts. Radiology 198:25–31

Boyle JR, Gibbs PJ et al. (2003) Predicting outcome in ruptured abdominal aortic aneurysm: a prospective study of 100 consecutive cases. Eur J Vasc Endovasc Surg 26(6):607–611

Brown LC, Powell JT (1999) Risk factors for aneurysm rupture in patients kept under ultrasound surveillance. Ann Surg 230:289–296

Bush RL, Lin PH, Lumsden AB (2003) Endovascular management of abdominal aortic aneurysms. J Cardiovasc Surg (Torino) 44(4):527–534

Greenberg R (2003) The Zenith AAA endovascular graft for abdominal aortic aneurysms: clinical update. Semin Vasc Surg 16(2):151–157

Kibbe MR, Matsumura JS (2003) The Gore Excluder US multicenter trial: analysis of adverse events at 2 years. Semin Vasc Surg 16(2):144–150

Lin PH, BR, Katzman JB, Zemel G, Puente OA, Katzen BT, Lumsden AB (2003) Delayed aortic aneurysm enlargement due to endotension after endovascular abdominal aortic aneurysm repair. J Vasc Surg 38(4):840–842; 840–842

Matsumura JS, Chaikof EL (1999) Anatomic changes after endovascular grafting for aneurysmal disease. Semin Vasc Surg 12(3):192–198

Matsumura JS, Katzen BT et al. (2001) Update on the bifurcated EXCLUDER endoprosthesis: phase I results. J Vasc Surg 33(2 Suppl):S150–153

Matsumura JS, Brewster DC et al. (2003) A multicenter controlled clinical trial of open versus endovascular treatment of abdominal aortic aneurysm. J Vasc Surg 37(2):262–271

May J, White GH, Yu W et al. (1998) Concurrent comparison of endoluminal versus open repair in the treatment of abdominal aortic aneurysms: Analysis of 303 patients by life table analysis. J Vasc Surg 27:213–220

Moore WS, Matsumura JS et al. (2003) Five-year interim comparison of the Guidant bifurcated endograft with open repair of abdominal aortic aneurysm. J Vasc Surg 38(1):46–55

Parodi JC, Palmaz JC et al. (1991) Transfemoral intraluminal graft implantation for abdominal aortic aneurysms. Ann Vasc Surg 5(6):491–499

Prisant LM, Mondy JS 3rd (2004) Abdominal aortic aneurysm. J Clin Hypertens (Greenwich) 6(2):85–89

Scott RA, Ashton HA, Kay DN (1991) Abdominal aortic aneurysm in 4237 screened patients: prevalence, development and management over 6 years. Br J Surg 78:1122–1125

Spurgeon D (2004) US screening programme shows high prevalence of aortic aneurysm. BMJ 328(7444):852

Zarins CK (2003) The US AneuRx Clinical Trial: 6-year clinical update 2002. J Vasc Surg 37(4):904–908

CHAPTER 18

Endarterectomy of the Abdominal Aorta and Its Branches

Rajabrata Sarkar, Louis M. Messina

INTRODUCTION

The application of endarterectomy, or direct removal of a lesion from within an artery, was the first operation performed to restore flow in arterial occlusive disease. Dos Santos performed the first endarterectomy in a superficial femoral artery and termed the operation "disobliteration" and noted the critical role that the anticoagulant heparin had in his success. Jack Wylie at the University of California at San Francisco (UCSF) performed the first successful endarterectomy in the United States for occlusive disease of the abdominal aorta soon thereafter, and went on to report a significant series of these pioneering operations. This established a tradition of endarterectomy at UCSF which has evolved to treat occlusive lesions throughout the arterial system.

Occlusive disease of the abdominal aorta and its branches can have a variety of clinical presentations ranging from silent but progressive ischemic nephropathy to the striking and acute crisis of intestinal infarction. Endarterectomy of these vessels was the first procedure developed to relieve ischemia, and it remains the standard in terms of effectiveness and durability against which newer methods of revascularization should be compared.

Occlusive atherosclerotic lesions of the mesenteric branches of the aorta, namely the celiac axis, and superior and inferior mesenteric arteries, usually present with intestinal angina, or postprandial abdominal pain, which leads to fear of eating and progressive weight loss. Misdiagnosis is common, largely due to the rarity of mesenteric occlusive disease relative to other common causes of abdominal pain, and patients are often subjected to lengthy but fruitless evaluations to establish a cause for their persistent symptoms. Without revascularization, the intestinal ischemia will worsen, often resulting in fatal intestinal infarction when mesenteric arterial thrombosis supervenes on the worsening stenosis. Mesenteric arterial occlusion is usually limited to the aortic ostia and the first few centimeters of the mesenteric vessel; it is thus amenable to transaortic endarterectomy. Occlusive disease which extends further into the superior mesenteric artery requires a counterincision in the superior mesenteric artery to remove the extension of plaque which ends at the first superior mesenteric artery branch.

Renal artery occlusive disease causes renovascular hypertension and ischemic nephropathy. The most common cause of renal artery occlusive disease is atherosclerosis; rarer causes include developmental stenosis and fibromuscular dysplasia. Primary aortorenal atherosclerosis is often suitable for endarterectomy, whereas the other causes of renal artery stenosis are treated with different forms of revascularization.

Occlusive disease of the infrarenal aorta and iliac arteries presents as claudication of the calves, thighs and buttocks but may also cause erectile dysfunction in men and occasionally manifest as either acute or chronic limb-threatening ischemia. Despite the widespread popularity of aortofemoral bypass and angioplasty/stenting, aortoiliac endarterectomy remains an excellent option in selected patients. Aortoiliac endarterectomy does not require use of prosthetic graft material and thus avoids the risk of graft infection. In men with suspected vasculogenic impotence, endarterectomy allows direct revascularization of occluded internal iliac arteries. Aortoiliac endarterectomy is recommended for patients with occlusive lesions limited to the aorta and common iliac arteries.

Three anatomic features of atherosclerotic plaques allow safe and effective application of surgical endarterectomy. These features are: (1) the localized nature of atherosclerotic plaques with respect to the layers of the arterial wall, (2) the focal distribution of plaques at areas of turbulent flow within the vascular system, and (3) the surprising tensile strength of the residual outer media and adventitia that remains after endarterectomy.

Atherosclerotic plaques are localized to the intima and inner media of the arterial wall, and this allows development of an endarterectomy plane between the plaque and the non-diseased layers of the arterial wall that leaves sufficient strength in the remaining artery to withstand pulsatile arterial pressure. The presence of pre-aneurysmal change or degeneration of the arterial wall characterized by focal dilatations is a contraindication to the application of the endarterectomy as the weakened residual layers of the arterial wall are at risk for rupture.

The localized distribution of plaques at points of turbulent blood flow (low shear stress) and arterial bifurcations is also essential for the success of endarterectomy, as it allows smooth and tapered development and termination of the endarterectomy in selected areas of the artery. Atherosclerotic plaques of aortic branch vessels usually involve the aortic ostia and terminate shortly within the branch vessel. This distribution allows endarterectomy via a transaortic approach for major branches of the abdominal aorta (renal and mesenteric vessels). The flow pattern and shear stress changes at the aortic bifurcation are more complicated, and atherosclerosis originating in the aortic bifurcation often extends past the common iliac arteries to the iliac bifurcations. Thus aortoiliac endarterectomy requires both a transaortic and a transiliac approach for complete access to these lesions.

Endarterectomy of the abdominal aorta and its branches combines several specific endarterectomy techniques, based on the surgical exposure, and the type and extent of the target lesion. Open endarterectomy uses a longitudinal arteriotomy for complete visualization of the target lesion, as in carotid endarterectomy. Semi-closed endarterectomy is done through a transverse arteriotomy placed at either end of the target lesion and involves retrograde extraction of plaque from the intervening unopened segment of the artery. This technique is used in aortoiliac endarterectomy (see below) and avoids the use of the lengthy patch required to close a longitudinal arteriotomy the length of the lesion. Extraction endarterectomy is done either antegrade or retrograde through a distant arteriotomy without direct visualization of the lesion, and is utilized in endarterectomy of the hypogastric artery.

Endarterectomy of the abdominal vessels has several attractive features in comparison to bypass grafting. When there are occlusive lesions of multiple arteries, such as combined mesenteric and renal occlusive disease, endarterectomy is quicker and can often be accomplished with less visceral ischemia than sequential bypass grafting to multiple vessels, particularly multiple renal arteries on one side. The avoidance of prosthetic material is important in situations where there is potential contamination with bacteria (i.e. ischemic bowel). In comparison to aortofemoral bypass grafting, aortoiliac endarterectomy avoids the use of femoral incisions and their associated higher infection rates and other problems such as lymphoceles and graft pseudoaneurysms.

Figure 1: Transaortic Mesenteric Endarterectomy: Medial Visceral Rotation

Exposure of the proximal abdominal aorta and its branches is best obtained through a left-to-right medial visceral rotation, which can be performed through a midline transperitoneal approach. An alternative incision is a bilateral subcostal incision with lateral extension to the midaxillary line. The decision to use a bilateral subcostal versus a midline incision is largely influenced by the patient's body habitus, with the subcostal incision generally providing better exposure in patients with a wide costal angle. Following abdominal exploration, the lateral peritoneal attachment of the left colon is mobilized, and the plane in the retroperitoneum is developed anterior to the left kidney. The retroperitoneal dissection is then extended cephalad along the aorta behind the pancreas and the spleen. Attention is then turned to the upper abdomen, where the peritoneum overlying the esophagus and supraceliac aorta is incised, followed by division of the lateral diaphragmatic attachments of the esophagus and spleen, which allows these structures to be gently retracted to the right. Division of the splenic attachments to diaphragm and lateral abdominal wall prior to placing medial or upward tension on the spleen is critical to avoid injury to the splenic capsule. Rotation of the spleen, pancreas and small bowel medially is then possible with careful packing of moistened laparotomy sponges between these organs and the blades of a self-retaining retractor system. Although the marked displacement of the pancreas and spleen anteriorly and medially is maintained by a self-retaining retractor system, the surgeon must be constantly vigilant to the amount of traction placed on these organs as the exposure develops, to prevent postoperative pancreatitis or splenic injury resulting in splenectomy.

Figure 1

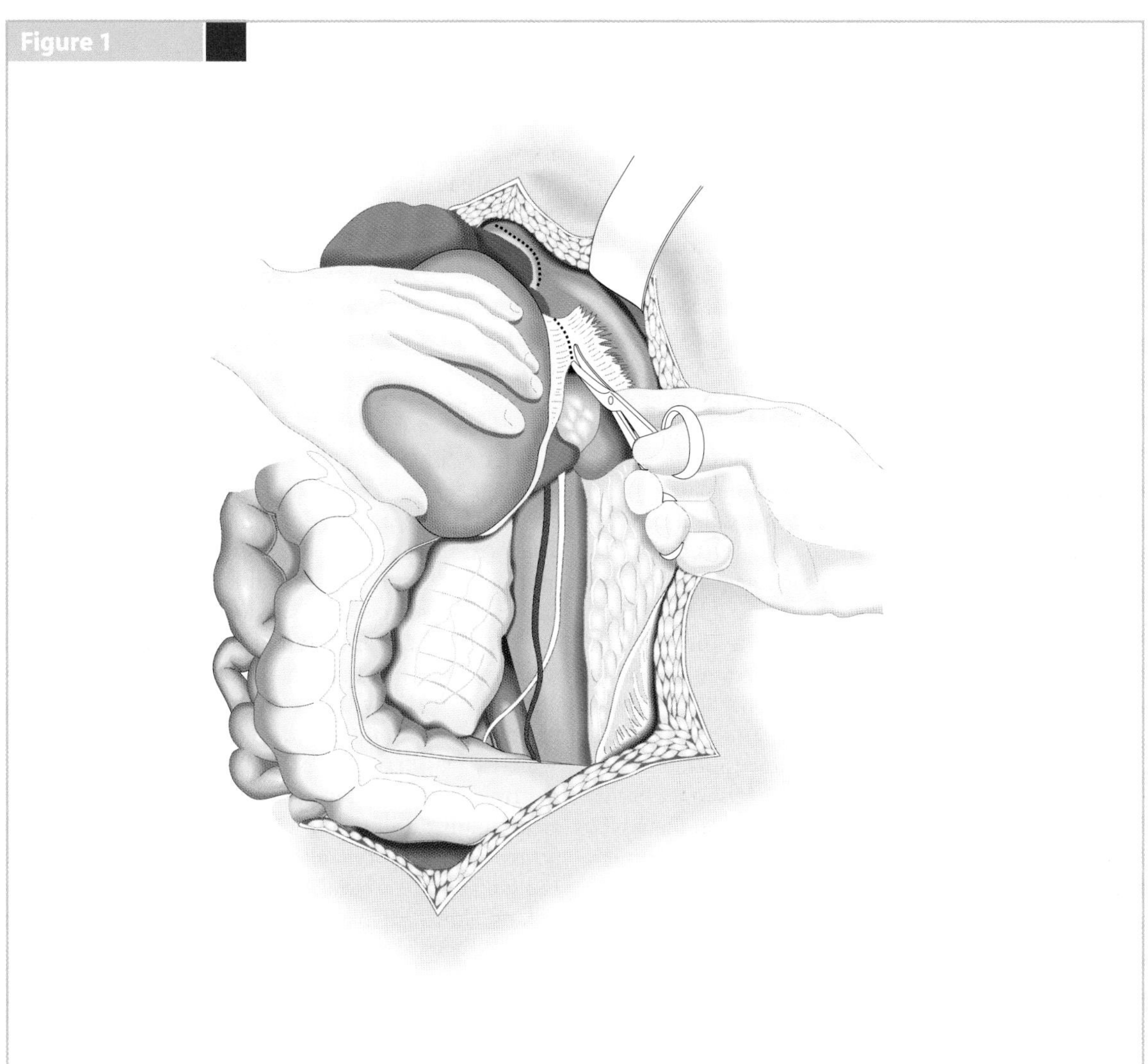

Figure 2: Transaortic Mesenteric Endarterectomy: Paravisceral Aortic Exposure

Following medial visceral rotation of the viscera as described above, aortic exposure is commenced by division of the tissue overlying the anterior surface of the infrarenal aorta, with care taken to avoid injury to the inferior mesenteric artery. A critical step in achieving exposure of the paravisceral aorta is full mobilization of the left renal vein. This vessel is encountered by continuing the dissection on the anterior surface of the infrarenal aorta in a cephalad direction. Complete mobilization of the left renal vein requires division of its three branches, the left gonadal vein, the left adrenal vein and the ascending lumbar vein which enters on the posterolateral and inferior aspect. For exposure of the paravisceral aorta the renal vein is mobilized caudad, and early division of the adrenal vein prevents tearing of this branch upon later retraction. Complete dissection of the left renal vein from the renal hilum to the junction with the vena cava allows the vein to be easily suspended with plasma tubing and retracted to allow exposure of the underlying aorta. Following these maneuvers, dissection is continued cephalad along the paravisceral aorta with division of the ganglionic tissue overlying the anterolateral surface of the aorta around the base of the mesenteric arteries. The median arcuate ligament and left crus of the diaphragm are divided to allow exposure of the supraceliac aorta.

The aorta must be mobilized circumferentially to allow clamping of lumbar arteries in the segment of the planned endarterectomy. The lumbar arteries on the right side of the aorta at the levels of the mesenteric vessels are particularly prone to injury during circumferential dissection. Following satisfactory mobilization of the paravisceral aorta, the mesenteric arteries are sharply dissected free from their overlying neural and connective tissue. The superior mesenteric artery is isolated to beyond its first major branch, usually the inferior pancreaticoduodenal artery. The dissection of the celiac axis must be carried out so that the individual branches of the celiac axis are free for clamping. Both the superior mesenteric artery and the celiac axis must be circumferentially mobilized from the surrounding adherent tissues to allow these vessels to be invaginated into the aorta during the critical portion of the subsequent endarterectomy. If renal artery endarterectomy is to be done concurrently, the renal arteries are dissected free for a length of several centimeters to allow the artery to be similarly prolapsed into the aorta during the transaortic endarterectomy. Adequate exposure and mobilization of the right renal artery often requires lateral mobilization of the vena cava, which can be facilitated by division of the lumbar veins on the left side of the vena cava to allow sufficient rotation and lateral retraction of the cava to expose the mid and distal portions of the right renal artery.

Figure 2

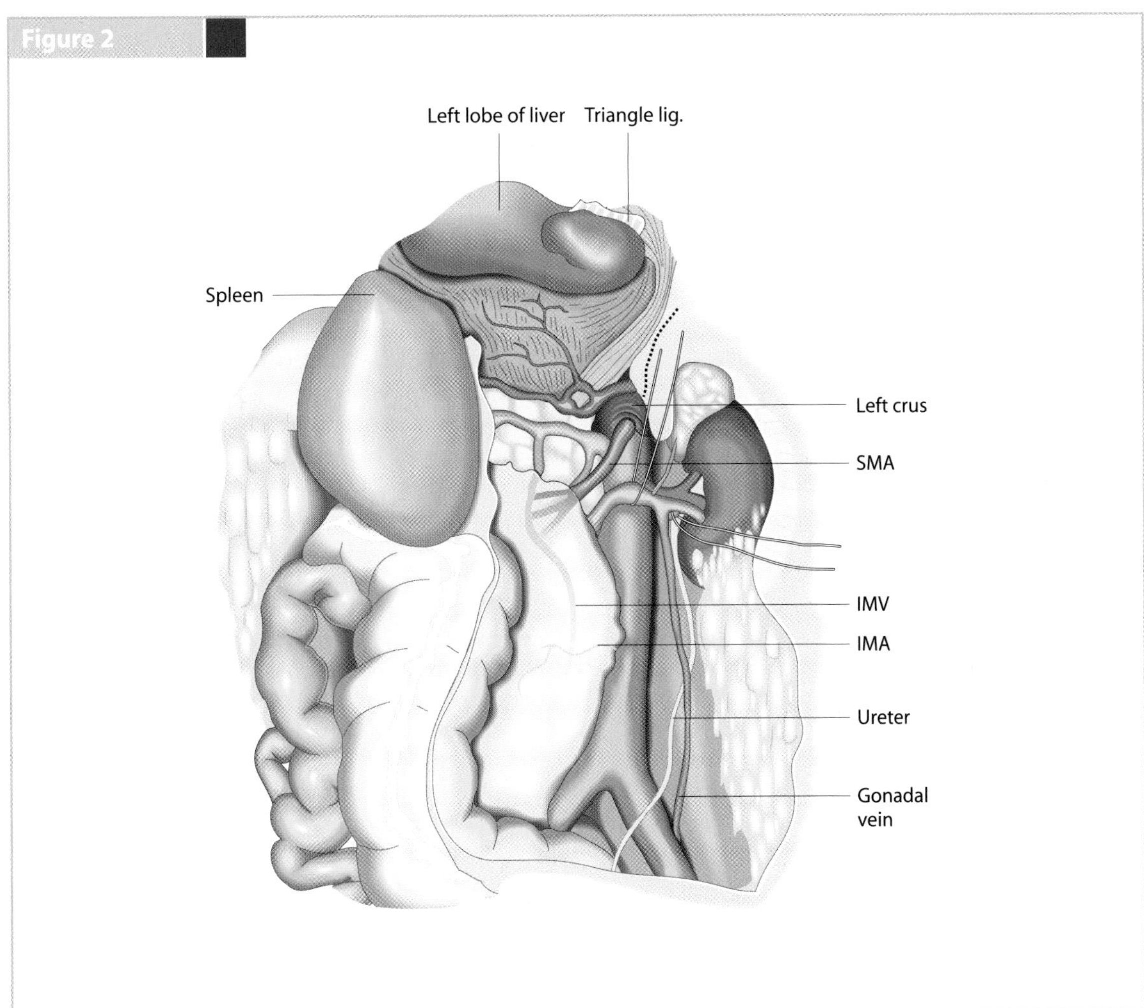
Left lobe of liver
Triangle lig.
Spleen
Left crus
SMA
IMV
IMA
Ureter
Gonadal vein

Figure 3: Transaortic Mesenteric Endarterectomy: Exposure/Clamping

Palpation of the mesenteric vessels is done to confirm that disease is limited to the proximal several centimeters and is thus suitable for endarterectomy. The finding of more extensive disease, usually in the superior mesenteric artery, may be better treated with aortovisceral bypass grafting, which can be easily performed from the same exposure. Following satisfactory exposure and mobilization of the aorta and target branch vessels, systemic heparinization is achieved and mannitol is administered to establish an osmotic diuresis and as a free radical scavenger. The renal arteries, superior mesenteric artery and branches of the celiac axis are individually clamped as shown, followed by vertical clamps on the supraceliac and infrarenal aorta. Lumbar arteries are controlled with bulldog clamps to prevent backbleeding (Fig. 3). The proximal aortic clamp must be sufficiently above the celiac axis so that the aortotomy can be created and opened without undue tension. An anterolateral aortotomy is made in a trapdoor fashion to allow elevation of a anterior aortic flap which allows direct visualization of the anterior orifices of the mesenteric vessels (Fig. 4). If endarterectomy is to be limited to the mesenteric vessels, the end of the aortotomy is tailored around the base of the superior mesenteric artery. If endarterectomy of the renal vessels is also planned, the aortotomy is extended straight down the anterior surface of the aorta to the infrarenal aorta.

The establishment of the proper endarterectomy plane is critical to the success of the procedure. It is easiest to establish this on the free edge of the aortotomy flap, which is adjacent to the orifices of the mesenteric vessels. The atherosclerotic plaque is often thickest here, and this facilitates establishment of the plane in the outer medial layer of the aorta. Gentle traction on the plaque coupled with sweeping of the pliable aortic wall away from the lesion is used to free the plaque from the aorta circumferentially around each mesenteric orifice (Fig. 4). The plaque is transected at the base of the flap prior to commencing the endarterectomy within the mesenteric vessel itself. Eversion endarterectomy of each vessel is done by moving the clamp on the mesenteric vessel towards the aorta, which prolapses the vessel into the aorta. The proper dissection and mobilization of each vessel as described previously is essential to the success of this maneuver. As the mesenteric vessel is invaginated into the aorta, the end of the plaque becomes visible and a tapered endpoint can be established under direct vision (Fig. 4). The prolapsed lumen of the mesenteric vessel is carefully inspected and irrigated to reveal any flaps or plaque fragments, and backbleeding is assessed prior to flushing with heparinized saline. If endarterectomy is to be limited to the mesenteric vessels, the aortotomy is closed following the endarterectomy of the celiac axis and superior mesenteric artery.

Figure 4: Combined Mesenteric and Renal Endarterectomy (Multiple Panels)

If a concurrent renal endarterectomy is to be done, the endarterectomy is continued cephalad to remove a cylinder of aortic plaque below the level of the renal arteries. Eversion endarterectomy of each renal artery is done in a fashion similar to the mesenteric vessels, and it is possible to remove a single sleeve of aortic atherosclerotic plaque with multiple renal ostial extensions. If graft replacement of the infrarenal aorta is planned for occlusive disease, the aortotomy is ended in the proximal infrarenal aorta to allow placement of an infrarenal aortic clamp caudad to the end of the aortotomy. This allows perfusion of the viscera and kidneys during reconstruction of the infrarenal aorta.

Following either transaortic mesenteric endarterectomy or combined mesenteric/renal transaortic endarterectomy, the aortotomy is closed with a continuous 4-0 suture, after backbleeding each of the clamped vessels. Flow is restored gradually to the viscera, kidneys and infrarenal aorta in close coordination with the anesthesiologists to ensure there is a precipitous fall in blood pressure upon declamping. Flow is restored first to the infrarenal aorta, followed by the renal arteries and lastly to the mesenteric vessels.

Figure 3

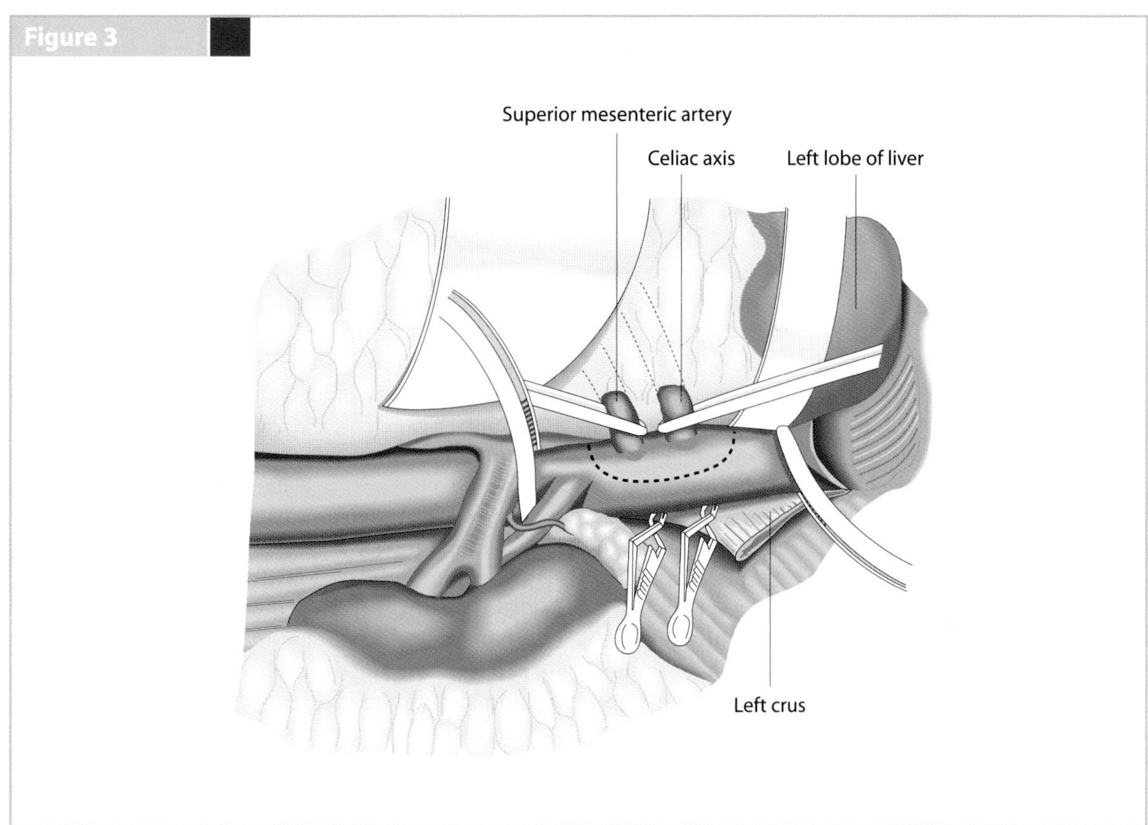

Figure 4

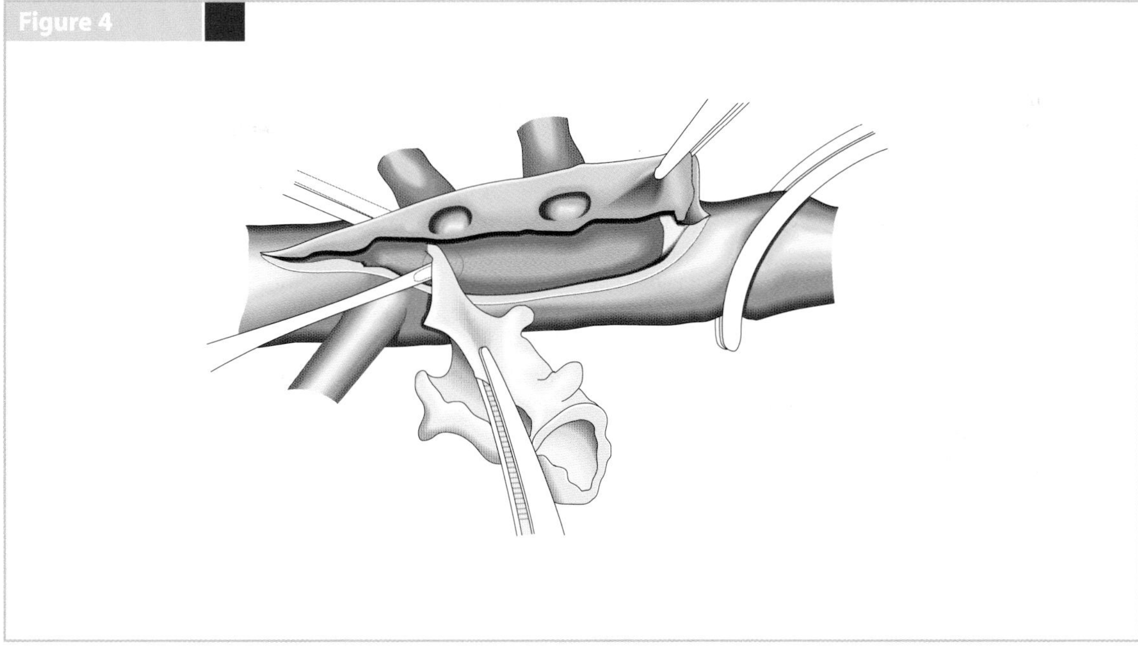

Figure 5: Superior Mesenteric Artery Arteriotomy (Separate Arteriotomy in SMA, Two Panels)

A complete occlusion of the superior mesenteric artery is usually associated with a tapered thrombus attached to the distal aspect of the occluding plaque, and extending to either the first or second branch of the superior mesenteric artery, where collateral flow reenters to supply the distal mesenteric circulation. Complete occlusion should be discernable preoperatively on the lateral aortogram, and is confirmed by palpation of the vessel. This tail of thrombus should be removed with the plaque and requires particular care to ensure that thrombus fragments are not left behind.

If it is evident that residual chronic thrombus or plaque remains distal to the transaortic endarterectomy specimen, then a separate longitudinal arteriotomy is made in the superior mesenteric artery prior to reestablishing antegrade flow in this vessel (Fig. 5). This can be done after restoring flow to the celiac axis and distal aorta by clamping the proximal superior mesenteric artery prior to restoring flow in the aorta and other splanchnic vessels. This sequence allows timely restoration of perfusion of the liver and kidneys while allowing further meticulous work on the superior mesenteric artery without the time pressure associated with complete supraceliac clamping.

A longitudinal arteriotomy is made in the superior mesenteric artery to allow complete removal of any residual plaque or chronic thrombus and careful inspection of the endarterectomy endpoint if there is any question of its adequacy as previously visualized from the transaortic approach. Although a transverse arteriotomy can be more easily closed primarily without narrowing the mesenteric vessel, the advantage of a longitudinal arteriotomy is that it can be extended as needed to visualize the end of the thrombus. Closure with a patch (either autologous or prosthetic) is often required to prevent narrowing (Fig. 5).

A similar strategy is used if the intraoperative completion duplex scan demonstrates a significant flap of either the celiac axis or the superior mesenteric artery. Flow is restored to the kidneys and the other mesenteric vessel while selective clamping is used to isolate the mesenteric vessel that requires attention. A transverse arteriotomy is made just distal to the flap (as marked on the outside of the vessel by the duplex scan) and a new endpoint established under direct vision and the proximal flap removed.

Figure 5

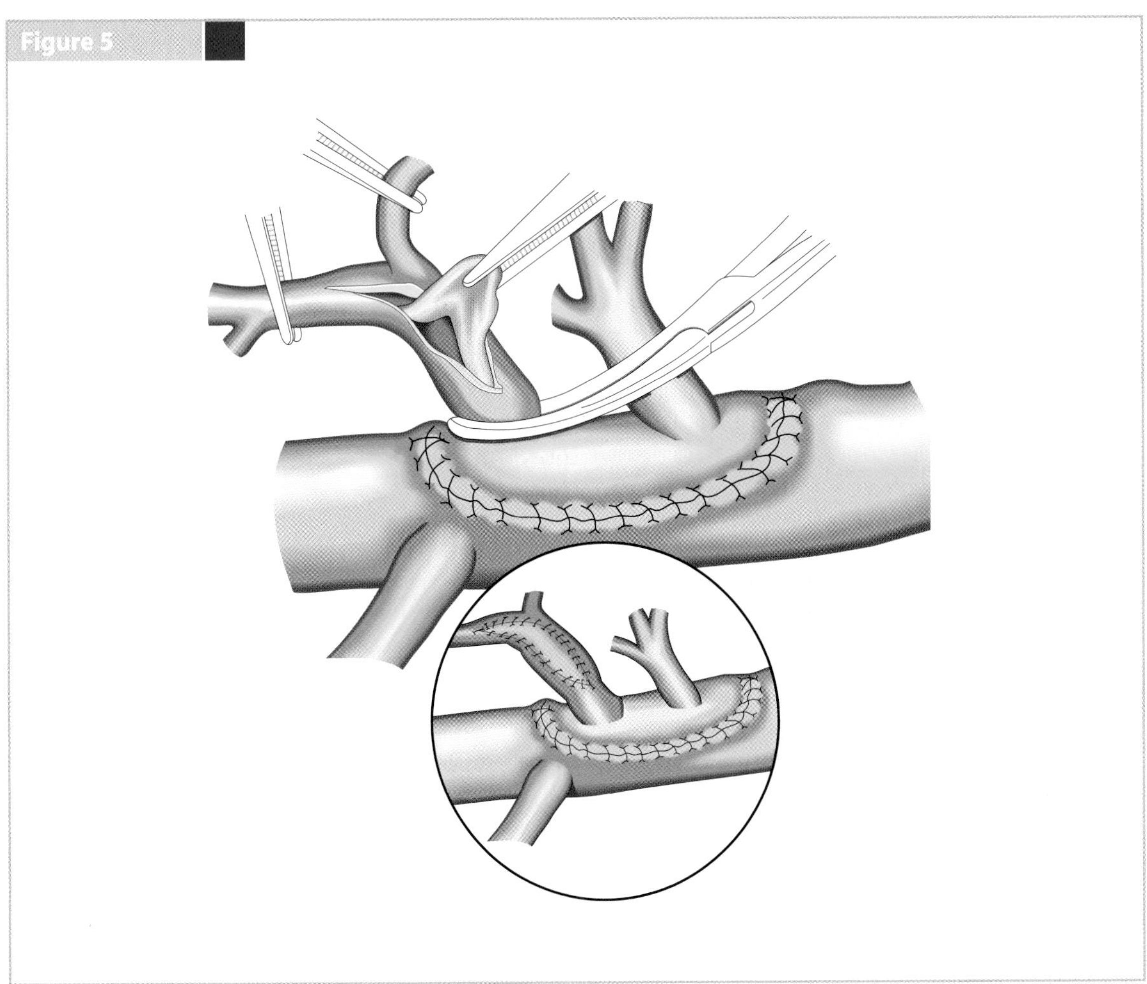

Figure 6: Transaortic Renal Endarterectomy: Infracolic Exposure

For atherosclerotic occlusive disease isolated to the renal arteries, transaortic endarterectomy is an efficient means of renal revascularization and can readily be combined with replacement of the infrarenal aorta for either occlusive or aneurysmal disease. Disease patterns that are favorable for transaortic endarterectomy include proximal stenoses that are essentially extensions of aortic atherosclerotic plaque and the absence of disease extending throughout the main renal arteries and into branches. The major contraindication, as is the case for any endarterectomy, is aneurysmal or other degeneration of either the pararenal aorta or the renal arteries. Multiple renal arteries are not a contraindication to endarterectomy and indeed are often treated most expeditiously by endarterectomy rather than complex sequential bypass grafting.

If the aorta immediately below the renal arteries is aneurysmal, the renal endarterectomy is done through the transected neck of the aorta as described below. If the juxtarenal aorta is free of disease and can be clamped below the renal arteries leaving sufficient space for the endarterectomy, the renal endarterectomy is done through an anterior longitudinal aortotomy which is closed prior to reconstruction of the infrarenal aorta. In either case, proper exposure of the pararenal aorta and renal arteries is critical to the successful execution of transaortic renal endarterectomy.

Optimal exposure is achieved through an transperitoneal infracolic approach to the aorta, with mobilization of the duodenum and small bowel to the right side of the abdomen (see Fig. 9). The retroperitoneum is opened vertically over the infrarenal aorta, and dissection is carried cephalad to the left renal vein. Complete mobilization of the left renal vein is essential to the exposure of the pararenal aorta. Division of the three branches and mobilization of the left renal vein to the caval junction is done as described above after medial visceral rotation. In contrast to exposure of the paravisceral aorta where the renal vein is retracted caudad, for infracolic exposure of the pararenal aorta it is important to divide the left gonadal and ascending lumbar veins (along with the adrenal vein) to allow for subsequent cephalad retraction. Division of the diaphragmatic crura which encase the pararenal aorta is done on either side of the aorta to allow anterior mobilization and dissection of the aorta. The renal arteries are dissected free to the first major branch to allow prolapsing the vessel into the aortic lumen during the inversion endarterectomy as described above. Division of the lumbar veins allows lateral mobilization of the vena cava to facilitate dissection of the right renal artery. The distance between the renal arteries and superior mesenteric artery is variable and may not be adequate for aortic clamping without impinging on the renal orifices. It is important that the proximal aortic clamp be placed sufficiently distant from the renal arteries to allow a segment of suprarenal aorta to be manipulated during the eversion endarterectomy. If the suprarenal aorta below the superior mesenteric artery is not adequate for this, the aorta above this vessel is exposed to allow aortic clamping immediately above the superior mesenteric artery (Fig. 7). The ganglionic tissue overlying the aorta in the region of the superior mesenteric artery is excised, and an aortic clamp can also be placed vertically at the base of the superior mesenteric artery and angled upward to clamp the aorta and the superior mesenteric artery.

Figure 6

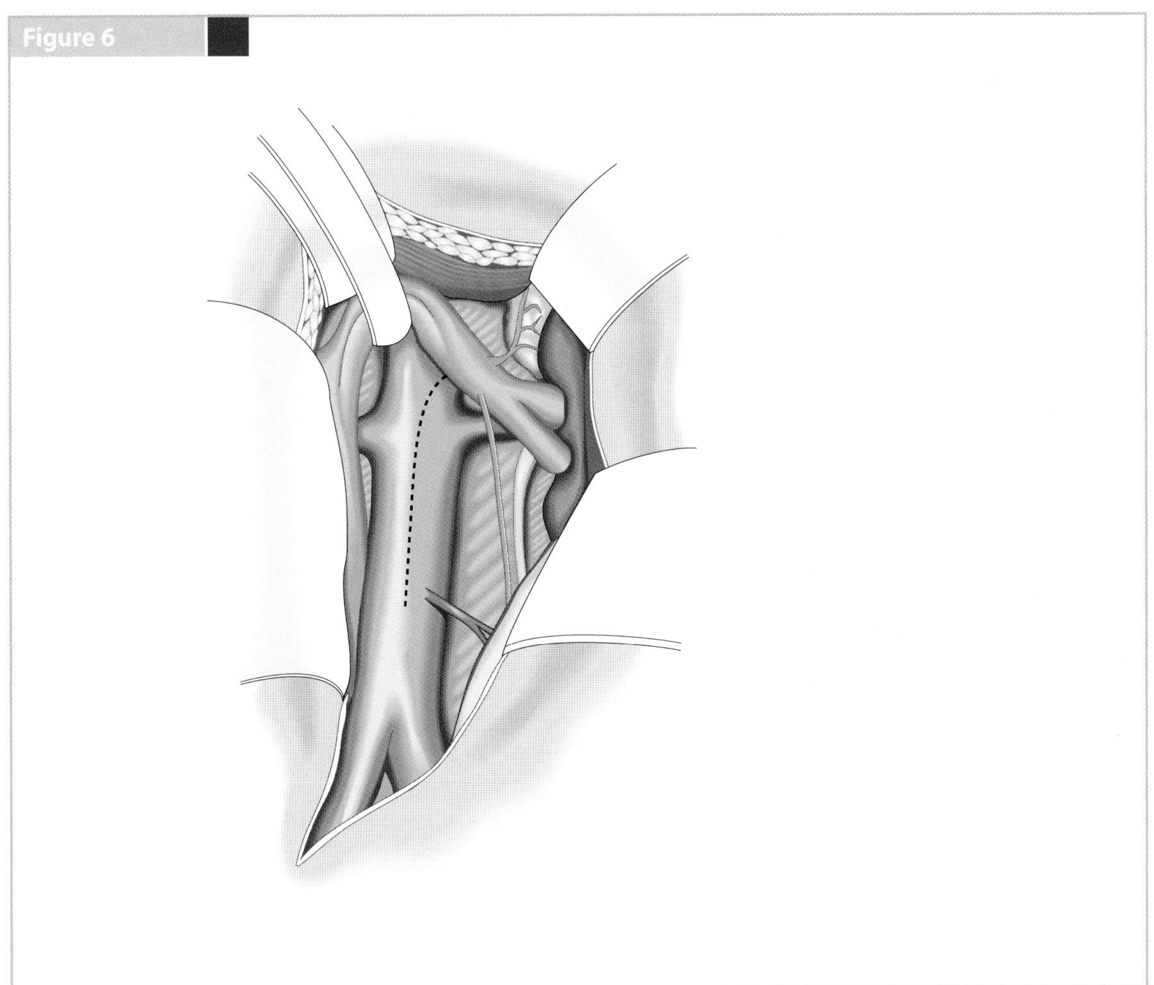

Figure 7: Transaortic Renal Endarterectomy: Vertical (Multiple Panels)

Following exposure and mobilization of the pararenal aorta, the renal arteries and infrarenal aorta are clamped after administration of heparin and mannitol and a continuous infusion of the selective renal vasodilator fenoldopam is started. The suprarenal aorta and superior mesenteric artery are clamped last, and lumbar arteries are clamped to prevent backbleeding. A longitudinal arteriotomy is made on the anterior surface of the aorta and the renal arteries are flushed with ice-cold lactated Ringer's solution and then reclamped. If the distance between the renal arteries and the superior mesenteric artery is limited, the longitudinal aortotomy is curved to the left of the superior mesenteric artery. The endarterectomy plane between the plaque and aortic wall is developed as described above for mesenteric endarterectomy. The plaque is freed circumferentially from the aorta around the renal orifice prior to performing the eversion endarterectomy of the renal artery (Fig. 7). The plaque is sharply transected in the aorta first inferiorly above the infrarenal aortic clamp and then superiorly just below the orifice of the superior mesenteric artery; leaving the plaque attached to the vessel only in the renal artery (Fig. 7). The clamp on the renal artery is pushed towards the aorta to prolapse the vessel into the aorta and allow direct visualization of the endpoint of the endarterectomy as the end of the plaque emerges in the invaginated renal artery. The renal artery wall is carefully pushed away from the plaque with a Halle dural elevator in a circumferential fashion as the renal artery is progressively pushed into the aorta. Following completion of the endarterectomy, the cut edges of the remaining aortic plaque are inspected and beveled as needed to prevent emboli or an origin for thrombosis. The renal arteries are unclamped to allow backbleeding and the endarterectomy site carefully irrigated free of debris. The aortotomy is closed with a continuous non-absorbable suture and the infrarenal and suprarenal aorta are flushed (with the renal arteries clamped) prior to completion of the closure. The endarterectomy is assessed with intraoperative duplex scanning and significant technical defects (large intimal flaps, areas of increased velocity) are corrected immediately. If replacement of the infrarenal aorta is needed for either occlusive or aneurysmal disease, flow is restored to the renal arteries and the infrarenal clamp maintained to allow graft replacement below it.

Figure 7

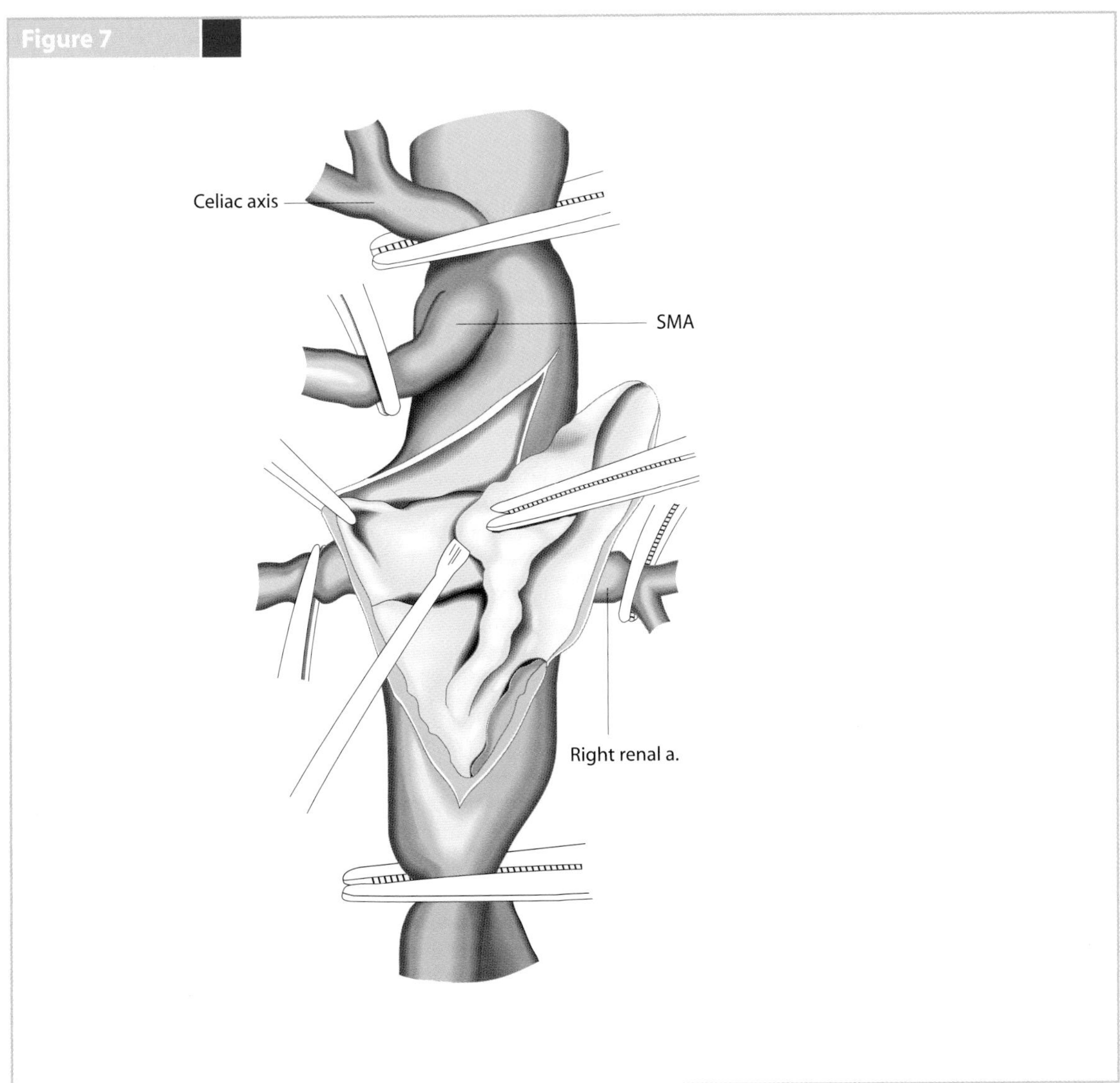

Figure 8: Transaortic Renal Endarterectomy (Via Transected Aorta)

If there is not sufficient length of aorta between the renal arteries and a juxtarenal aneurysm, then the transaortic renal endarterectomy is done through the orifice of the transected aorta. This is technically more demanding than when done through a longitudinal aortotomy, and is associated with a longer period of renal ischemia as flow is restored to the kidneys after completion of both the endarterectomy and the anastomosis of the graft to the juxtarenal aorta. Exposure of the pararenal aorta and renal arteries for this technique is essentially the same as described above for transaortic renal endarterectomy (Fig. 6); however, with large juxtarenal aneurysms there may not be enough space above the aneurysm to allow placement of an aortic clamp between the aneurysm and the renal arteries. In such cases distal vascular control is obtained below the aneurysm, and clamping of the renal arteries and suprarenal aorta is performed as described above (Fig. 7). If the aneurysm can be clamped proximally, considerable time can be saved in terms of renal ischemia as the renal endarterectomy can be performed immediately without having to first open the aneurysm and oversew vessels.

A critical step in the successful execution of transaortic renal endarterectomy through the transected aorta is to mobilize the pararenal aorta sufficiently to allow the transected aortic neck to be turned anteriorly so that the surgeon is looking down the aortic lumen. In addition to circumferential dissection of the renal arteries and pararenal aorta as described above, including division of the diaphragmatic crura, this requires division and ligation of the one or two pairs of lumbar arteries in this region that tether the back of the aorta to the posterior tissues of the retroperitoneum. Division of these vessels, coupled with sharp dissection of the para-aortic neural tissue around the aorta, allows the divided end of the juxtarenal aorta to be turned upwards towards the surgeon. As in transaortic endarterectomy done through a vertical aortotomy, it is critical that the suprarenal aortic clamp be placed sufficiently proximal so that there is no distortion of the renal orifices and an adequate section of suprarenal aorta is free to allow eversion endarterectomy to be performed without undue tension on the aortic wall (Fig. 8). This may require the suprarenal clamp to be placed at or above the superior mesenteric artery, depending on the distance between the renal arteries and the superior mesenteric artery. The clamp can usually be placed underneath the renal vein so that it is retracted out of the field.

Prior to clamping, heparin and mannitol are administered as a bolus and Fenoldopam infusion is begun. Following clamping below the aneurysm (or if possible between the aneurysm and the renal arteries), the renal arteries and suprarenal aorta are clamped. The aorta is transected approximately 5 mm below the renal arteries and the renal orifices are flushed with ice-cold lactated Ringer's solution for renal preservation. The transected juxtarenal aorta is turned anteriorly so that the surgeon can easily look down the aortic lumen beyond the renal artery orifices. If the renal vein is not retracted cephalad by the aortic clamp as described above, the divided aorta can often be transposed anterior to the left renal vein temporarily for the performance of the endarterectomy. The development of the endarterectomy plane of the aortic neck is often easiest to begin posteriorly, where the plaque is often thickest. A sleeve of aortic intima extending above the renal artery orifices is freed prior to directing attention to the renal endarterectomy (Fig. 8). The plaque is transected superiorly above each renal orifice, and can also be divided anteriorly and posteriorly to create two halves of aortic intima which can be more easily manipulated for each renal endarterectomy. Prolapsing each renal artery into the aortic lumen, coupled with gentle traction on the plaque, allows progressive visualization of the eversion endarterectomy and the development of the endpoint in the invaginated renal artery lumen as described above in Fig. 7. The endarterectomy site is carefully irrigated with heparinized saline and any debris or intimal fragments are removed. Each renal artery is transiently unclamped to allow backbleeding. A suitable aortic graft is then sewn to the transected aorta with non-absorbable monofilament suture. Following completion of the anastomosis, the suprarenal aortic clamp is opened to flush any debris from either the aortic clamp or the anastomosis out through the open graft with the renal arteries still clamped to prevent renal artery embolism. Finally the renal arteries are unclamped and a soft jaw clamp is placed on the graft immediately below the anastomosis to restore renal perfusion. Intraoperative duplex scanning is used to assess the endarterectomy as described above, and significant technical defects are corrected immediately. The remainder of the infrarenal aortic reconstruction (for either aneurysmal or occlusive disease) is performed in the standard fashion, with the distal aortic or iliac anastomosis completed after perfusion is restored to the kidneys.

Figure 8

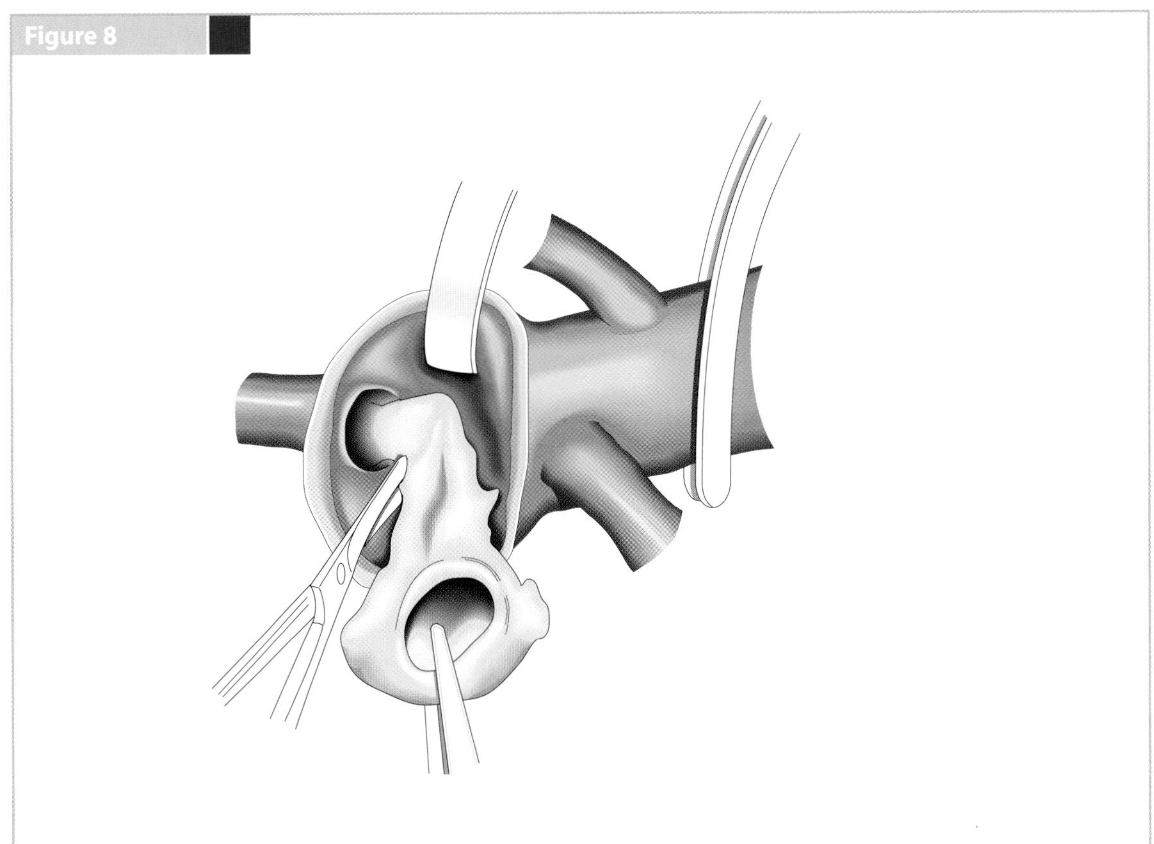

Figure 9: Aortoiliac Endarterectomy: Exposure

Exposure for aortoiliac endarterectomy is easily established through a vertical midline transperitoneal incision. The transverse colon is retracted cephalad out of the abdominal cavity and the small bowel is retracted to the patient's right side, respectively, to provide infracolic exposure of the aorta. The retroperitoneum overlying the aorta is opened vertically on the right side of the aorta to preserve parasympathetic nerves important in erectile function in men and avoid injury to the inferior mesenteric artery or its branches. Complete circumferential mobilization of the infrarenal aorta, iliac arteries and branches, including the lumbar arteries, is needed for aortoiliac endarterectomy, and minimal manipulation is essential during the mobilization to prevent embolization of atherosclerotic plaque or thrombus from within these diseased vessels. Palpation of the external iliac arteries and preoperative angiography allows determination of the extent of plaque in the external iliac arteries. Usually dissection and mobilization of the proximal half of the external iliac artery is sufficient. Lumbar arteries and the inferior mesenteric artery are dissected sufficiently to allow placement of bulldog clamps. If the angiogram demonstrates either occlusion or significant stenoses affecting the hypogastric arteries, these vessels must also be mobilized and dissected past their first bifurcation to allow extraction endarterectomy.

After satisfactory exposure and systemic heparinization, the external iliac and hypogastric arteries are clamped followed by clamping of the aorta below the renal arteries. If the preoperative angiogram demonstrates thrombus extending close to the renal arteries, infrarenal clamping may cause extrusion of the thrombus cephalad with resulting embolism to the renal arteries. Such thrombus is present when the infrarenal aorta is occluded, and the exposure and dissection should be extended to the pararenal aorta to allow temporary clamping of the suprarenal aorta and the renal arteries. Once the juxtarenal thrombus has been removed through the aortotomy, the suprarenal clamp can be replaced by an infrarenal clamp allowing perfusion of the renal arteries during the remainder of the procedure.

Figure 10: Aortoiliac Endarterectomy: Aortotomy and Endarterectomy

The aorta is opened longitudinally on the right side and an endarterectomy plane is developed circumferentially in the aorta which frees a sleeve of plaque from the aortic wall. Opening the aorta on the right side allows better visualization of the orifice of the inferior mesenteric artery on the inside of the anterior aortic wall, which usually requires an eversion endarterectomy as part of the removal of the aortic plaque. The plaque is sharply transected with a pair of scissors at the upper aspect where it is thinner near the renal arteries. The endarterectomy is done in a standard fashion and stops at the aortic bifurcation where the aortotomy (but not the plaque) ends. The endarterectomy of the aortic bifurcation is continued in a semi-closed fashion as far as possible through the aortotomy.

Figure 9

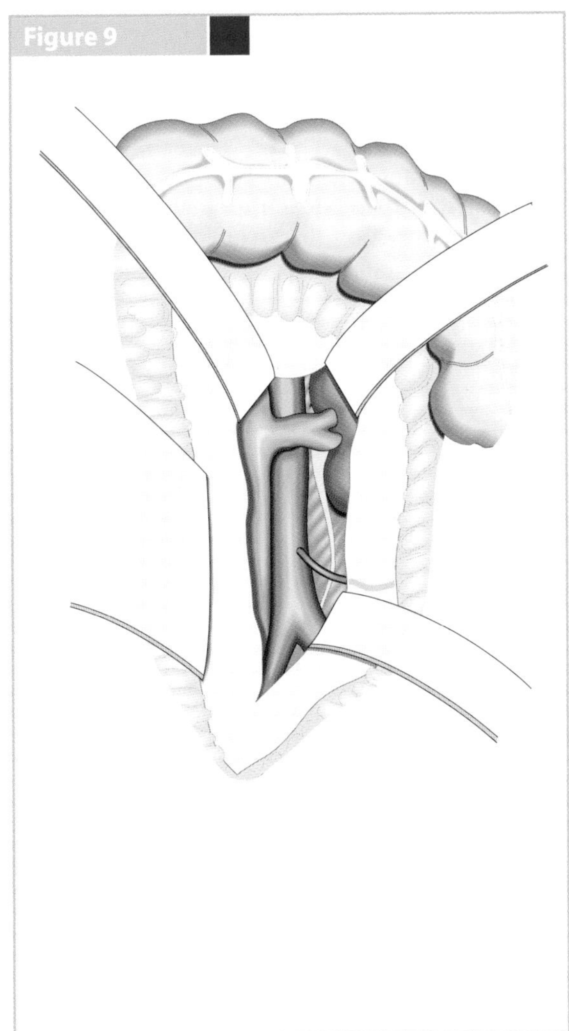

Figure 10

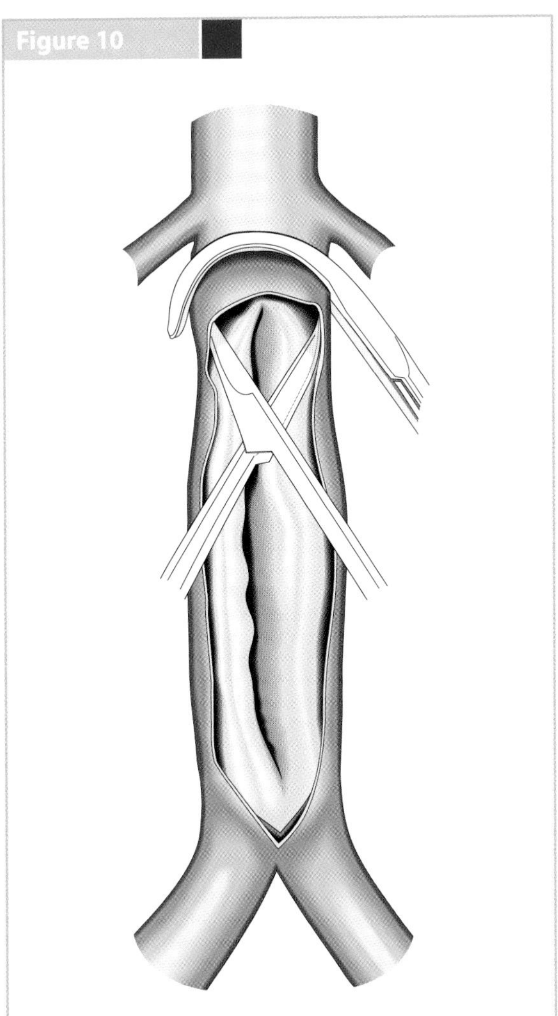

Figures 11–13: Aortoiliac Endarterectomy: Exposure/Aortotomy

The distal aspect of the plaque is treated through a transverse arteriotomy in the external iliac artery just distal to the iliac artery bifurcation. A Beaver blade is used to create a smooth endpoint at the end of the plaque and the atheroma in the intervening segment of common iliac artery is freed by passing either looped strippers proximally or manually by the use of a conventional or powered oscillating endarterectomy device (Fig. 12). Once the plaque is freed at the endpoint and circumferentially in the common iliac artery, it is then reflected back up through the common iliac artery and brought out through the aortotomy above (Fig. 13).

Figure 11

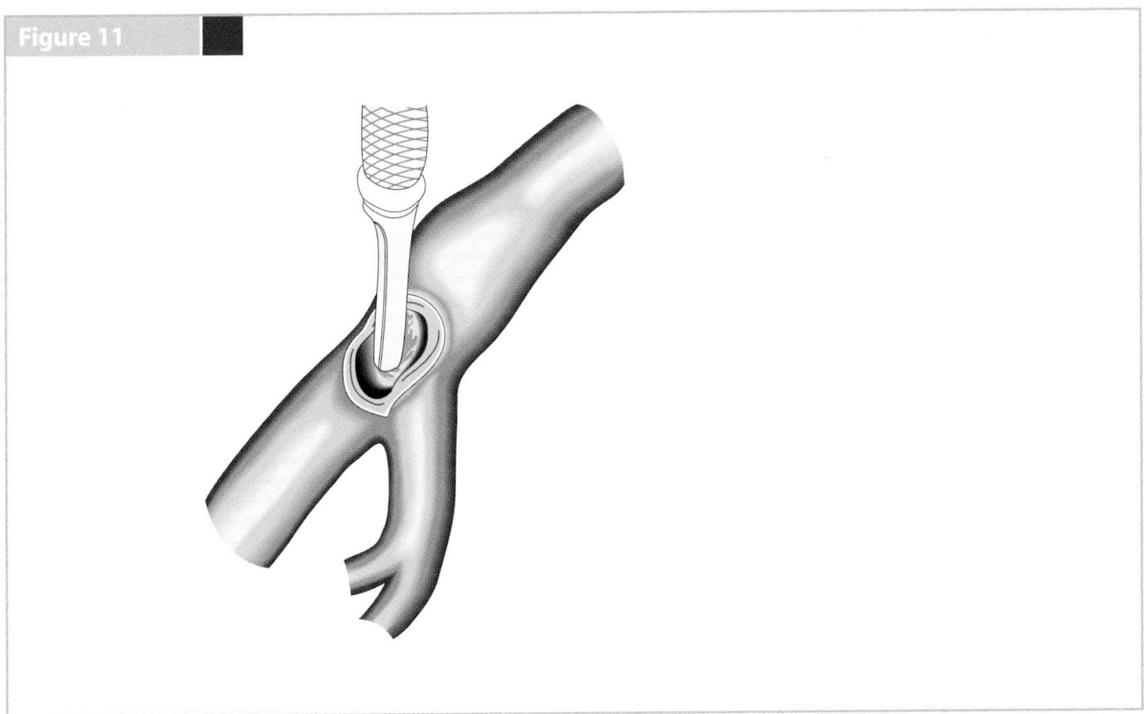

Figure 12

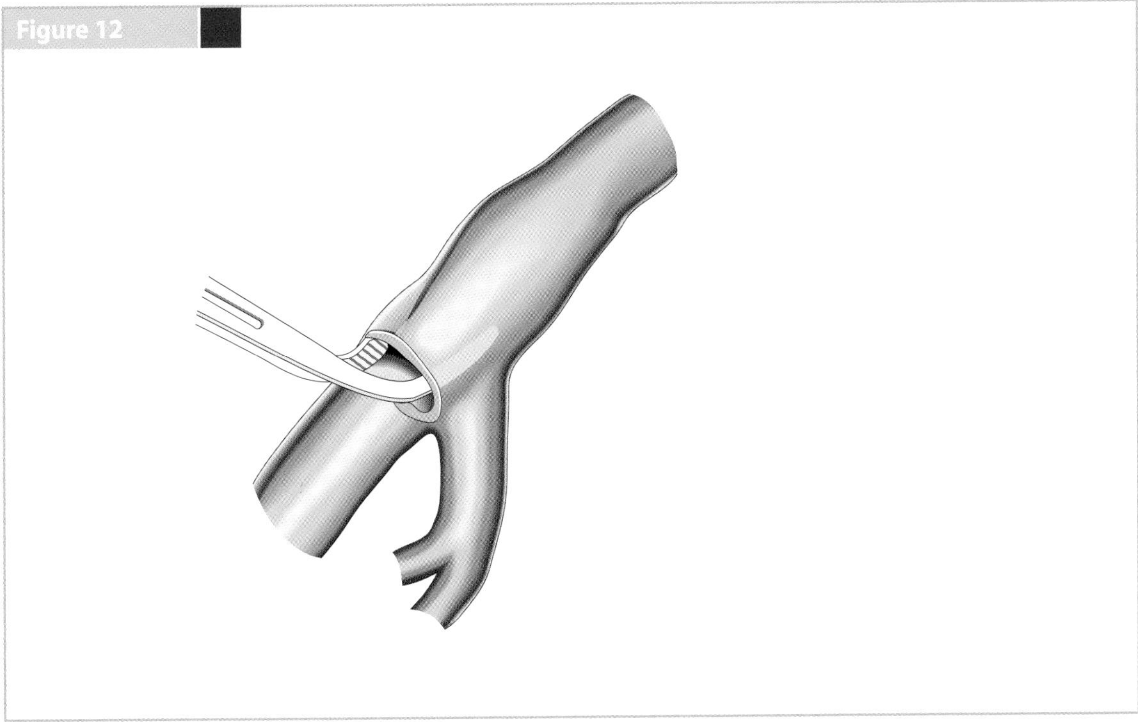

Figure 13

Figure 14: Aortoiliac Endarterectomy: Closure of Arteriotomy

If the disease extends beyond the iliac bifurcation into the external iliac artery, the endpoint in the external iliac artery is achieved under direct visualization through a second transverse arteriotomy in the external iliac artery just beyond the palpable extent of the plaque. A Beaver blade is used at the end of the plaque to create a smooth transition to the remaining intima, and this end of the plaque can be reflected back and delivered through either the common iliac arteriotomy or the aortotomy. Extension of disease into the external iliac artery is often associated with significant extension of the plaque into the internal iliac artery, and an extraction endarterectomy is performed of the internal iliac artery through the opening in the common iliac artery. The plaque is first freed circumferentially from the underlying arterial wall by dissection from the arteriotomy at the iliac bifurcation, and then removed through this same arteriotomy. Angled extraction clamps designed especially for this maneuver are available, and external palpation of the internal iliac artery to guide the extraction endarterectomy is essential for complete removal of the plaque.

The aortotomy is closed with continuous sutures and the iliac arteriotomies are closed with interrupted sutures to prevent narrowing. The endarterectomy is assessed immediately with intraoperative duplex scanning. Significant technical defects are corrected immediately, and the retroperitoneum is closed with continuous absorbable suture. Oral antiplatelet agents are started on the first postoperative day and postoperative anticoagulation is not routinely used.

Figure 13

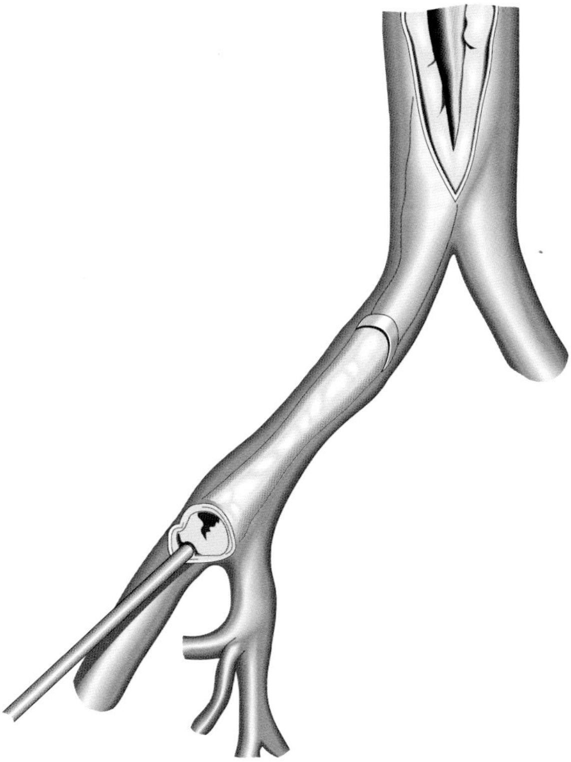

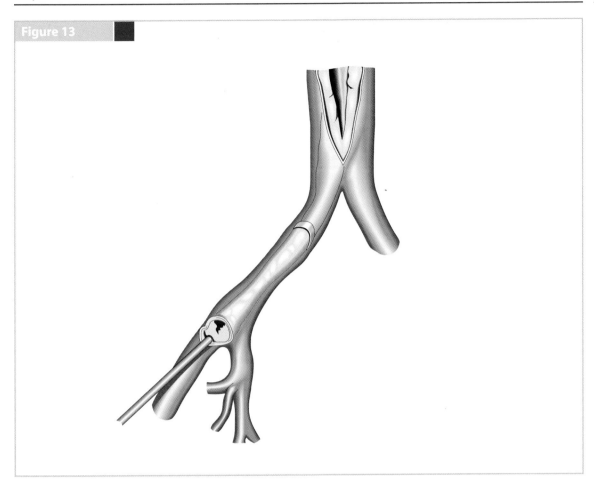

Figure 14

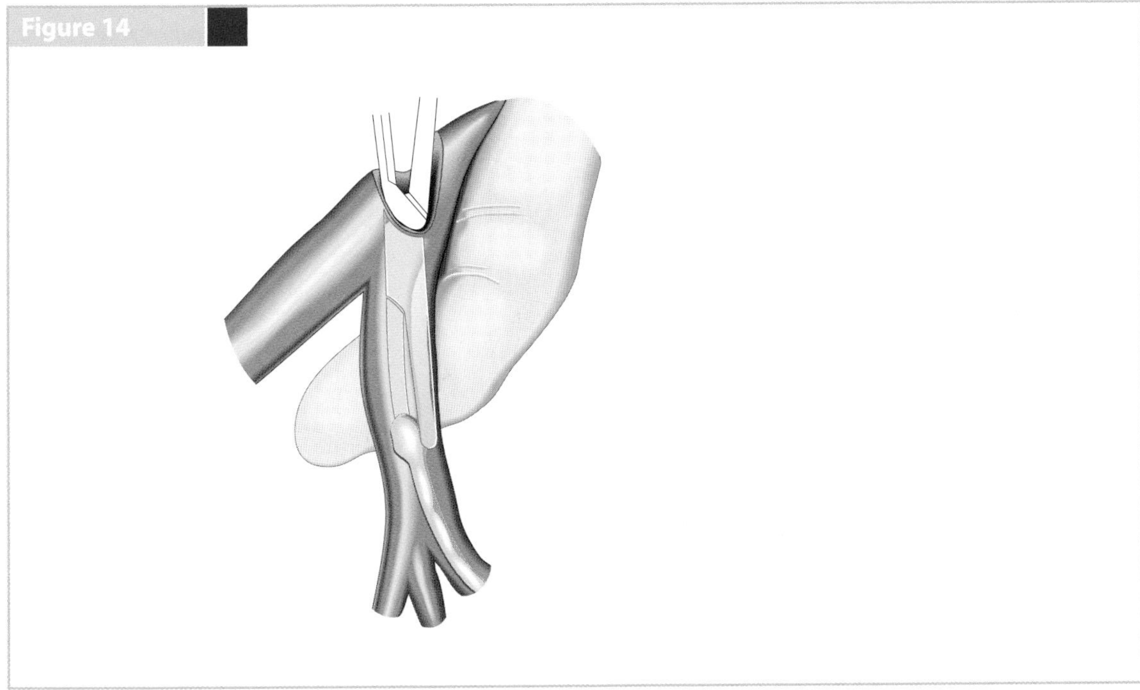

CONCLUSION

Endarterectomy remains an effective and durable means of revascularization for the abdominal aorta and its branches, and is the technique of choice for proximal disease involving multiple branch vessels. Although technically demanding, the speed and efficiency of transaortic endarterectomy is particularly applicable to the renal and mesenteric vessels where prolonged clamp times cause detrimental visceral and renal ischemia. Although most commonly utilized in referral centers with large experiences with aortic surgery, the need for endarterectomy does not appear to be decreasing. The natural history of mesenteric and renal artery occlusive disease suggests that an aggressive approach is warranted in most symptomatic patients, and the presence of significant splanchnic vessel disease in patients undergoing reconstruction of the infrarenal aorta for aneurysm or occlusive disease suggests that familiarity with endarterectomy is important for the aortic surgeon in the future.

Endarterectomy of the abdominal aorta or its major branches requires careful preoperative assessment, meticulous attention to intraoperative technical detail, and careful postoperative care. Patients who undergo prolonged clamping of the supraceliac aorta are susceptible to postoperative transient pulmonary dysfunction, which in the elderly patient with preexisting lung disease may require mechanical ventilation for the first 48 h after surgery. Maintenance of postoperative blood pressure in the normal range is critical for all patients undergoing arterial endarterectomy, as hypotension may predispose to thrombus formation and hypertension to significant suture line bleeding. In patients who have undergone endarterectomy of the mesenteric or renal vessels, an imaging study of the reconstruction is performed prior to discharge from the hospital to document the revascularization and establish a baseline for the future. This is particularly useful should the patient develop recurrent symptoms as comparison with later studies is valuable in determining if symptoms are due to recurrent ischemia and to plan any further interventions. The imaging modality previously used exclusively was contrast arteriography; however, the improvements in magnetic imaging technology have allowed the use of magnetic resonance angiography (MRA) to largely supplant invasive studies for studying proximal aortic branch vessels. MRA is particularly useful in patients undergoing renal endarterectomy who have chronic renal insufficiency, as it eliminates the danger of contrast nephropathy in these high risk patients. Endarterectomy has evolved from being the first technique for basic aortic revascularization to an optimal technique for treating complex patterns of occlusive disease involving both the aorta and its critical branch vessels.

REFERENCES

Jean-Claude JM, Reilly LM, Stoney RJ, Messina LM (1999) Pararenal aortic aneurysms: the future of open aortic aneurysm repair. J Vasc Surg 29:902–912

Sarkar R (2002) Evolution of the management of mesenteric occlusive disease. Cardiovasc Surg 10:395–399

Schneider DB, Schneider PA, Reilly LM, Ehrenfeld WK, Messina LM, Stoney RJ (1998) Reoperation for recurrent chronic visceral ischemia. J Vasc Surg 27:276–284

Stoney RJ, Schneider DB, Sarkar R (2001) Surgery of the celiac and superior mesenteric arteries. In: Baker RJ, Fischer JE (eds) Mastery of surgery, 4th edn. Lippincott, Williams and Wilkins, Baltimore

18

CHAPTER 19

Bypass Procedures for Mesenteric Ischemia

Tina R. Desai, Bruce L. Gewertz

INTRODUCTION

Acute or chronic mesenteric ischemic syndromes result from interruption of mesenteric blood flow. Specific symptoms depend on the nature, degree, and duration of blood flow interruption as well as individual differences in specific mesenteric anatomy and collateral development. Typically, elderly patients with multiple atherosclerotic comorbidities are more frequently affected by acute syndromes; patients with chronic mesenteric ischemia symptoms are more frequently younger (mean age of 58) and female (60%) (Moawad et al. 1997). Both groups of patients manifest a high incidence of smoking, hypertension, coronary artery disease and cerebrovascular disease.

Operative treatment of mesenteric ischemia may consist of antegrade or retrograde mesenteric bypass procedures. In acutely ischemic patients, bypass is utilized if other procedures such as embolectomy fail or are not suitable. These patients are often gravely ill and may manifest hemodynamic instability, coagulation abnormalities, and systemic toxicity from necrotic bowel. Under these circumstances, the bypass is necessarily limited by the patient's status, often originating from the infrarenal aorta or iliac vessels and including revascularization of at least one mesenteric artery (most often the superior mesenteric artery). Usually it is preferable to perform the bypass first, and reevaluate bowel viability after revascularization. Resection of grossly necrotic segments is necessary at the time of the original operation, but every effort is made to preserve viable intestine. Adjunctive evaluations such as intraoperative observation under a Woods lamp after fluorescein injection, Doppler interrogation of mesenteric end vessels, or second look operations after 24–48 h may be required. When bypass is combined with bowel resection or when the viability of intestinal segments is in question, bypass with autologous conduit is recommended.

Patients with chronic mesenteric ischemia are offered revascularization to alleviate symptoms of chronic postprandial abdominal pain, food fear, weight loss and malnutrition, and to prevent the onset of acute mesenteric ischemia, which is preceded by chronic symptoms in 20–50% of cases (Kaleya and Boley 1995). Preoperative evaluation should exclude other causes of abdominal pain with abdominal radiographs, upper and lower gastrointestinal contrast studies, endoscopy or computed tomography as indicated by the patient's symptoms. Duplex ultrasonography by an experienced technician is a useful screening tool for chronic mesenteric ischemia but arteriography including a lateral view of the aorta and selective mesenteric views is necessary for definitive diagnosis and operative planning. In these patients, revascularization of two of the three mesenteric vessels is generally recommended. We prefer antegrade bypass originating from the supraceliac aorta because this segment is usually free of atherosclerotic disease and grafts to both the celiac and superior mesenteric arteries (SMAs) can be performed from this location with an excellent lie tunneled in the retropancreatic position. However, retrograde bypasses or endarterectomy may be utilized in selected cases.

Preoperative preparation for mesenteric bypass depends on the acuity of symptoms, existing comorbidities and the magnitude of procedure. Further evaluation for coronary artery disease and pulmonary disease should be performed in symptomatic or high risk patients. The procedures are performed with the patient under general anesthesia. Supplemental epidural anesthetic may be advantageous in selected patients. An arterial line and central venous monitoring and resuscitation catheters are placed in most patients in the operating room. Patients are positioned supine. Placement of a towel roll behind the upper back may be useful in larger patients to allow better exposure of the retroperitoneum.

Figure 1: Anterior Exposure for Antegrade Mesenteric Bypass

Antegrade mesenteric bypass arising from the supraceliac aorta is the procedure of choice in elective revascularizations. Bypass can be performed easily to both the celiac and superior mesenteric arteries from this approach while avoiding the problem of kinking seen in retrograde bypasses. Access to the abdominal cavity is most frequently obtained via a midline incision in cases of acute mesenteric ischemia. This approach allows maximal exposure for abdominal exploration and facilitates bowel resection should it prove necessary. An alternative bilateral subcostal incision may be used in cases of chronic mesenteric ischemia where an antegrade bypass is planned. Exposure of the supraceliac aorta begins with mobilization of the left lobe of the liver and retraction of the stomach and esophagus to the left. The lesser sac is entered by opening the gastrohepatic ligament. The right crus of the diaphragm is divided to expose the supraceliac aorta, which is almost always free of atherosclerotic disease. Exposure of an adequate length of aorta (usually 4–6 cm) is essential to allow placement of clamps and performance of the proximal anastomosis. This can be accomplished by continued cephalad dissection along the anterior surface of the aorta into the mediastinum. Caudad dissection with retraction of the superior border of the pancreas exposes the origin of the celiac artery. This artery is typically encased with dense fibrous and neural tissue which must be divided to allow assessment of the patency of the vessel. Typically, exposure to the branch point of the left gastric, splenic and common hepatic arteries is necessary to allow enough room for the distal anastomosis even if this is performed to the celiac artery proper. In these emaciated patients, the exposure of the supraceliac aorta and celiac artery from this approach is surprisingly easy. Occasionally with longer segment stenoses or occlusions, the distal anastomosis is positioned at the common hepatic artery which is exposed in the lesser omentum. Although the left gastric artery can be ligated if necessary for exposure, all attempts are made to preserve collateral flow in the setting of mesenteric ischemia.

Figure 2: Exposure of the Superior Mesenteric Artery

The SMA is exposed at the root of the small bowel mesentery. The most proximal segment of this vessel can be exposed by retracting the small bowel to the right, dividing the ligament of Treitz, and mobilizing the fourth portion of the duodenum. The SMA and vein are found just inferior to the fourth portion of the duodenum at the base of the mesentery. Care must be taken to avoid injury to the fragile mesenteric venous branches as an adequate length of SMA is dissected. This approach to the SMA is preferred because it provides the largest caliber vessel to accept the distal anastomosis and because kinking of a retropancreatically tunneled graft is minimized in this location.

Alternatively, the SMA can also be exposed by reflecting the transverse colon up and retracting the small bowel down. The artery is exposed on the anterior surface of the small bowel mesentery where its caliber is smaller than the more proximal position. Care must be taken in this location to avoid kinking of an antegrade graft positioned in a retropancreatic tunnel.

Figure 1

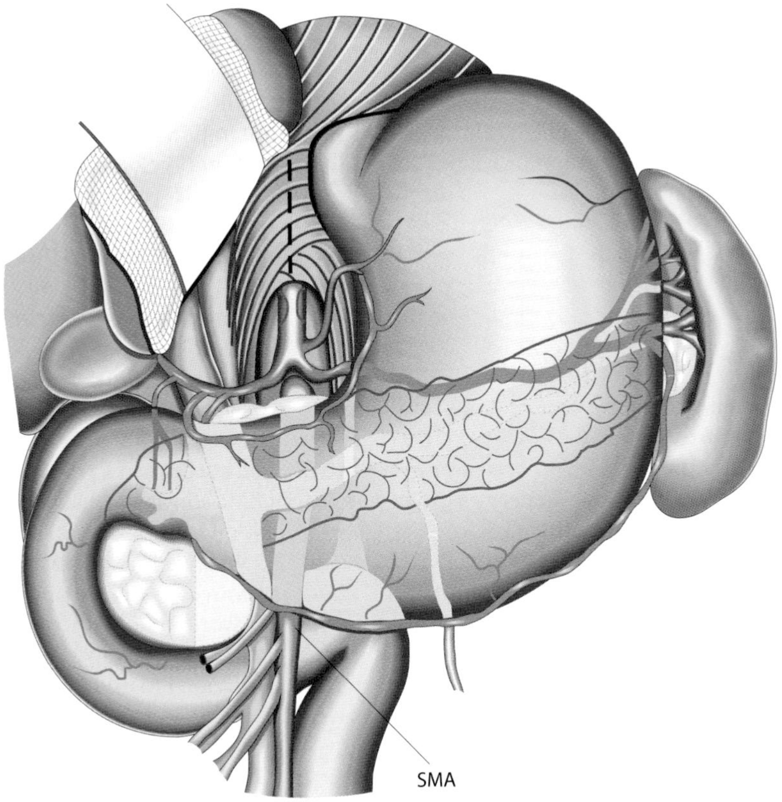

SMA

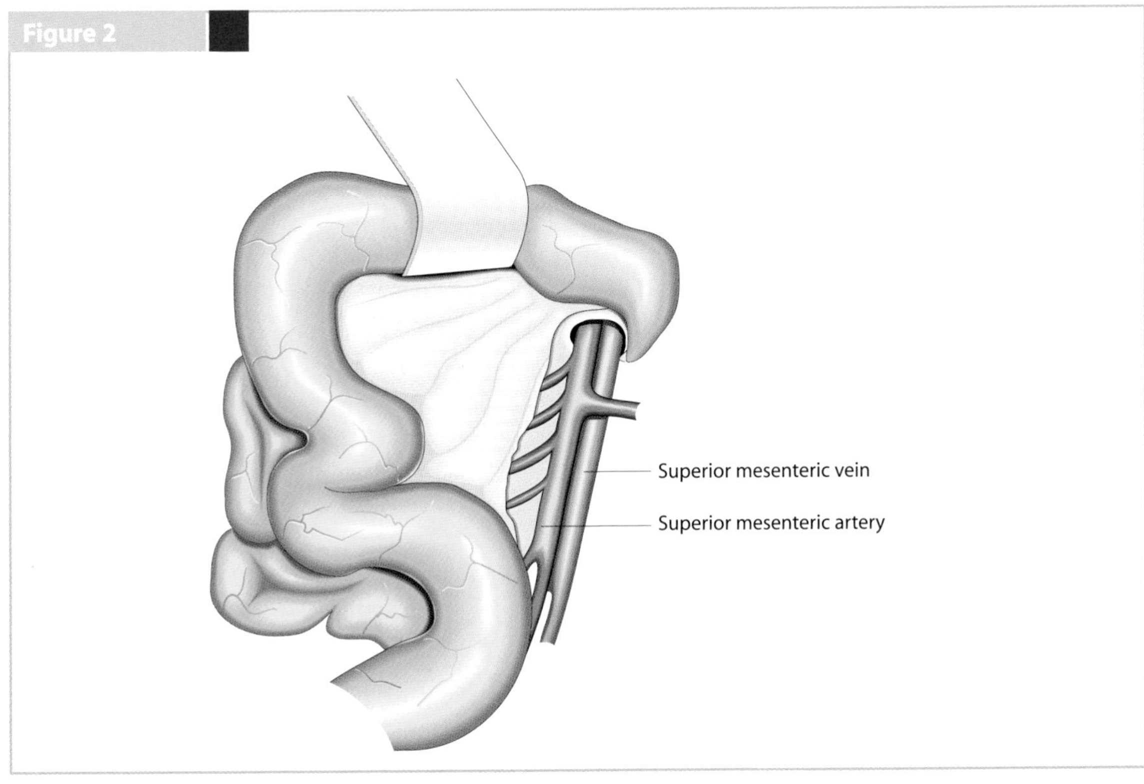

Figure 2

Figure 3, 4: Antegrade Celiac/SMA Bypass Via Retropancreatic Tunnel

Revascularization of both the celiac and superior mesenteric arteries is preferred in the setting of chronic mesenteric ischemia. This is best accomplished using a bifurcated prosthetic graft which provides excellent antegrade revascularization of both vessels while minimizing the tendency to kink. Once the supraceliac aorta, celiac artery, and SMA have been exposed, a retropancreatic tunnel to the SMA in the base of the small bowel mesentery is created using blunt finger dissection to the left of the aorta (Fig. 3).

After systemic heparinization, the aorta is clamped with either a partial occlusion clamp or proximal and distal clamps. The bifurcated graft (usually 12×6 mm size) is trimmed such that it has a short common trunk. An end-to-side anastomosis is performed to the supraceliac aorta with 5-0 monofilament continuous suture, leaving adequate distal length between the end of the anastomosis and the position of the celiac anastomosis to prevent kinking. One limb of the bifurcated graft is anastomosed end to side to the celiac artery and the other limb is tunneled through the retropancreatic tunnel to the superior mesenteric artery. Both distal anastomoses are performed with continuous 6-0 monofilament suture (Fig. 4).

When the celiac stenosis is short, a single bypass graft from supraceliac aorta to the SMA can be performed. The arteriotomy is started in the celiac artery at the level of the celiac stenosis and extended into the aorta. The proximal anastomosis will incorporate this arteriotomy and will serve as a patch for the celiac stenosis. The graft is tunneled in a retroperitoneal plane and the distal anastomosis is constructed to the SMA. This may avoid kinking that can be encountered in a graft from the supraceliac aorta to the proximal celiac artery. In the patient with acute mesenteric ischemia who requires an antegrade bypass, we occasionally revascularize only the SMA from this approach via a retropancreatic tunnel.

An alternative exposure to the supraceliac aorta and mesenteric vessels can be performed through a **medial visceral rotation**. This approach should selectively be applied to patients who have origin stenoses of the celiac and superior mesenteric arteries and is often used when a transaortic endarterectomy is planned. It allows extensive access to the visceral, juxtarenal, and infrarenal abdominal aorta, but exposure to visceral branch vessels or the right renal artery is limited. Once the abdomen is entered, the left colon, spleen, and left kidney are mobilized to expose the abdominal aorta. The left crus of the diaphragm is divided to allow adequate proximal exposure. The celiac and superior mesenteric artery origins are exposed. If an aortic endarterectomy is not thought to be feasible, a local endarterectomy of the celiac origin can be performed to allow a single graft to the SMA to originate from this site. Otherwise, a bifurcated graft as described for the anterior approach can be utilized from the supraceliac aorta. From this retroperitoneal approach, tunneling of the graft is not necessary.

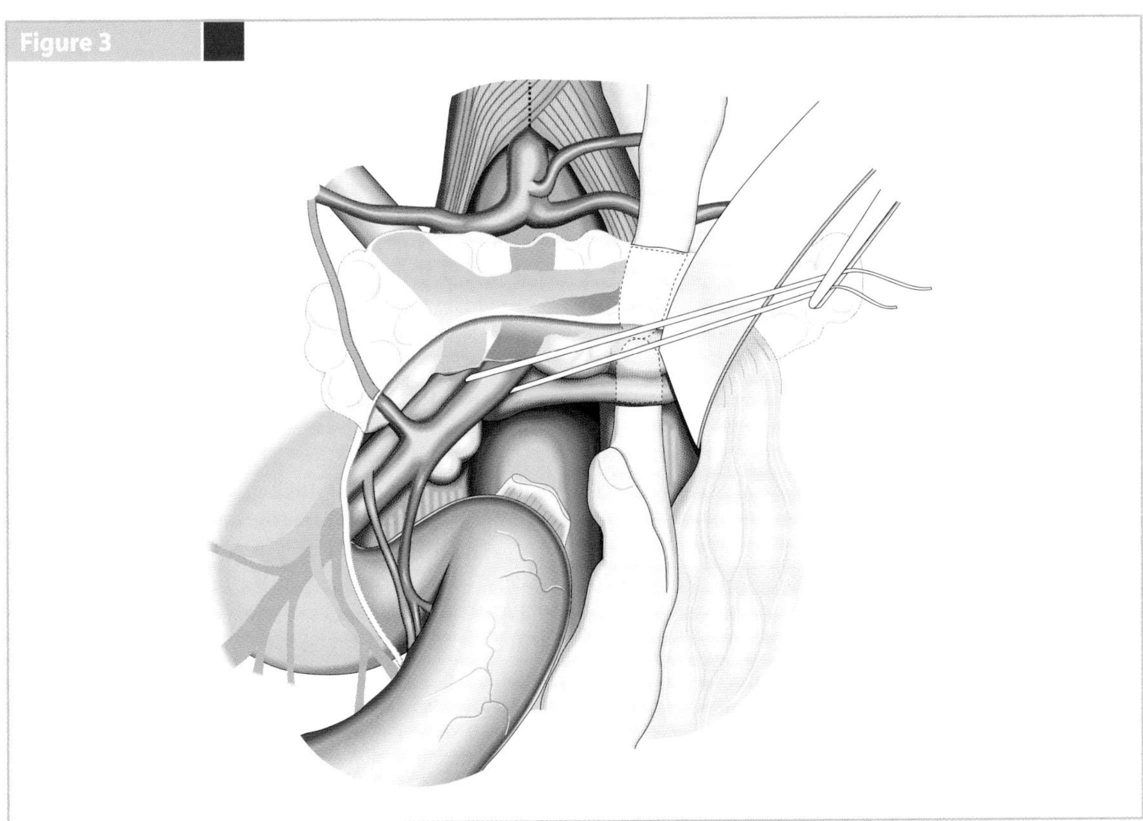

Figure 3

Figure 4

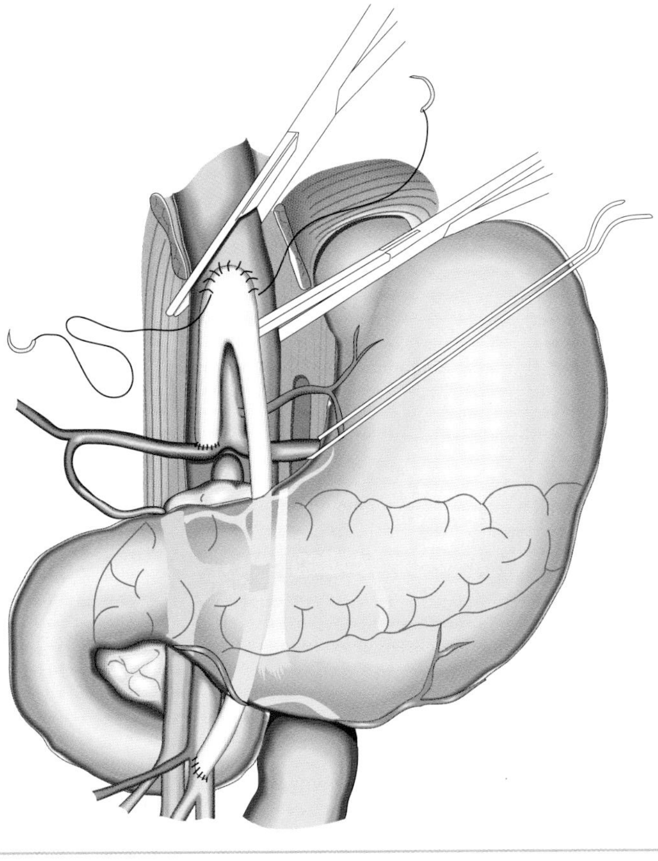

Figure 5A, B: Retrograde Mesenteric Bypass

Retrograde aorto-superior mesenteric artery bypass (Fig. 5A) is most commonly applied in patients with acute mesenteric ischemia and in patients in whom SMA thrombectomy/embolectomy has been unsuccessful. This bypass can also be utilized in patients with chronic mesenteric ischemia who cannot tolerate supraceliac clamping. The infrarenal aorta is easily exposed by division of the ligament of Treitz and mobilization of the fourth portion of the duodenum. With cephalad retraction of the transverse colon and retraction of the small bowel to the right, the infrarenal aorta is dissected along an adequate length to allow proximal anastomosis (4–6 cm). A reversed saphenous vein graft is utilized in the acute setting while a prosthetic graft is an option in chronic cases. An end-to-side proximal anastomosis is performed to the aorta with 5–0 monofilament suture. The SMA is exposed at the root of the mesentery as previously described and an end-to-side distal anastomosis is performed with 6-0 monofilament suture. The short graft between the infrarenal aorta and proximal SMA is prone to kinking when the bowel is returned to its normal position, especially if a vein graft is used. Performing the proximal anastomosis last to a position on the aorta that provides a satisfactory lie of the graft may minimize this problem. Use of externally supported PTFE is another alternative to prevent kinking. A celiac artery graft (Fig. 5B) can also originate from this location. The distal anastomosis is typically performed to the hepatic artery in the porta hepatis. The graft may be routed behind the pancreas (Fig. 4) or in the bed of a medial visceral rotation. Care must be taken to insure adequate lie of the graft to avoid kinking.

Figure 5A

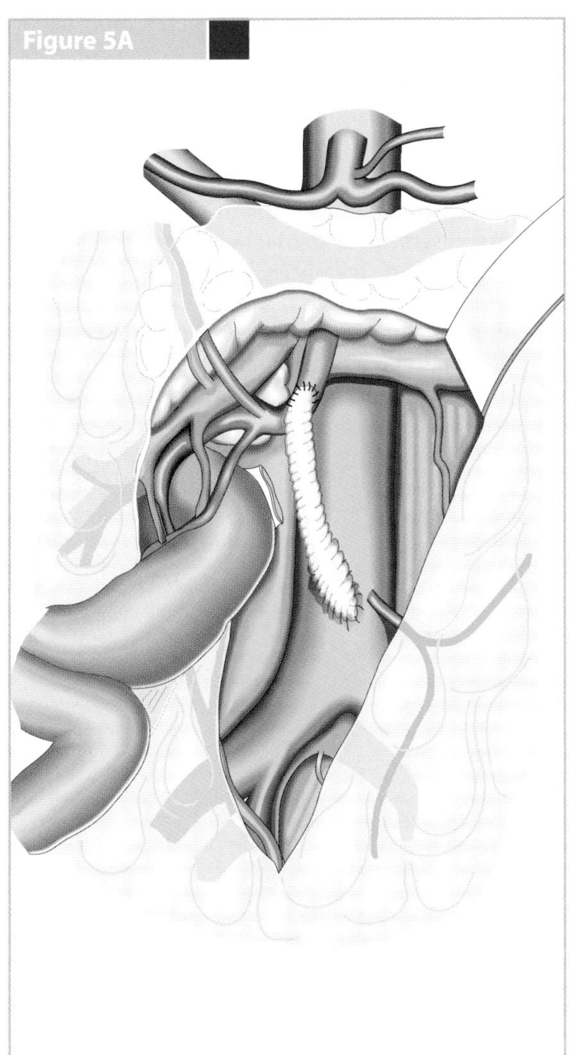

Figure 5B

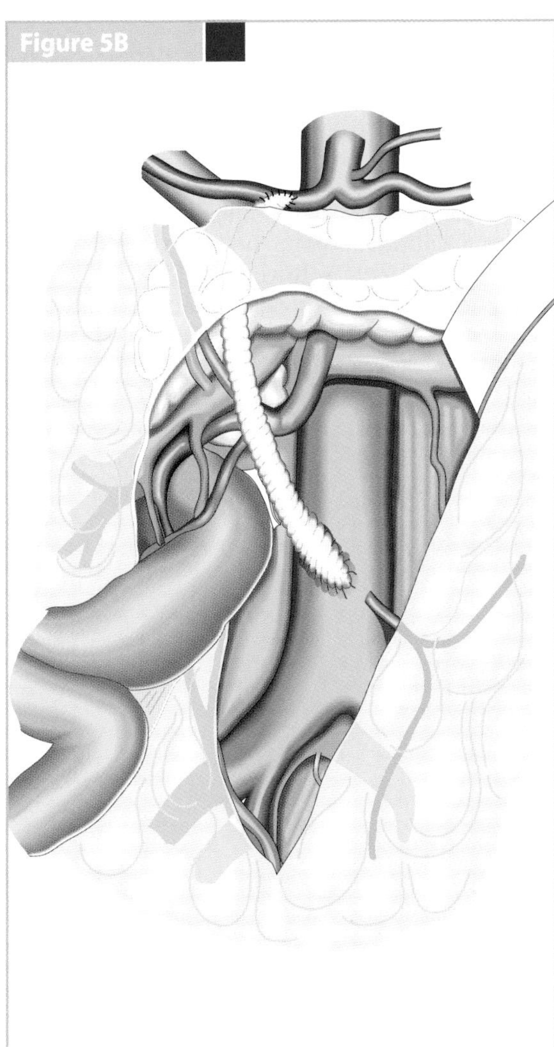

Figure 6: Retrograde Mesenteric Bypass: Iliac Artery Origin

Occasionally, the supraceliac and infrarenal aorta are both unsuitable for a proximal anastomosis. If inflow is compromised, retrograde mesenteric bypass may be performed in conjunction with replacement of the infrarenal aorta. In this setting, the infrarenal graft can serve as the inflow to the SMA alone or to both the SMA and celiac arteries. If inflow is preserved in the setting of a supraceliac and infrarenal aorta which is not suitable for a proximal anastomosis or if the patient cannot tolerate aortic clamping, the iliac artery can be used as an inflow source. The right or left common iliac artery is dissected along adequate length to allow a proximal anastomosis. After systemic heparinization, the artery is clamped and a proximal anastomosis performed with 5-0 monofilament suture in a running fashion. Prosthetic graft can be used if the patient has chronic symptoms and in the absence of bowel necrosis or contamination. Otherwise, reversed saphenous vein is used. A long bypass with a wide turn into the SMA will prevent kinking of this graft. The intestines must be returned to their normal position in the abdominal cavity when measuring the length of the graft to assure an adequate lie.

Figure 6

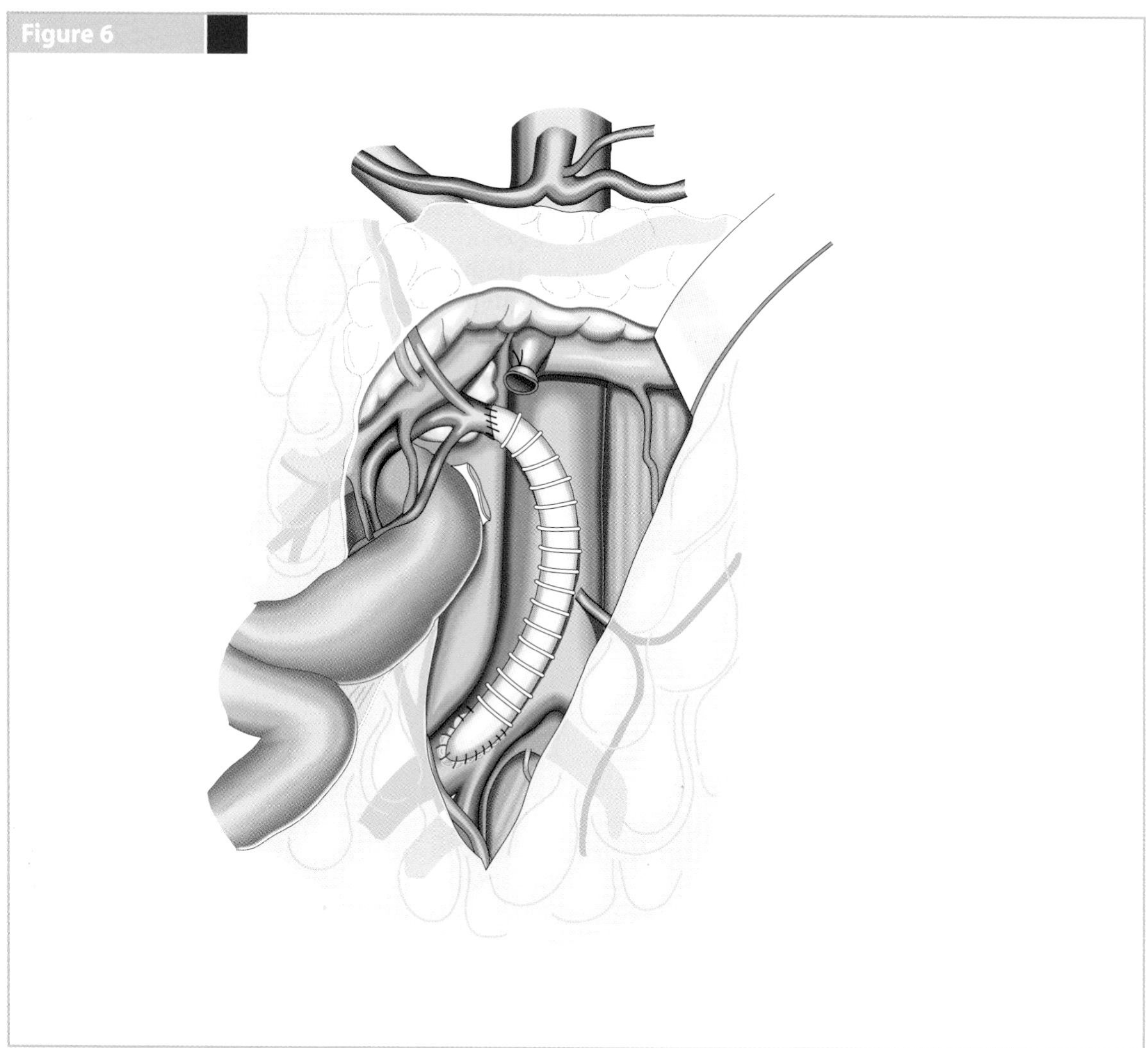

CONCLUSION

Because most clinical series of patients undergoing mesenteric bypass procedures for chronic ischemia include fewer than 50 patients, limited conclusions can be drawn from these studies. Nonetheless, acceptable morbidity and mortality rates can be achieved. In most institutions, mortality rates of 5–7% are reported for this complex procedure in patients with multiple comorbidities (Harward et al. 1993; Johnston et al. 1995). Complications from the procedure are related to concomitant coronary artery disease and to early graft occlusions. Overall 5-year survival in these patients ranges from 50% to 71% (Calderon et al. 1992; Christensen et al. 1994; Moawad et al. 1997).

Overall results with mesenteric bypass procedures for acute or chronic ischemia are exemplified by our recent experience at The University of Chicago (Moawad et al. 1997). Of 24 consecutive patients treated with mesenteric revascularization, all had involvement of the SMA, while 21 of the 24 had additional celiac artery involvement. Seventeen antegrade and seven retrograde bypass procedures were performed. Five-year primary patency was 78% as documented by duplex scan or arteriography. No patient with a patent graft experienced recurrent symptoms.

Most clinicians agree that recurrence is less likely when more than one mesenteric vessel is revascularized. Hollier and colleagues (Hollier et al. 1981) support these conclusions in their series of 56 mesenteric bypasses. Patients with complete revascularization of multivessel disease yielded a late recurrence rate of 11% versus 50% in patients who only had one vessel bypassed. These conclusions are also supported by the experience of McAfee and colleagues (McAfee et al. 1992) and Zelenock and associates (Zelenock et al. 1980).

Although technical factors may support the use of antegrade bypasses to provide an optimal inflow source and graft lie, series attempting to compare antegrade and retrograde bypass procedures have failed to find a difference in long-term patency. Likewise, patency of prosthetic and vein reconstructions have been indistinguishable. McMillan and colleagues (McMillan et al. 1995) used duplex and angiography to follow grafts in 25 patients after mesenteric bypass. In patients who survived for longer than 1 month, graft patency was 89% at a mean follow-up of 35 months. Their study confirmed equivalent patency regardless of type of conduit or orientation of bypass.

The morbidity and mortality of patients undergoing bypass for acute mesenteric ischemia remain high. The duration of the ischemic episode, the underlying lesion, and the patient's cardiovascular comorbidity are the most important determinants of outcome. In a report of 90 patients by Klempnauer and associates (Klempnauer et al. 1997), 31 patients survived and were discharged from the hospital. In this group of patients who survived their initial procedure, cumulative 5-year survival was 50%. Patients who suffered mesenteric arterial thrombosis demonstrated the worst survival rate.

REFERENCES

Calderon M, Reul GJ, Gregoric ID et al. (1992) Long-term results of the surgical management of symptomatic chronic intestinal ischemia. J Cardiovasc Surg (Torino) 33:723–728

Christensen MG, Lorentzen JE, Schroeder TV (1994) Revascularisation of atherosclerotic mesenteric arteries: experience in 90 consecutive patients [see comments]. Eur J Vasc Surg 8:297–302

Harward TR, Brooks DL, Flynn TC, Seeger JM (1993) Multiple organ dysfunction after mesenteric artery revascularization. J Vasc Surg 18:459–467; discussion 467–469

Hollier LH, Bernatz PE, Pairolero PC, Payne WS, Osmundson PJ (1981) Surgical management of chronic intestinal ischemia: a reappraisal. Surgery 90:940–946

Johnston KW, Lindsay TF, Walker PM, Kalman PG (1995) Mesenteric arterial bypass grafts: early and late results and suggested surgical approach for chronic and acute mesenteric ischemia. Surgery 118:1–7

Kaleya RN, Boley SJ (1995) Acute mesenteric ischemia. Crit Care Clin 11:479–512

Klempnauer J, Grothues F, Bektas H, Pichlmayr R (1997) Long-term results after surgery for acute mesenteric ischemia. Surgery 121:239–243

McAfee MK, Cherry KJ Jr, Naessens JM et al. (1992) Influence of complete revascularization on chronic mesenteric ischemia. Am J Surg 164:220–224

McMillan WD, McCarthy WJ, Bresticker MR et al. (1995) Mesenteric artery bypass: objective patency determination. J Vasc Surg 21:729–740; discussion 740–741

Moawad J, McKinsey JF, Wyble CW, Bassiouny HS, Schwartz LB, Gewertz BL (1997) Current results of surgical therapy for chronic mesenteric ischemia. Arch Surg 132:613–618; discussion 618–619

Zelenock GB, Graham LM, Whitehouse WM Jr et al. (1980) Splanchnic arteriosclerotic disease and intestinal angina. Arch Surg 115:497–501

CHAPTER 20 Renal Artery Bypass

James C. Stanley, Peter K. Henke

INTRODUCTION

Operative treatment of patients with renovascular occlusive disease has become somewhat standardized. Although newer diagnostic tests and refined indications for therapeutic interventions have contributed to better surgical results, salutary outcomes have been influenced most by the proficient performance of properly chosen primary procedures by experienced surgeons. The procedures are tailored to the subgroups of renal artery disease.

Arteriosclerotic occlusive disease is the most common cause of renovascular hypertension. Nearly 65% of these stenoses represent aortic spillover lesions. Another 30% of these stenoses present as focal eccentric or concentric narrowings intrinsic to the proximal 1.5 cm of the renal artery, and the remaining 5% occur as isolated narrowings within the segmental vasculature. Renal artery bypass has been the most widely applied procedure in treating these patients.

Arterial dysplasia is the second most common cause of renovascular hypertension and the most common cause of renal artery stenotic disease in hypertensive children and young women. Dysplastic lesions in adulthood are categorized into three groups: medial fibrodysplasia, perimedial dysplasia and intimal fibroplasia. Medial fibrodysplasia, usually presenting as serial stenoses with intervening mural aneurysms, is the most frequently encountered dysplastic lesion. This type of stenotic disease usually affects the middle and distal thirds of the main renal artery with extension into segmental vessels in 20% of cases. Renal artery bypass is often quite complex and encompasses a variety of surgical options in this group of patients. Children having dysplastic developmental stenoses of their renal artery ostia are usually treated by reimplantation procedures, with bypass reconstructions being less common.

Autologous saphenous vein grafts are usually preferred for renal artery bypass reconstructions in adults. Autologous internal iliac artery grafts are favored for use in pediatric-aged patients because of aneurysmal changes occurring in vein grafts of children. The internal iliac artery may also be used in adult reconstructions. Autologous vein and artery grafts should be carefully procured, gently handled, and cautiously irrigated with heparinized blood containing papaverine prior to implantation, to minimize endothelial cell damage. Synthetic grafts of fabricated Dacron or expanded Teflon (polytetrafluoroethylene, PTFE), are often used with equivalent results for arteriosclerotic main renal artery reconstructive procedures. However, synthetic grafts are less compliant and technically more difficult to use when revascularizations involve small dysplastic arteries.

Figure 1A, B

Good surgical exposure is an essential element for successful performance of all renal arterial reconstructions. Preference is given to a transverse supraumbilical abdominal incision extending from the opposite midclavicular line to the posterior-axillary line on the side of the renal artery reconstruction. Such a transverse incision provides a distinct technical advantage in the greater ease of handling instruments parallel to the longitudinal axis of the renal artery during complex procedures. Exposure is facilitated by placing a rolled pack under the lumbar spine so as to accentuate the patient's lumbar lordosis. Alternatively, midline vertical incisions are favored by some surgeons. After the peritoneal cavity has been entered, the intestines are retracted to the opposite side of the abdomen. In small adults, children, and infants, exposure of the renal vasculature is more easily obtained if the intestines are displaced outside the confines of the abdominal cavity. Containment of the viscera in a plastic bag avoids organ desiccation and heat loss.

The right renal vascular pedicle, aorta, and inferior vena cava are exposed by incising the lateral parietes from the hepatic flexure to the cecum, then reflecting the overlying right colon, duodenum and pancreas medially, with an extended Kocher-like maneuver. Dissection of the renal artery is facilitated by retraction of the renal vein, which should be freed carefully from surrounding tissues, with its adrenal and ureteric branches being ligated and transected. In certain cases of right-sided ostial atherosclerosis, it is often possible to retract the vena cava laterally and dissect the proximal renal artery without the necessity for exposing the more distal renal artery.

The left renal vascular pedicle is exposed using a similar retroperitoneal approach, with medial reflection of the viscera, including the left colon. This provides better visualization of the mid and distal renal vessels, compared with exposure gained through the posterior retroperitoneum at the root of the mesocolon and mesentery. Adequate exposure of the left renal artery usually requires mobilization of the overlying renal vein, which is facilitated by ligation and transection of its gonadal and adrenal branches.

Figure 1A

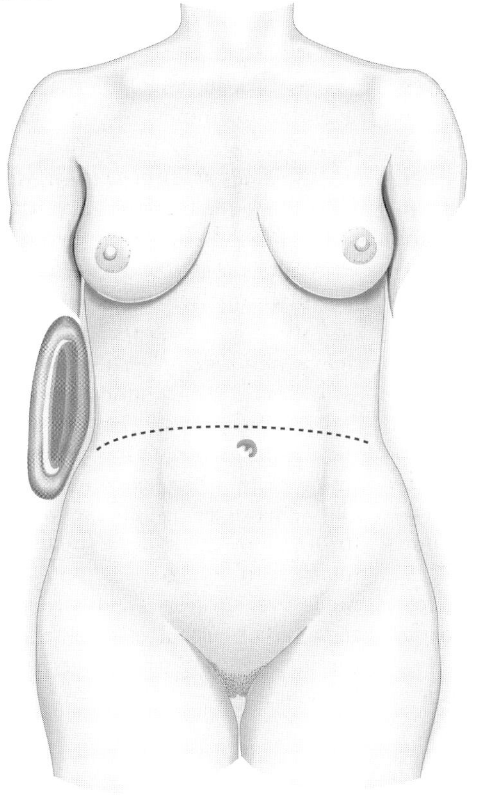

Figure 1B

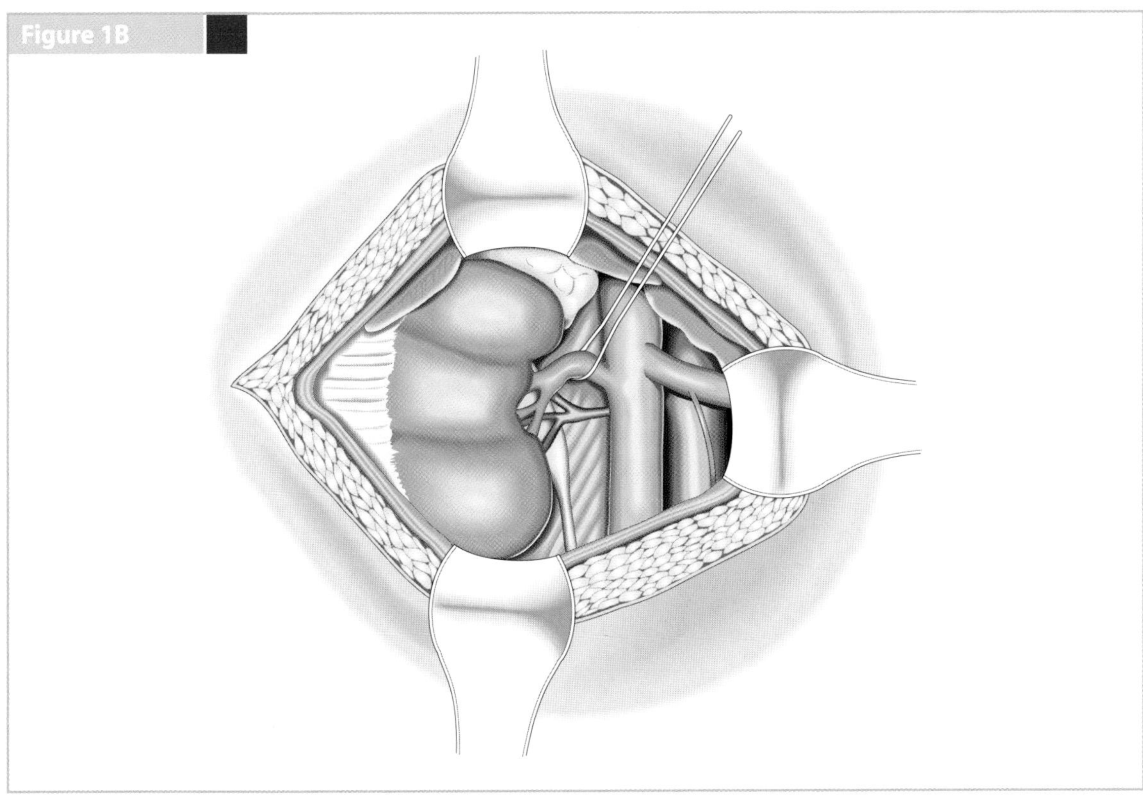

Figure 2

The infrarenal aorta is dissected about its circumference below the origin of the renal arteries with care taken not to inadvertently injure nearby vessels. Ligation and transection of the lumbar veins and arteries may be undertaken without consequence when necessary. A side-biting vascular clamp is used to partially occlude the aorta after systemic anticoagulation is obtained by intravenous administration of sodium heparin, 100–150 units/kg. A lateral aortotomy is created, with its length approximately two to three times the chosen graft's diameter. It is not necessary to remove an ellipse of aortic tissue as part of such an aortotomy, although some surgeons prefer the use of an aortic punch to create a circular aortotomy. The aortotomy in the arteriosclerotic subgroup of patients should be cautiously performed so as not to create a plane within the diseased media that might result in a later dissection. Localized aortic endarterectomies are not favored in this setting. When completing the graft-to-aortic anastomosis, sutures should include the entirety of diseased intimal and medial tissues.

The most direct route for right-sided aortorenal grafts is in a retrocaval position originating from a lateral aortotomy. However, grafts are less likely to kink when arising from an anterolateral aortotomy and carried in front of the inferior vena cava. Grafts to the left kidney are almost always positioned behind to the left renal vein. The aortic clamp is often left in place during completion of the renal anastomosis, thus avoiding clamping the graft, which in the case of vein or arterial conduits might prove injurious.

Figure 2

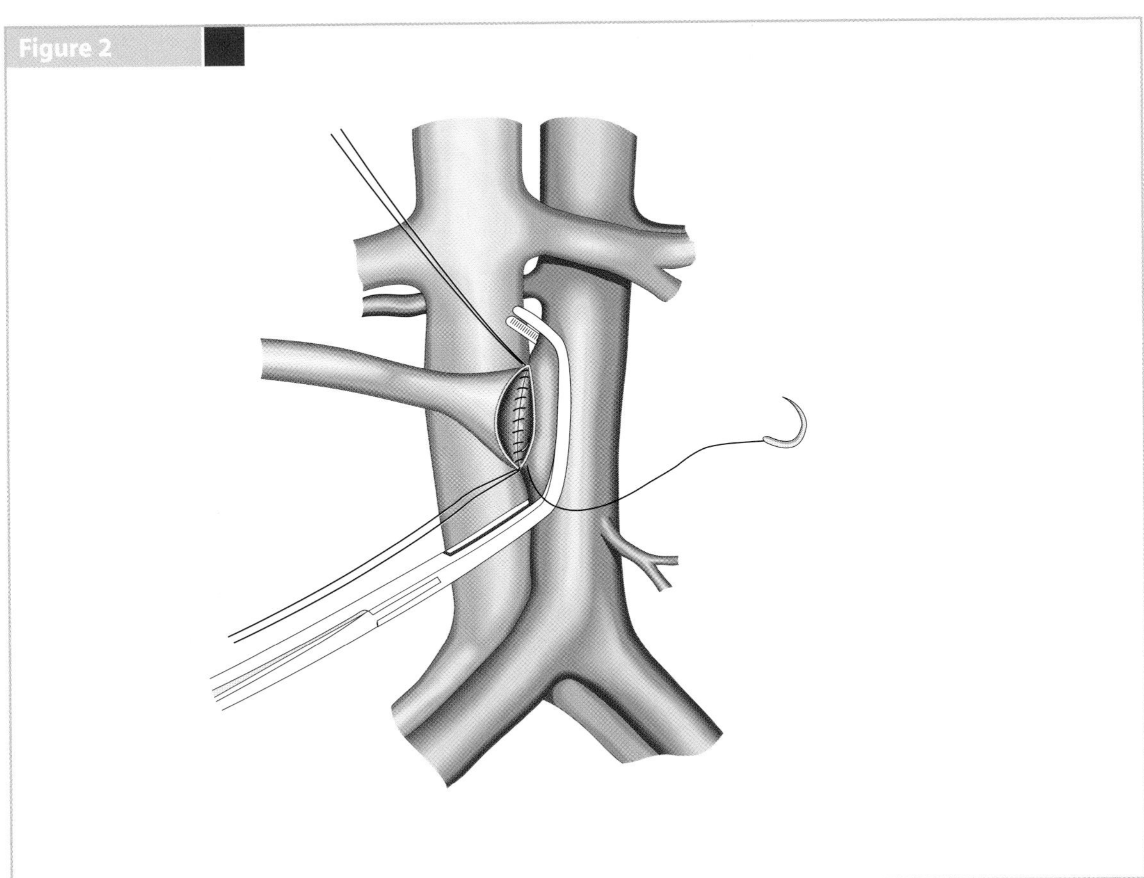

Figure 3A–C

The saphenous vein is the most commonly used conduit for aortorenal bypass procedures. The vein is excised with a branch included at its caudal end whenever possible. This branch is incised along its lumen adjacent to the parent vein so that a common orifice is created connecting it to the lumen of the main trunk. The generous circumference created by this branch patch maneuver lessens the likelihood of anastomotic narrowing and allows for a relatively perpendicular origin of the vein graft from the aorta. The same preparation technique involving the incision of branches may be used to prepare the internal iliac artery. Graft-to-aortic anastomoses are performed using 4-0 or 5-0 cardiovascular suture. In certain patients other sites of origin for renal grafts may be preferable, with the common iliac, splenic, and hepatic arteries being the most frequent. Grafts originating from these arteries function just as well as those arising from the aorta. Prosthetic grafts are often used if a concurrent aortoaortic, aortoiliac or aortofemoral graft is placed.

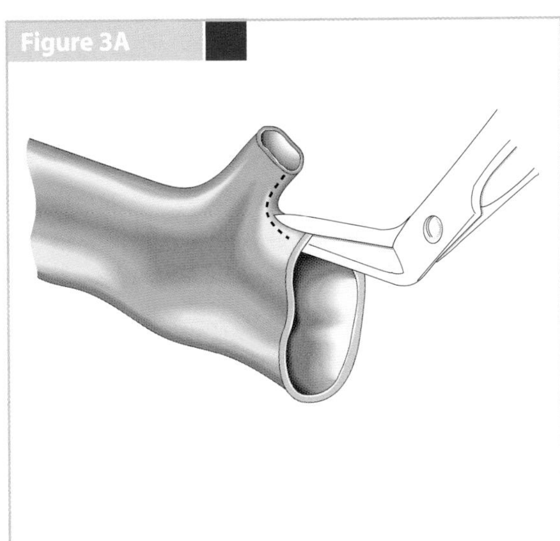
Figure 3A

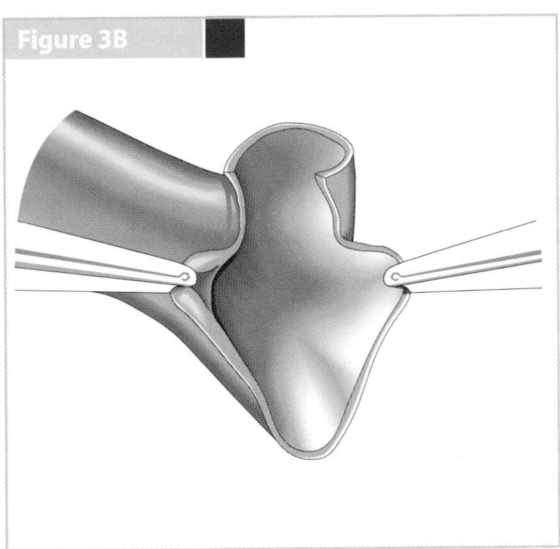
Figure 3B

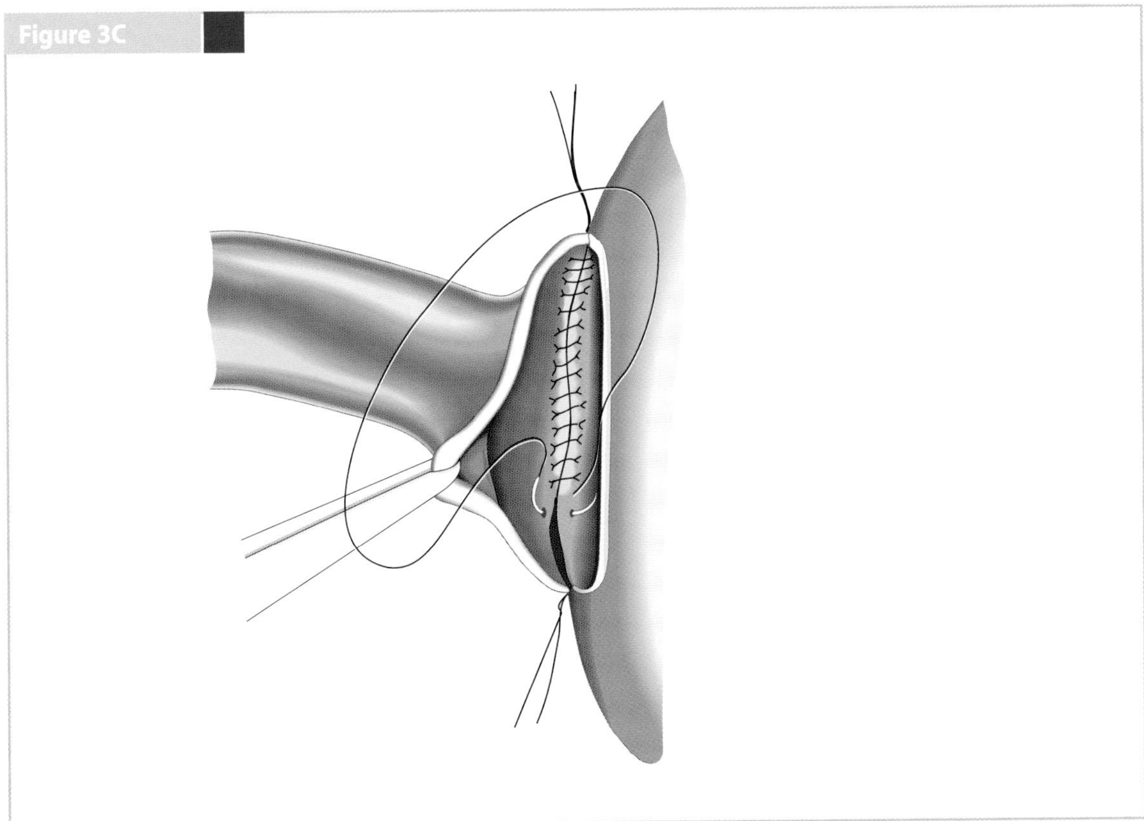
Figure 3C

Figure 4A–C

An end-to-end graft-to-renal artery anastomosis is favored over an end-to-side anastomosis. A sustained diuresis should be established by intravenous administration of 12.5 g of mannitol prior to interrupting antegrade renal artery blood flow. In most chronically ischemic kidneys, preformed collateral vessels usually provide enough blood flow to maintain kidney viability during the period of renal artery occlusion. Microvascular Heifetz clamps, developing tensions ranging from 30 to 70 g, are favored over conventional macrovascular clamps or elastic slings for occluding the renal vessels. They have less potential to cause arterial injury, and because of their very small size do not obscure the operative field.

The graft-to-renal artery anastomosis is facilitated by spatulation of the graft posteriorly and the renal artery anteriorly. This allows visualization of the artery's interior, such that inclusion of its intima with each stitch is easily accomplished. Stay sutures are placed at the apex of each spatulation, being continued to the tongue of the opposite vessel. In adults, the anastomosis is completed using a continuous 5-0 or 6-0 cardiovascular suture. In pediatric-aged patients, multiple interrupted 6-0 or 7-0 cardiovascular sutures are used to provide for later anastomotic growth. Spatulated anastomoses completed in this manner are ovoid and with healing are less likely to develop strictures.

After the aortic and renal anastomoses are completed, the vascular clamps are removed and antegrade renal blood flow is reestablished. Anticoagulation is reversed with slow intravenous administration of 1.5 mg of protamine sulfate for each 100 units of heparin given previously. Assessment of the reconstruction is undertaken by duplex scanning or flow evaluation with a directional Doppler.

Figure 4A

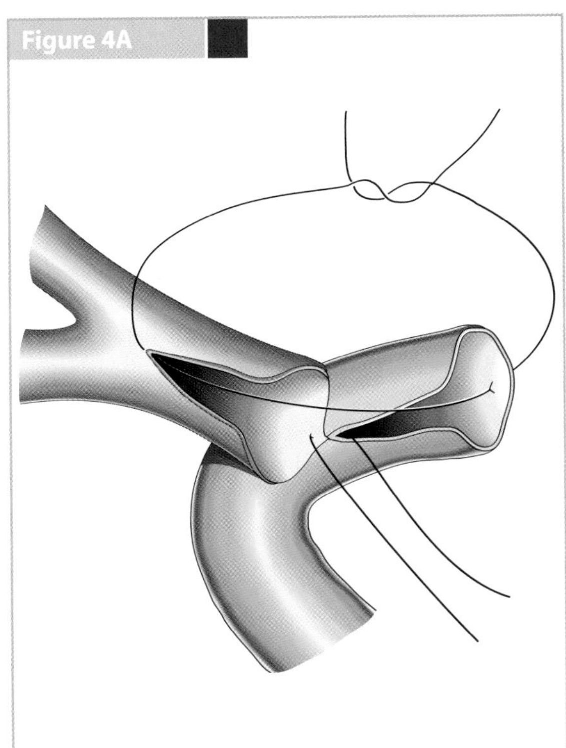

Figure 4B

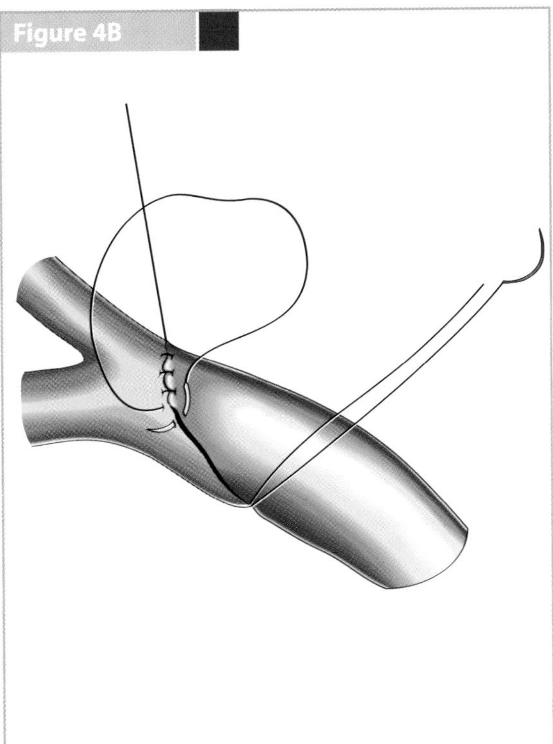

Figure 4C

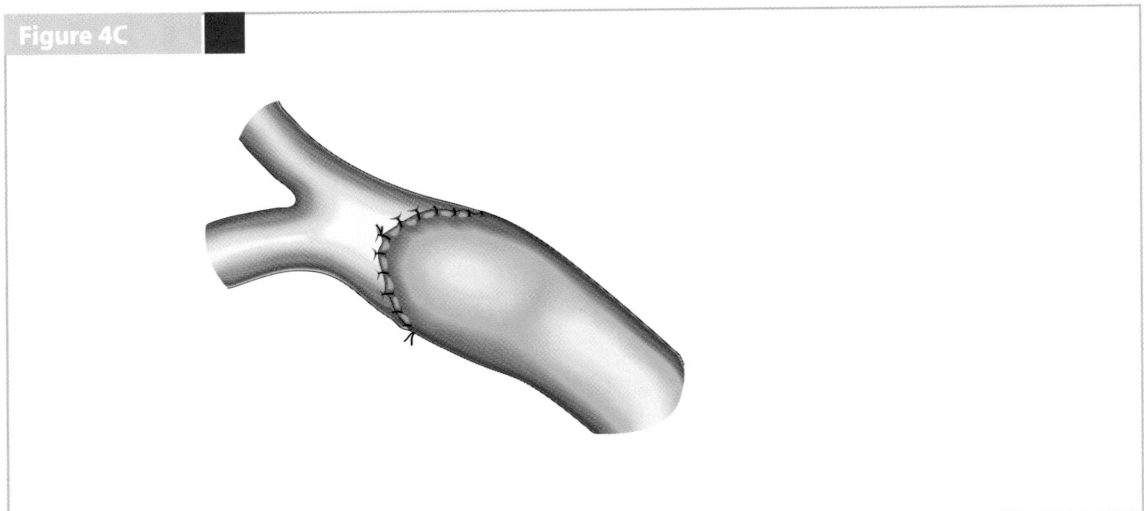

Figure 5A–C

Management of stenotic disease affecting multiple renal arteries or segmental branches often requires separate implantations of the renal arteries into a single conduit. This is usually accomplished with an end-to-side anastomosis of one artery into the side of the proximal graft, and an end-to-end anastomosis of the second artery to the distal graft. If a nonreversed branching segment of saphenous vein in which the valves have been cut or a hypogastric artery with branches is used for the bypass, construction of multiple end-to-end, graft-to-renal artery anastomoses may be undertaken.

In some patients it may be easier to perform an anastomosis of the involved arteries in a side-to-side manner, so as to form a single channel, with the graft then anastomosed to this common orifice. Surgeons should be prepared, preferably during preoperative planning, to perform ex vivo repairs with bench reconstruction of diseased vessels when complex segmental renal artery fibrodysplasia is not amenable to conventional in situ revascularization techniques.

Figure 5A

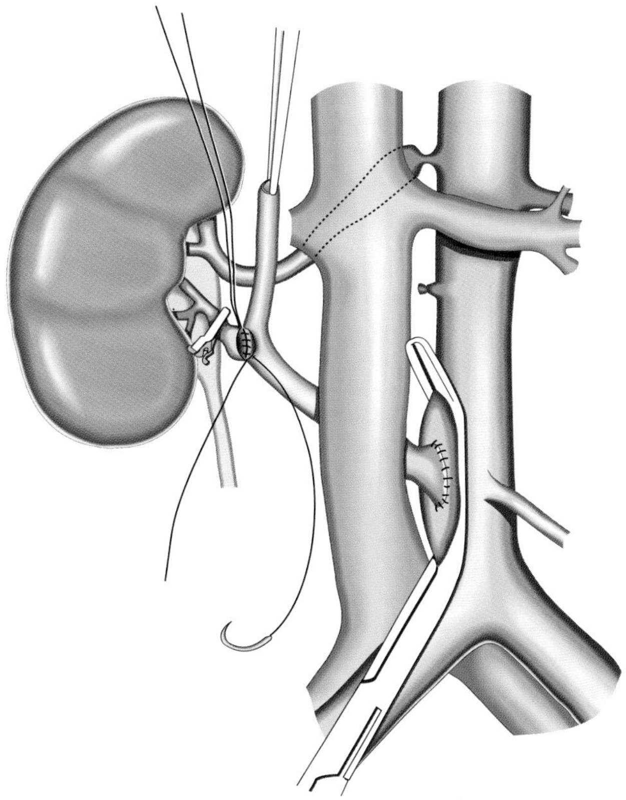

Figure 5B

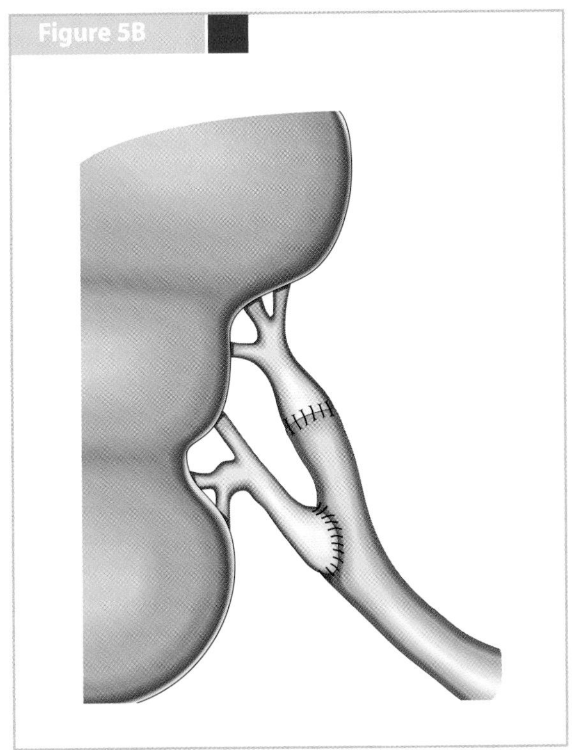

Figure 5C

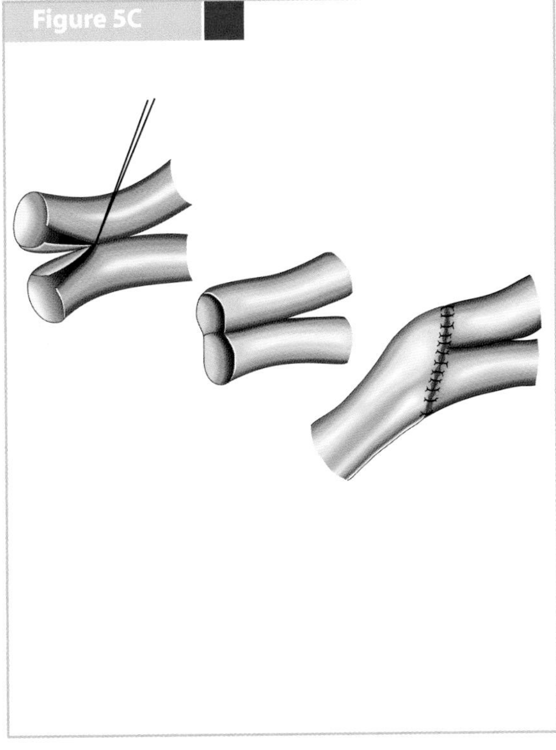

Figure 6

Splenorenal bypass is the most frequently performed alternative to an aortorenal bypass for patients with left-sided disease. This usually involves a direct end-to-end anastomosis of the splenic artery to the renal artery. Occasionally, this may necessitate placement of an interposition vein graft between the splenic and renal arteries. It is critical that preoperative lateral aortography confirms that a significant celiac artery stenosis does not exist in these circumstances.

The left renal artery is exposed by medial reflection of the viscera in a manner similar to that described for an aortorenal bypass. Such an extraperitoneal approach to the mid and distal renal vessels is preferred over exposure gained directly through an incision in the posterior retroperitoneum at the root of the mesocolon and mesentery. The renal artery should be mobilized for 2–3 cm beyond its aortic origin, so as to allow the artery to assume a gentle curve upward when anastomosed to the splenic artery.

Exposure of the splenic artery is performed after medial mobilization of viscera and exposure of the renal artery. The splenic artery can be palpated as it courses along the superior border of the pancreas a few centimeters above and anterior to the left renal artery. Because of tortuosity and calcification it may be difficult to mobilize the splenic artery for the anastomosis to the renal artery without buckling or kinking. Care in its positioning before completing an anastomosis is very important to insure a good technical result.

The splenic and renal arteries, or an interposition vein graft if used, should be spatulated so as to create an ovoid end-to-end anastomosis. Although some report end-to-side, splenic artery-to-renal artery reconstructions when significant size differences in these two arteries exist, this manner of anastomosis is not favored. Splenorenal bypasses in children are in disfavor, because of early thromboses, as well as late problems if celiac artery stenotic disease evolves as the child grows, a problem that may result in recurrent hypertension.

Figure 7

Hepatorenal bypass for right-sided renal artery disease in selected patients has become another accepted alternative to more conventional renal revascularization procedures. This usually requires interposition of a saphenous vein graft, originating from the common hepatic artery in an end-to-side manner, and anastomosed to the renal artery in an end-to-end fashion. Given the duality of the liver's blood supply from the hepatic artery and portal vein, one may consider direct use of the hepatic artery in reconstructions of the renal artery in patients without liver disease.

The right renal artery is usually exposed through an extraperitoneal approach similar to that for aortorenal bypasses (Fig. 1). The renal artery is usually dissected from its aortic origin to near the hilum, so as to provide sufficient length for it to gently curve upwards toward the hepatic circulation. This lessens the risk of kinking.

Exposure of the hepatic artery is best obtained through the lesser sac following incision of the hepatoduodenal ligament. Dissection of the common hepatic artery is performed first and continues distally until the gastroduodenal artery is identified. The distal common hepatic, gastroduodenal, and proper hepatic arteries are dissected about their circumference and encircled with vessel loops. The site for originating the vein graft depends upon the individual's anatomy. An inferior arteriotomy is usually made in the distal common hepatic artery, or occasionally at the origin of the gastroduodenal artery, which may be transected and ligated distally.

The vein is spatulated anteriorly and posteriorly to provide a generous patch for anastomosis to the hepatic artery in an end-to-side manner using a fine 6/0 or 7/0 cardiovascular suture. The graft is then carried behind the duodenum and anastomosed to the mobilized renal artery. Both the vein graft and renal artery should be spatulated so as to facilitate construction of an ovoid anastomosis. Synthetic prostheses have occasionally been used as grafts in these procedures, but they are not favored because of their proximity to the duodenum. In some patients the right renal artery is long enough to allow direct end-to-side reimplantation into the hepatic artery. In other patients a direct end-to-end gastroduodenal-renal artery anastomosis may be fashioned, especially when revascularizing segmental or small accessory right renal arteries.

Figure 6

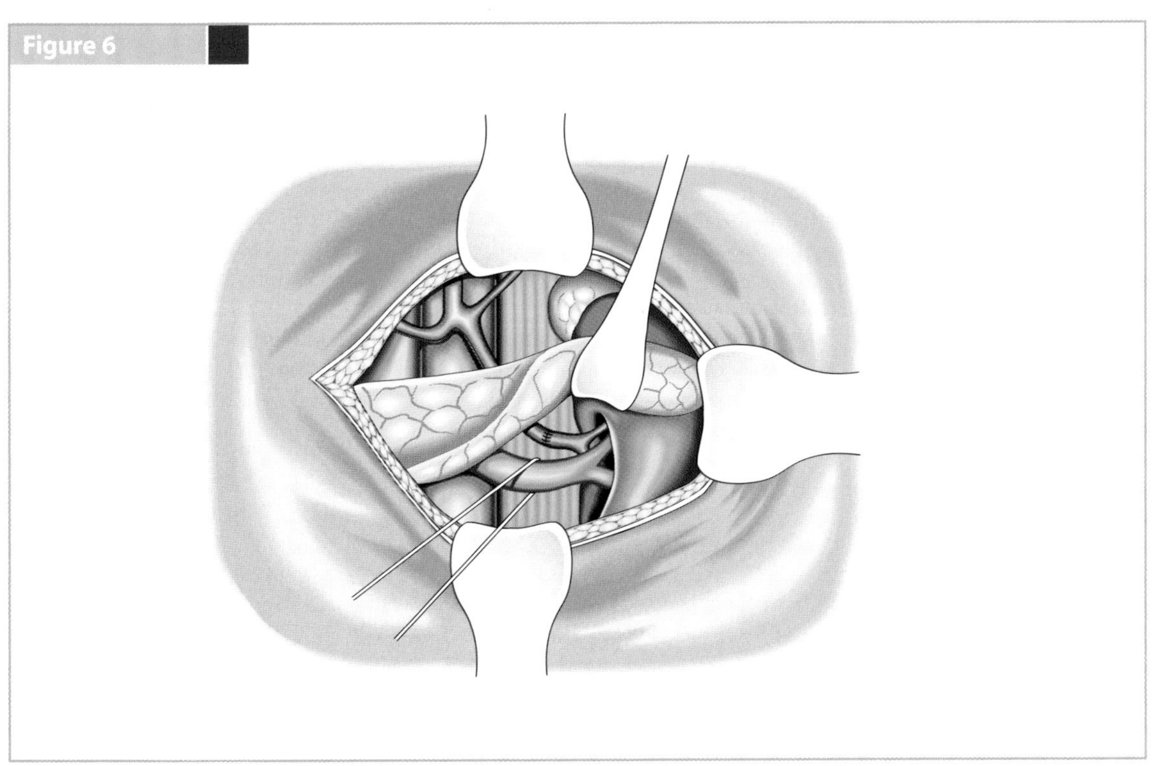

Figure 7

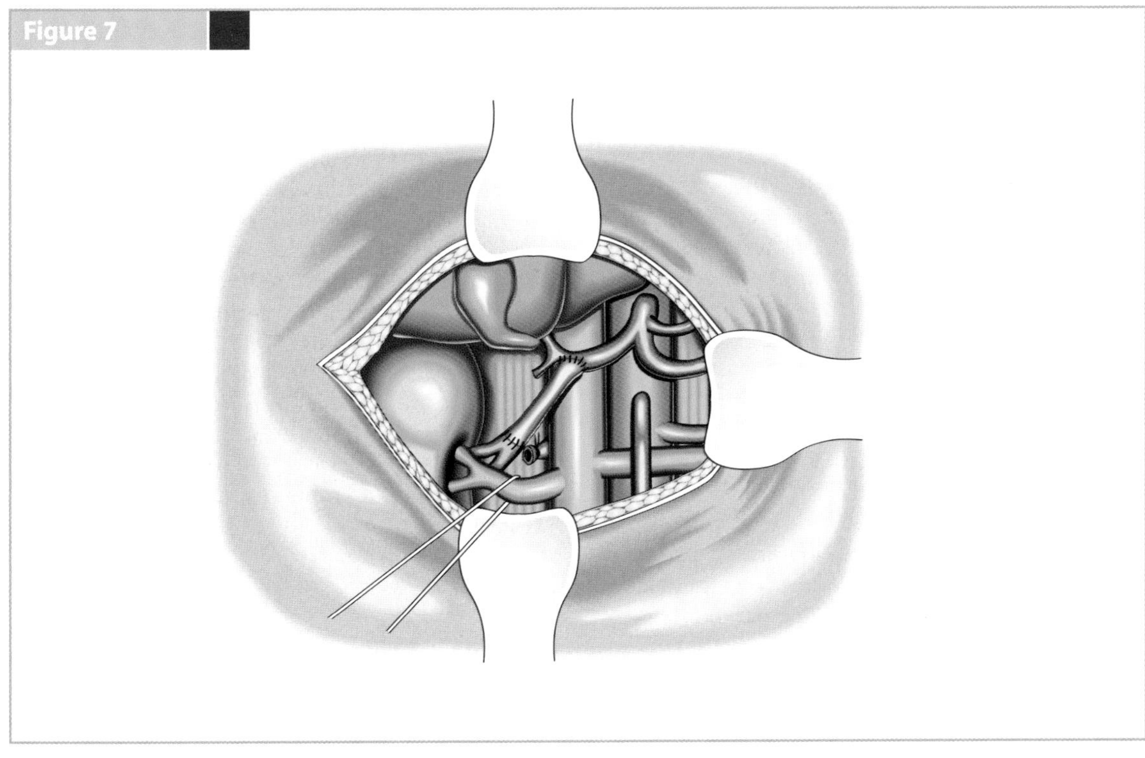

Figure 8

An iliorenal bypass using either an autologous saphenous vein or a synthetic graft should be considered in certain patients with a hostile aorta or upper abdomen that preclude a conventional aortorenal reconstruction, or a nonanatomic splenorenal or hepatorenal bypass.

Origination of an iliorenal graft is usually possible from the anterior or anterolateral surface of the proximal common iliac artery. At this site, even in severely arteriosclerotic iliac arteries, the vessel is often free of calcific plaque. The graft should be spatulated so as to create a generous hood at its end-to-side anastomosis to the iliac artery. The iliorenal graft is then positioned in the retroperitoneum alongside the aorta with a gentle curve at the level of the kidney, where it is anastomosed to the renal artery in an end-to-side fashion. Because dissection in the region of a previous anastomosis of an aortic graft may lead to troublesome complications, an iliorenal graft should originate from the limbs of aortoiliac or aortofemoral conduits rather than from the proximal infrarenal aorta or graft body itself.

Figure 8

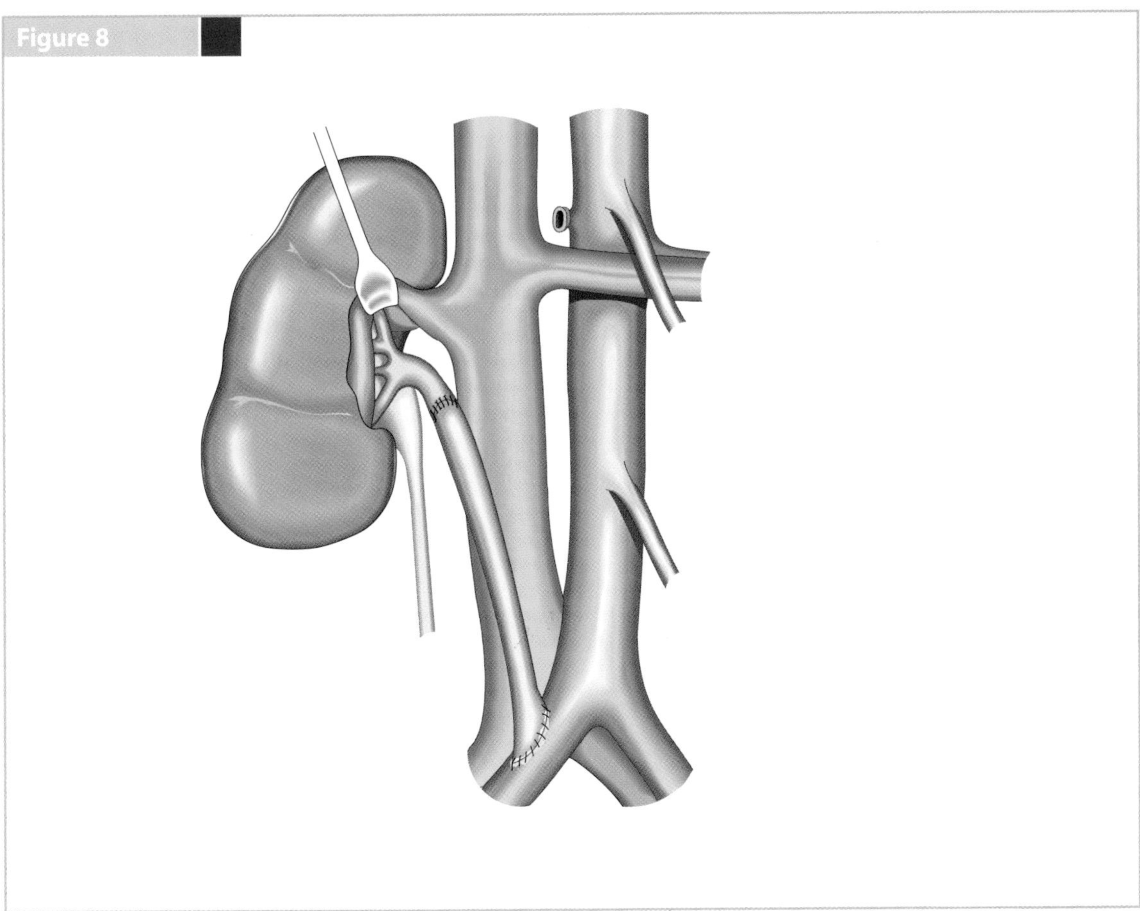

CONCLUSION

Operative therapy of renovascular hypertension is preferred in all pediatric patients and young adults. Similarly, it may be advantageous to pursue surgical therapy in select older patients with either fibrodysplastic or focal renal artery arteriosclerotic disease, especially in those with bilateral renal artery stenoses. The salutary results of bypass procedures in these patients are remarkably similar at most centers where large numbers of renovascular hypertensive patients are treated. Alternatives to conventional operative intervention, such as polypharmacy drug therapy or percutaneous transluminal angioplasty, must be judged in the light of excellent long-term operative results.

Beneficial responses in terms of controlling hypertension and stabilizing renal function following surgical intervention should be expected in 90–95% of patients with developmental or fibrodysplastic renovascular hypertension and in 70–80% of those treated for arteriosclerotic disease. These results represent standards of contemporary practice that reflect the two most important determinants of successful treatment – an accurate preoperative diagnosis and a properly executed operation. In regard to the latter, careful selection of an appropriate bypass procedure and deft skill at its performance are essential in providing an optimal surgical outcome.

SELECTED BIBLIOGRAPHY

Chibaro EA, Libertino JA, Novick AC (1984) Use of the hepatic circulation for renal revascularization. Ann Surg 199:406–411

Khauli RB, Novick AC, Ziegelbaum M (1985) Splenorenal bypass in the treatment of renal artery stenosis: Experience with sixty-nine cases. J Vasc Surg 2:547–551

Moncure AC, Brewster DC, Darling RC (1986) Use of the splenic and hepatic arteries for renal revascularization. J Vasc Surg 3:196–203

Novick AC, McElroy J (1985) Renal revascularization by end-to-end anastomosis of the hepatic and renal arteries. J Urol 134:1089–1093

Stanley JC (1997) Surgical treatment of renovascular hypertension. Am J Surg 174:102–110

Stanley JC, Zelenock GB, Messina LM (1995) Pediatric renovascular hypertension: A thirty-year experience of operative treatment. J Vasc Surg 21:212–227

Part V Lower Limb

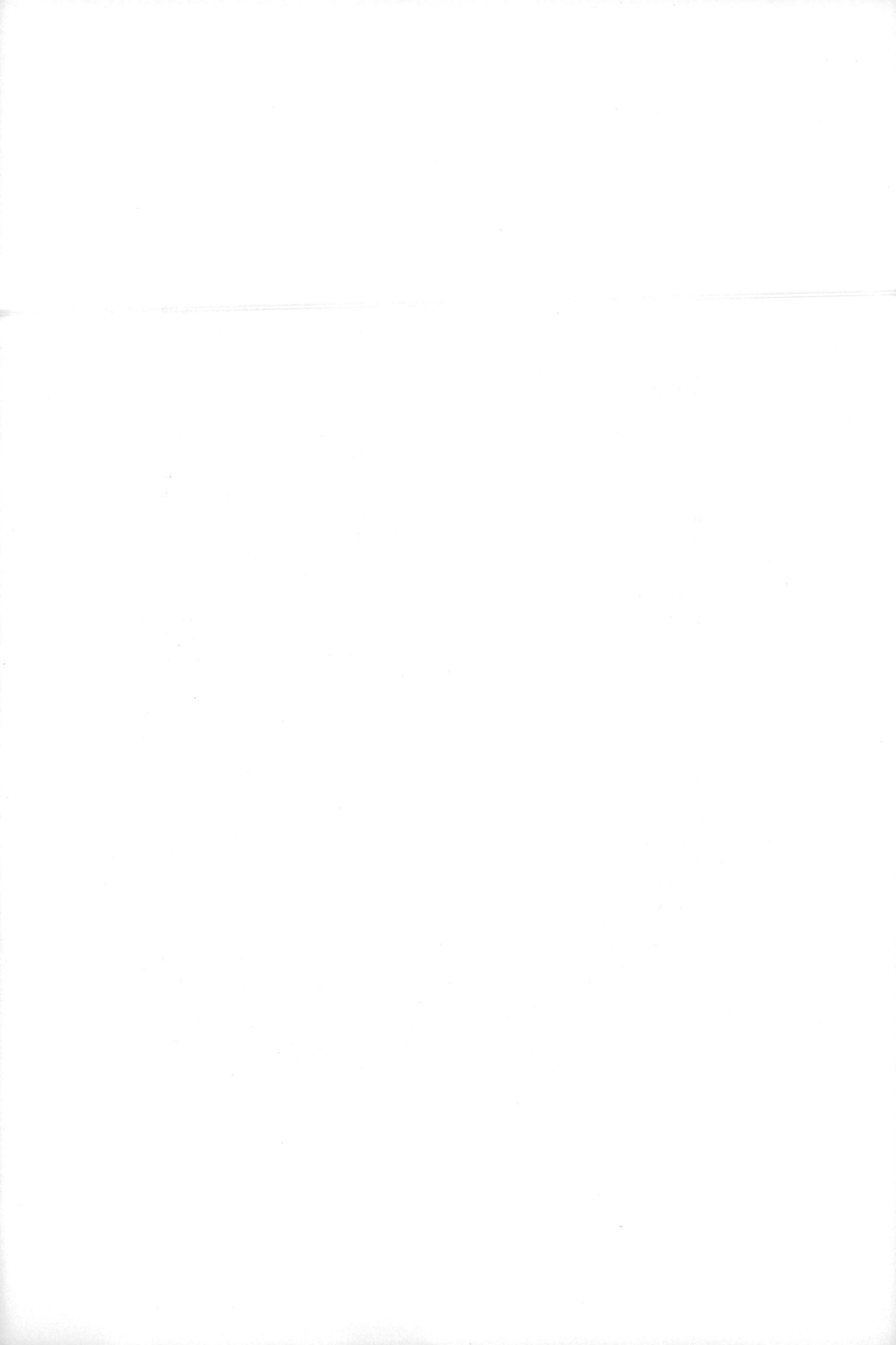

CHAPTER 21

Introduction to Lower Extremity Arterial Occlusive Disease

Jamal J. Hoballah

Lower extremity arterial occlusive disease (LEAOD) most commonly represents one of the manifestations of atherosclerosis. Atherosclerotic disease can affect various segments of the arterial tree. The presence of LEAOD suggests the likelihood of atherosclerotic disease elsewhere in the arterial tree. In the United States, it is estimated that 8.5 million individuals over the age of 60 suffer from LEAOD. Approximately 50% of individuals with LEAOD are asymptomatic, and 40% suffer from various degrees of claudication. The remaining individuals have critical limb ischemia manifested by rest pain or tissue loss in the form of non-healing ulcers and or gangrene.

Management of LEAOD includes risk factors modification and revascularization. The former is offered to all patients. The latter is selectively offered to those with disabling claudication and critical limb ischemia.

The pattern and degree of involvement will determine the type of revascularization offered. Patients may suffer from "inflow" aortoiliac disease, "outflow" infrainguinal disease or a combination of both. In the presence of both, correction of the inflow alone may be sufficient to address the symptoms.

In general, patients with localized iliac pathology are treated with endovascular interventions using balloon angioplasty/stenting techniques. Patients with unilateral iliac occlusion not amenable to endovascular therapy are treated using a femoro-femoral bypass or an iliofemoral bypass. In the presence of severe bilateral iliac or aortoiliac disease unyielding to endovascular therapy, an aortobifemoral bypass using an end-to-side or end-to-end configuration will be recommended. Aortoiliac endarterectomy is also an option although currently less frequently performed. In patients with poor medical condition, ascites or severe cardiopulmonary disease, an extra-anatomic approach using axillo-bifemoral bypasses is often recommended.

In patients with infrainguinal disease, the outcome of endovascular treatment is often limited and not long lasting. Bypasses represent the main option for revascularization and long-term patency. Profundoplasty is occasionally used to treat patients with rest pain and femoral bifurcation disease. When constructing a bypass, the general concept is to identify an inflow source, a target vessel and connect the two with a conduit. Currently, the best available conduit for infrainguinal bypasses is the greater saphenous vein. However, adjustments are needed to deal with the venous valves. One option is to turn the vein 180 degrees, resulting in a "reversed vein bypass." Alternatively the vein is kept in its original direction and a valvulotome is used to disrupt the valves. If only the proximal and distal ends of the vein are mobilized and the rest of the vein is kept undisturbed in its bed, the bypass is called an "in situ bypass." If the vein is harvested, the bypass is referred to as a "translocated" or "non-reversed vein bypass." In the absence of an adequate greater saphenous vein, other venous conduits may be used. These include the lesser saphenous, the cephalic and the basilic veins.

If a vein conduit is unavailable, prosthetic grafts can be used. Many surgeons use them preferentially when performing bypasses to the above knee popliteal artery. Prosthetic bypasses to the infrapopliteal levels are associated with patency rates significantly lower than those seen with vein bypasses. Adjunctive techniques have been proposed to improve the patency rates of infrageniculate prosthetic bypasses which include vein patches, vein cuffs and arteriovenous fistulae.

In the following chapters, the various open surgical methods used to manage lower extremity occlusive disease will be reviewed.

CHAPTER 22

Aortobifemoral Bypass

Jamal J. Hoballah, Ronnie Word, W. John Sharp

INTRODUCTION

With the advancement of endovascular interventions, a large portion of aortoiliac occlusive disease is now amenable to balloon angioplasty and stenting. Nevertheless, standard surgical revascularization with aortobifemoral bypasses remains an important mainstay of the treatment of aortoiliac occlusive disease. Aortobifemoral bypass is a procedure that has stood the test of time and can be performed with low mortality and morbidity and excellent long-term patency rates. It is ideally suited for patients with severe diffuse bilateral iliac occlusive disease involving long segments (greater than 5 cm) of external or common iliac artery disease. It may also be the only option besides extra-anatomic reconstruction in patients with bilaterally occluded iliac arteries, aortic occlusion or unsuccessful attempts at endovascular revascularization.

When constructing an aortobifemoral bypass, several technical issues need to be addressed. These issues relate to the aortic exposure, the site of proximal aortic control, the site of construction of the proximal anastomosis, the configuration of the proximal anastomosis (end to end versus end to side), the preservation of pelvic blood flow, the tunneling of the graft limbs, the femoral vessels' exposure, the site of the distal anastomoses and the need for any concomitant infrainguinal procedures.

PATIENT PREPARATION

The patient is placed supine on the operating table. The arms are usually placed at 80°. Normal bony prominences are padded. Appropriate intravenous, monitoring lines and catheters are placed. An epidural catheter can provide excellent postoperative pain relief allowing early ambulation. The patient's prepping starts at the nipple line. Although prepping to the mid thigh level may be sufficient, both lower extremities down to the toes can be included in the prepping and draping. The feet are placed in transparent sterile plastic bags and a sterile sheath is used to cover the extremities to the upper thigh levels. Prepping down to the toes provides easy access to the ankles and feet for the purpose of evaluating distal perfusion at the completion of the procedure. This will avoid struggling under the drapes to assess the pedal pulses or reprepping and draping if distal ischemic problems are discovered after the sterile drapes have been removed. Preoperative antibiotics are administered prior to skin incision. Whether to start by exposing the femoral vessels or the aorta remains controversial. The theoretical advantage of starting with the abdominal incision relates to minimizing the time of having open groin wounds for fear of groin infection. Its disadvantage relates to the fluid loss from the open abdomen during dissection of the femoral arteries.

Figure 1: Femoral Exposure

The femoral vessels are typically exposed through vertical groin incisions. A vertical skin incision is started in each groin midway between the pubic symphysis and the anterior superior iliac spine and extends for approximately 10–12 cm. The incision is deepened through the subcutaneous tissues with electrocautery. The encountered lymphatics are ligated and divided to prevent postoperative lymph leaks. The femoral sheath is incised and the common femoral artery is then exposed and sharply dissected circumferentially. The dissection is extended proximally to the inguinal ligament and distally to include the superficial femoral and profunda femoris arteries. The common femoral, superficial femoral and profunda femoris arteries are encircled with Silastic vessel loops. Minor branches of the common femoral artery are identified and spared. Antibiotic-soaked sponges are then placed in both groin wounds.

In overweight patients or in the presence of skin rashes and maceration in the inguinal crease, the femoral exposure can be achieved through a suprainguinal transverse incision similar to that used for inguinal hernia exposures. The inguinal ligament is exposed, mobilized and reflected cephalad. The femoral sheath is then incised and the femoral vessels are dissected. Should the need for an extended profundoplasty arise, distal extension in this exposure is challenging – hence its limitations.

Figure 1

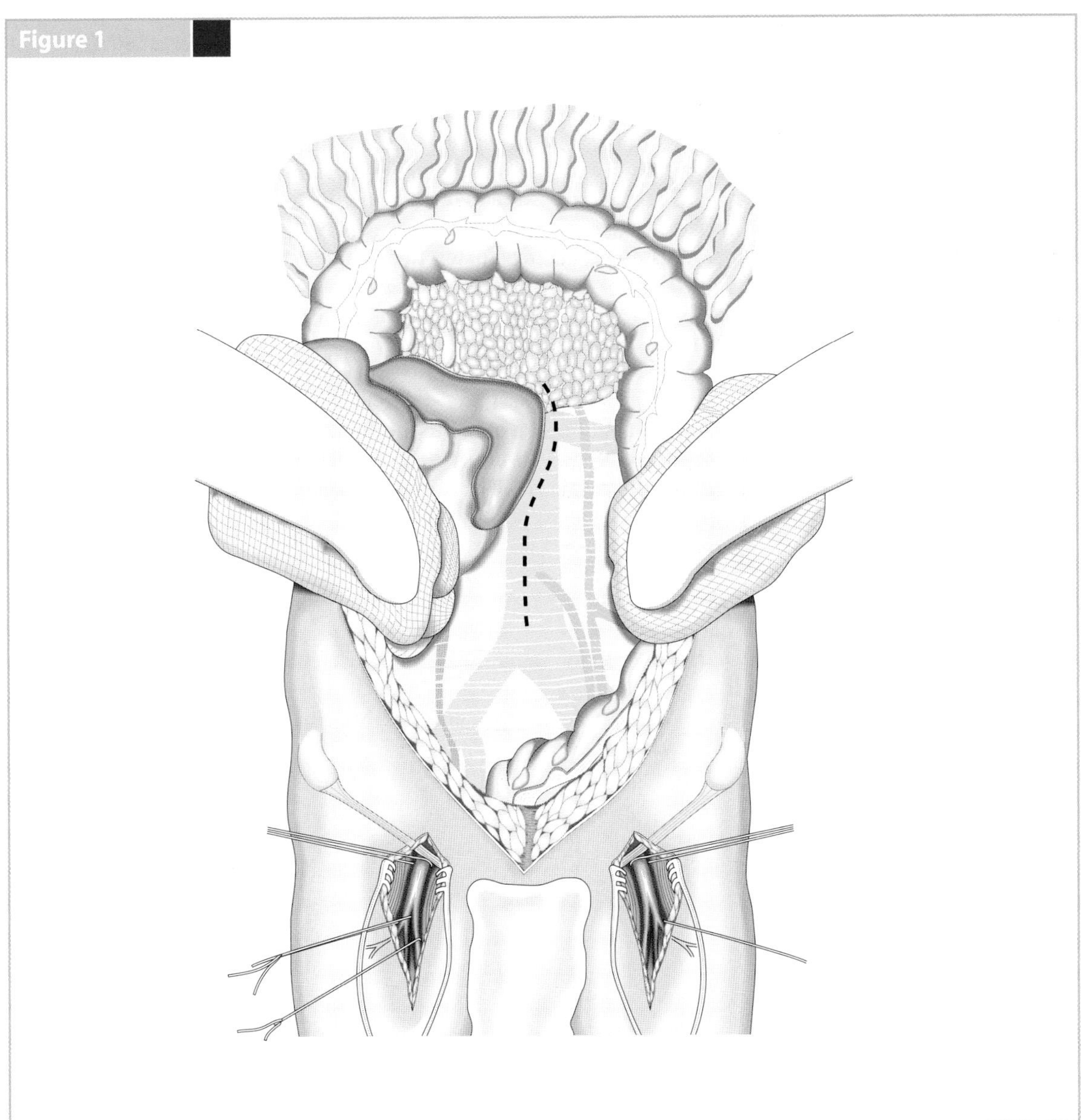

Figure 2: Aortic Exposure

The aorta is most commonly exposed through a midline transperitoneal incision extending from the xiphoid process to the pubis. After entering the peritoneal cavity, the abdomen is explored for unexpected findings. The transverse colon is then elevated anteriorly out of the wound, wrapped in a moist towel. A moist rolled lap pad is placed in the bed of the mesentery of the splenic flexure, which is retracted laterally and posteriorly. The remainder of the small bowel is then reflected to the right exposing the infrarenal aorta. The ligament of Treitz is incised and the distal fourth portion of the duodenum is mobilized off the aorta, allowing further exposure of the aorta and retraction of the small bowel to the right. The small bowel is then wrapped in a moistened towel and held in place using the fence blade of an Omni retractor.

The aorta is then exposed by incising its overlying retroperitoneum. The incision is continued proximally to the level of the left renal vein. The inferior mesenteric vein is encountered. It is frequently ligated and divided with no consequences to improve the exposure after ensuring that no meandering artery or arterial branches are included in the ligature. Lymphatic channels overlying the infrarenal aorta will be encountered. These lymphatics are ligated and divided to avoid any lymph leaks.

The infrarenal aorta is then sharply dissected and evaluated for adequacy of clamping. The dissection is carried for a 6-cm segment starting at the level of the left renal vein and extending towards the level of the inferior mesenteric artery (IMA). Autonomic nerve plexus around the IMA are preserved and dissection in the region of the aortic bifurcation is avoided to minimize the chances of sexual dysfunction.

The aorta can also be exposed through a retroperitoneal approach. This may be the ideal exposure in individuals with hostile abdomen from multiple previous surgery, presence of stomas, or marked obesity. The retroperitoneal exposure can be performed through a paramedian incision or more commonly through a left flank incision. The details of retroperitoneal aortic exposures are addressed in Chap. 16 (Geraghty and Sicard).

Figure 2

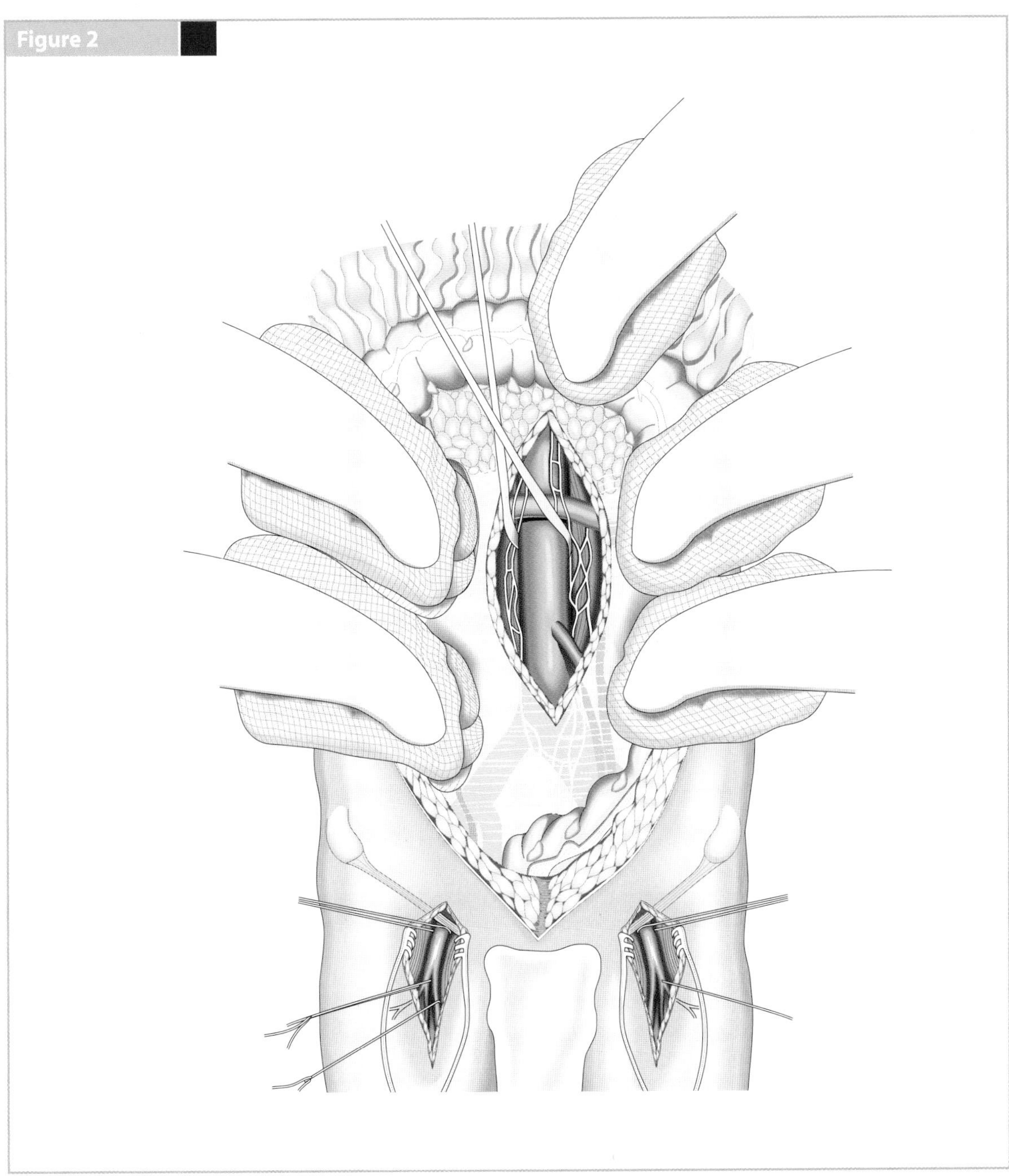

Figure 3: Site of Aortic Clamping

■ **Infrarenal Control.** The proximal control will be dictated by the extent of atherosclerotic disease identified intraoperatively. Typically, the aorta is clamped at the infrarenal level. The aortic segment just distal to the origin of the renal arteries is usually minimally affected by the atherosclerotic process and amenable to clamping. The aorta is carefully assessed between the thumb and the index finger for the presence of plaque. In the presence of a posterior plaque, the aortic clamp will be applied in a manner to appose the anterior aortic wall against the posterior wall. A clamp applied in a different manner could result in arterial wall injury at the clamp site or may not adequately control the blood flow through the aorta. In the presence of conditions that prohibit infrarenal clamping such as extensive plaques or juxtarenal occlusion, the options will include control at the suprarenal or supraceliac level.

■ **Suprarenal Control.** Suprarenal control can be very effective in patients with chronic aortic occlusion extending to the level of the renal arteries. In these patients, control of the renal arteries is necessary prior to suprarenal clamping to avoid significant embolization into the renal arteries. Exposure of the juxtarenal aorta typically requires full mobilization of the left renal vein. This is accomplished by carefully dividing its branches (gonadal, lumbar and adrenal). The lumbar branch is often short and wide and should be handled carefully to prevent venous injury and unpleasant bleeding. Once fully mobilized, the renal vein can be retracted cephalad or caudad exposing the renal arteries. The left and right renal arteries are identified at their origin from the aorta and encircled with Silastic vessel loops. The suprarenal aorta is sharply dissected and evaluated for adequacy of clamping. The clamp can be repositioned below the renal arteries after the arteriotomy is performed and the aortic plug removed or after constructing the proximal anastomosis.

Figure 4: Supraceliac Control

If the para/suprarenal aorta is felt to be inadequate for clamping, the supraceliac aorta is exposed and dissected. Supraceliac clamping has been reported to be safer than suprarenal or interrenal clamping and has been recommended as the preferred site for clamping when the infrarenal aorta is inadequate. To expose the supraceliac aorta, the triangular ligament of the liver is incised and the left lobe of the liver is mobilized to the right; the lesser omentum is incised and the stomach and the esophagogastric junction are retracted to the left; the presence of a nasogastric tube will help better identify the esophagus and avoid esophageal injury. The right crus of the diaphragm is identified and divided to enhance the exposure; the supraceliac aorta is sharply dissected and prepared for cross clamping.

Figure 3

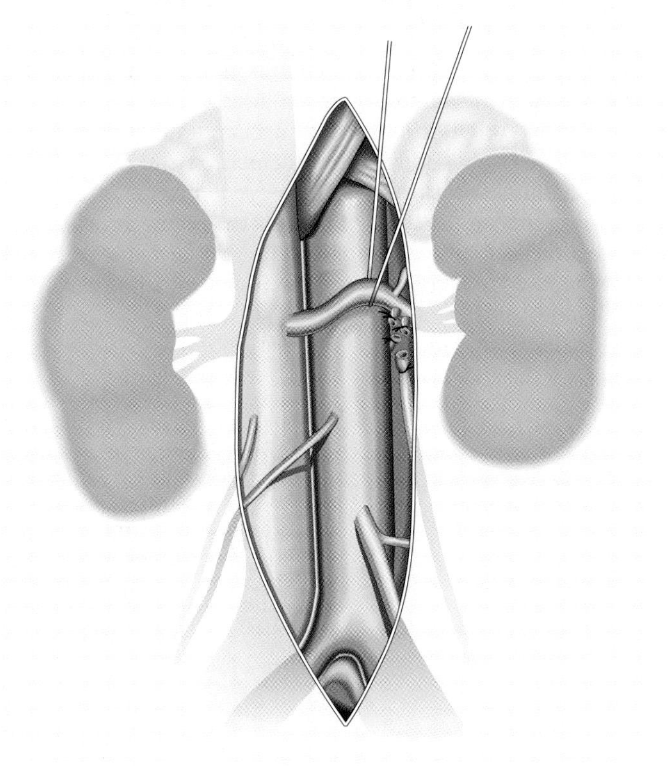

Figure 4

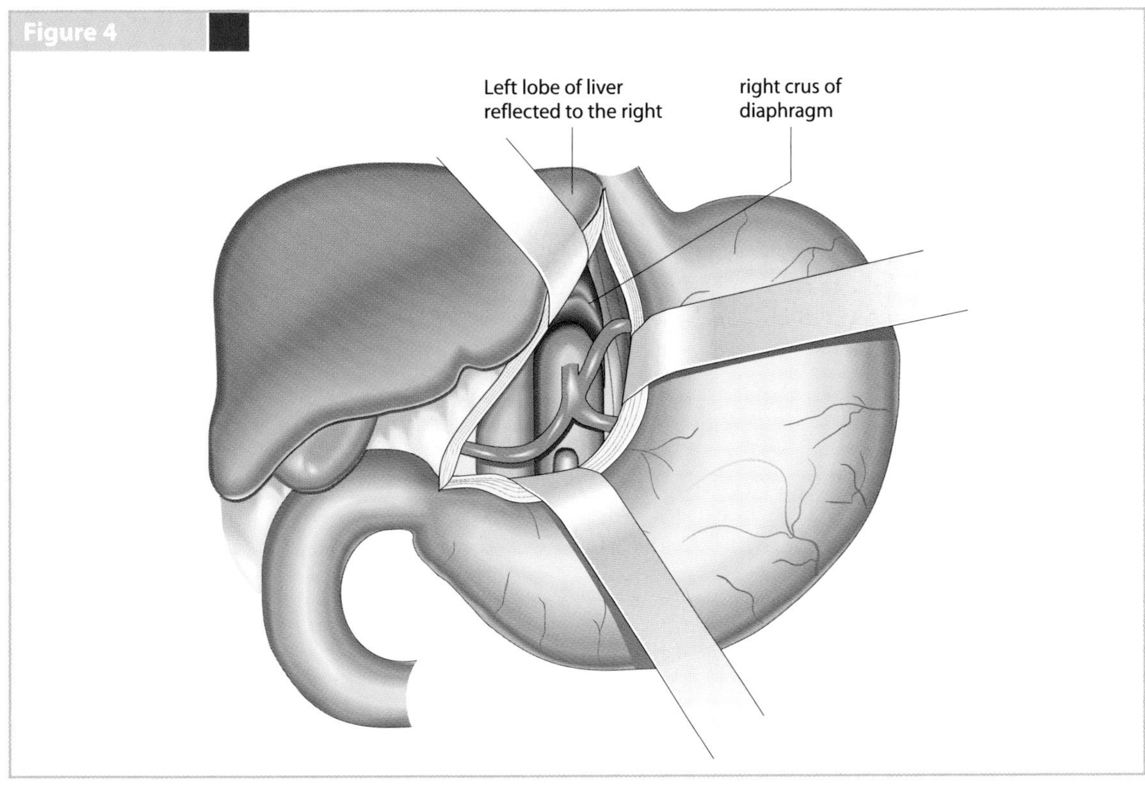

Figure 5: Tunneling

Once the aorta and femoral vessels are prepared for the construction of the anastomoses, tunneling is performed. The tunneling is performed such that the graft is lying posterior to the ureter to prevent any future entrapment of the ureter or complications such as hydronephrosis and graft-ureteric fistulae. Using gentle finger dissection a tunnel is started from the groin incision along the course of the common femoral and external iliac arteries. The second end of the tunnel is similarly created from the abdominal incision following the course of the common iliac artery. With an index finger placed from each end of the tunnel, gentle finger dissection is continued until both fingertips meet. A tunneling clamp is carefully introduced in the tunnel from the groin and an umbilical tape is retrieved to provide easy access to the tunnel at a later stage. The same is performed on the other side. Injury to an external iliac venous branch crossing over the external iliac artery can occur during tunneling. Identification, ligation and division of this vein branch prior to blunt finger tunneling can avoid this potential inconvenience.

ANTICOAGULATION

Once the tunneling is completed, heparin 75–100 units is administered intravenously. Heparin is usually allowed to circulate for 3–5 min prior to cross clamping to ensure adequate anticoagulation. During that period, the aortic graft is prepared for the anastomosis. The graft is transected leaving a short body segment measuring approximately 3–4 cm. This allows for easier coverage of the graft and decreases the chances of kinking of the tunneled limbs. If a concomitant aortorenal bypass or IMA reimplantation is contemplated, the graft is transected leaving a longer body segment to allow for clamping and creating an anastomosis in the graft body.

Figure 5

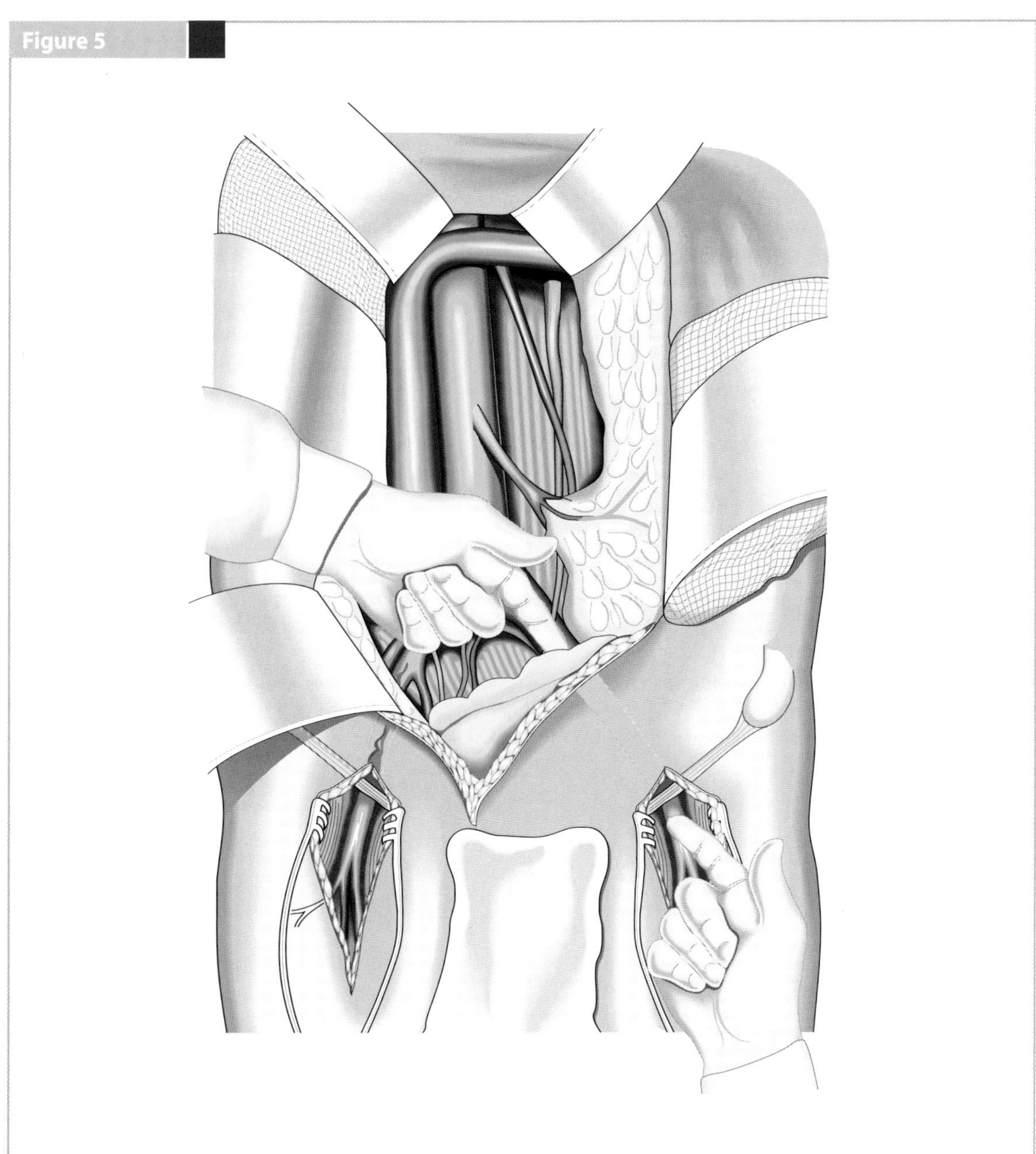

Figure 6A, B: The Site and Configuration of the Proximal Anastomosis

The aorta distal to the inferior mesenteric artery is usually extensively involved with the atherosclerotic process and should be avoided. The aorta between the inferior mesenteric artery and the renal arteries is an ideal site for constructing the proximal anastomosis, as it is usually the least diseased segment of the infrarenal aorta, and its involvement with disease of the proximal part is unlikely.

■ **Configuration of the Proximal Anastomosis and Preservation of Pelvic Perfusion.** There is no evidence to support a hemodynamic advantage of the end-to-end over the end-to-side configuration or vice versa. An end-to-side reconstruction is recommended when the preservation of the existing pelvic circulation is desired especially in the presence of external iliac occlusive disease that prohibits retrograde pelvic perfusion through the hypogastric vessels. The presence of aneurysmal dilatation of the infrarenal aorta will obviously preclude the construction of an end-to-side anastomosis. The extent of atherosclerotic disease and calcification can make the construction of an end-to-side anastomosis impossible, necessitating transecting the infrarenal aorta. One challenge with the end-to-side configuration is identifying adequate periaortic tissue to cover the protruding graft especially in thin patients. Inferior mesenteric revascularization should be considered when there is significant concern that the available reconstruction has deprived the pelvis of essential pelvic perfusion.

THE GRAFT MATERIAL

Polyester grafts are likely to be the most commonly used prosthetic aortic graft. At the University of Iowa, we have routinely used PTFE aortic grafts for our aortobifemoral reconstructions and have not witnessed any significant troublesome needle hole bleeding.

Figure 6A

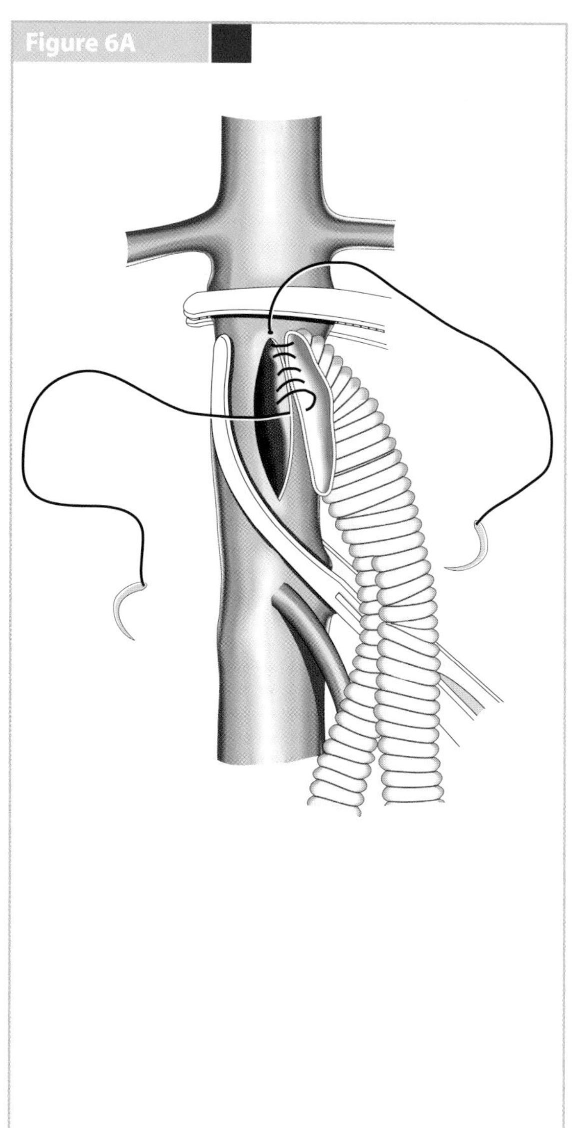

Figure 6B

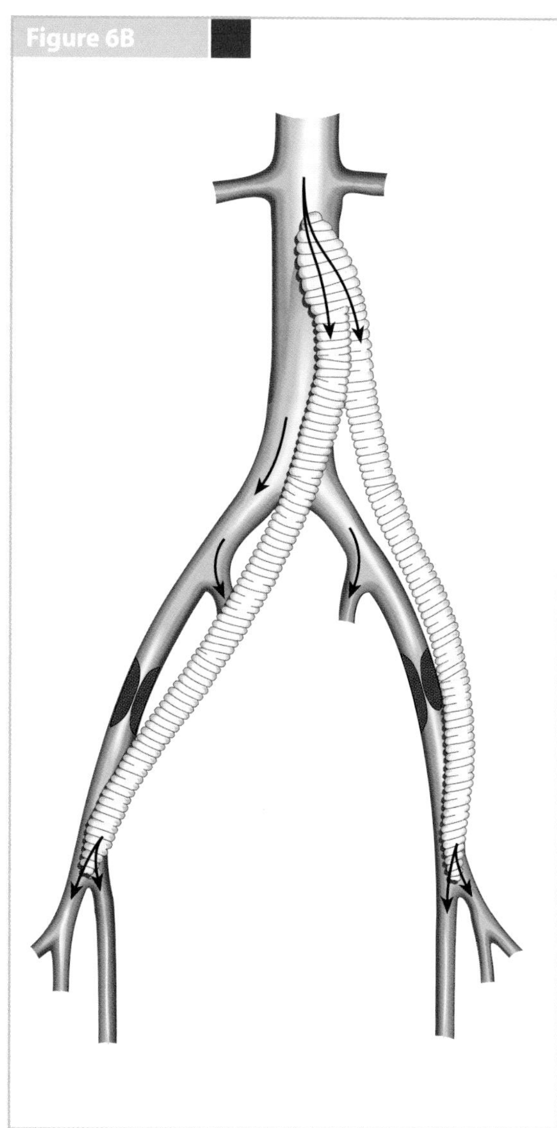

Figure 7: Construction of the Proximal Anastomosis

The aortic clamp is applied at the selected clamp site. Distal control is typically achieved by applying a clamp on the distal aorta. It is not uncommon to find the distal aorta extensively involved with disease, necessitating clamping at the iliac level. If an end-to-end anastomosis is being performed, the aorta is transected 3 cm distal to the level of the renal vein. A small segment of the distal aorta may be excised to allow the short body of the graft to lie without significant anterior angulation. This could facilitate the graft coverage with periaortic tissue. The distal aortic end is oversewn with a running 3-0 Prolene suture. In the presence of severe calcifications, a localized endarterectomy of the distal aortic end may facilitate its closure. The proximal anastomosis is constructed using a 3-0 Prolene suture. Localized endarterectomy may also be necessary if the calcifications are such that the needle cannot penetrate the aortic wall.

If an end-to-side anastomosis is being performed, a longitudinal arteriotomy is created in the anterior aortic wall. The aortic lumen is irrigated with heparinized saline solution and all debris removed.

The anastomosis is constructed in running fashion with 3-0 Prolene sutures using a parachute or anchor technique. At the completion of the suture line, the sutures are tied, and the anastomosis checked for hemostasis. Suture line bleeding is controlled with interrupted mattress sutures. Needle hole bleeding is controlled with the topical application of Gelfoam soaked with thrombin.

Attention is then focused on the femoral anastomoses.

Figure 7

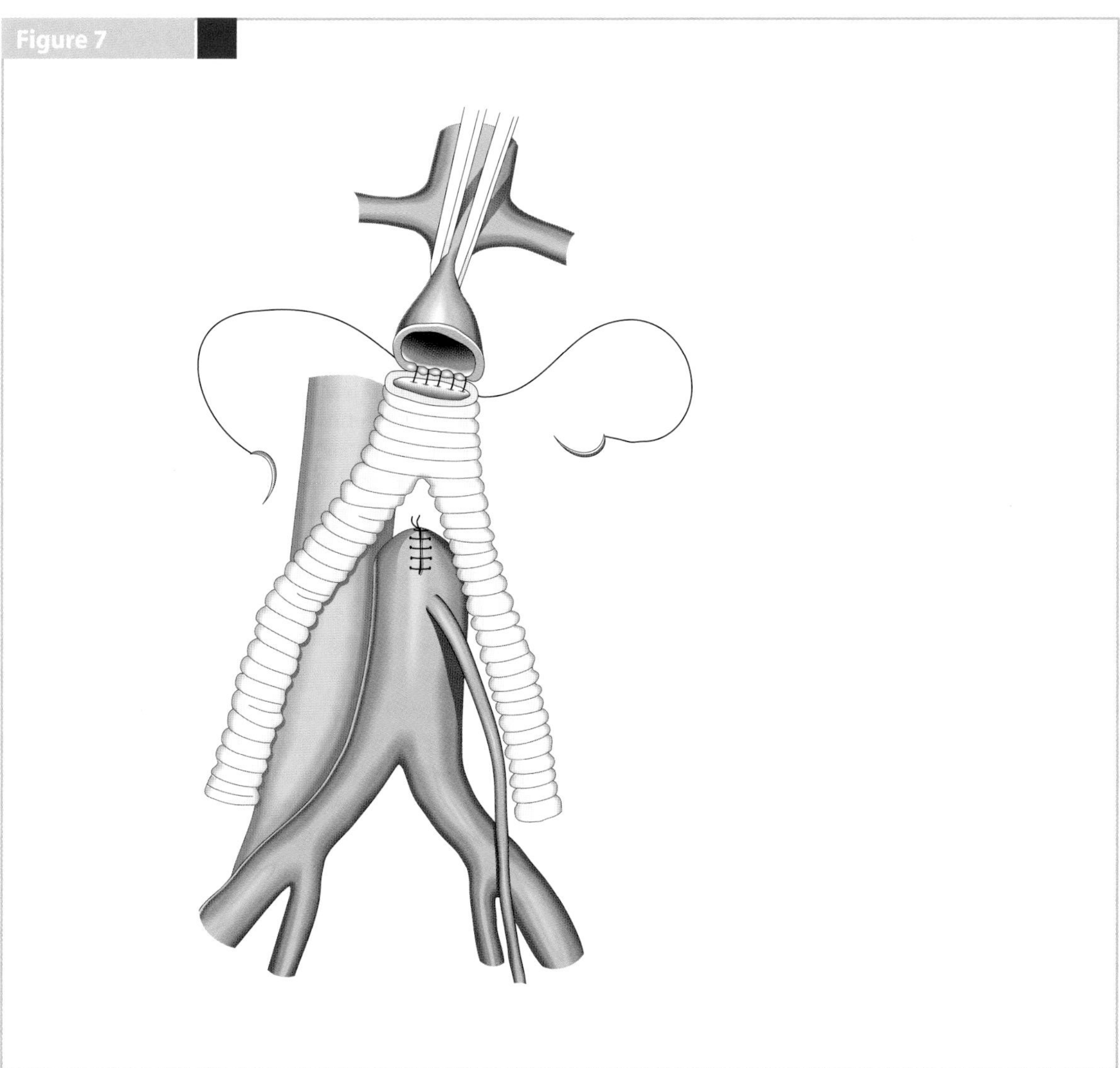

Figure 8: The Distal Anastomosis

One limb of the graft is then passed in the preformed tunnel posterior to the ureter, maintaining alignment and avoiding any kinks. The common femoral, superficial femoral and profunda femoris arteries are cross clamped. The distal anastomosis is usually carried at the level of the common femoral artery. In the presence of significant disease at the level of the common femoral bifurcation, the arteriotomy is started in the common femoral artery and extended into the superficial femoral or profunda femoris artery in the configuration that maximizes distal revascularization. It is essential to ensure flow into the profunda femoris artery to ensure long-term patency of that graft limb should the superficial femoral artery occlude in the future. Some surgeons routinely fashion the anastomosis into the profunda to ensure an unobstructed flow into it. In the presence of extensive atherosclerotic plaque in the common femoral artery, an endarterectomy may be necessary. Often, the external iliac artery at the level of the epigastric branch is soft with minimal plaque. Using a Freer elevator, the plaque in the common femoral artery is elevated and circumferentially dissected. The plaque is transected proximally at the level of the epigastric artery origin. The plaque is elevated and feathered at the distal end in the profunda femoris artery. Very rarely, the plaque extends very distally in the profunda femoris artery necessitating an extended profundoplasty. This will require further distal exposure of the profunda femoris artery. Alternatively, the plaque is transected and tacking sutures at the distal endpoint are placed to prevent lifting of the plaque when flow is resumed. The graft limb is sized with the graft distended and then transected. The anastomosis is then performed with 5-0 Prolene running suture. Prior to completing the anastomosis, the distal clamps are released allowing for backbleeding of the superficial and profunda femoris arteries. The aortic clamp is released for forward flushing of the graft. The anastomosis is copiously irrigated with heparinized saline solution. The clamps are then released allowing flow into the profunda femoris artery first followed by the superficial femoral artery. The Doppler signals in the right superficial femoral and profunda femoris arteries are then checked to ensure good flow.

The procedure is then repeated on the opposite side.

An additional distal revascularization is rarely needed in conjunction with an aortobifemoral bypass. In the presence of combined aortoiliac and infrainguinal occlusive disease, a simultaneous infrainguinal bypass may be considered if the aortofemoral bypass is felt to be inadequate to heal the tissue loss in the foot. If an additional infrainguinal bypass is needed, originating the graft from the superficial femoral or profunda femoris artery rather than the aortofemoral graft limb may be desired.

Figure 9: Perigraft Coverage

Reinspection of all the suture lines is performed to ensure adequate hemostasis.

The field is usually irrigated with antibiotic solution although the scientific evidence for the benefit of such irrigation is lacking. The surrounding periaortic tissue is used to cover the graft. If such tissue is inadequate, an omental flap is developed and used to provide coverage of the graft. A simple technique is to base the omental flap on the left gastroepiploic artery, thus preventing retrocolic tunneling and preserving a significant part of the anterior omentum. A tongue of omentum based on the left omental artery is created. The flap is gently folded over the transverse colon mesentery and placed over the aortic prosthesis. The flap is then secured in place with a running 3-0 silk suture.

Figure 8

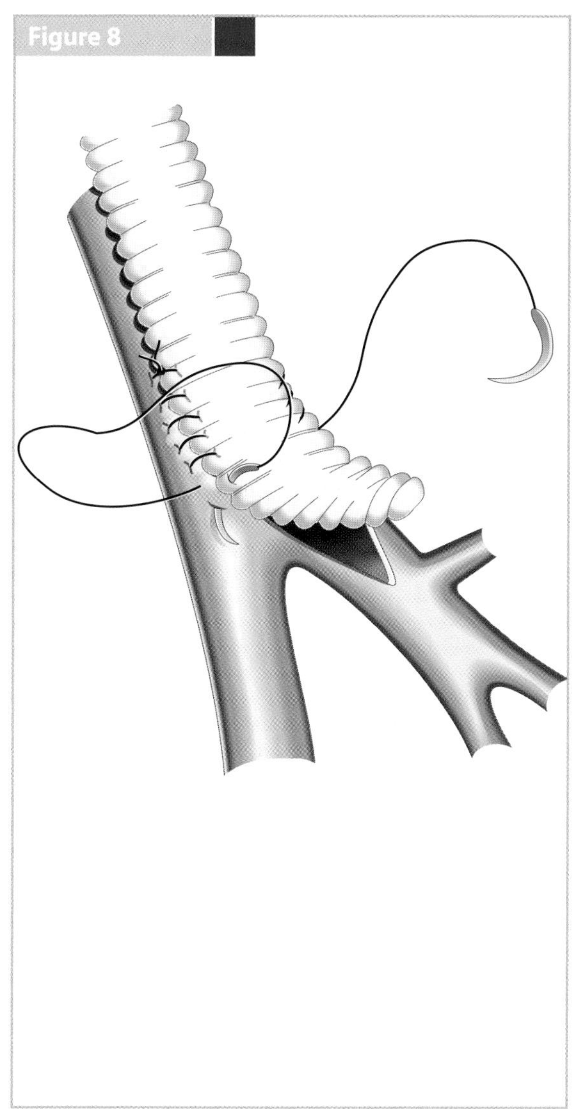

Figure 9

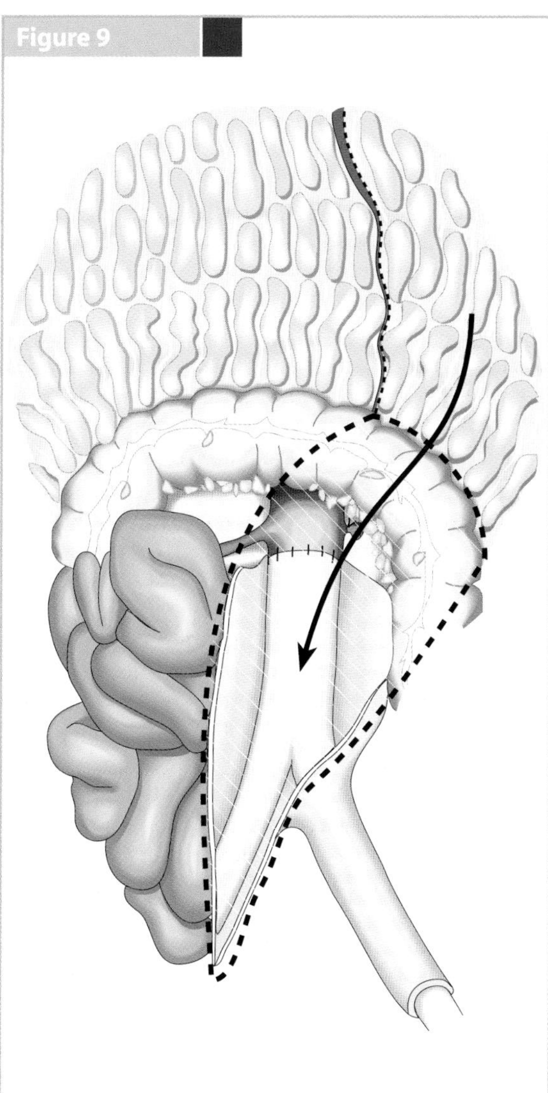

INCISIONS CLOSURE

The bowel is then placed back in the anatomical position. Abdominal wall closure is then performed with running or interrupted #1 Prolene sutures. The soft tissues in the groin are closed over the graft limbs in two layers of 3-0 Vicryl. The skin edges are opposed with skin staples. The peri-incisional prep and drape are cleaned and dried, followed by 4×4 gauze and silk tape. The feet are inspected and the pedal vessels are evaluated for presence of palpable pulses or Doppler signals.

CONCLUSION

Despite advances in endovascular technology, revascularization using an aortobifemoral bypass remains a very effective and durable method for treating severe aortoiliac occlusive disease. Advances in laparoscopy and vascular stapling could further decrease the morbidity of this procedure without negatively impacting its excellent long-term patency rates.

CHAPTER 23

Extra-anatomic Revascularization

Jamal J. Hoballah, Joseph S. Giglia

INTRODUCTION

In the presence of severe unilateral iliac occlusive disease that is not amenable to endovascular therapy, revascularization can be accomplished via an extra-anatomic route by performing a crossover femoro-femoral bypass originating from the contralateral limb. The donor limb should not suffer untoward effects from the extra-anatomic revascularization even in the presence of infrainguinal disease unless proximal hemodynamic stenoses were missed or left untreated. If the donor inflow is marginal due to the presence of proximal disease in its iliac system, endovascular therapy is used to correct the proximal pathology. This can be performed a few days prior to the extra-anatomic revascularization, typically when the pathology is identified on preoperative angiography. Alternatively, the endovascular therapy can be performed simultaneously during the construction of the femoro-femoral bypass especially if magnetic resonance angiography or CT angiography was used for preoperative evaluation.

If endovascular therapy was unsuccessful at correcting the pathology in the donor iliac artery, an aortobifemoral bypass will become necessary. Alternatively, revascularization can be achieved via an axillobifemoral bypass especially in the presence of conditions that prohibit an aortic procedure. These conditions include severe uncorrectable coronary artery disease, severe COPD, ascites, a hostile abdomen due to multiple previous laparotomies or stomas.

Another useful though infrequently used extra-anatomic revascularization is the trans-obturator foramen bypass. This bypass is especially useful when the common femoral artery is associated with infection, tumor or postradiation changes. The inflow source can be the aorta, iliac arteries or a non-infected limb of an aortofemoral bypass.

Figure 1: Femoro-Femoral Bypass

Although a femoro-femoral bypass can be performed using local anesthesia with conscious sedation, this procedure is usually performed with the patient under general or regional anesthesia and positioned supine. The prepping and draping involves both groins and usually extends from mid thighs to the umbilicus. Prepping and draping should be extended to the nipple line or the clavicle if there are any concerns regarding the adequacy of the donor arterial system that could result in conversion to an aortobifemoral or axillobifemoral bypass.

■ **Femoral Artery Exposure.** The femoral artery is exposed through a standard vertical incision. On the donor site, the incision is placed directly over the femoral pulsation. On the recipient site, anatomic landmarks are used to guide the incision. The incision is started halfway between the pubic symphysis and the anterior superior iliac spine. A vertical incision on the recipient site allows for distal extension for more distal exposure of the profunda femoris artery. In overweight individuals or in the presence of inflamed skin or rash in the groin, a transverse skin incision can be used to expose the femoral vessels.

The skin incision is deepened through the subcutaneous tissue and fat, exposing the femoral sheath. Any crossing lymphatic channels are ligated and divided to prevent lymph leak. The common femoral artery is exposed and circumferentially dissected. Similarly the dissection is extended distally to involve the superficial femoral artery and the profunda femoris artery. The site for constructing the anastomosis is selected based on the preoperative angiogram and the intraoperative findings. A soft and pliable segment of the artery is chosen.

■ **Tunneling.** A subcutaneous tunnel between both femoral arteries is created. The graft should ideally be lying on the anterior rectus sheath. The tunnel is started with sharp dissection in the deep subcutaneous tissue exposing the external oblique fascia. This allows the development of adequate soft tissue for coverage of the graft in the groin. The tunnel is further developed bluntly with the index fingers or by using a curved C shaped tunneler.

Figure 1

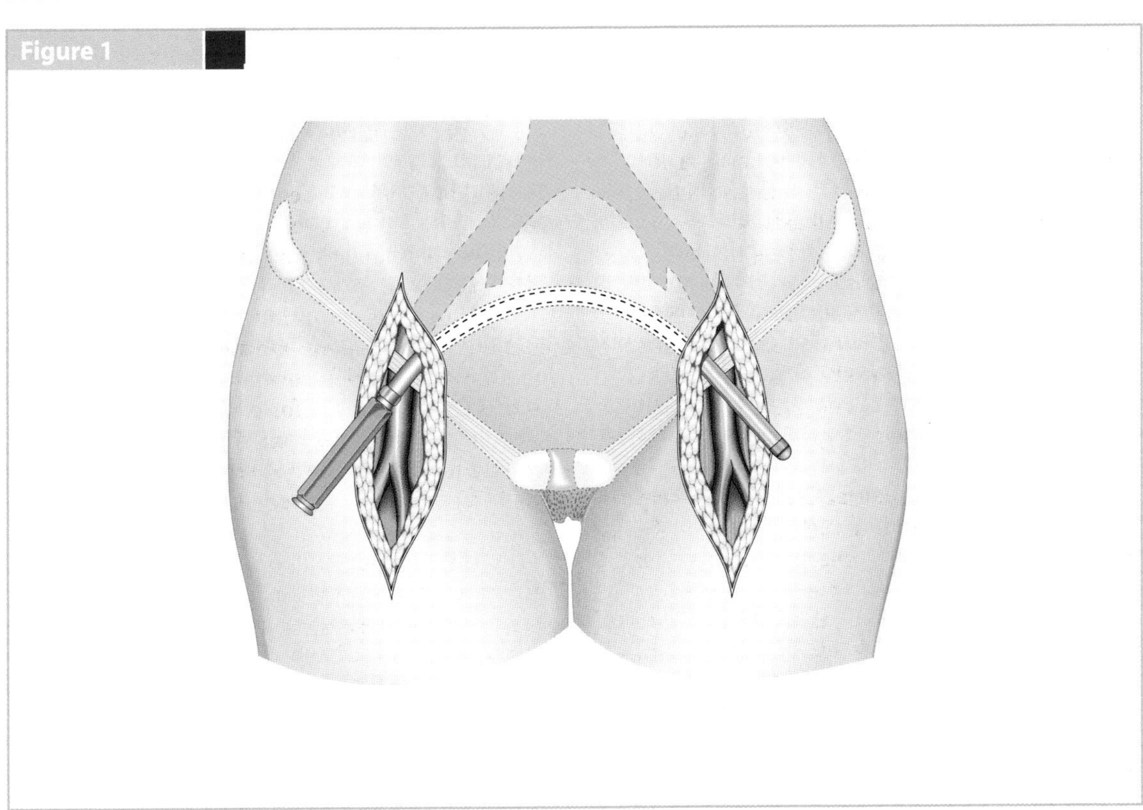

Figure 2A–C: Construction of the Proximal (Donor) Anastomosis

If the common femoral artery is free of any significant disease, a 1–1.5 cm arteriotomy is started in its anterior wall, extending towards the origin of the superficial femoral artery. An arteriotomy in the most distal part of the common femoral artery allows for a gentle C curve in the graft without kinking or angulation. Occasionally extension of the arteriotomy into the superficial femoral or profunda femoris artery is needed to eliminate any kinks especially when the common femoral artery has a high bifurcation close to the inguinal ligament level. If the arteriotomy in the donor femoral artery needs to be extended proximally into the external iliac artery, a gentle C configuration will be hard to achieve and a kink will become apparent after passing the graft in the tunnel. To avoid the kink, the arteriotomy will be closed with a patch and the proximal anastomosis is created in the most distal part of the patch. Alternatively, the external iliac artery is dissected and mobilized by lifting or dividing the inguinal ligament. The arteriotomy is created in the most proximal part of the femoral artery and extended towards the external iliac artery. The femoro-femoral bypass will then follow a lazy S configuration. The more proximal the donor anastomosis is constructed in the external iliac artery, the gentler the curvature of the lazy S configuration.

Figure 2A

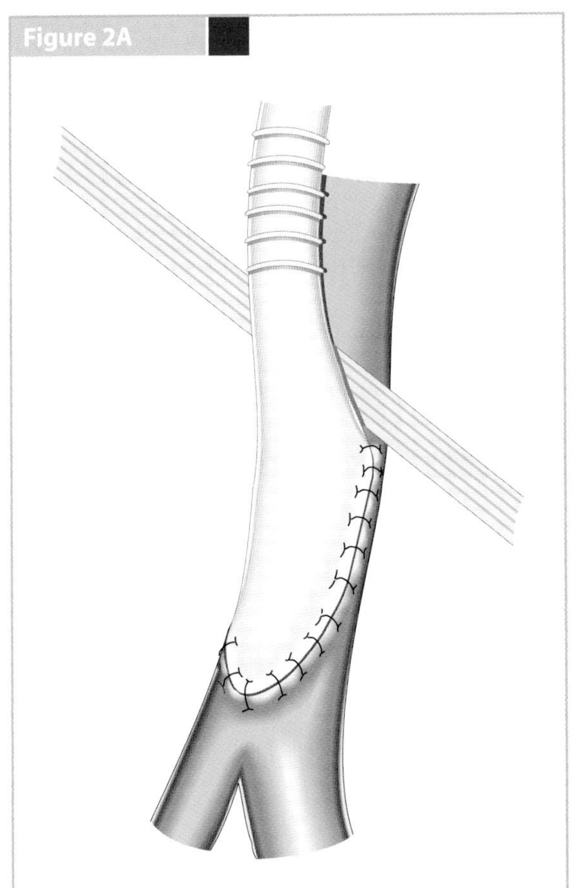

Figure 2B

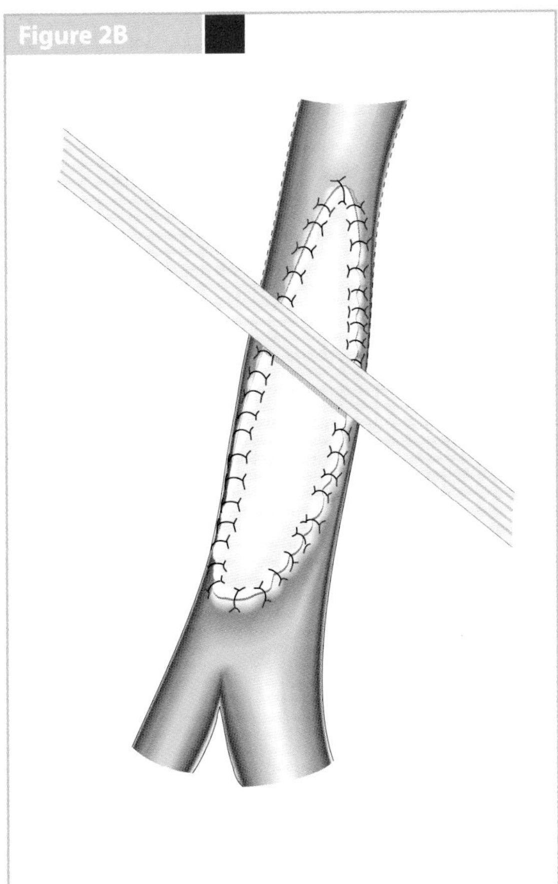

Figure 2C

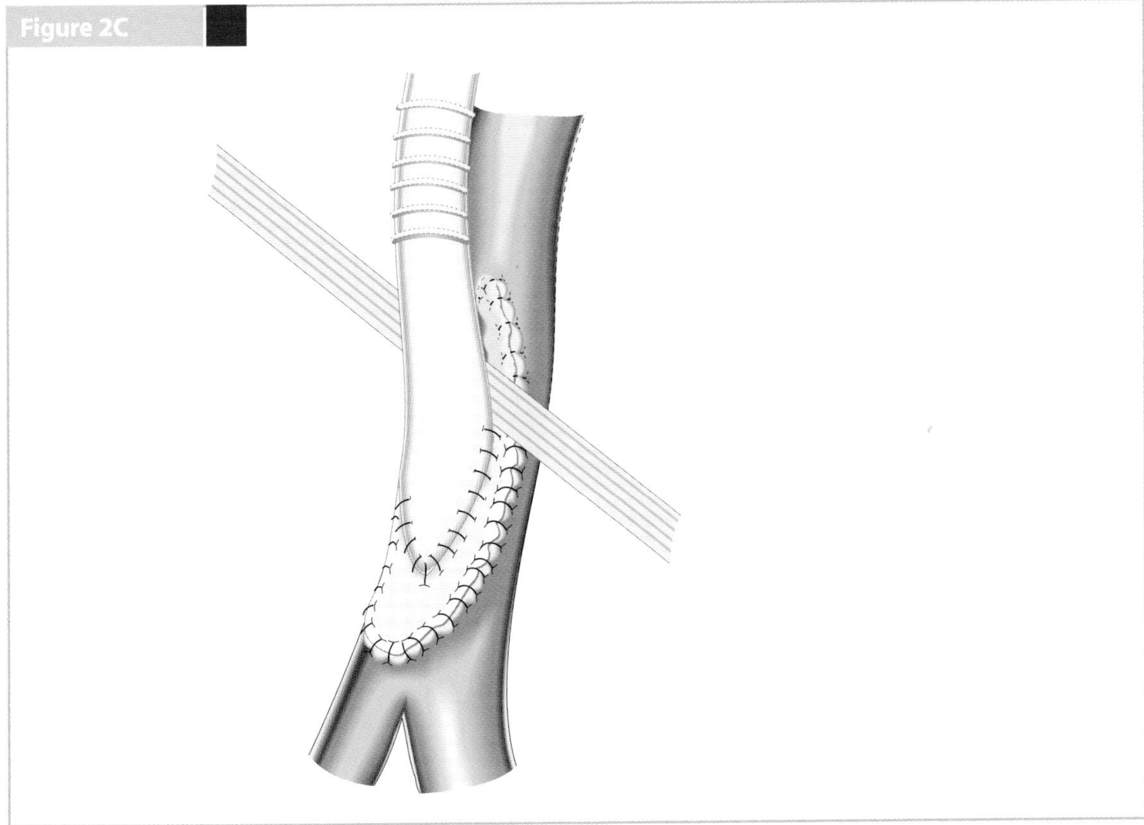

Figures 3A–D, 4: Construction of the Distal Anastomosis

Similar to the proximal anastomosis, the placement and shape of the arteriotomy are essential to prevent any kink. An arteriotomy extending into the external iliac artery should be avoided as it will invariably result in a kink. The distal anastomosis is often carried at the distal part of the common femoral artery. In the presence of significant disease at the level of the common femoral bifurcation, the arteriotomy is started in the distal common femoral artery and extended into the superficial femoral or profunda femoris artery in the configuration that maximizes distal revascularization. Occasionally a localized endarterectomy is necessary at the common femoral artery.

It is essential to ensure flow into the profunda femoris artery to improve long-term patency of the graft should the superficial femoral artery occlude in the future (Fig. 4). This may require an extended profundoplasty.

WOUND CLOSURE

The groin incisions are closed in layers. Typically, two layers of subcutaneous tissue are closed each with a running absorbable suture. It is important to provide good soft tissue coverage over the graft. It is also important to avoid including the greater saphenous vein in the soft tissue closure in the distal part of the wound. The skin is closed with staples or subcuticular closure.

Figure 3A

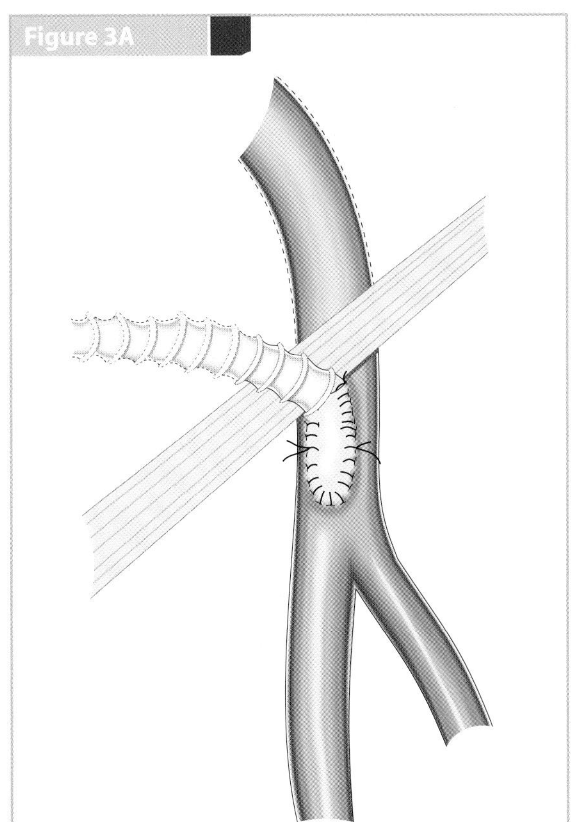

Figure 3B

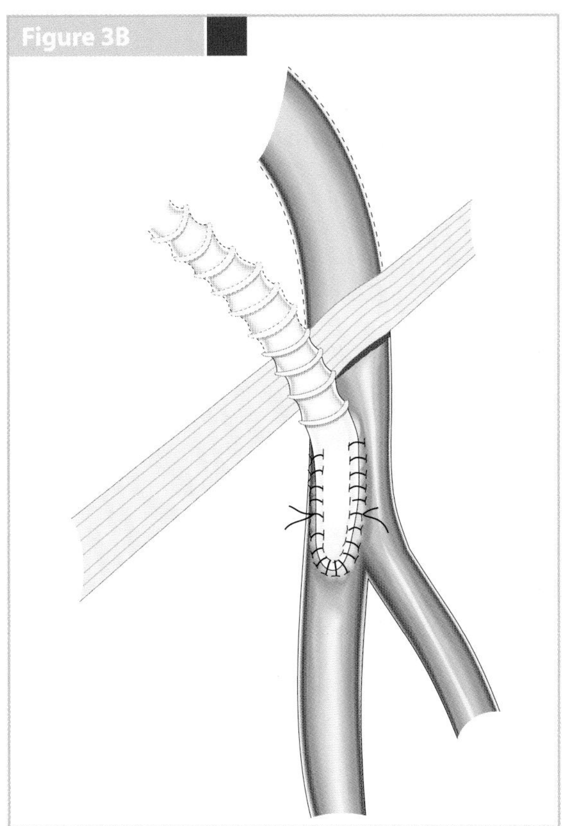

Figure 3C

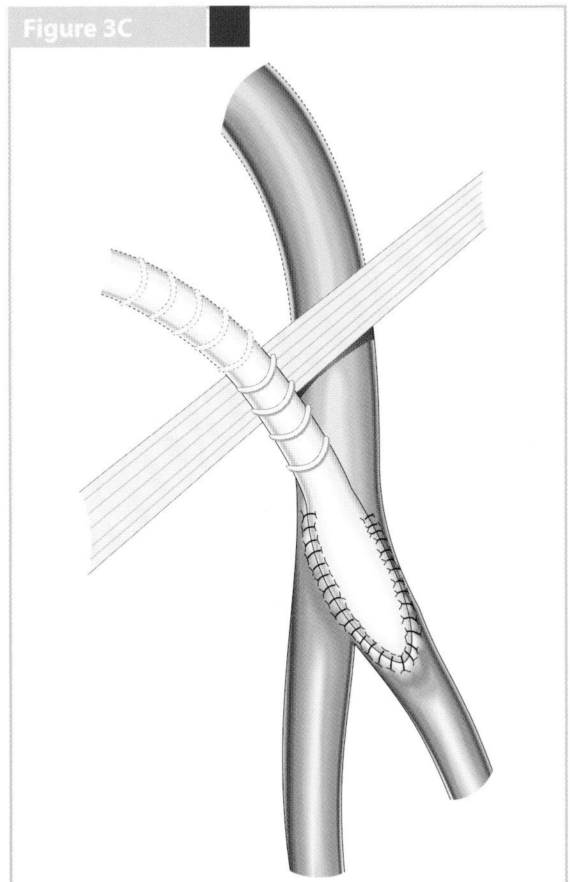

Figure 3D

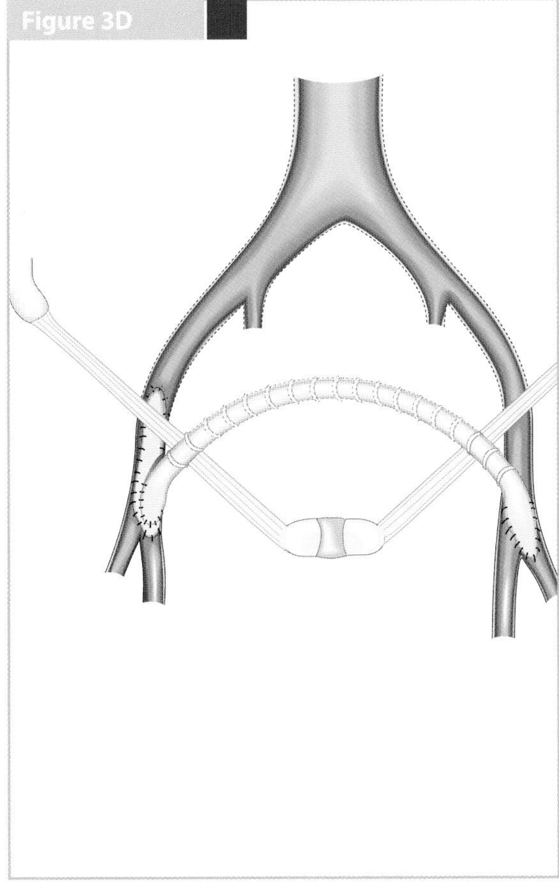

Figure 4

AXILLOFEMORAL/BIFEMORAL BYPASS

Although an axillofemoral bypass has been performed using local anesthesia, it is usually performed with the patient under general anesthesia. The prepping and draping starts from the mid thighs and extends cephalad to include both groins, abdomen, chest and shoulder of the donor upper arm. The entire donor upper extremity is prepped and included in the field to allow various movements of the upper extremity. This also allows for inspection of the graft with various arm positions. The upper arm is usually placed on the patient's side. If the arm is extended on an arm board it will result in tension of the pectoralis muscle during the exposure.

Most often, the right axillary artery is used since the left subclavian artery has a higher incidence of orificial stenosis. Nevertheless, the donor vessel should be evaluated preoperatively to ensure the absence of significant proximal stenosis. This typically includes measurements of the arm pressure or duplex evaluation of the axillary artery and its waveform analysis. When the symptoms are limited to one extremity and in the presence of severe coronary artery disease and comorbid conditions where an expedient procedure is needed, an axillofemoral rather than axillobifemoral bypass is created. Otherwise, an axillobifemoral bypass is typically constructed. One of the reasons often cited for the construction of an axillobifemoral bypass, even when the symptoms are limited to one side, is the increased flow rates in the axillofemoral part of the graft due to the addition of the crossover limb. However, whether an axillobifemoral bypass has a better patency rate than an axillofemoral bypass remains debatable.

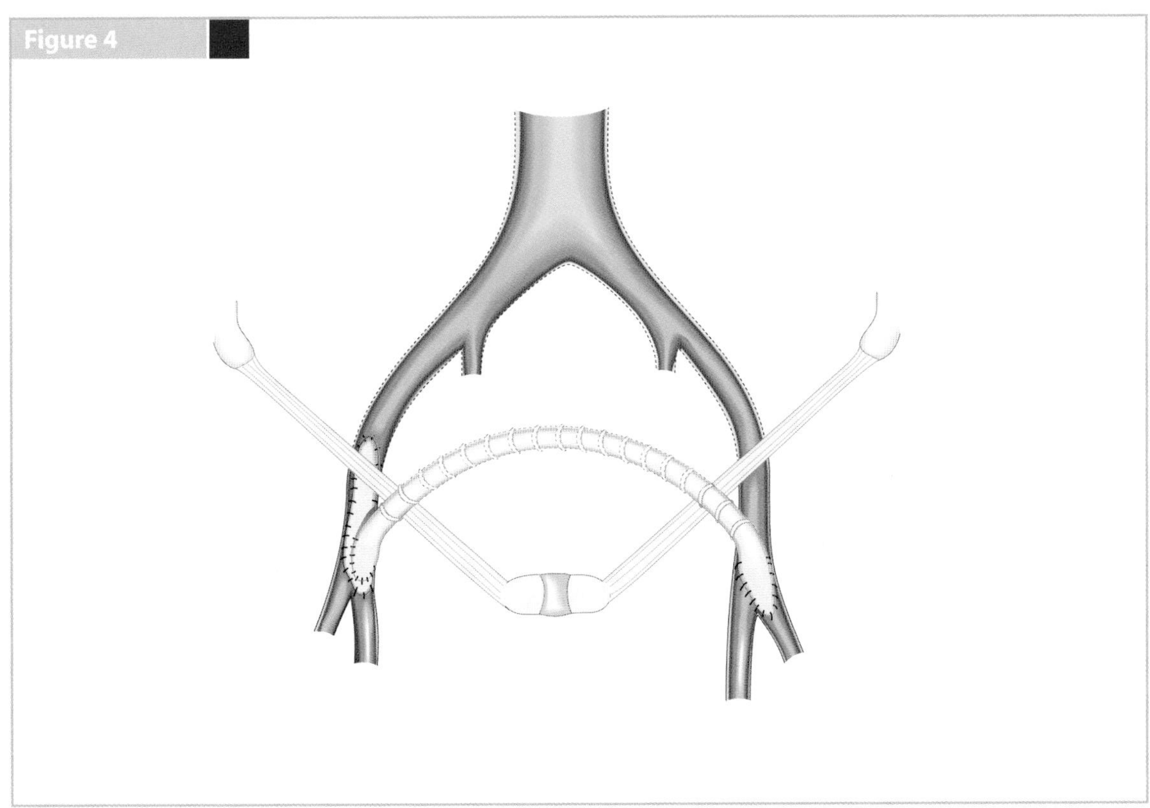
Figure 4

Figure 5: Procedure

■ **Axillary Artery Exposure.** The axillary artery is exposed through a 10-cm infraclavicular incision placed two finger breadths inferior and parallel to the clavicle. The incision is deepened to expose the pectoralis major muscle. The exposure of the axillary artery can be enhanced by dividing the pectoralis minor partially or completely. The pectoralis muscle is split along its fibers and a self-retaining retractor is used to provide access to the axillary artery. The axillary vein and artery are then visualized along with the brachial plexus. The axillary vein may need to be mobilized cephalad and anteriorly to better expose the axillary artery. Alternatively the axillary vein is mobilized caudad, often necessitating division of the venous tributaries including the cephalic vein to enhance the exposure. The first part of the axillary artery is the preferred segment for constructing the proximal anastomosis. Extensive mobilization of the axillary artery has been reported to be associated with a Y angulation of the axillofemoral bypass that could predispose the graft for failure or distal embolization.

■ **Femoral Artery Exposure.** The femoral artery is exposed through a standard vertical incision. Anatomic landmarks are used to guide the incision. The incision is started halfway between the pubic symphysis and the anterior superior iliac spine. The skin incision is deepened through the subcutaneous tissue and fat exposing the femoral sheath. Any crossing lymphatic channels are ligated and divided to prevent lymph leak. The common femoral artery is exposed and circumferentially dissected. Similarly the dissection is extended distally to involve the superficial femoral artery and the profunda femoris artery. The same is done on the other side.

■ **Axillofemoral Tunneling.** Between the infraclavicular and the inguinal incisions, the tunnel is created anterior to the chest wall and posterior to the pectoralis major muscle. A long tunneler (Gore-Tex or Impra Kelly-Wick) is introduced from the groin incision and advanced medial to the anterior superior iliac spine. The tunneler is further advanced and guided to lie on the chest wall along the mid-axillary line. A counterincision may be needed at the nipple line to ensure tunneling posterior to the pectoralis major muscle in the pectoral region. The tunneling should be done carefully to avoid pushing the tunneler's head into the abdominal or pleural cavity. If the graft is constructed to treat an infection in the femoral area, the graft is tunneled lateral to the anterior superior iliac spine to avoid any contacts with the infected or contaminated groin. In this situation, the femoral incision is usually lateral to the sartorius muscle.

■ **Femoro-femoral Tunneling.** A subcutaneous tunnel between both femoral arteries is created. The graft should ideally be lying on the anterior rectus sheath. The tunnel is started with sharp dissection in the deep subcutaneous tissue exposing the external oblique fascia. This allows the development of adequate soft tissue for coverage of the graft in the groin. The tunnel is further developed bluntly with the index fingers or by using a curved C shaped tunneler.

Figure 5

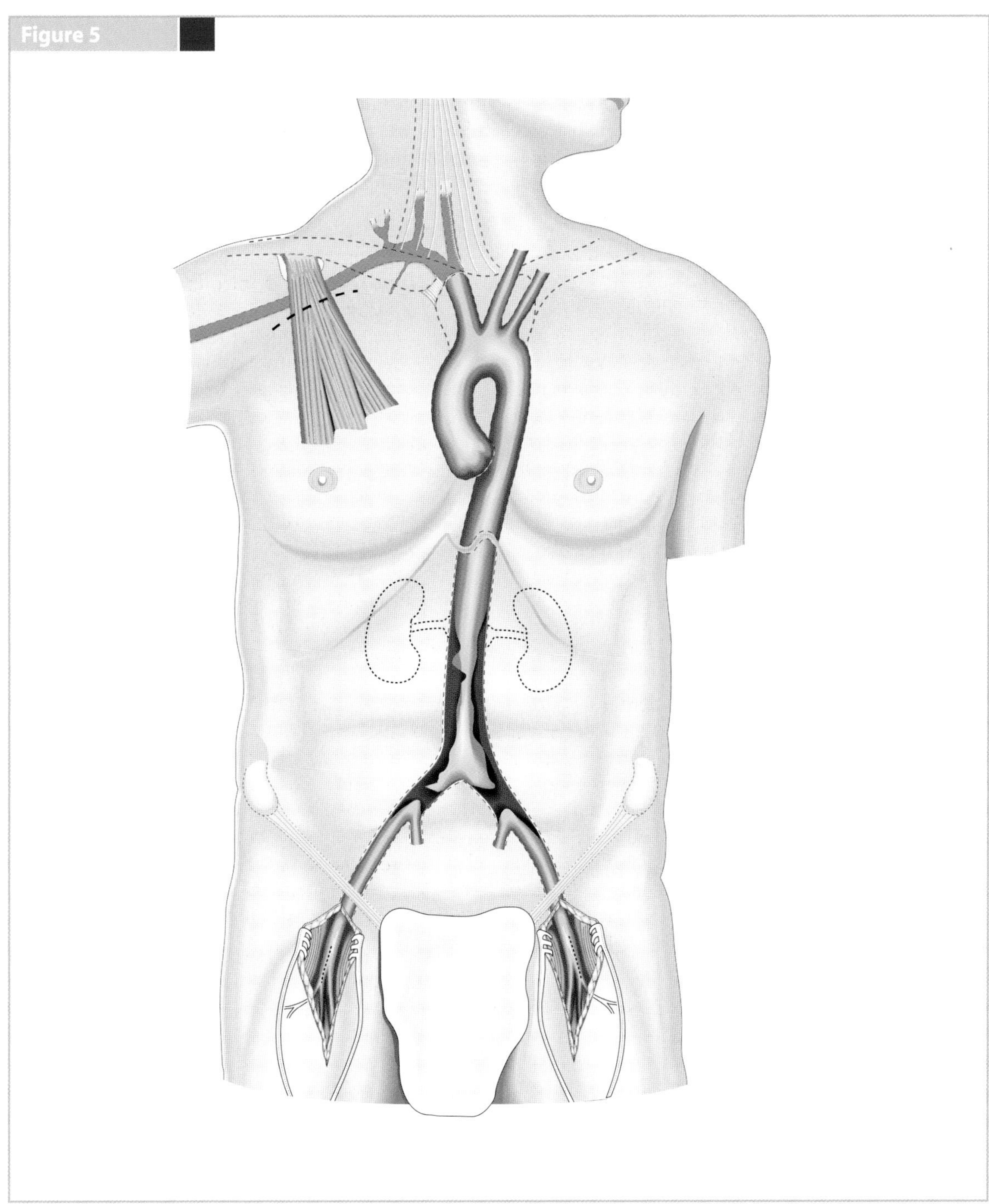

Figure 6A, B: Construction of the Axillary Anastomosis

After passing the grafts in the tunnels, heparin is administered and the anastomoses are constructed. The axillary anastomosis is constructed on the anterior aspect or the anteroinferior aspect of the axillary artery using a 5-0 running Prolene suture. Creating the anastomosis on the most proximal part of the axillary artery allows for the development of a gentle curve in the proximal graft to avoid kinks or tension with shoulder and upper arm extensions.

Figure 6A

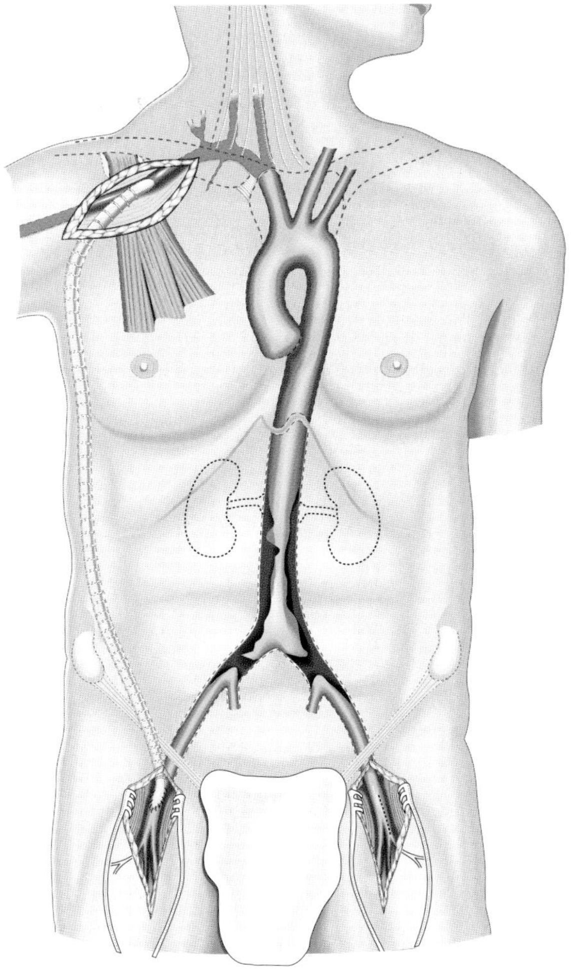

Figure 6B

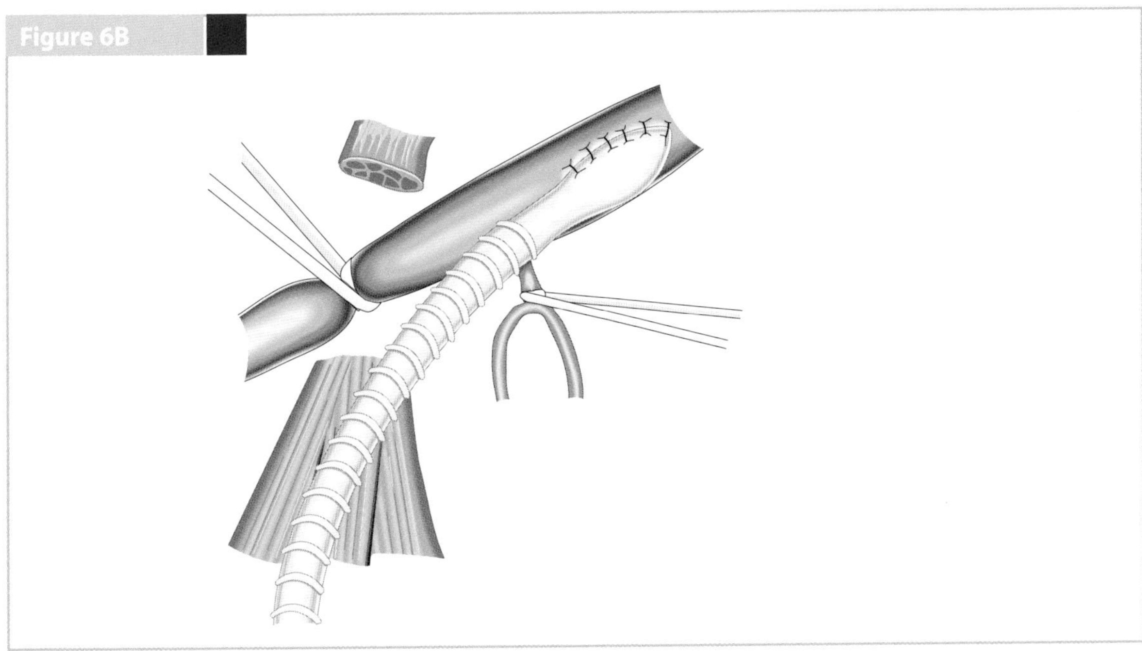

Figure 7A, B: Construction of the Femoral Anastomoses

The site for constructing the anastomosis is selected based on the preoperative angiogram and the intraoperative findings. A soft and pliable segment of the artery is chosen. The construction of the femoral anastomosis and the femoro-femoral crossover graft can follow numerous configurations. In one common configuration, the axillofemoral anastomosis is conducted to the selected site in the common, superficial or profunda femoris artery. The crossover femoro-femoral bypass can originate from the distal part of the axillofemoral bypass in a C, S or H configuration. The proximal femoro-femoral anastomosis can also originate from the femoral artery proximal or distal to the axillofemoral anastomosis. Alternatively, a femoro-femoral bypass is first constructed and the axillofemoral anastomosis is constructed to the hood of the proximal anastomosis of the femoro-femoral bypass.

■ **Wound Closure.** The axillary wound is closed with one layer of absorbable suture to approximate the pectoralis muscle fascia. The subcutaneous tissue in the inguinal incisions is closed with two layers of absorbable sutures. The skin is closed with staples.

Figure 7A

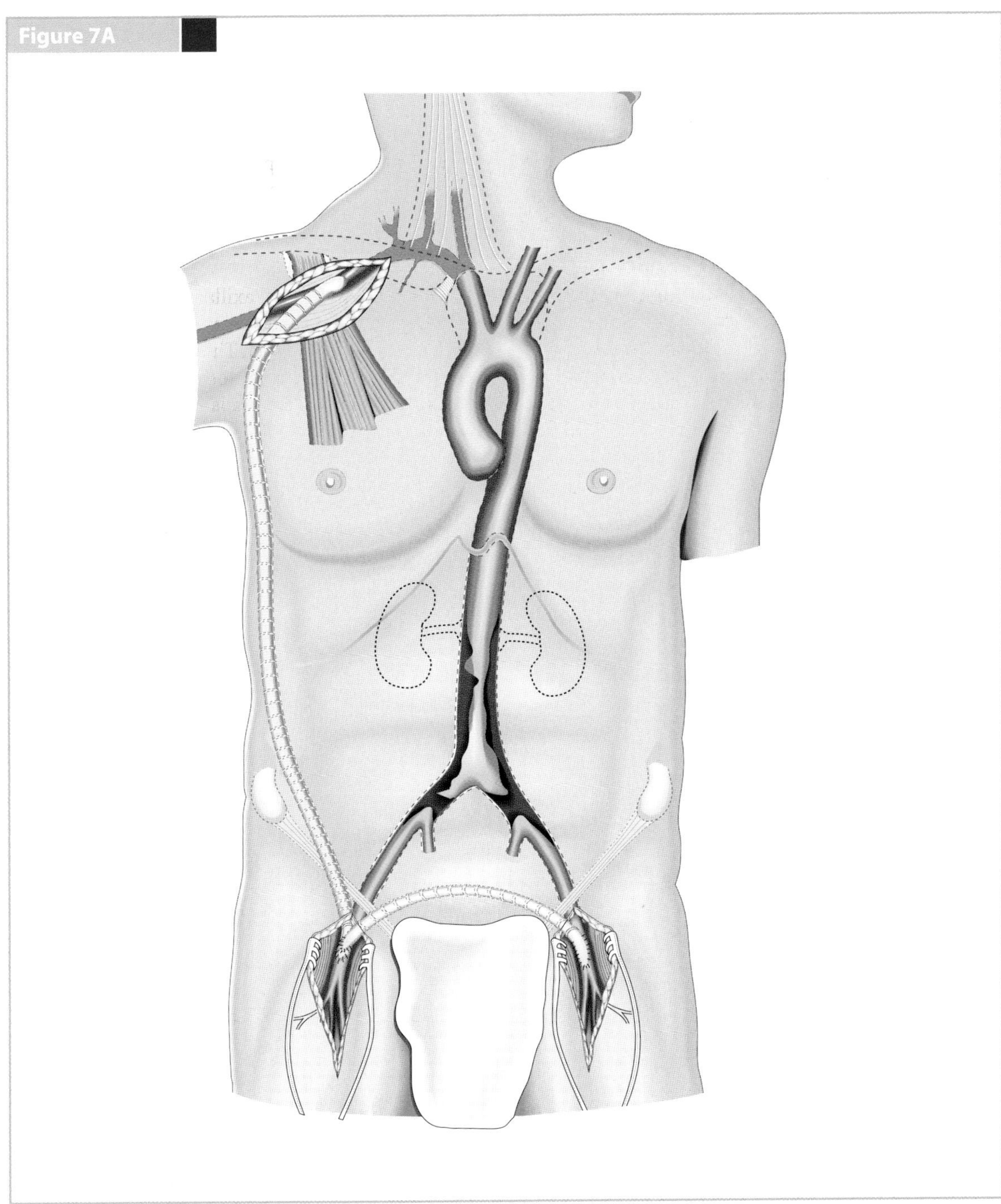

Figure 7B

Figure 7B

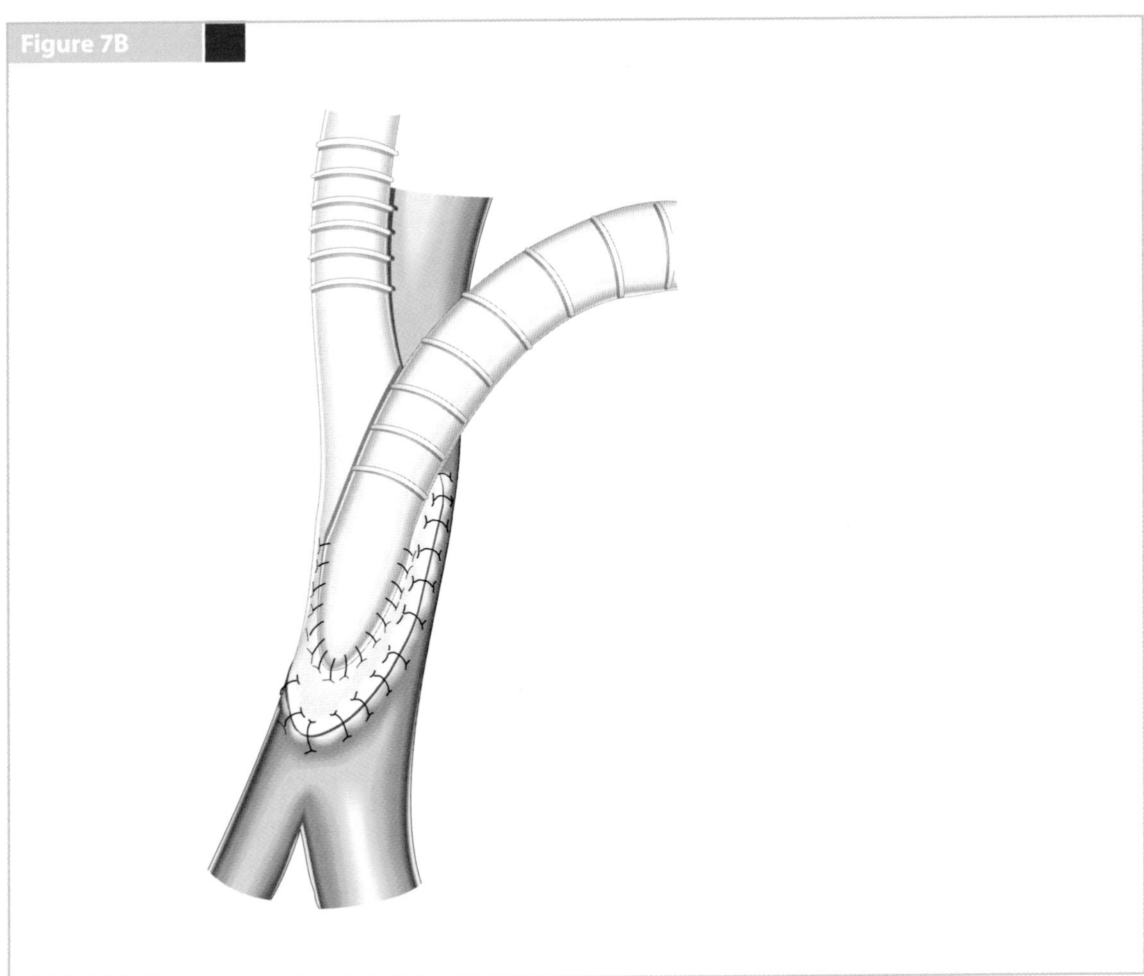

Figure 8A, B: Trans-Obturator Foramen Bypass

Aortofemoral or iliofemoral bypass tunneled via the obturator foramen can be performed when the common femoral artery is associated with infection, tumor, or postradiation arteritis. It is uniquely useful in patients with an aortobifemoral bypass suffering from localized infection at the femoral anastomosis with sparing of the intra-abdominal graft limb. In this situation, the aortic graft is preserved. The proximal part of the graft limb is used as an inflow for the new bypass which will be tunneled through the obturator foramen down to the lower extremity avoiding the femoral infection.

■ **Preparation of the Inflow and Target Sites.** General or epidural anesthesia is utilized. The involved femoral region is covered with an impervious adherent dressing prior to prepping and draping the abdomen, both groins and the entire lower extremity. The involved side is elevated on a bump and the table is rotated toward the contralateral side. The distal target is exposed via medial thigh incision. While the distal anastomosis can be performed to a branch of the profunda femoris, it is typically done to the superficial femoral or popliteal artery. The aorta or proximal common iliac artery is exposed via a midline incision or an oblique lower quadrant incision. If a graft is present at this level it is examined for signs of infection (fluid, lack of incorporation). Infection at this level requires an alternative inflow source. The graft, if present, is clamped, transected and suture ligated distally. The distal end is advanced and the track is closed with absorbable suture. The inflow source (aorta, iliac artery, or proximal graft) is then prepared for an anastomosis.

■ **Tunneling Through the Obturator Foramen (Fig. 8).** The obturator membrane is located by identifying the inferolateral portion of the pubic symphysis. The anteromedial portion of the obturator membrane is then exposed using a combination of blunt and electrosurgical dissection. Care is taken to avoid the obturator neurovascular bundle which courses through the posterolateral portion of the membrane. Figure 8A, once exposed, the extremely tough membrane is incised sharply, creating an adequate opening for passage of a tunneling device. A tunnel is created between the inflow and target sites in either an antegrade or retrograde fashion posterior to the adductor longus and brevis muscles and anterior to the adductor magnus. Figure 8B, a prosthetic graft of the appropriate size is advanced through the tunnel. Following systemic anticoagulation the proximal and distal anastomoses are created using standard techniques. Both wounds are closed in layers.

If the operation is being performed for femoral infection both incisions are covered with adherent occlusive dressings and isolated with surgical drapes before the femoral region is exposed. The femoral artery pathology is then treated as appropriate.

Figure 8A

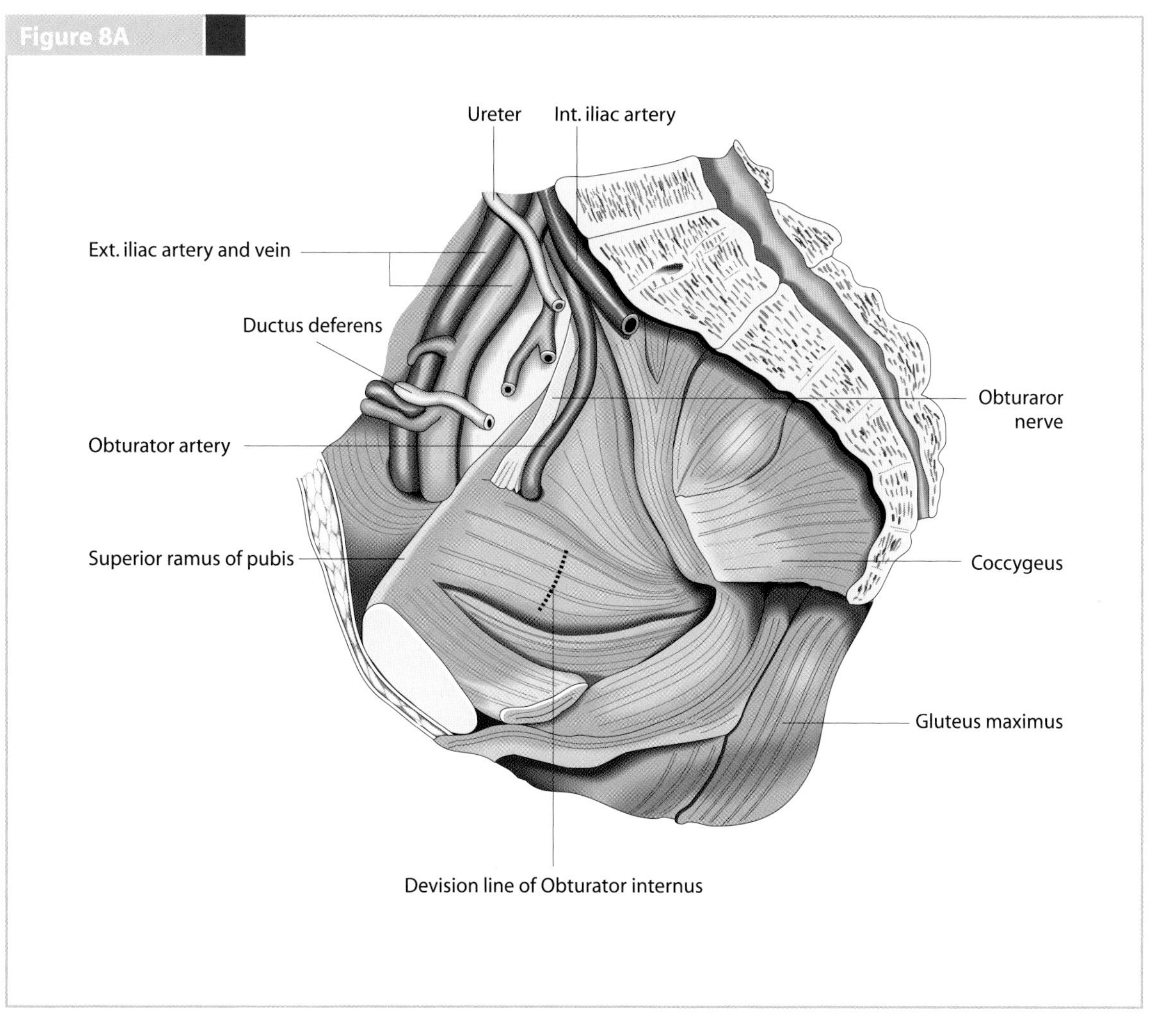
Ureter
Int. iliac artery
Ext. iliac artery and vein
Ductus deferens
Obturaror nerve
Obturator artery
Superior ramus of pubis
Coccygeus
Gluteus maximus
Devision line of Obturator internus

Figure 8B

Figure 8B

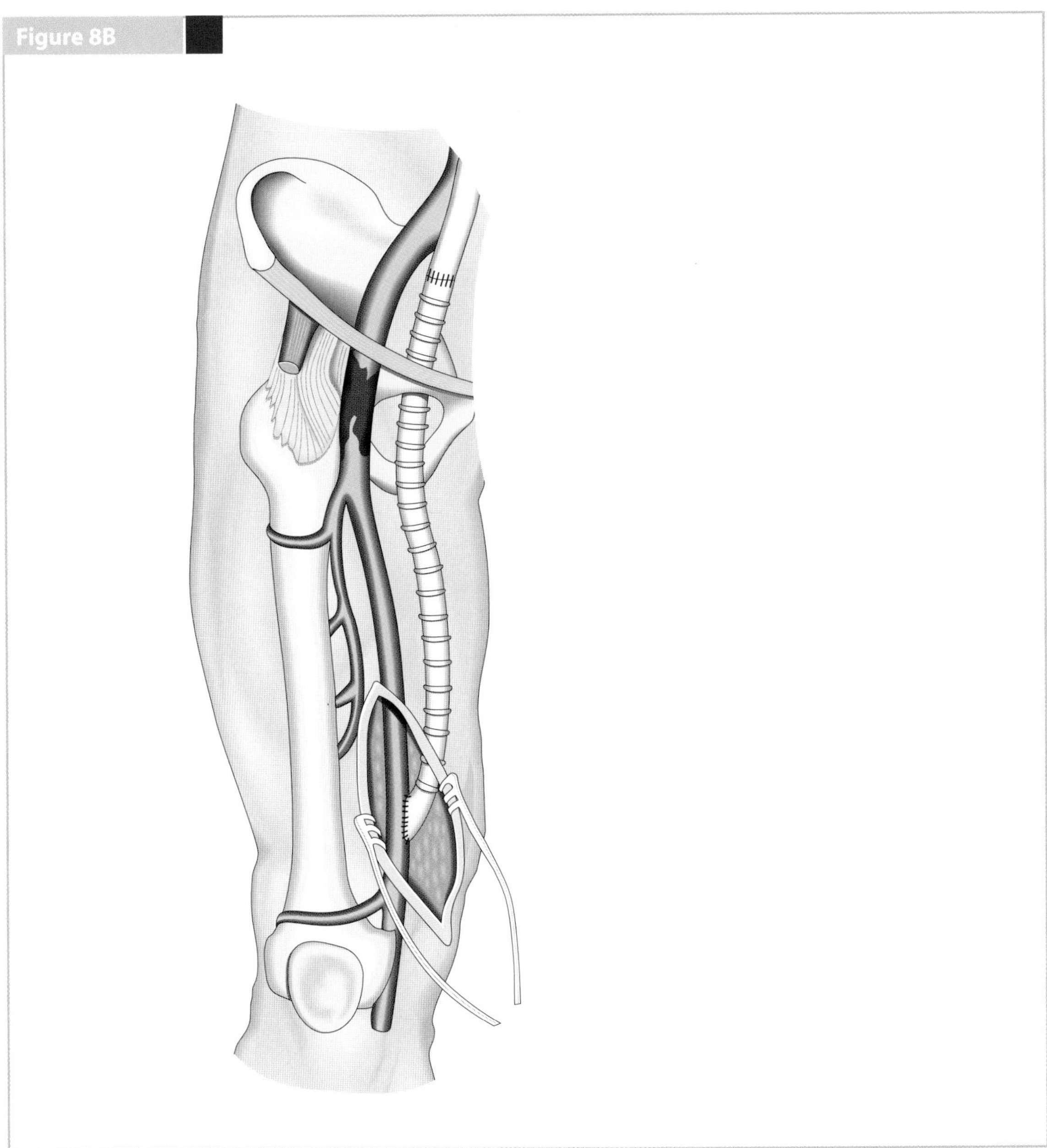

CONCLUSION

Extra-anatomic revascularizations are very useful when dealing with graft infections, scarring or patients with significant co-morbid medical conditions. Although their patency rates are usually lower than those observed with other direct anatomic revascularizations, they remain an essential part of the vascular surgeon's armamentarium.

CHAPTER 24

Descending Thoracic Aorta to Femoral Artery Bypass

Joseph J. Fulton, Blair A. Keagy

INTRODUCTION

Use of the descending thoracic aorta as an inflow source for treatment of aortoiliac occlusive disease was first described in 1961 (Blaisdell 1961; Sevenson et al. 1961). These initial reports were attempts to find an alternative inflow supply when conditions prohibited use of the infrarenal aorta. Upon the heels of these publications, the use of the less complex axillofemoral bypass for extra-anatomic aortoiliac reconstruction was developed and popularized, diminishing interest in the use of the thoracic aorta. During recent years, experience has accumulated and the indications, surgical technique, and excellent results of descending thoracic aorta to femoral artery bypass have been characterized.

INDICATIONS

Bypass from the descending thoracic aorta to one or both of the femoral arteries is indicated in situations when transabdominal aortic reconstruction is impossible, inadvisable, or overtly hazardous. Hostile abdominal conditions include previous or current inflammatory or infected abdominal disease, previous abdominal operations, radiation therapy, complex ventral hernia, or presence of abdominal wall stomas. The descending thoracic aorta may be a more desirable inflow source in those patients with a severely atherosclerotic or hypoplastic infrarenal aorta. Unusual anatomic constraints, such as a horseshoe kidney, in which exposure of the intra-abdominal aorta may be difficult are also indications. Contraindications include aneurysmal or severe atherosclerotic disease of the descending thoracic aorta, prior left thoracotomy, or left lung parenchymal or pleural disease.

Figures 1–4: Surgical Technique

The use of an epidural catheter placed preoperatively reduces the intraoperative need for inhalational agents and systemic narcotics and provides excellent postoperative analgesia. After general anesthesia and placement of a double-lumen endotracheal tube, the patient is positioned with the left hemithorax elevated to a 45- to 65-degree angle, with the left arm positioned to the right, secured in an arm rest to avoid left brachial plexus injury, and a roll is positioned under the right axilla (Fig. 1). The left scapula and thoracic spine should be included in the operative field to allow a full thoracotomy if necessary. The pelvis is placed as flat as possible to allow access to bilateral groins, and pillows are placed under the knees to prevent hyperextension. The legs are secured to the table to allow for safe lateral rotation of the table.

Bilateral vertical groin incisions exposing the femoral arteries are made first to minimize the time the left pleural cavity is exposed. While the right groin exposure is below the inguinal ligament, the left groin incision is extended cephalad 5–10 cm above the inguinal ligament. With division of the left internal oblique and transversus muscles parallel to the direction of the muscle fibers, the left retroperitoneal space anterior to the iliac vessels is entered. This space is later used for tunneling of the graft between the left chest and both groins. The groin incisions are then packed with antibiotic solution-soaked sponges.

A limited left posterolateral thoracotomy is performed through the eighth or ninth intercostal space. The latissimus dorsi muscle is spared by developing superior and inferior skin flaps to allow posterior retraction of the muscle. This maneuver limits postoperative pain. The left lung is deflated, the inferior pulmonary ligament is taken down to the level of the inferior pulmonary vein and the lung is retracted superiorly. To allow exposure of the distal descending thoracic aorta, the diaphragm is retracted inferiorly, avoiding injury to the underlying spleen and visceral organs. The pleura is incised approximately 6 cm longitudinally over the distal aorta, just proximal to the diaphragm. The aorta is palpated, and a site with minimal atherosclerotic disease is selected for the site of proximal anastomosis. The distal descending thoracic aorta is mobilized from the parietal pleura to allow for placement of a partial occluding clamp. Intercostal arterial branches are carefully preserved. Circumferential control of the aorta is optional but not necessary.

After the proximal and distal anastomotic sites have been dissected, a retroperitoneal tunnel from the left pleural cavity to the left suprainguinal preperitoneal space is created. For this purpose, the diaphragm is mobilized approximately 5 cm from its posterior attachments. Using blunt finger dissection, a retroperitoneal plane is developed posteromedial to the spleen, posterior to the kidney, and anterior to the psoas muscle. Simultaneously, using the opposite hand from the left suprainguinal preperitoneal space, blunt dissection is carried upward, crossing over the external iliac vessels onto the anterior surface of the psoas muscle up to the level of the retroperitoneal space (Fig. 2).

Figure 1

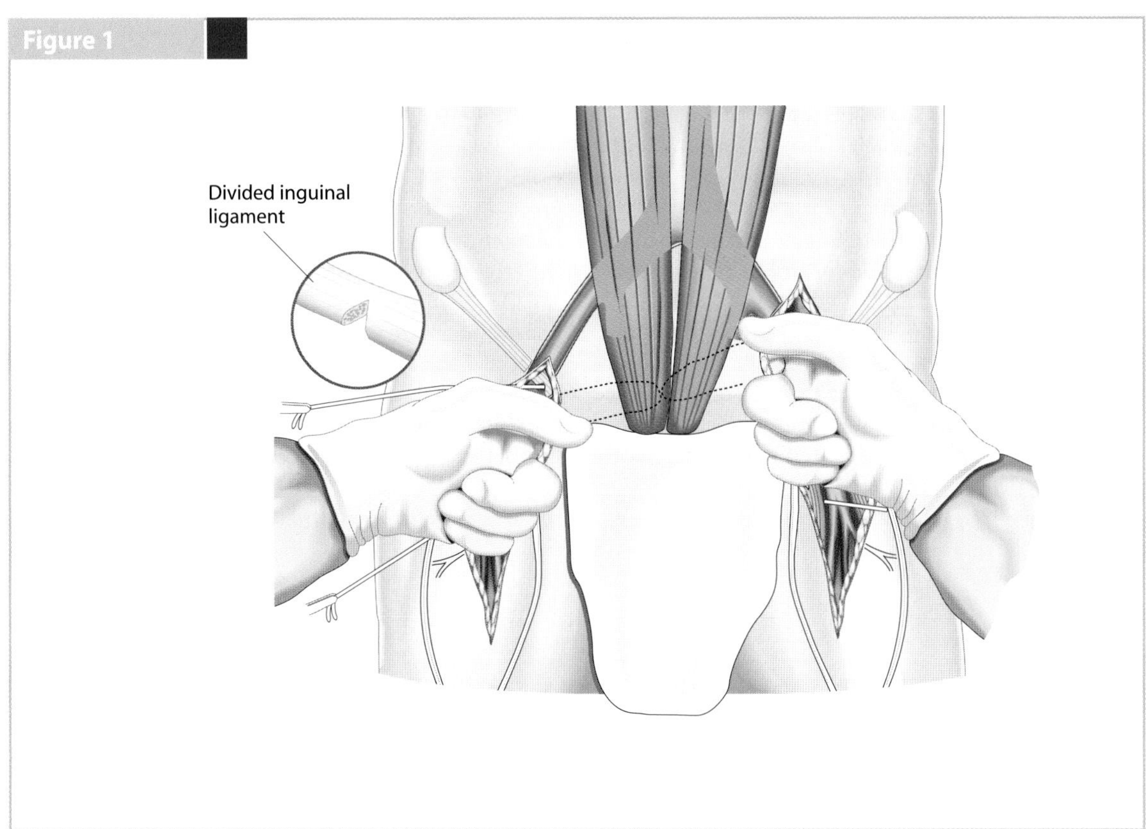

Figure 2

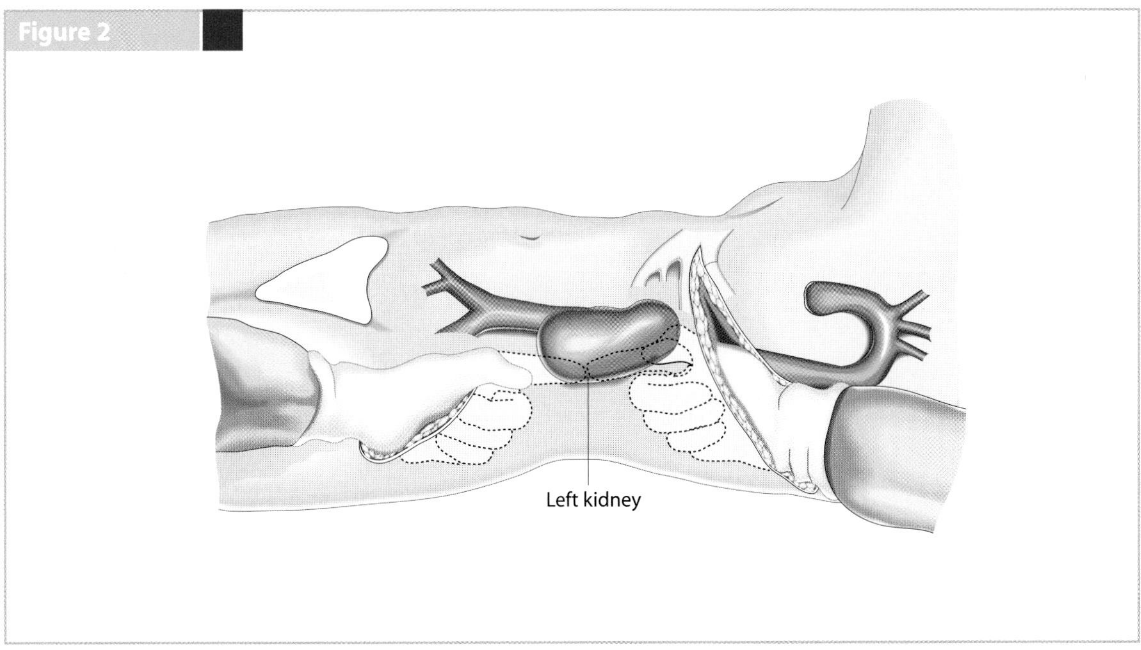

Figures 3, 4

Next, a crossover tunnel is made between the left suprainguinal preperitoneal space and the right groin, posterior to the rectus muscle and anterior and cephalad to the bladder (Fig. 3).

After systemic heparinization, a partially occluding aortic clamp is used for control of the distal descending thoracic aorta, verified by use of a handheld continuous-wave Doppler probe, which maintains perfusion to the spinal cord and to the renal and visceral vessels during proximal anastomosis. The proximal end of a bifurcated graft is beveled, and anastomosis to the distal descending thoracic aorta is performed.

The graft is tunneled between the left chest and left suprainguinal preperitoneal space. From this location, the left limb of the graft is tunneled to the left groin over the iliac vessels and under the inguinal ligament, and the right limb of the graft is directed to the right groin posterior to the rectus muscles through the previously formed tunnel (Fig. 4). Distal anastomoses are performed between each limb of the graft and the femoral arteries. A thoracostomy tube is placed in the left pleural space, and the left lung is reinflated under direct vision. Thoracotomy and groin incisions are closed in standard fashion. A closed suction drain is left subcutaneously to drain the space under the skin flaps.

Figure 3

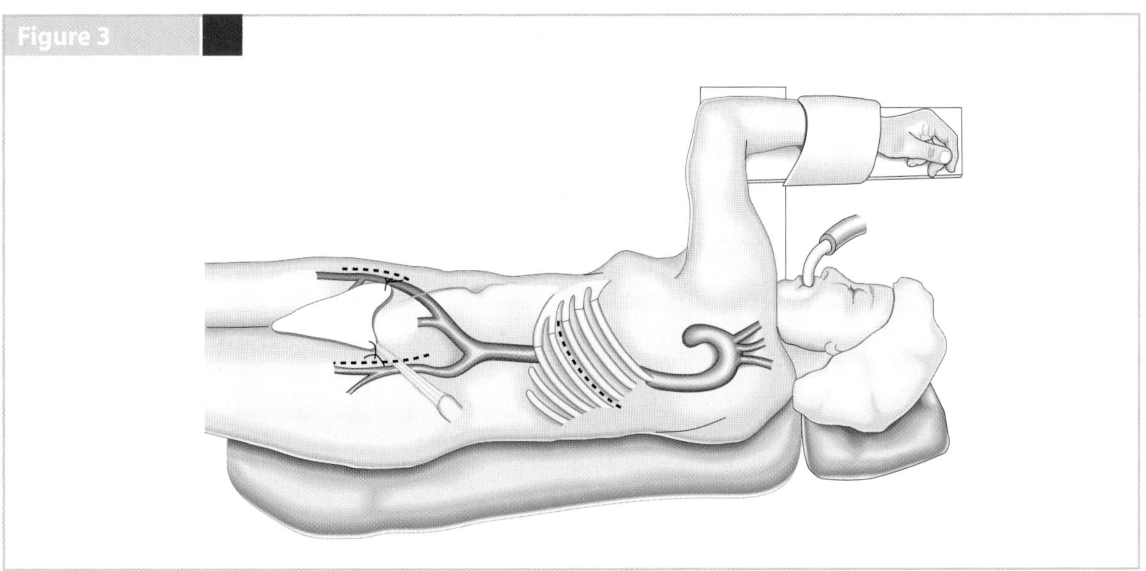

Figure 4

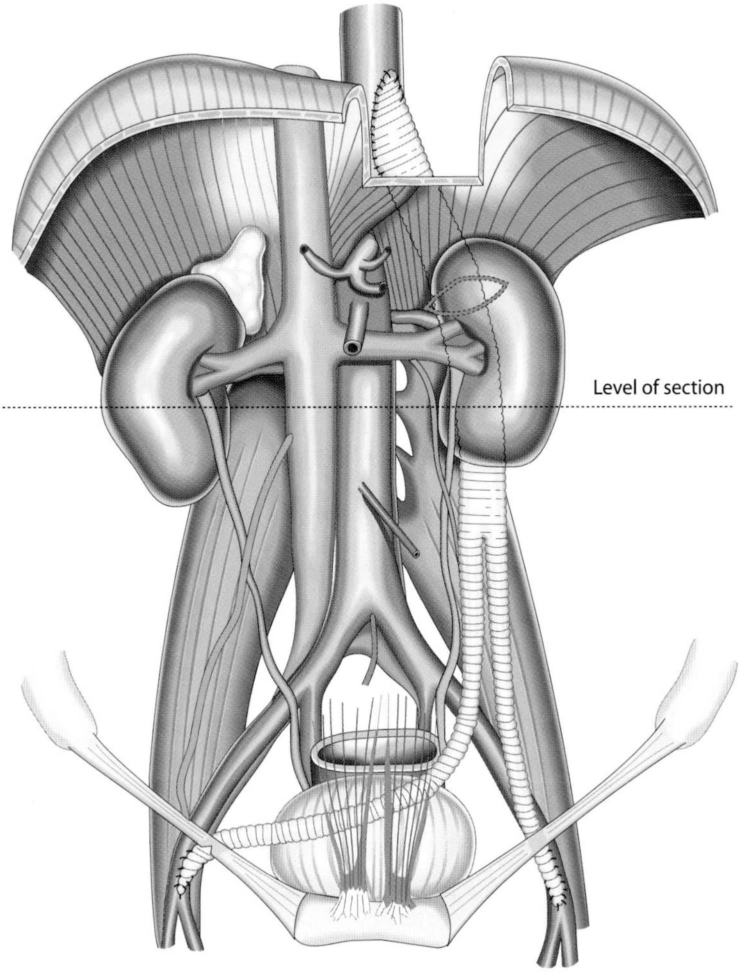

Level of section

CONCLUSION

Descending thoracic aorta to femoral artery bypass has excellent long-term results, with 5-year patency rates of 76–86% and a major complication rate comparable with aortofemoral bypass grafting (Criado and Keagy 1994; Feldhaus et al. 1985; McCarthy et al. 1993). At the University of North Carolina, 50 descending thoracic aorta to femoral artery bypass operations have been performed between 1983 and 1997 (Passman et al. 1999). Overall operative mortality was 4% with a perioperative complication rate of 16%. There were no episodes of renal failure or spinal cord ischemia associated with the operation. Cumulative life-table 5-year primary patency, secondary patency, limb salvage, and survival were 79%, 84%, 93%, and 67% respectively.

REFERENCES

Blaisdell FW (1961) Extraperitoneal thoracic aorta to femoral bypass. Am J Surg 102:83–85

Criado E, Keagy BA (1994) Use of the descending thoracic aorta as an inflow source in aortoiliac reconstruction: indications and long-term results. Ann Vasc Surg 8:38–47

Feldhaus RJ, Sterpetti AV, Shultz RD et al. (1985) Thoracic aorta-femoral bypass: indications, technique, and late results. Ann Thorac Surg 40:588–592

McCarthy WJ, Mesh CL, McMillan WD et al. (1993) Descending thoracic aorta-to-femoral artery bypass: ten years experience with a durable procedure. J Vasc Surg 17:336–348

Passman MA, Farber MA, Criado E et al. (1999) Descending thoracic aorta to iliofemoral artery bypass: a role for primary revascularization for aortoiliac occlusive disease? J Vasc Surg 29:249–258

Sevenson JK, Sauvage LR, Harkins HN (1961) A bypass homograft from thoracic aorta to femoral arteries for occlusive vascular disease. Am Surg 27:632–637

CHAPTER 25

Introduction to Infrainguinal Revascularization

Jamal J. Hoballah

Infrainguinal revascularization is typically performed for disabling claudication or critical limb ischemia manifested by rest pain, ischemic ulcerations or gangrene. The superficial femoral artery is among the first infrainguinal vessels to be affected by the atherosclerotic process, typically starting at the level of the adductor canal. The atherosclerotic process can also affect the infrapopliteal vessels with variable sparing of the distal tibial or pedal vessels, a pattern typically noted in diabetic patients. Endovascular treatment and endarterectomy have a limited role in the management of infrainguinal occlusive disease especially when the infrainguinal pathology is diffuse in nature and involves the tibial vessels. Endovascular therapy can be useful in patients with focal superficial femoral artery disease and limited life expectancy. In most other patients, lasting revascularization is best achieved using bypasses. The basic principles of constructing an infrainguinal bypass are:

1. Identifying an arterial segment that can serve as a dependable source of blood inflow
2. Identifying an arterial segment that can serve as the target vessel through which new blood flow can be received and distributed into the ischemic leg
3. Connecting the inflow artery and target vessels together with a conduit
4. Constructing the shortest bypass possible
5. Adhering to a postoperative duplex surveillance protocol especially for vein bypasses to identify failing bypasses and revising them before thrombosis

The ideal infrainguinal conduit is yet to be found. The best results have been achieved with the great saphenous vein. Nevertheless, the conduit of choice when constructing bypasses to the suprageniculate popliteal artery (above knee popliteal artery) remains controversial. When vein and PTFE bypasses to the above knee popliteal artery were analyzed in prospective randomized trials, the patency rates were comparable at 4 years and showed superiority of the vein bypasses thereafter. When a bypass to the above knee popliteal artery fails, the next revascularization is typically to an infrageniculate level. Prosthetic bypasses to the infrageniculate level have significantly lower patency rates than vein bypasses. Proponents of the preferential use of prosthetic grafts to the above knee level propose saving the great saphenous vein for later use when the above knee bypass fails. They prefer to start with a PTFE to the above knee level followed by vein to the infrageniculate level rather than starting with a vein to the above knee level and a PTFE bypass to the infrageniculate level. The proponents of preferential use of vein to the above knee popliteal artery reject the previous argument citing that a second revascularization may not be necessary if the vein bypass with better patency rate is used first. Furthermore the great saphenous vein may be damaged during the above knee prosthetic bypass. Clearly this is a very debatable issue and the choice should be individualized. When the greater saphenous vein is unavailable or inadequate, an autogenous conduit is still the preferred conduit especially when the bypass is intended to cross the knee joint. The autogenous conduit alternatives to the great saphenous vein include the short saphenous vein, the cephalic or basilic veins and the superficial femoral vein. The short saphenous and the arm veins are especially suitable for use as a short bypass, or when revising failing grafts by performing jump or interposition grafts or vein patch angioplasty. When autogenous conduits are unavailable, infrainguinal bypasses are usually constructed using PTFE, umbilical veins, or cadaveric cryopreserved veins.

The number of potential variations in the construction of an infrainguinal bypass is unlimited. When using a vein conduit, the variations include the creation of an in situ bypass versus a reversed or non-reversed vein bypass. When using a prosthetic bypass, various adjunctive procedures have been devised to improve the patency of prosthetic bypasses to the infrageniculate vessels. These techniques which include vein patches or collars and creation of adjunctive arteriovenous fistulae add to the possible variations. Furthermore, blood vessels can typically be exposed through more than one approach. Except for the anterior tibial artery and occasionally the peroneal artery, most infrainguinal vessels are typically exposed through a medial approach. Tunneling of the graft also adds to the possible variations in infrainguinal reconstructions. To provide a comprehensive description of the possible variations in infrainguinal reconstructions the various exposures of the infrainguinal vessels and a sample of various bypasses procedures will be described.

The selected sample procedures are:

- Common femoral to above knee popliteal prosthetic bypass
- Common femoral to below knee popliteal bypass with reversed great saphenous vein
- Common femoral to posterior tibial/peroneal artery in situ bypass
- Profunda femoris to anterior tibial bypass with non-reversed great saphenous vein
- Common femoral to peroneal artery prosthetic bypass with an adjunctive vein collar/AV fistula

CHAPTER 26

Exposure of the Lower Extremity Arteries

Christopher T. Bunch, Jamal J. Hoballah

INTRODUCTION

The arteries of the lower extremity can be exposed through various approaches. Familiarity and comfort with the various exposures at different levels in the lower limb are essential to optimal revascularization.

Figure 1: The Common Femoral Artery

■ **Medial Infrainguinal Approach.** The common femoral artery and its bifurcation are typically approached through a vertical skin incision placed over the femoral pulse. If the femoral pulse is weak or nonpalpable, calcification in the common femoral artery can aid in identifying its location. A calcified femoral artery can often be palpated by rolling one's fingers gently over its expected anatomic position, which is at a point midway between the symphysis pubis and the anterior superior iliac spine. If the saphenous vein is visualized during subcutaneous dissection, it is spared and a more lateral course is sought. Encountering nerves, however, signals the need to dissect more medially, the dissection being more lateral than the actual location of the femoral artery. Encountered lymphatics are ligated and divided to avoid postoperative lymph leaks. The femoral sheath is identified and incised, exposing the common femoral artery. As the common femoral artery is dissected distally, a change in the caliber of the exposed artery will mark the transition from the common femoral to the superficial femoral artery with the profunda femoris artery originating on the posterolateral aspect. The superficial femoral artery can be further exposed and dissected distally by extending the incision distally.

■ **Exposure Through a Transverse Suprainguinal Incision.** An alternative approach to the common femoral artery is through a suprainguinal transverse incision placed two finger-breadth's superior to the inguinal ligament. This incision is comparable to an inguinal hernia incision and can be used in the presence of macerated skin in the inguinal crease. The incision is deepened through the subcutaneous tissue and Scarpa's fascia until the inguinal ligament is identified. The inguinal ligament is mobilized and freed along its length to allow retraction superiorly. The femoral sheath is identified and is then incised longitudinally exposing the common femoral artery. Because exposure of the superficial and profunda femoris arteries will be limited, the potential need for extended profundaplasty or other reconstructions distal to the common femoral artery bifurcation may preclude this approach.

Figure 1

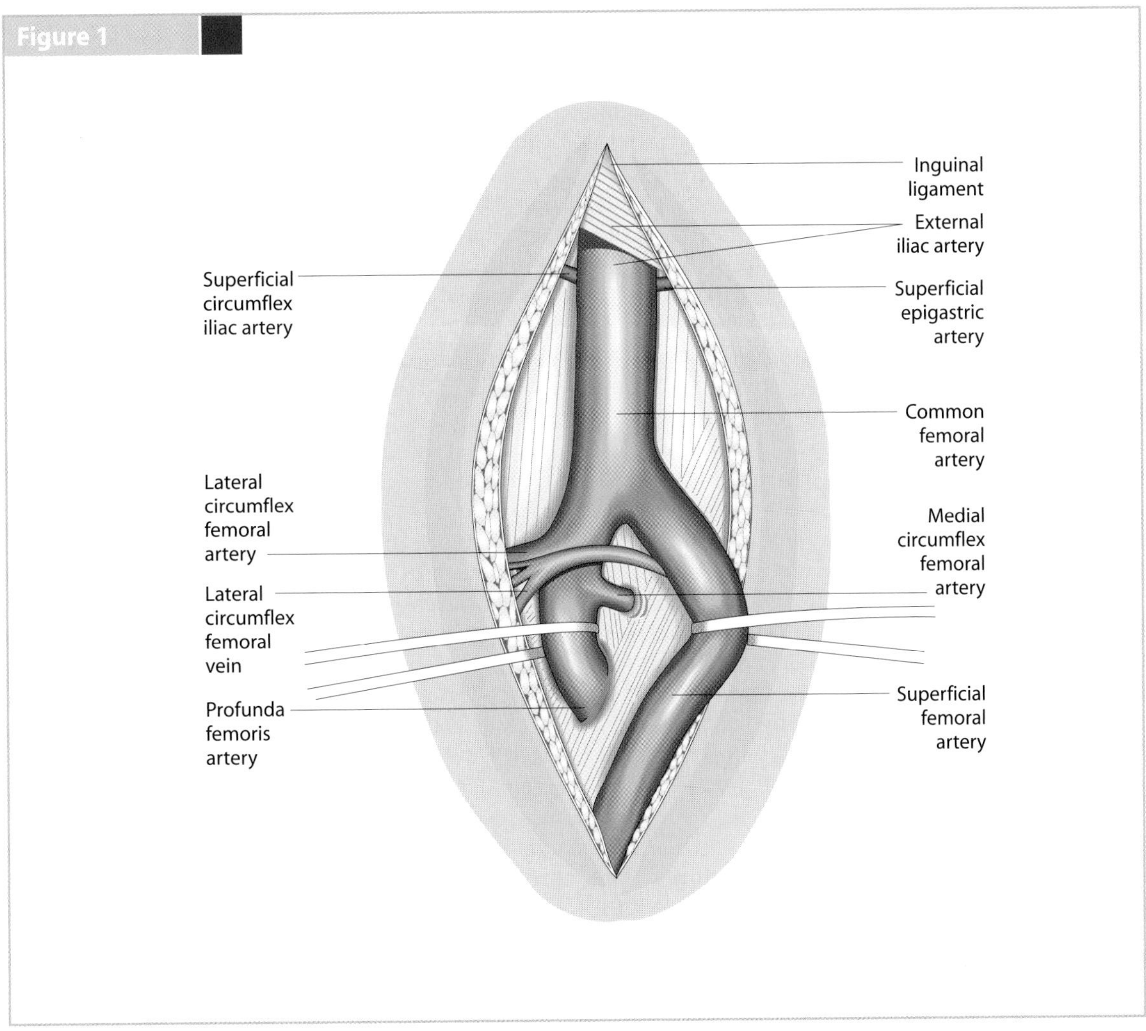
Inguinal ligament
External iliac artery
Superficial circumflex iliac artery
Superficial epigastric artery
Common femoral artery
Lateral circumflex femoral artery
Medial circumflex femoral artery
Lateral circumflex femoral vein
Profunda femoris artery
Superficial femoral artery

Figure 2: Lateral Approach

A lateral approach can also be used to approach the common femoral artery (Bridges and Gewertz 1980). In the presence of infection on the medial aspect of the groin in the vicinity of the site where the usual vertical incision is performed, radiation or severe scarring, a lateral approach becomes very useful. The sartorius muscle is an important landmark for the lateral approach. A vertical incision is made approximately 6–8 cm lateral to the femoral pulse. The incision is deepened through the subcutaneous tissues exposing the fascia lata. Incising the fascia lata will expose the lateral border of the sartorius muscle. The dissection is then continued posterior to the sartorius muscle in the direction of the femoral vessels. The exposure is enhanced by mobilization of the proximal part of the sartorius muscle which often necessitates transection of its first two segmental arterial branches. The femoral sheath is identified from beneath the sartorius muscle as the dissection is carried medially. The femoral sheath is incised along its lateral border exposing the common femoral artery. Extending the incision distally will allow for exposure of the superficial and profunda femoris arteries.

■ **Technical Tips During Redo Procedures.** The exposure of the femoral vessels during redo procedures may be challenging. The exposure may be facilitated by identifying and encircling the superficial femoral artery underneath the sartorius muscle a few centimeters distal to its origin, and then continue the dissection proximally. The dissection is started on the medial aspect to minimize the chances of injuring the origin of the profunda femoris artery. The medial dissection is extended proximally to the level of the inguinal ligament where circumferential dissection of the common femoral or external iliac artery is performed to allow proximal control. The dissection is then continued on the lateral aspect starting at the inguinal ligament and progressing distally to identify and control the profunda femoris artery. In the presence of dense scarring, the profunda femoris artery may be more safely controlled from within by occlusing it with a Fogarty catheter once the arteriotomy is created. Dissection with a #15 blade can be very useful in dense scarring.

Occasionally severe calcification in the common femoral artery precludes the safe application of a vascular clamp. In this situation, the dissection is extended underneath the inguinal ligament. This will often identify a soft segment in the external iliac artery just proximal to the origin of the superficial iliac circumflex and superficial epigastric branches. More proximal exposure of the external iliac artery can be obtained by dividing the inguinal ligament and applying deep retractors.

Figure 2

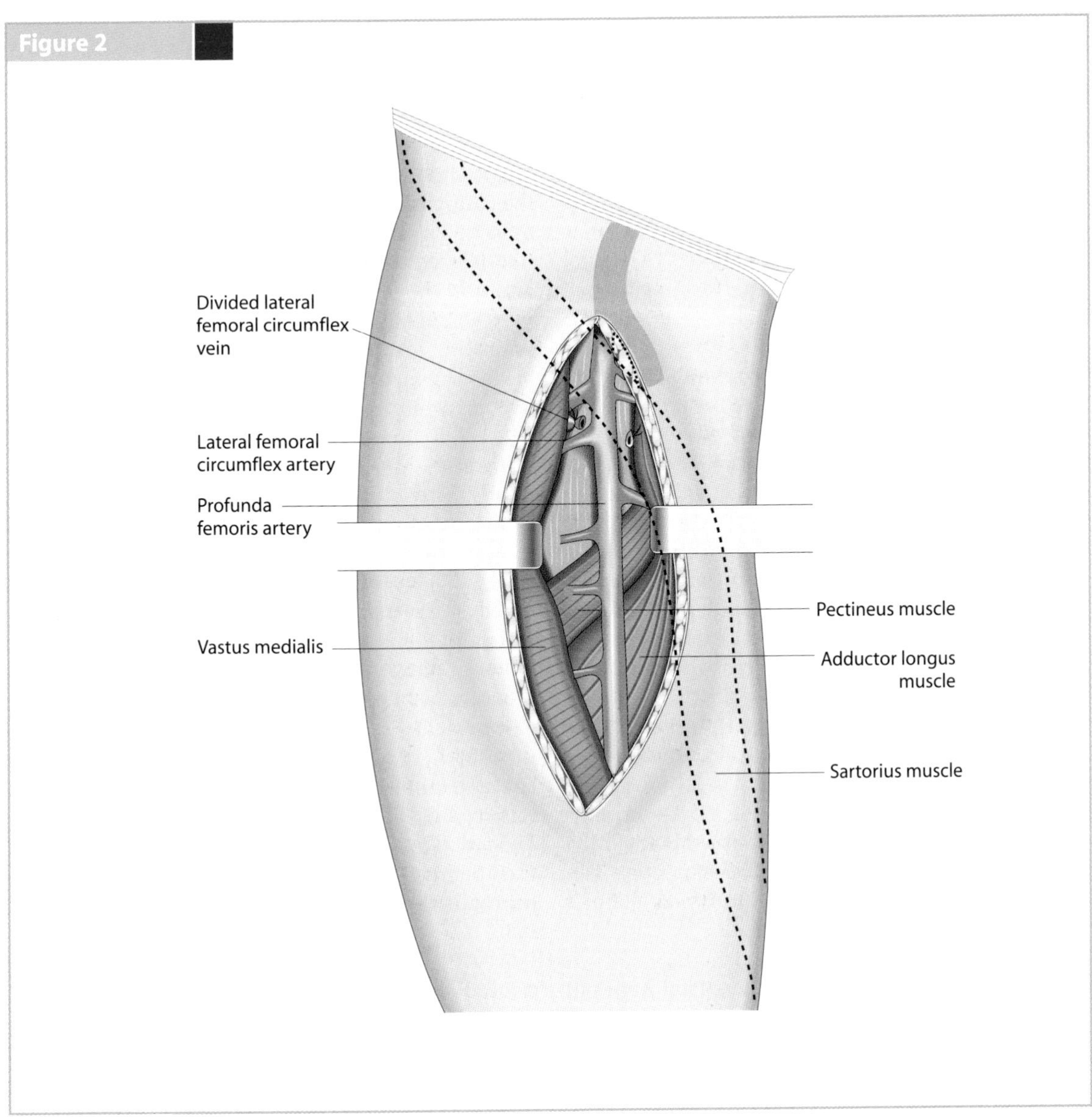
Divided lateral femoral circumflex vein
Lateral femoral circumflex artery
Profunda femoris artery
Vastus medialis
Pectineus muscle
Adductor longus muscle
Sartorius muscle

Figure 3: The Profunda Femoris Artery

The profunda is divided arbitrarily into three zones when describing surgical exposures. The origin to just distal to the lateral femoral circumflex artery is termed the proximal zone. The region from the lateral femoral circumflex artery to the end of the femoral triangle is termed the middle zone. The distal zone usually includes the second perforating branch and begins after the femoral triangle.

■ **Medial Approach to the Proximal Profunda Femoris Artery.** The proximal zone of the profunda femoris artery is typically approached by exposing the common femoral artery distally and dissecting along its lateral and posterior aspect to expose the origin of the profunda femoris artery (see Fig. 1). It is important to dissect the common femoral bifurcation circumferentially to identify any posterior branches originating at that level and avoid unexpected retrograde bleeding from these branches upon creating an arteriotomy. Venous branches cross the profunda femoris shortly after its origin from the common femoral artery. The first large venous branch is usually the lateral femoral circumflex vein, which crosses over the profunda femoris artery to join the more medial superficial femoral vein (Fig. 1). These veins should be divided in order to expose the profunda femoris artery further distally. The dissection can continue distally, following the profunda femoris artery and its branches for 5–8 cm.

■ **Medial Approach to the Mid and Distal Zones of the Profunda Femoris Artery.** The middle and distal zones of the profunda femoris artery can be exposed without exposing the common femoral bifurcation (Nunez et al. 1988). A 10–12 cm skin incision over the medial aspect of the sartorius muscle lower in the thigh allows for exposure of the middle and distal zones of the profunda femoris artery (Nunez et al. 1988). The superficial femoral artery and vein are retracted anteriorly and laterally with the sartorius with minimal dissection. The dissection is then continued posteriorly towards the femur through a longitudinal incision in the fibrous layer between the adductor longus muscle and the vastus medialis muscle. Palpation of the pulse or Doppler localization is used to identify the target profunda femoris artery in this deep location. An accompanying vein may be encountered prior to final exposure of the artery in this region. Dissection and mobilization of the accompanying vein will expose the profunda femoris artery.

■ **Lateral Approach to the Profunda Femoris Artery.** The initial dissection of the profunda femoris artery laterally is identical to that of the approach to the common femoral artery discussed above (Fig. 2). The sartorius muscle is freed on its lateral aspect and retracted medially. The superficial femoral artery lies in a plane posterior and medial to the sartorius muscle. By incising the connective tissue layer that extends from the adductor longus to the vastus medialis, the profunda femoris artery can be exposed in a plane also deep to the sartorius. The lateral femoral circumflex is often first identified in this region, the accompanying vein of which can be divided. The lateral femoral circumflex artery can then be traced proximally to its vessel of origin, the profunda femoris artery (Fig. 2) (Naraysingh et al. 1984).

■ **Medial Approach to the Superficial Femoral Artery in the Upper Thigh.** The superficial femoral artery lies posterior to the sartorius muscle in the upper thigh. The inferior border of the sartorius muscle is approached through a vertical skin incision, with care to avoid the great saphenous vein. Once the muscular fascia is incised exposing the sartorius muscle, the muscle is retracted laterally exposing the underlying superficial femoral artery and vein.

Figure 3

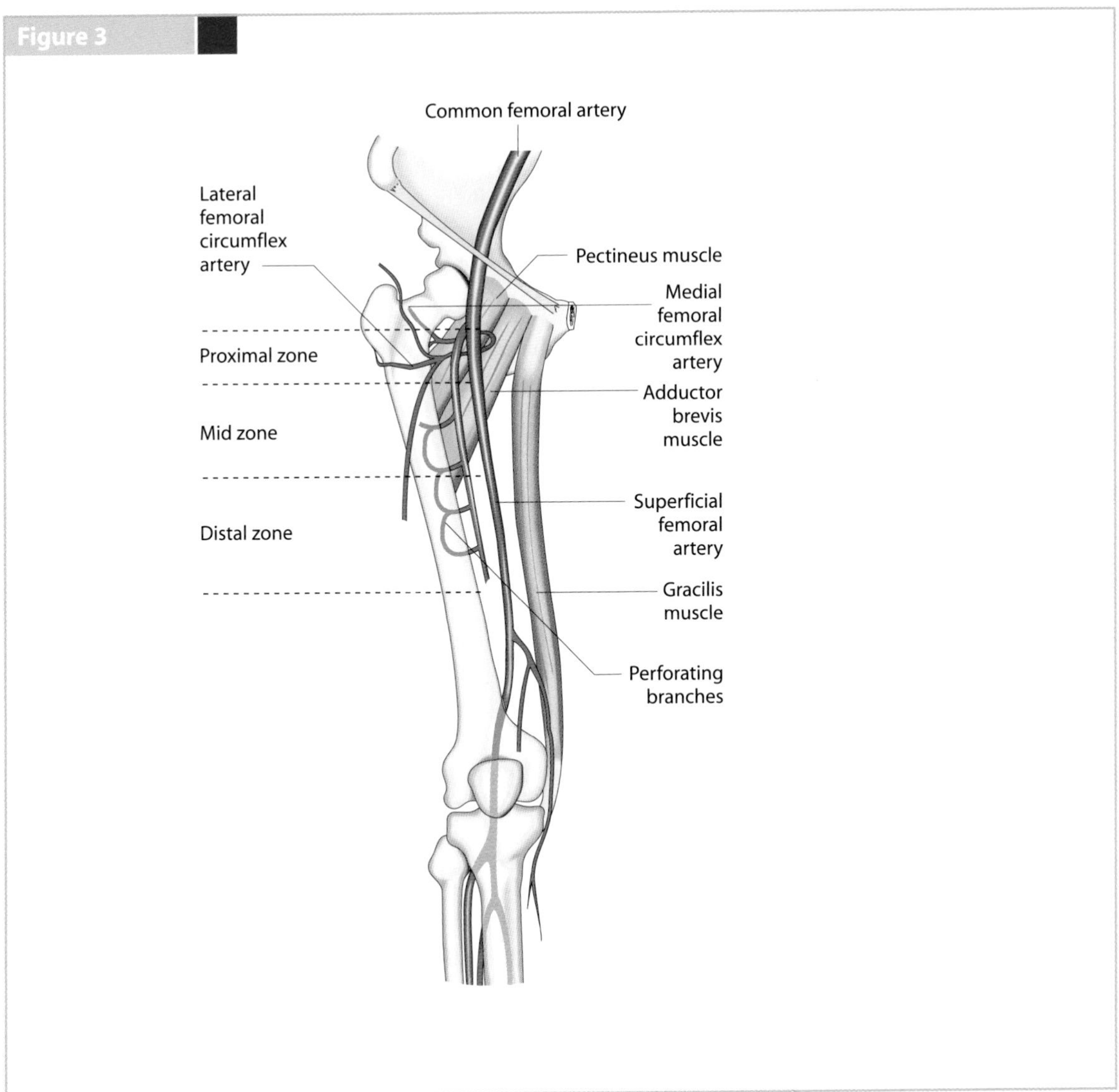
Common femoral artery
Lateral femoral circumflex artery
Pectineus muscle
Medial femoral circumflex artery
Proximal zone
Adductor brevis muscle
Mid zone
Distal zone
Superficial femoral artery
Gracilis muscle
Perforating branches

Figure 4: The Popliteal Artery

■ **Medial Approach to the Suprageniculate Popliteal Artery.** Along the anterior border of the distal sartorius muscle, a longitudinal skin incision is performed from the knee joint to a point 10–12 cm proximal to the knee joint. If the great saphenous vein is being harvested, this incision can be used to access the popliteal artery in its deeper plane. After descending through the subcutaneous tissue, the fascia is incised between the adductor tendon that lies anteriorly and the sartorius muscle that lies posteriorly. Self-retaining retractors are replaced to a deeper plane such that the adductor tendon and sartorius are spread apart exposing the popliteal fossa. A rolled towel under the proximal thigh helps to slightly bend the knee and allow gravity to retract the posterior popliteal fossa from the anterior portion. This improves exposure whereas placing the towel under the knee can hinder it. In patients with atherosclerotic disease, the hard, calcified popliteal artery can be palpated in the popliteal fossa regardless of patency. The proximal extent of exposure from this standard incision is the adductor canal. Near the adductor hiatus, care should be taken to avoid injury to the exiting great saphenous nerve. The nerve runs along an anterior course to the subcutaneous plane to join and parallel the great saphenous vein. The knee joint marks the inferior extent of this exposure.

Figure 5: Lateral Approach to the Suprageniculate Popliteal Artery

An alternate approach to the suprageniculate popliteal artery is via a lateral approach (Hoballah et al. 1996; Padberg 1998; Veith et al. 1987). At a level 1 cm posterior to the iliotibial tract, a 10–12 cm longitudinal incision is made from the knee joint superiorly. The deep fascia is incised allowing for separation of the iliotibial tract and biceps femoris muscles and visualization of the above knee popliteal artery. Proximal exposure with this approach extends to the distal superficial femoral artery by incising the adductor magnus muscle.

Figure 4

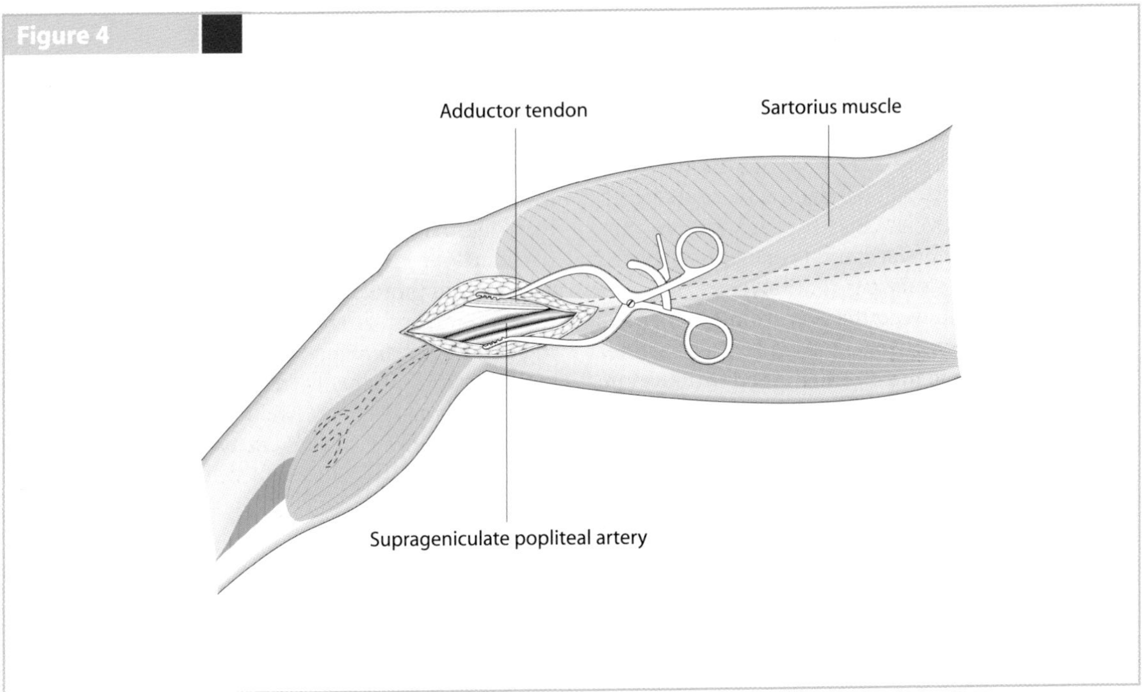
Adductor tendon
Sartorius muscle
Suprageniculate popliteal artery

Figure 5

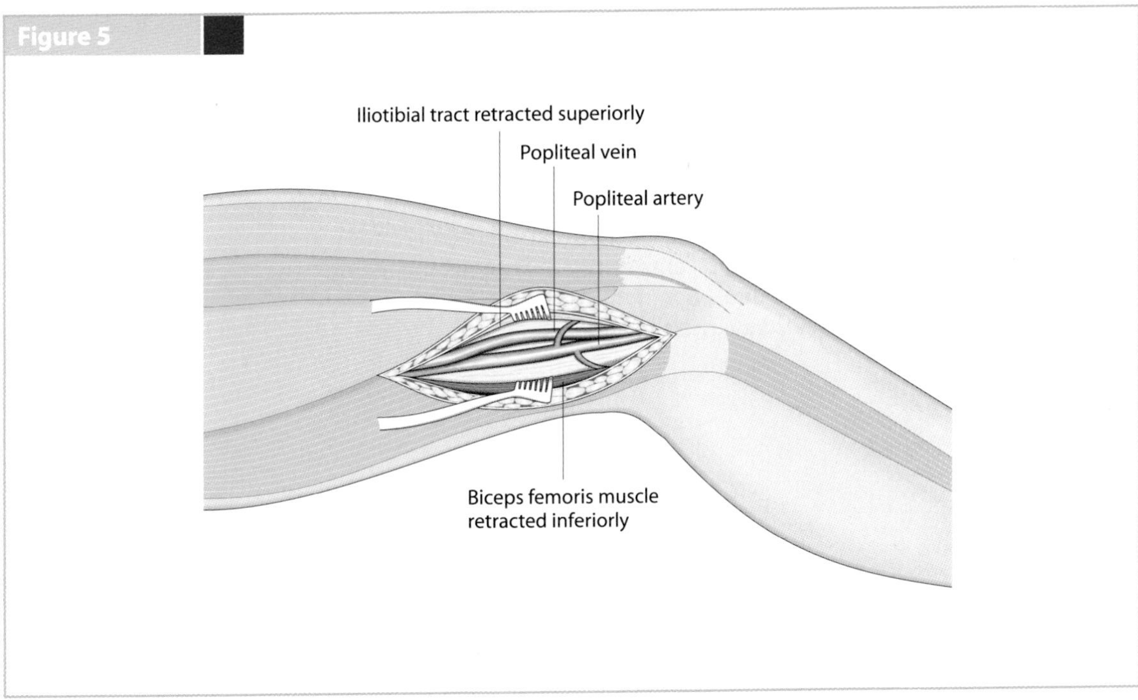
Iliotibial tract retracted superiorly
Popliteal vein
Popliteal artery
Biceps femoris muscle
retracted inferiorly

Figure 6: Medial Approach to the Infrageniculate Popliteal Artery

A 10–12 cm longitudinal skin incision is made from the level of the knee joint distally. The incision is deepened through the subcutaneous tissue to the underlying muscular fascia with care to avoid the greater saphenous vein. Once through the muscular fascia, the fascia is incised and the popliteal space is entered. Using a sweeping motion with the index finger, the space between the posterior gastrocnemius muscle and the anterior soleus muscle is dissected. Self-retaining retractors are positioned with the knee bent slightly to retract the gastrocnemius muscle posteriorly and laterally to better expose the popliteal space. Frequently, the tendons of the semimembranosus and semitendinosus muscles are identified superiorly in the incision and divided to enhance the exposure. The soleus muscle typically overlies the popliteal artery at the level of its trifurcation. The dissection beneath the soleus in the areolar tissue plane identifies the popliteal neurovascular bundle. The popliteal vein lies anterior to the popliteal artery, and often is seen in duplicate surrounding the popliteal artery. Separation of the popliteal vein from the popliteal artery allows encircling of the artery with a silastic vessel loop. Gentle traction on the vessel loop assists in extending the dissection proximally and distally.

Figure 7

Exposure of the proximal crural vessel region at and below the popliteal artery bifurcation typically requires dividing the overlying proximal soleus muscle. A right angle clamp placed underneath the soleus muscle guides the transection of the muscle using electrocautery to both prevent injury to the underlying structures and hold the muscle for controlled transection and hemostasis. As the dissection under the soleus progresses, soleal veins superficially and the anterior tibial vein may be seen crossing the anterior tibial artery. These veins may need to be divided in order to allow for the exposure of the origin of the anterior tibial artery and the origin of the tibioperoneal trunk. The anterior tibial artery can be further exposed for up to 1–2 cm by incising the interosseous membrane and the muscular fibers beneath it.

Figure 6

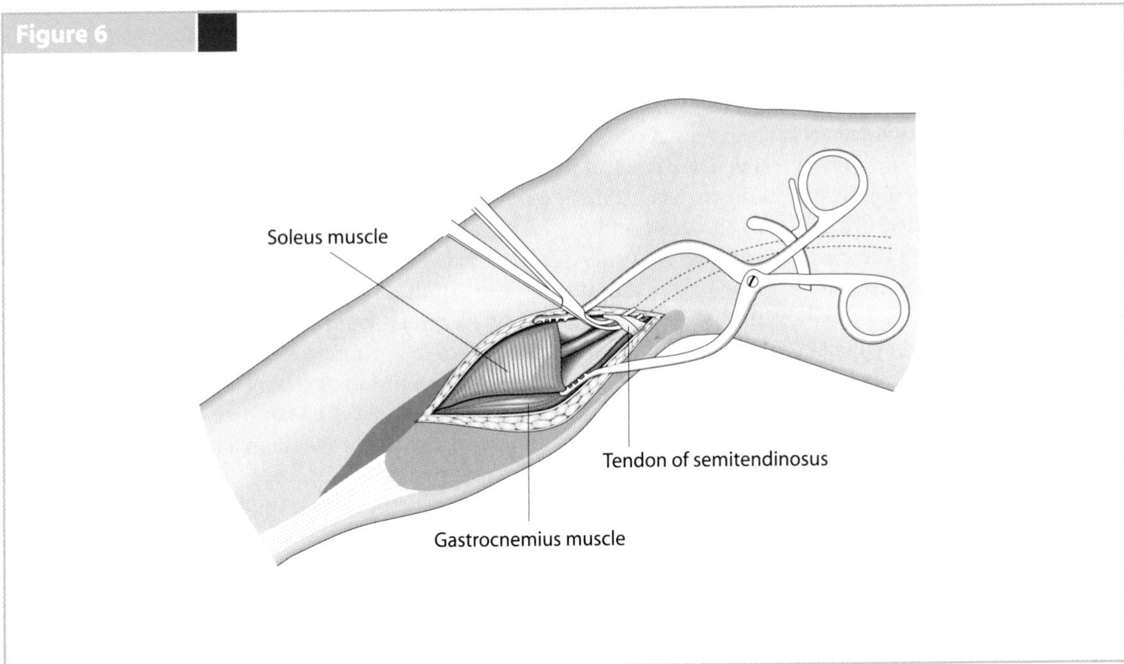
Soleus muscle
Tendon of semitendinosus
Gastrocnemius muscle

Figure 7

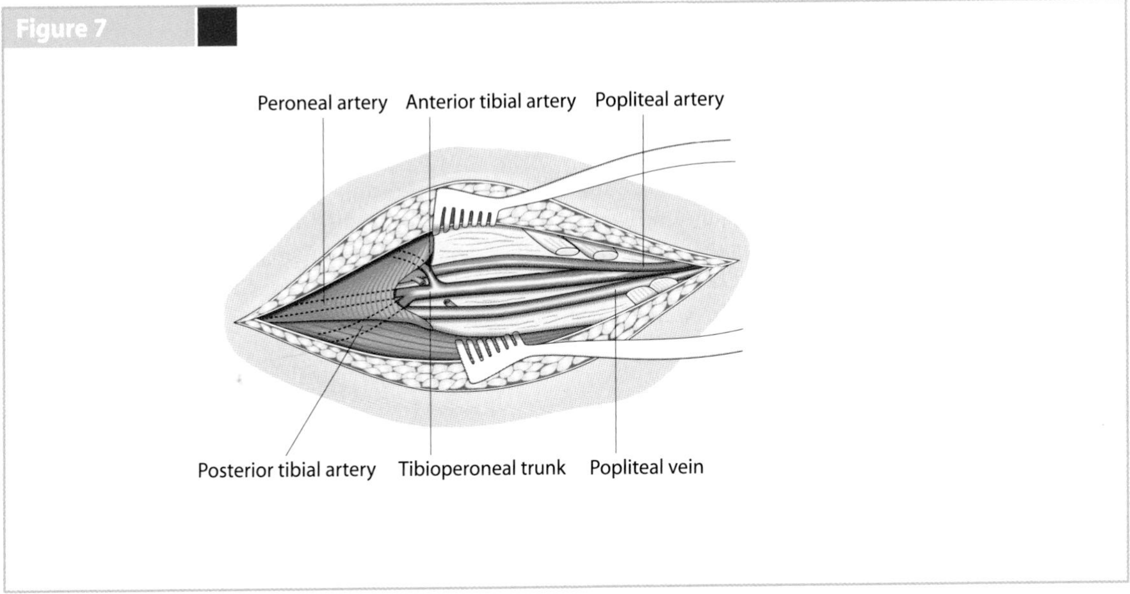
Peroneal artery
Anterior tibial artery
Popliteal artery
Posterior tibial artery
Tibioperoneal trunk
Popliteal vein

Figure 8: Lateral Approach to the Infrageniculate Popliteal Artery

The lateral approach more commonly used to expose the popliteal artery involves resection of the proximal fibula (Danese and Singer 1968; Dardik et al. 1974; Usatoff and Grigg 1997). A 10–12 cm longitudinal incision is extended distally from the head of the fibula (Fig. 8). During the dissection within the subcutaneous tissue the peroneal nerve is identified as it crosses over the neck of the fibula and is gently dissected and mobilized arteriorly. The fibular periosteum is circumferentially exposed, incised and elevated off the fibula. A right angle clamp is carefully passed under the fibula and, using controlled blunt dissection, the posterior fibular attachments can be scraped from the fibula, which is transected approximately 6–8 cm distal to its neck. The proximal segment is lifted with a bone grasper and the attachments of the fibula are further divided. The proximal part of the fibula is removed exposing the popliteal fossa. The popliteal artery can be palpated and dissected; however, the tibial nerve is usually identified by inspection or palpation crossing the below-knee popliteal artery from lateral to medial and is separated from it by the popliteal vein. More distal dissection provides an excellent exposure of the proximal crural vessels. Exposure of the infrageniculate popliteal artery via a lateral approach sparing the proximal fibula has also been described. This exposure is usually more limiting than the proximal fibula resection.

Figure 9: Posterior Approach to the Popliteal Artery

A posterior approach can be used to expose the popliteal artery. Such an approach requires having the patient in a prone position. The incision measures 12–14 cm starting along the medial aspect of the distal thigh, and continuing to the lateral proximal leg in a gentle "S" fashion. The incision is deepened through only the subcutaneous tissues to expose the popliteal fascia. The tibial nerve is usually encountered first and is protected with the common peroneal nerve. Next, the popliteal vein is dissected and retracted, exposing the popliteal artery. This approach provides a good exposure of the perigeniculate popliteal artery. Proximal exposure is limited by the biceps femoris muscle laterally and the hamstring muscles medially. Exposure of the distal part of the popliteal artery is limited by the heads of the gastrocnemius muscle. Retractors placed to spread these muscle groups from midline aid in further proximal and distal exposure. Ultimately, the soleus muscle distally and the limited spread of the hamstrings will limit the extent of this dissection.

Figure 8

Common peroneal nerve
Anterior tibial artery
Venae comitantes
Fibula
Popliteal artery
Tibioperoneal trunk
Popliteal vein

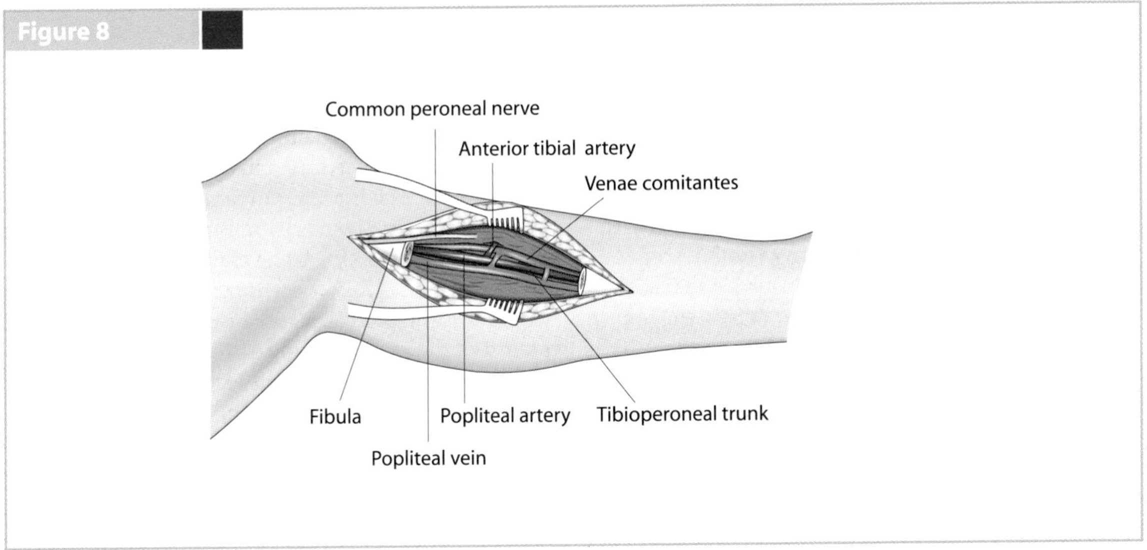

Figure 9

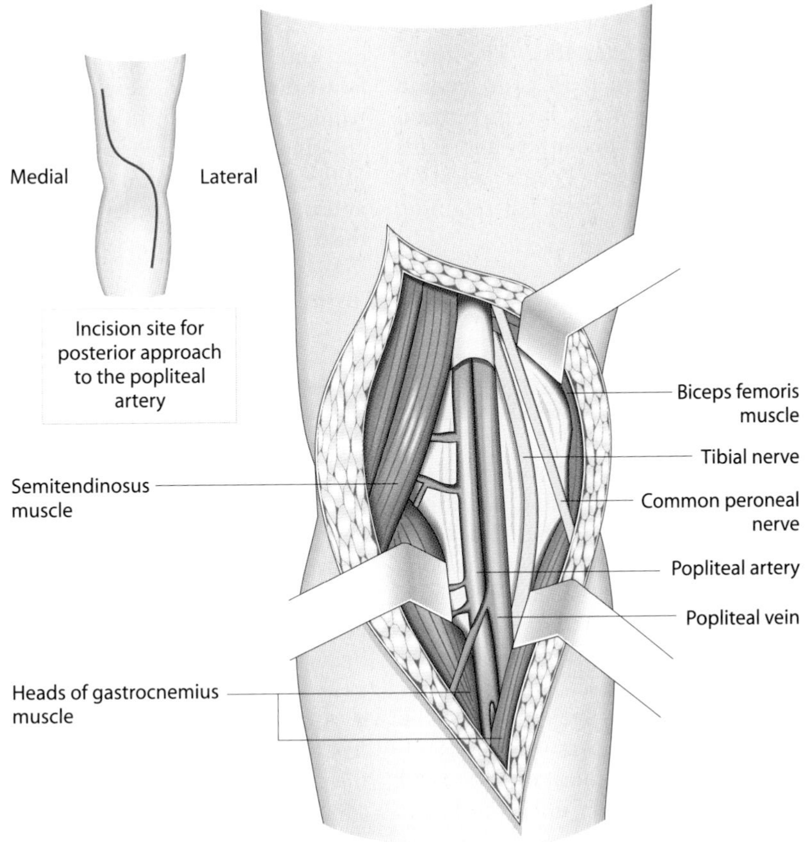

Medial
Lateral
Incision site for posterior approach to the popliteal artery
Semitendinosus muscle
Heads of gastrocnemius muscle
Biceps femoris muscle
Tibial nerve
Common peroneal nerve
Popliteal artery
Popliteal vein

Figure 10: The Anterior Tibial Artery

■ **Medial Approach to the Anterior Tibial Artery.** A lateral approach is typically used for exposure of the anterior tibial artery. However, as mentioned above, the proximal 1–2 cm of the anterior tibial artery can be exposed from a medial approach by exposing the distal popliteal artery and incising the interosseous membrane (Dardik et al. 1985). In order to assist in the exposure of the anterior tibial artery through a medial approach, digital pressure applied to the skin overlying the anterolateral compartment displaces the anterior tibial artery medially. This exposure has limited value due to the anterior tibial artery's depth from this angle.

■ **Lateral Approach to the Anterior Tibial Artery.** The typical approach to the anterior tibial artery starts with a 10–12 cm longitudinal incision parallel to the tibia. The incision starts 2 cm inferior to the tibial plateau and can be extended as needed. The fascia is likewise incised longitudinally. The anterior tibialis muscle is broadly attached to the tibia at its origin and is the first muscle to be seen. Next, the extensor digitorum muscle is identified. The longitudinal cleft between these two muscles is entered using gentle blunt dissection. Deep in this portion of the dissection, the anterior tibial artery and veins and peroneal nerve will be seen. Proper selection and placement of appropriately sized self-retaining retractors will aid in this dissection.

■ **Lateral Approach to the Anterior Tibial Artery in the Lower Leg.** In the lower leg, the anterior tibial artery is more superficial partly due to its position between the tendinous portions of the extensor muscles. An exposing incision is made 10–12 cm long and parallel to the tibia. The tibialis anterior tendon lies close to the tibia, and, inferiorly, the tendon of the extensor hallucis longus muscle can be seen. The tendon of the extensor hallucis longus muscle crosses over and defines the distal extent of the anterior tibial artery as the tendon progresses from lateral to medial to attach on the great toe.

Just above the ankle, the anterior tibial artery is exposed by a short longitudinal incision with retraction of the extensor digitorum longus muscle laterally and the extensor hallucis longus muscle medially.

■ **The Tibioperoneal Trunk: Medial Approach.** The tibioperoneal trunk is exposed by the same approach used to expose the infrageniculate popliteal artery and then extending the dissection distally (Fig. 7). A right angle clamp is placed posterior to the soleus muscle and anterior to the popliteal artery. The soleus muscle is divided longitudinally exposing the tibioperoneal trunk. Care is taken to gently dissect the tibial veins crossing over the tibioperoneal trunk and the origins of the peroneal artery and posterior tibial artery. The anterior tibial and other crossing veins often cover the origin of the tibioperoneal trunk. Dissection distal to these crossing veins avoids the need to encircle and divide these vulnerable structures.

Figure 11: The Posterior Tibial Artery

■ **Approach to the Posterior Tibial Artery in the Upper Leg.** A 10–12 cm longitudinal skin incision is made 2 cm posterior to the edge of the tibia. Once the incision is deepened through the subcutaneous tissue, the anterior fascia of the soleus muscle is exposed. This fascia and the soleus muscle fibers are divided along the length of the incision exposing the posterior fascia of the soleus muscle. The posterior fascia is then incised with care to avoid injury to the underlying vascular bundle (Imparato et al. 1973). After the fascia is incised, inspection at that level will reveal one muscle attached to the tibia: the flexor digitorum longus muscle (FDL). The second muscle posterior to FDL is the flexor hallucis longus muscle (FHL). The posterior tibial artery and veins are usually lying in the groove between the FDL and the FHL muscles. The tibialis posterior muscle will be lateral to the posterior tibial vascular bundle.

The exposure of the posterior tibial artery below the middle of the leg is similar to the more proximal exposure. However, at the lower level of the leg, the soleus muscle is usually attenuated. The posterior tibial artery and veins will be seen between the tendons of the flexor digitorum longus muscle and the flexor hallucis longus muscle.

■ **Approach to the Posterior Tibial Artery at the Ankle.** An 8–10 cm skin incision is performed at the ankle. The incision is deepened through the subcutaneous tissue until the flexor retinaculum is identified. The flexor retinaculum is divided and the posterior tibial artery is identified between the tendons of the flexor digitorum longus and the flexor hallucis longus.

Figure 10

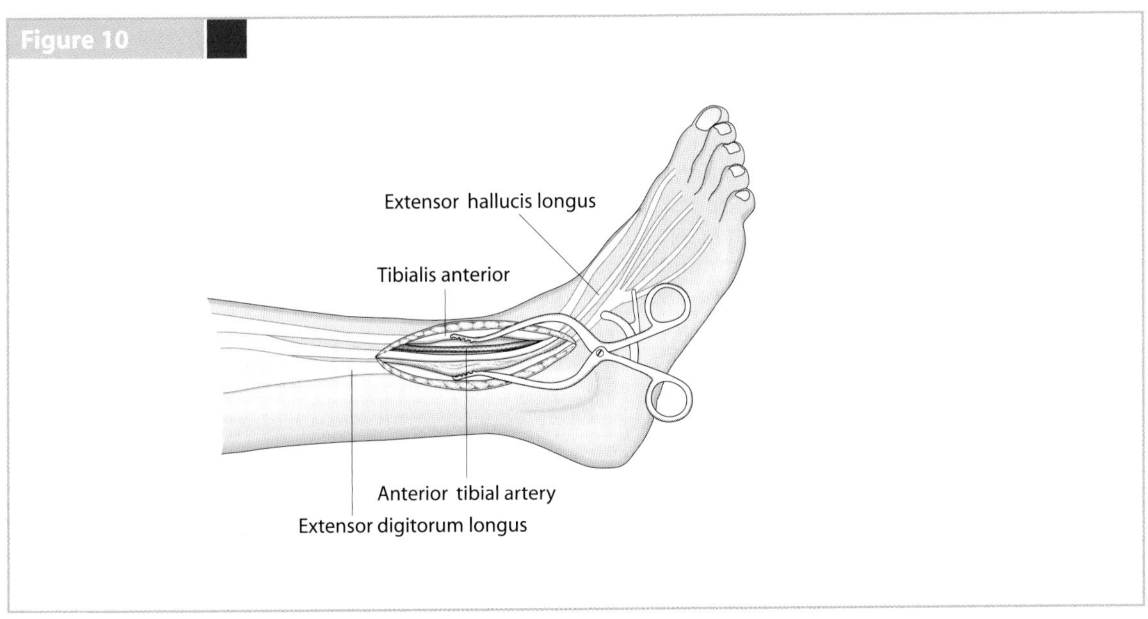

Figure 11

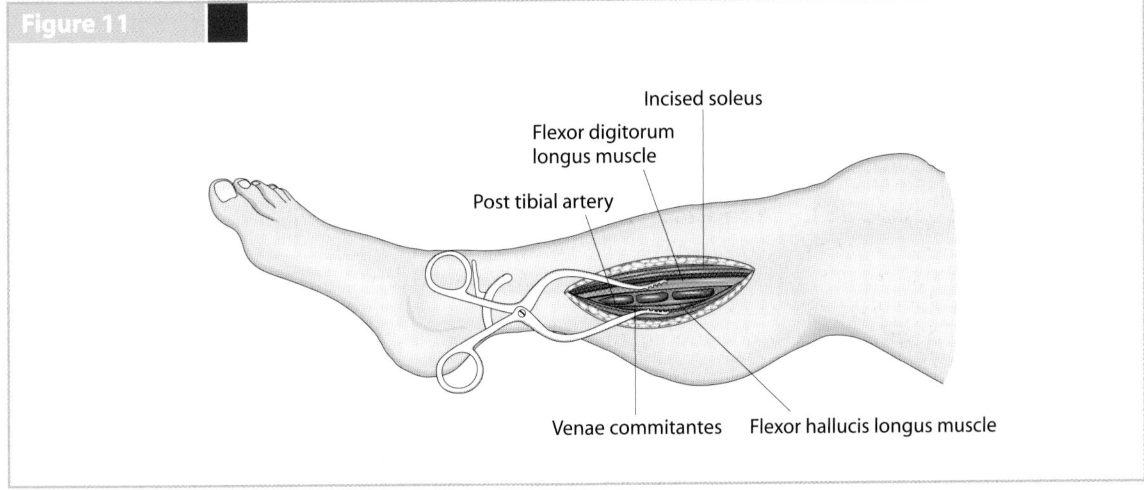

Figure 12: Medial Approach to the Peroneal Artery

The peroneal artery is exposed from a medial incision in the upper leg by initially exposing the posterior tibial neurovascular bundle as described above (Dardik et al. 1979; Minken and May). In the upper leg, the posterior tibial neurovascular bundle can be retracted anteriorly along with the flexor digitorum longus muscle (Fig. 12). In the mid and lower leg, the posterior tibial neurovascular bundle with the flexor hallucis longus muscle can be retracted inferiorly. The dissection is then continued towards the fibula in the intermuscular septum: the tissue plane between the posterior tibialis muscle and the flexor hallucis longus muscle. Deep in the wound, a fascial layer will be identified, incision of which will usually expose the veins surrounding the peroneal artery. Further dissection and mobilization of these veins posteriorly will expose the peroneal artery. This usually requires division of and one or more of these delicate venae comitantes crossing over the peroneal artery.

The exposure of the peroneal artery distally is limited in those with large leg diameters due to obesity or significant musculature. A lateral approach should be considered in these situations.

Figure 13: Lateral Approach to the Peroneal Artery

While the lateral approach to the distal peroneal artery is more superficial, it also requires resection of the distal fibula. This approach to the peroneal is ideal in redo procedures and difficult anatomic situations. An 8–10 cm longitudinal skin incision centered over the distal fibula starts the exposure. If the proximal part of the peroneal artery is also to be exposed, care should be taken to avoid injury to the peroneal nerve as it crosses the neck of the fibula. Once the incision is deepened, the periosteum is elevated circumferentially clearing the fibula of all tissue attachments. A right angle clamp is passed underneath the fibula and one end of a Gigli saw is drawn under the bone. Before transsection of the bone above and below, it is important to completely clear the tissues from the fibula to avoid injury to the underlying peroneal vessels. Under the medial periosteum of the resected fibula lies the peroneal artery and vena comitantes. While somewhat more complicated, this approach allows for excellent exposure of the peroneal artery, including distally, especially in redo operations.

Figure 12

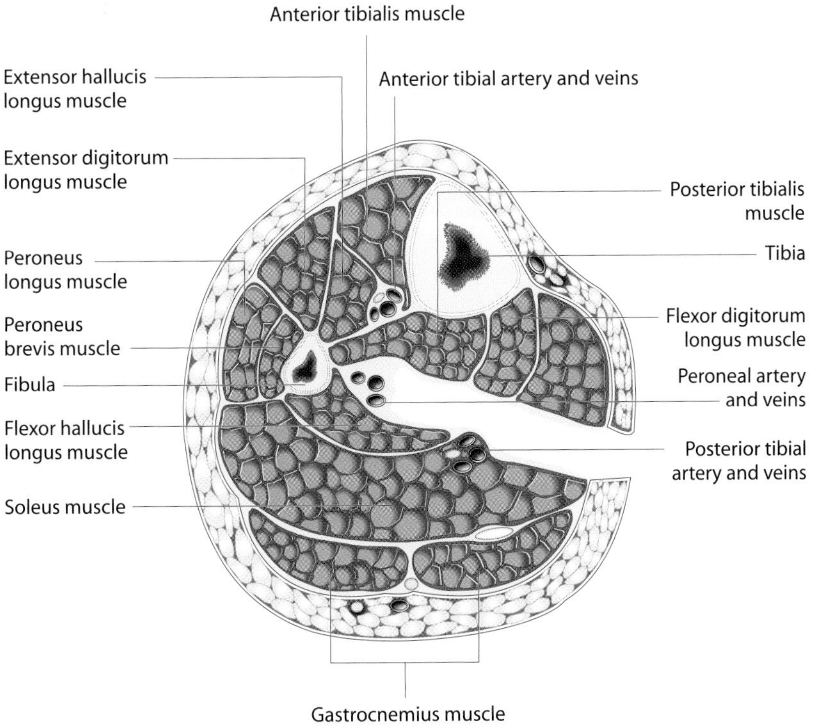

Anterior tibialis muscle
Extensor hallucis longus muscle
Anterior tibial artery and veins
Extensor digitorum longus muscle
Posterior tibialis muscle
Peroneus longus muscle
Tibia
Flexor digitorum longus muscle
Peroneus brevis muscle
Peroneal artery and veins
Fibula
Flexor hallucis longus muscle
Posterior tibial artery and veins
Soleus muscle
Gastrocnemius muscle

Figure 13

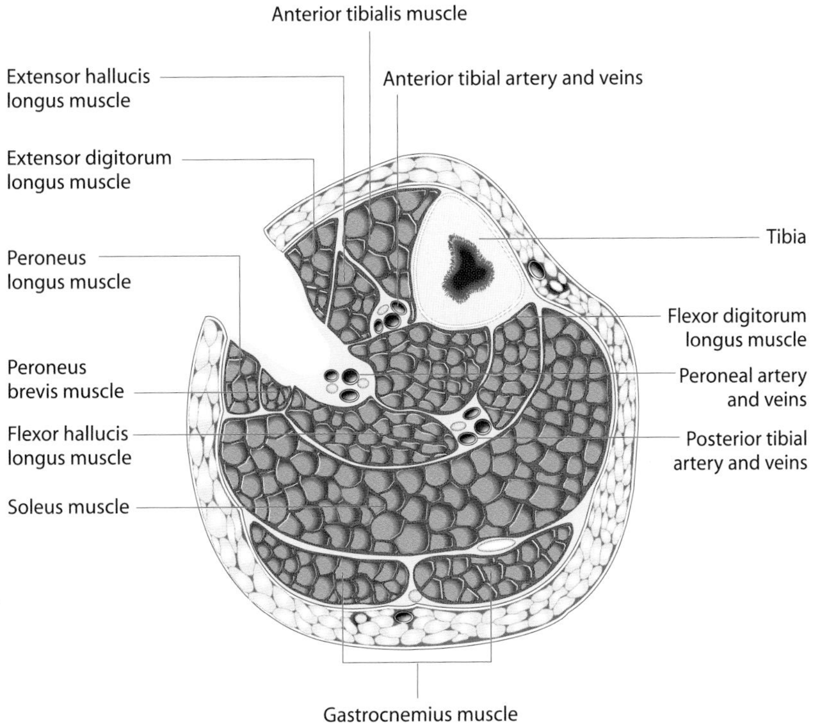

Anterior tibialis muscle
Extensor hallucis longus muscle
Anterior tibial artery and veins
Extensor digitorum longus muscle
Tibia
Peroneus longus muscle
Flexor digitorum longus muscle
Peroneus brevis muscle
Peroneal artery and veins
Flexor hallucis longus muscle
Posterior tibial artery and veins
Soleus muscle
Gastrocnemius muscle

Figure 14: The Plantar Arteries

A 6–8 cm skin incision is performed between the medial malleolus and the calcaneus bone. After deepening the incision through the subcutaneous tissue, the flexor retinaculum is identified. The flexor retinaculum is incised exposing the posterior tibial artery, which is usually surrounded by the tendinous sheath of the flexor digitorum longus superiorly and the flexor hallucis longus inferiorly. The posterior tibial artery is followed distally until it bifurcates into the medial and lateral plantar arteries (Ascer et al. 1985). The lateral plantar artery can be further exposed by dividing the overlying muscles, mainly the abductor hallucis and the flexor digitorum brevis muscles.

Figure 15: The Dorsalis Pedis Artery

Exposure of the dorsalis pedis artery is usually performed through a longitudinal incision placed directly over the vessel. The location of the dorsalis pedis can also be mapped preoperatively using duplex ultrasonography to avoid flap creation. However, some surgeons prefer to create a curved incision placed medial to the vessel and then create a skin flap. This technique is proposed to avoid having the graft and the anastomosis directly under the skin suture line, which can be prone to nonhealing problems that could result in graft exposure at the anastomotic site. The retinaculum is identified and incised exposing the dorsalis pedis artery and its surrounding veins. Alternatively, the dorsalis pedis artery can be exposed beyond the flexor retinaculum in the first metatarsal space.

Figure 14

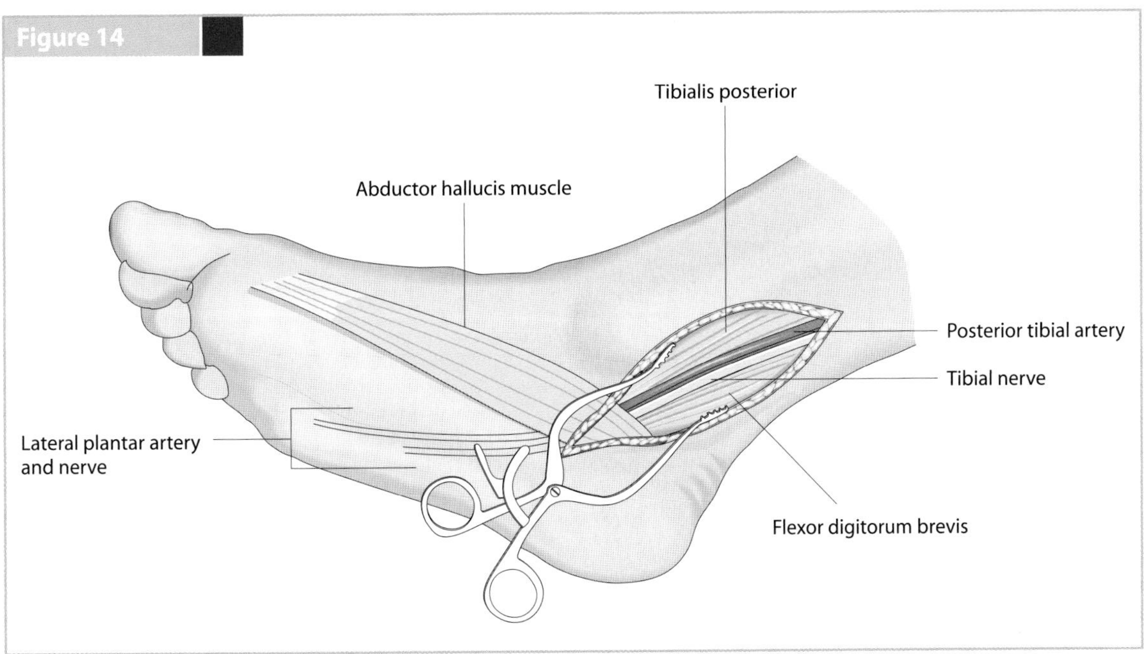

Figure 15

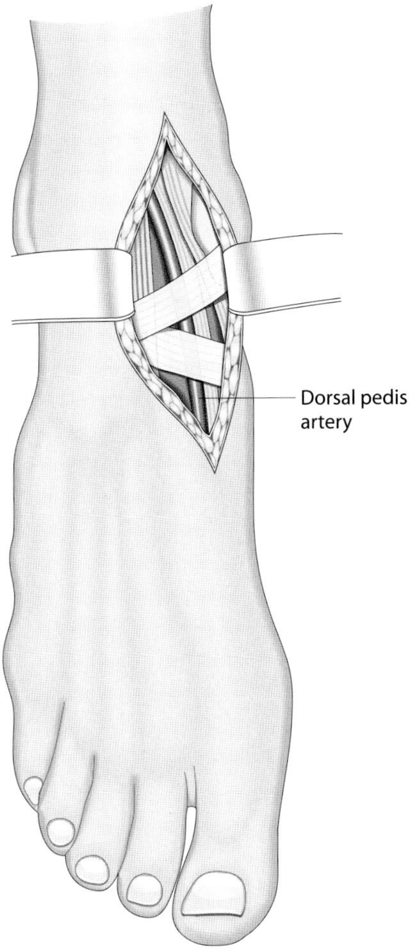

Dorsal pedis artery

CONCLUSION

Experience with the various exposures of the major arteries of the lower extremity and their branches is crucial to successful lower limb revascularization especially in the presence of scarring or infection.

REFERENCES

Ascer E, Veith F, Gupta S (1985) Bypasses to plantar arteries and other tibial branches: An extended approach to limb salvage. J Vasc Surg 8:434

Bridges R, Gewertz BL (1980) Lateral incision for exposure of femoral vessels. Surg Gynecol Obstet 150:733

Danese CA, Singer A (1968) Lateral approach to the trifurcation popliteal artery. Surgery 63:588–590

Dardik H, Dardik I, Veith FJ (1974) Exposure of the tibioperoneal arteries by a single lateral approach. Surgery 75:377–382

Dardik H, Ibrahim IM, Dardik II (1979) The role of the peroneal artery for limb salvage. Ann Surg 189:189–198

Dardik H, Elias S, Miller N et al. (1985) Medial approach to the anterior tibial artery. J Vasc Surg 2:743

Hoballah JJ, Chalmers RT, Sharp WJ et al. (1996) Lateral approach to the popliteal and crural vessels for limb salvage. Cardiovasc Surg 4:165–168

Imparato AM, Kim GE, Chu DS (1973) Surgical exposure for reconstruction of the proximal part of the tibial artery. Surg Gynecol Obstet 136:453–455

Minken SL, May AG (1969) Use of the peroneal artery for revascularization of the lower extremity. Arch Surg 99:594–597

Naraysingh V, Karmody AM, Leather RP, Corson JD (1984) Lateral approach to the profunda femoris artery. Am J Surg 147:813–814

Nunez AA, Veith FJ, Collier P, Ascer E, Flores SW, Gupta SK (1988) Direct approaches to the distal portions of the deep femoral artery for limb salvage. J Vasc Surg 8:576–581

Padberg FT Jr (1998) Lateral approach to the popliteal artery. Ann Vasc Surg 2:397–401

Usatoff V, Grigg M (1997) Letter to the Editor: A lateral approach to the below-knee popliteal artery without resection of the fibula. J Vasc Surg 26:168–170

Veith FJ, Ascer E, Gupta SK, Wengerter KR (1987) Lateral approach to the popliteal artery. J Vasc Surg 6:119–123

CHAPTER 27

Femoral to Above Knee Popliteal Prosthetic Bypass

Jamal J. Hoballah, Christopher T. Bunch, W. John Sharp

INTRODUCTION

Various choices are available when selecting a prosthetic bypass to the above knee popliteal artery. The choices include the material, the size and the external support. Whether to use polytetrafluoroethylene (PTFE), polyester graft or human umbilical vein is a matter of surgeon's preference since none of these grafts has been proven to offer a significant patency advantage over the other. However, the use of larger diameter grafts (8 mm) has been shown to be associated with better patency rates than smaller diameter grafts. Although there is no strong evidence to support using externally supported grafts to the above knee popliteal artery, our preference has been to use 8-mm PTFE ringed grafts to decrease the possibility of kinking during tunneling. Newer PTFE grafts with various features such as carbon lining or heparin coated and specially designed cuffs continue to be introduced into the market. Whether they will provide better patency rates is yet to be proven.

Figure 1: Common Femoral to Above Knee Popliteal Prosthetic Bypass

The patient is placed supine on the operating table. The arms are tucked in or placed at 80°. Normal bony prominences are padded. A Foley catheter is placed under sterile technique. The patient's lower abdomen and both lower extremities are circumferentially prepped and draped in the usual sterile fashion. Preoperative antibiotics are administered prior to skin incision.

■ **Exposure of the Inflow Vessel.** A vertical skin incision overlying the common femoral artery pulse is made. The incision is deepened through the subcutaneous tissues with electrocautery. The encountered lymphatics are ligated and divided. The common femoral artery is then exposed and sharply dissected circumferentially. The dissection is extended proximally to the inguinal ligament and distally to include the superficial femoral and profunda femoris arteries. The common femoral, superficial femoral and profunda femoris arteries are encircled with Silastic vessel loops. Minor branches of the common femoral artery are identified and spared.

■ **Exposure of the Outflow Vessel: Suprageniculate Popliteal Artery.** A 10–12 cm longitudinal skin incision is performed on the medial aspect of the thigh along the anticipated anterior border of the sartorius muscle. The skin incision is deepened through the subcutaneous tissue exposing the adductor tendon anteriorly and the sartorius muscle posteriorly. The fascia between these two muscles is incised and the popliteal fossa entered (Fig. 1). A self retaining retractor is placed deeper in the wound and the popliteal artery is palpated and exposed. A 2-cm segment of the popliteal artery is sharply dissected.

Figure 2: Tunneling

A subfascial or subsartorial tunnel is created using a Zepplin, Kelly-Weck or Gore-Tex tunneler. The tunneler is introduced from the above knee incision starting in a subfascial or subsartorial plane and advanced gently towards the femoral area. The tunneler is guided to exit at the level of the femoral bifurcation.

Figure 1

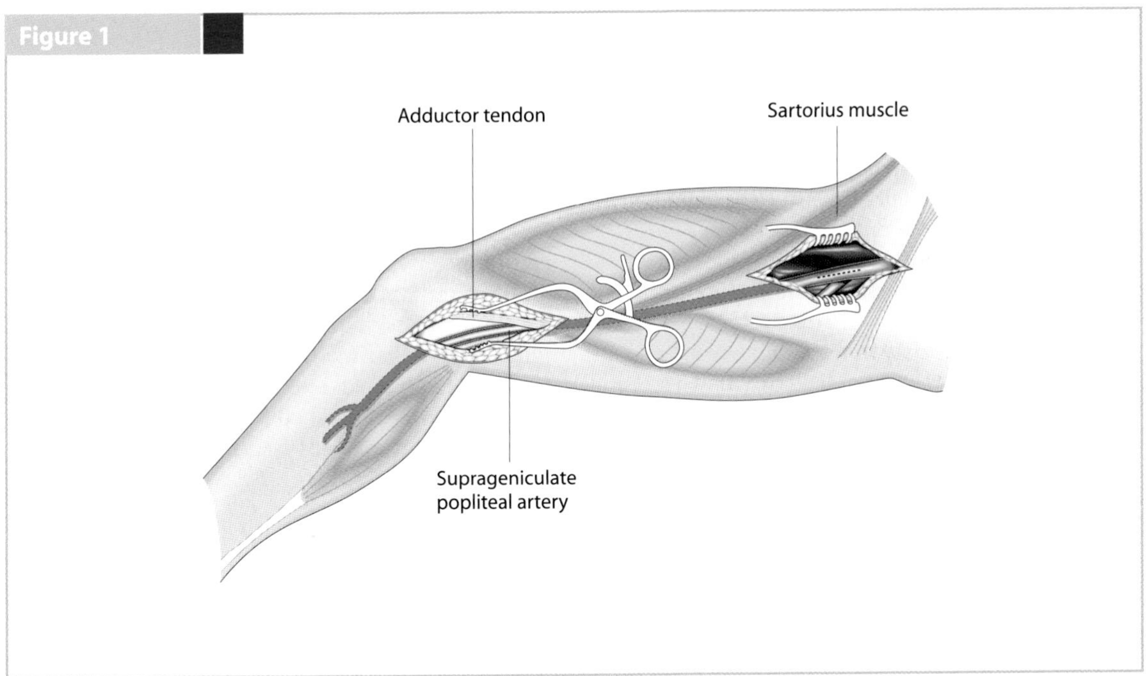

Figure 2

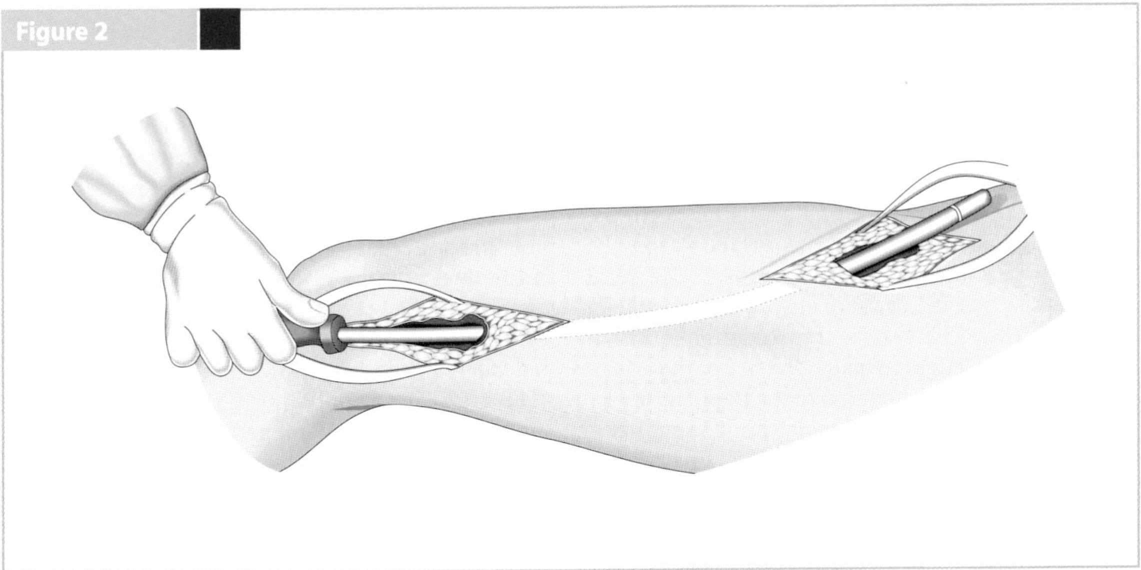

Figure 3: Construction of the Proximal Anastomosis

The PTFE graft is passed through the tunnel avoiding any twists, and 5000 units of heparin are given intravenously and allowed to circulate for approximately 5 min. The common femoral artery is palpated to determine the presence of plaque and the least traumatic way of applying a vascular clamp. The profunda and superficial femoral arteries are occluded by applying Yasargil clips or soft bulldog clamps. A longitudinal arteriotomy in the common femoral artery is performed and extended with Potts scissors for 1 cm. An 8-mm PTFE graft reinforced with rings is used and its end fashioned to match the femoral arteriotomy. The proximal anastomosis is constructed between the PTFE graft and the femoral arteriotomy with a running 5-0 Prolene suture. Prior to completing the suture line, a Fogarty clamp is applied on the PTFE graft just distal to the proximal anastomosis. Backbleeding of the profunda and superficial femoral arteries and forward flushing of the common femoral artery is performed. The lumen of the anastomosis and the common femoral artery are irrigated with heparinized saline solution. The anastomosis is completed and checked for hemostasis. Needle hole bleeding is controlled with the application of Gelfoam soaked with thrombin.

Figure 4A, B: Construction of the Distal Anastomosis

Atraumatic vascular clamps/bulldogs/Yasargil clips or vessel loops are placed proximally and distally on the dissected popliteal artery. A 1-cm arteriotomy is created in the medial wall of the popliteal artery. Occasionally the popliteal artery is heavily calcified and complete transaction of the popliteal artery with the construction of an end-to-end anastomosis may be necessary to construct the anastomosis. The graft alignment is checked again to ensure the absence of any twist. The PTFE graft is transected obliquely at the appropriate length to match the size of the arteriotomy. The distal anastomosis to the popliteal artery is constructed with a running 5/6-0 Prolene suture. A parachute technique may facilitate the construction of the anastomosis especially if the popliteal artery is deep in the wound. Prior to completing the suture line, backbleeding, forward flushing and irrigation of the anastomosis with heparinized solution is performed. The anastomosis is then completed and checked for hemostasis. A 20G angiocatheter may be introduced into the PTFE graft near the proximal anastomosis and an intraoperative arteriogram is performed. The angiocatheter is removed and its puncture site repaired with a 6-0 Prolene suture. The suture lines and the wounds are then rechecked for hemostasis. The pedal vessels are then checked for the presence of palpable pulses or Doppler signals that augment with compressing and releasing the PTFE graft. The wounds are all irrigated with antibiotic solution. The subcutaneous tissue in the groin wound is closed in two layers of 3-0 Vicryl suture. The fascia overlying the sartorius muscle is approximated with 3-0 Vicryl suture. The skin is closed with staples.

Figure 3

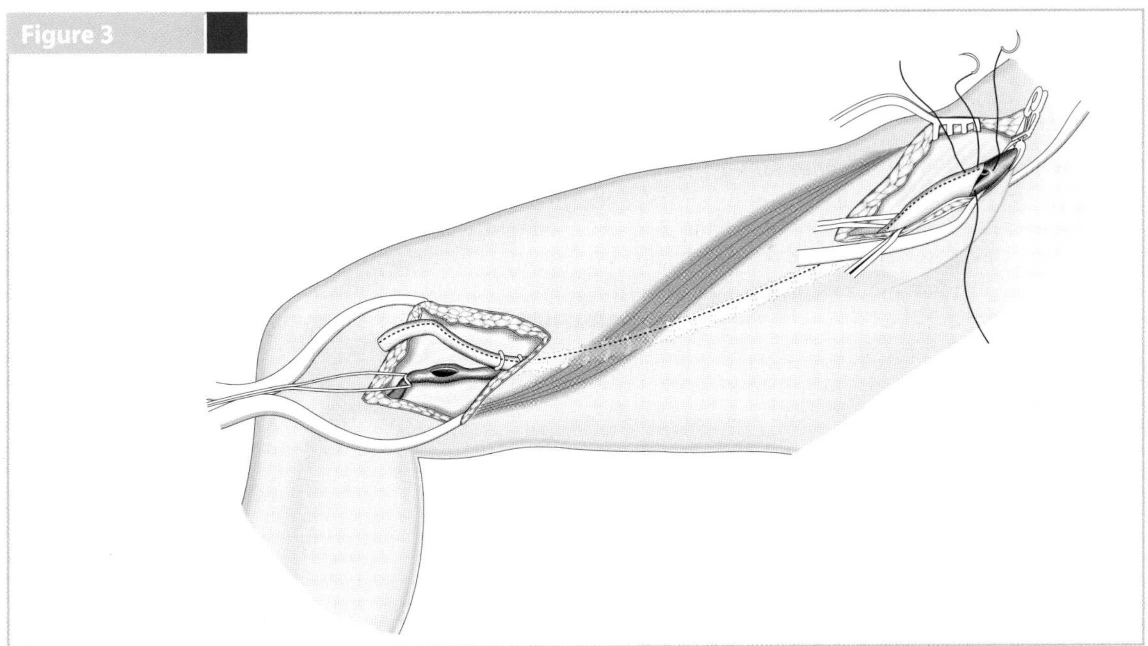

Figure 4A

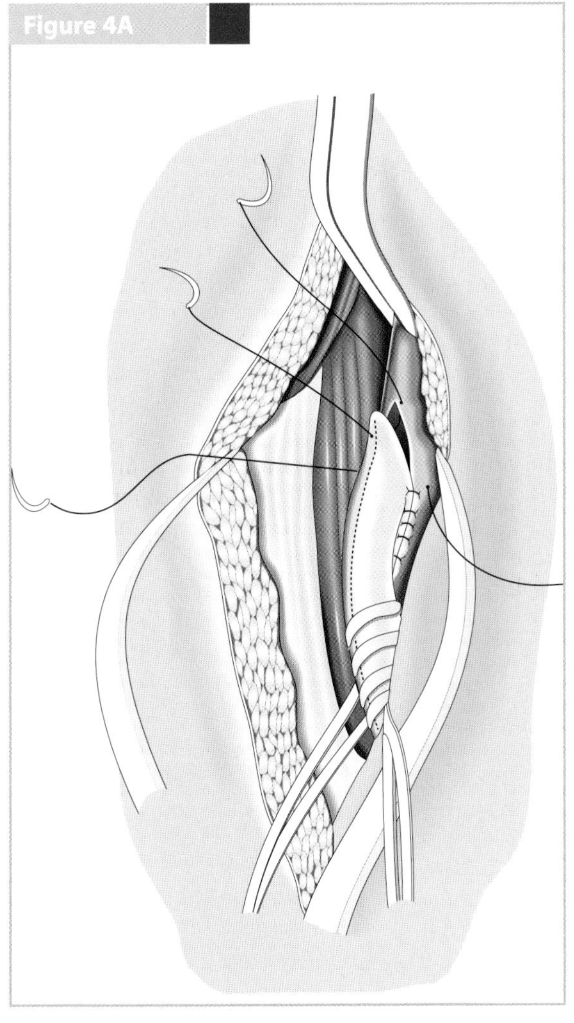

Figure 4B

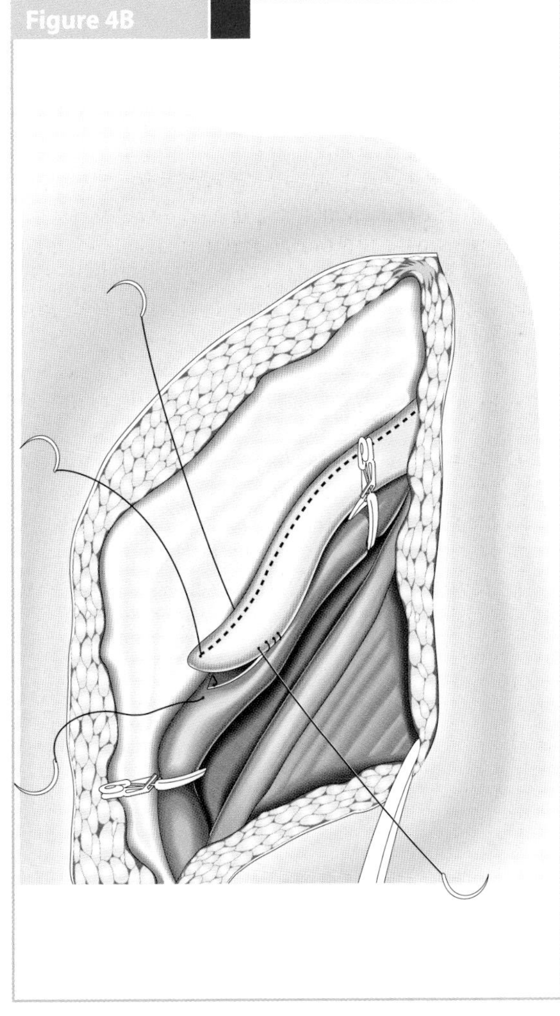

CONCLUSION

The primary patency rate of prosthetic above knee femoropopliteal bypasses is approximately 80% at 1 year and 60% at 4 years. The secondary patency rate increases to 90% at 1 year and 70–80% at 4 years. The value of postoperative color duplex surveillance in improving the patency rate of prosthetic grafts remains debatable. Although duplex surveillance can identify failing grafts, a large portion of these prosthetic bypasses fail despite having no abnormality identified on their last duplex surveillance. All patients should be placed on antiplatelet therapy. Routine anticoagulation with coumadin has not been proven to be advantageous and is recommended only in patients with known or suspected hypercoagulable states.

CHAPTER 28

Femoral to Below Knee Popliteal Bypass with Reversed Great Saphenous Vein

Jamal J. Hoballah, Christopher T. Bunch, W. John Sharp

INTRODUCTION

The patient is placed supine on the operating table. The arms are placed at 80°. Normal bony prominences are padded. After placement of the appropriate line and induction of anesthesia, a Foley catheter is placed under sterile technique. The patient's lower abdomen and both lower extremities are circumferentially prepped and draped. The great saphenous vein has been assessed preoperatively by duplex ultrasound and its location mapped with ink. Preoperative antibiotics are administered prior to skin incision.

Figure 1: Inflow Vessel Exposure

A vertical curvilinear skin incision overlying the common femoral artery is made extending down the upper medial thigh along the preoperatively mapped great saphenous vein. The incision is deepened through the subcutaneous tissues with electrocautery. The encountered lymphatics are ligated and divided. The common femoral artery is then exposed and sharply dissected circumferentially. The dissection is extended proximally to the inguinal ligament and distally to include the superficial femoral and profunda femoris arteries. The common femoral, superficial femoral and profunda femoris arteries are encircled with Silastic vessel loops. Minor branches of the common femoral artery are identified and spared.

■ **Great Saphenous Vein Exposure.** The great saphenous vein is identified. The vein is exposed from the saphenofemoral junction to the mid/lower leg through one continuous incision or through multiple incisions separated by skin bridges. The vein may also be dissected and harvested endoscopically. A side branch in the most distal aspect of the vein is identified. A blunt needle is inserted into that branch to allow for infusion of a dextran-heparin-papaverine solution into the saphenous vein during its mobilization. The great saphenous vein is then fully mobilized and its tributaries ligated with 3-0 silk ties.

■ **Target Vessel Exposure: Infrageniculate Popliteal Artery.** A 10–12 cm longitudinal incision is performed through the bed of the mobilized great saphenous vein below the knee 1–2 cm posteromedial and parallel to the tibia exposing the fascia. The fascia is incised and the popliteal space is entered. A self retaining retractor is applied retracting the gastrocnemius muscle posteriorly and laterally. The tendons of the semimembranosus and semitendinosus muscles are encountered in the most proximal part of the incision and often need to be divided to further facilitate the exposure. The popliteal vein is identified. The popliteal vein is mobilized posteriorly exposing the popliteal artery. A 2-cm segment of the popliteal artery is sharply dissected circumferentially. The infrageniculate popliteal artery is often sandwiched between the main popliteal vein and a deeper smaller duplicate popliteal vein. The popliteal artery is assessed for the construction of the distal anastomosis.

Figure 2: Tunneling

A 5-cm longitudinal incision is performed on the medial aspect of the thigh along the anticipated anterior border of the sartorius muscle through the bed of the saphenous vein in the subcutaneous tissue exposing the adductor tendon anteriorly and the sartorius muscle posteriorly. The fascia between these two muscles is incised and the above knee popliteal fossa entered. A tunnel is created bluntly between the heads of the gastrocnemius muscle connecting the infrageniculate popliteal space with the suprageniculate popliteal space. A subsartorial or subfascial tunnel is created between the suprageniculate popliteal artery and the femoral artery using a Zepplin, Kelly-Wick or Gore-Tex tunneler.

Figure 1

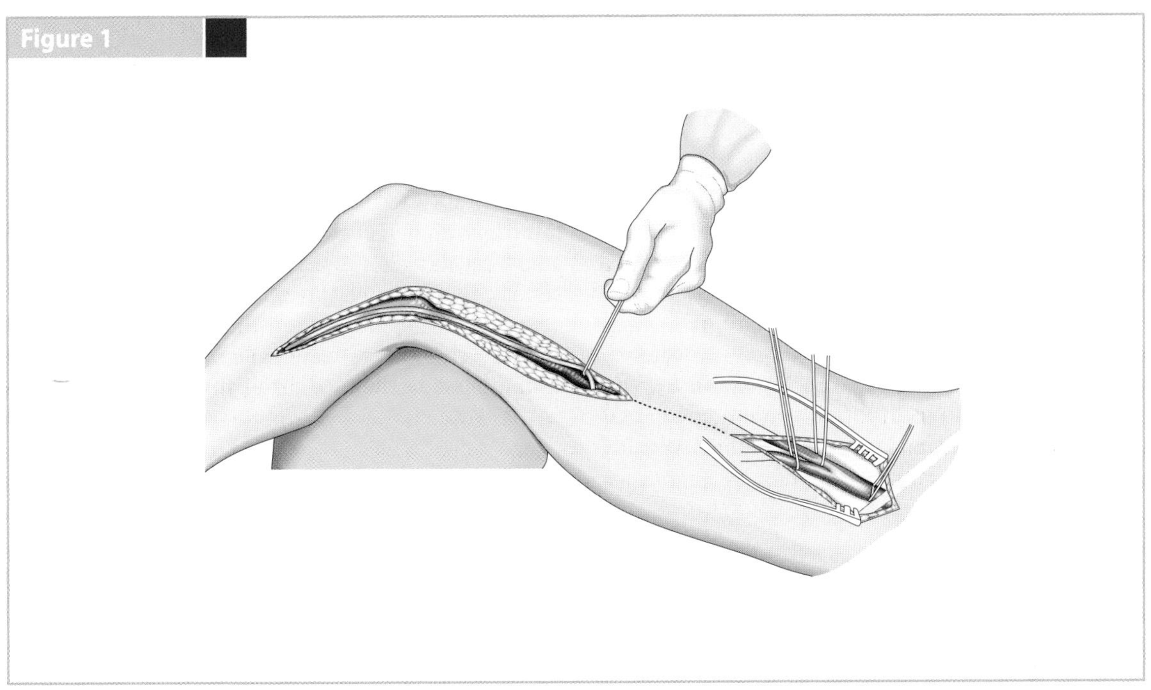

Figure 2

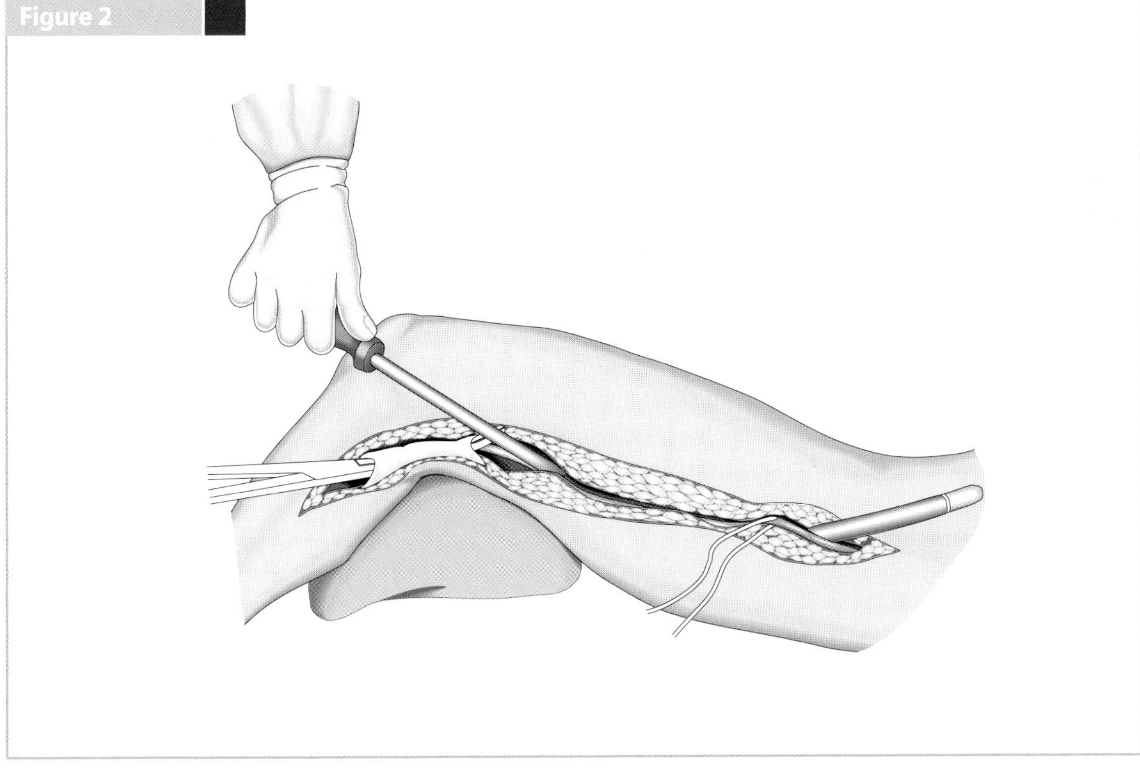

Figure 3: Construction of the Proximal Anastomosis

Five thousand units of heparin are given intravenously. The saphenous vein is transected at the saphenofemoral junction and its stump suture ligated with 2-0 silk suture. The distal end is double ligated and transected. The common femoral artery, profunda, and superficial femoral artery are clamped. A longitudinal arteriotomy in the common femoral artery is performed and extended with Potts scissors for 1 cm. The vein is then reversed and its distal end is incised along its posterior wall. If possible the venotomy is created to incorporate a side branch creating a T-junction shape. The proximal anastomosis is constructed between the spatulated vein and the femoral arteriotomy with a running 5-0/6-0 Prolene suture. Prior to completing the suture line, backbleeding, forward flushing and irrigation of the anastomosis with heparinized solution is performed. The anastomosis is completed and checked for hemostasis. The flow through the vein is checked to ensure its pulsatility. The end of the vein is ligated with a 2-0 silk tie. The vein is rechecked for hemostasis. The vein is passed distended through the tunnel avoiding any twists.

Figure 4, 5: Construction of the Distal Anastomosis

Atraumatic vascular clamps/bulldogs/Yasargil clips are placed proximally and distally on the dissected or vessel loops popliteal artery. A 1-cm arteriotomy is created in the anterior wall of the popliteal artery. Occasionally the popliteal artery is heavily calcified and complete transaction of the popliteal artery with the construction of an end-to-end anastomosis may be necessary to construct the anastomosis. The graft alignment is checked again to ensure the absence of any twist. The vein is transected at the appropriate length and spatulated along its posterior wall to match the size of the arteriotomy. The distal anastomosis to the popliteal artery is constructed with a running 5/6-0 Prolene suture. A parachute technique may facilitate the construction of the anastomosis especially if the popliteal artery is deep in the wound. Prior to completing the suture line, backbleeding, forward flushing and irrigation of the anastomosis with heparinized solution is performed. The anastomosis is then completed and checked for hemostasis. A 20G angiocatheter may be introduced into the vein near the proximal anastomosis and an intraoperative arteriogram performed. The angiocatheter is removed and its puncture site repaired with a 6-0 Prolene suture. The suture lines and the wounds are then rechecked for hemostasis. The pedal vessels are then checked for the presence of palpable pulses or Doppler signals that augment with compressing and releasing the vein graft. The wounds are all irrigated with antibiotic solution. The subcutaneous tissue in the groin wound is closed in two layers of 3-0 Vicryl suture. The fascia overlying the sartorius muscle and the fascia below the knee are approximated with 3-0 Vicryl suture. The skin is closed with staples.

Figure 3

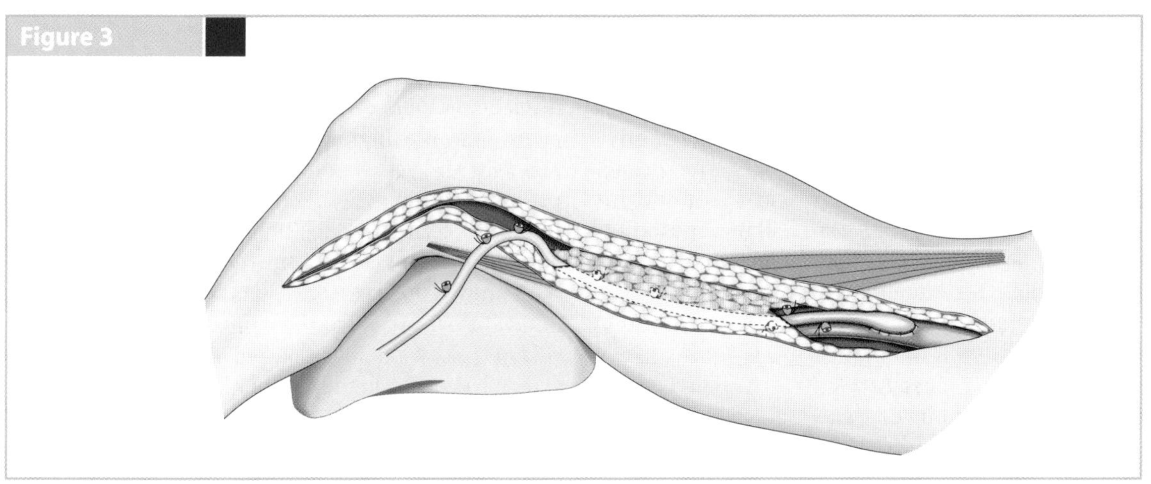

Figure 4

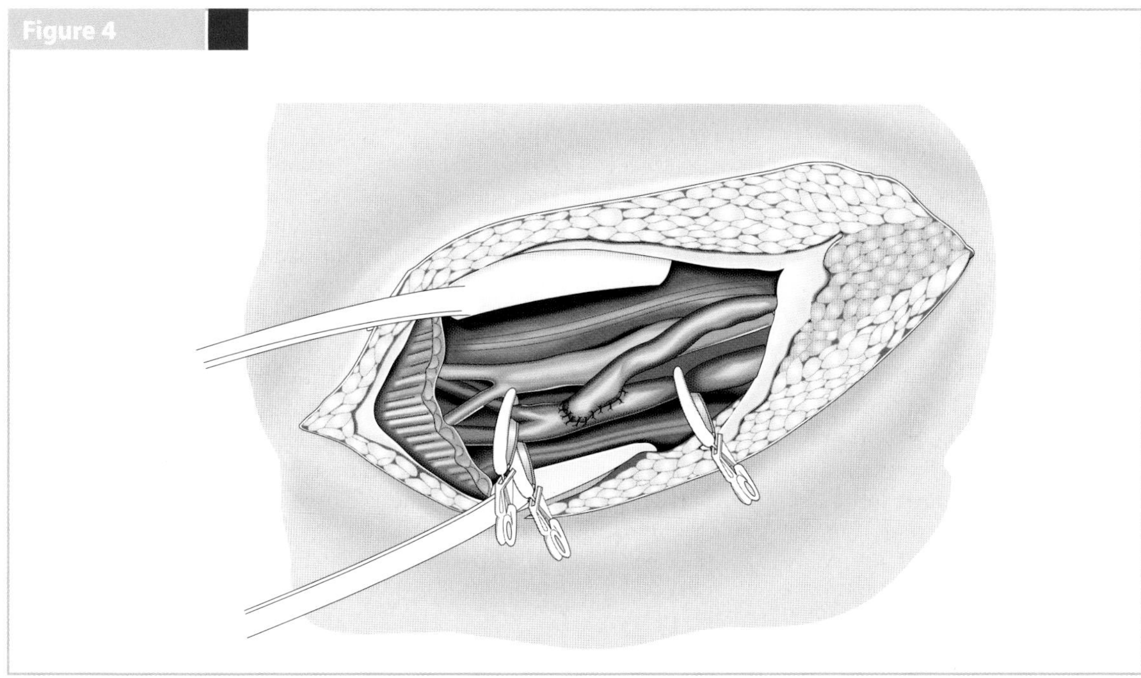

Figure 5

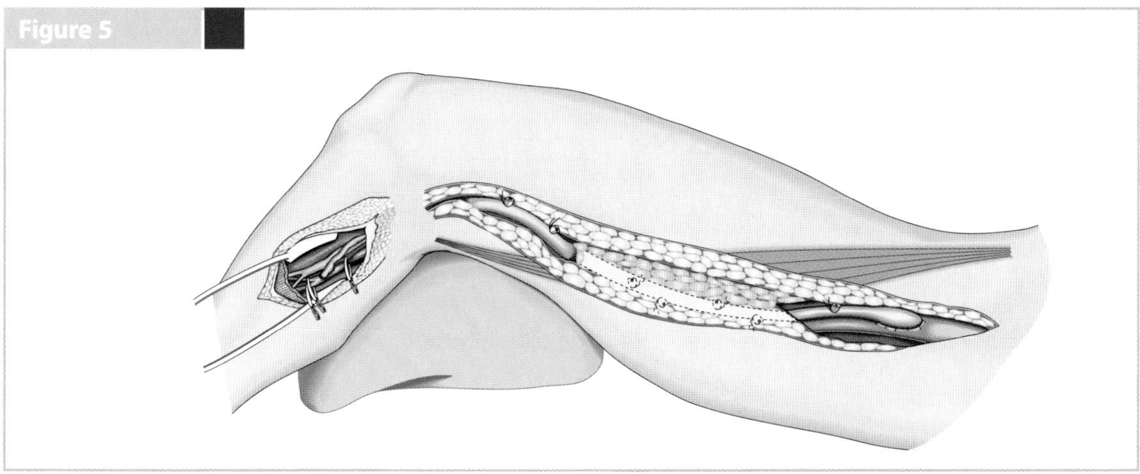

CONCLUSION

The primary patency rate of reversed saphenous vein below knee femoropopliteal bypasses is approximately 85% at 1 year and 75% at 4 years. The secondary patency rate increases to 95% at 1 year and 70–80% at 4 years. Postoperative surveillance is essential to identify failing bypasses that can be salvaged prior to occlusion. Our surveillance protocol consists of physical examination, ankle brachial index and color duplex surveillance at 1 month postoperatively then every 3 months in the 1st year, every 6 months in the 2nd year and yearly thereafter. All patients should be placed on antiplatelet therapy. Routine anticoagulation with coumadin has not been proven to be advantageous and is recommended only in patients with known or suspected hypercoagulable states.

CHAPTER 29

Femoral to Posterior Tibial/Peroneal Artery In Situ Bypass

Jamal J. Hoballah, Christopher T. Bunch, W. John Sharp

INTRODUCTION

The hallmark of in situ bypasses is to leave the vein in its bed, in situ, to minimize the damage and ischemia that can occur during vein harvesting. Furthermore it provides for a better size match between the bypass and the target infrapopliteal vessels. The disadvantages include the risk of trauma from the valvulotomy and a higher incidence of wound complications. Wound complications increase the vulnerability of the vein bypass to thrombosis, desiccation and disruption if it becomes exposed. Various methods have been devised to construct an in situ bypass. Similarly various valvulotomes are available to disrupt the valves, and various techniques are available to occlude the venous branches which if left alone can progress to become arteriovenous fistulae.

The procedure described here is the preferred method used at the University of Iowa. This method involves exposing the entire vein, arterializing the vein, using the retrograde Mills valvulotome to disrupt the valves under direct vision and constructing the distal anastomosis.

The patient is placed supine on the operating table. The arms are placed at 80°. Normal bony prominences are padded. The anesthesia team places the appropriate lines, and regional/general anesthesia is induced. A Foley catheter is placed under sterile technique. The patient's lower abdomen and both lower extremities are circumferentially prepped and draped in the usual sterile fashion. Preoperative antibiotics are administered prior to skin incision.

Figure 1: Exposure of the Target Vessel

Our preference is to start by exposing the target vessel as this will help determine the length of vein needed and any modifications in the selection of the site of the proximal anastomosis. A 10–12 cm vertical skin incision is performed overlying the preoperatively mapped greater saphenous vein at the level chosen for the construction of the distal anastomosis. The saphenous vein is identified and protected. The incision is deepened through the subcutaneous tissue exposing the underlying fascia. The fascia is incised exposing the soleus muscle. The soleus muscle is incised with the electrocautery along its attachment down to its posterior deep fascia. This fascia is incised exposing the flexor muscles. Gentle blunt dissection between these two muscles is performed and a self retaining retractor is placed deeper in the wound exposing the posterior tibial artery and veins. If the target vessel is the peroneal artery, the posterior tibial vascular bundle is then retracted anteriorly and the dissection continued toward the fibula along the intermuscular septum exposing the peroneal vessels. The peroneal vein is identified and mobilized exposing the peroneal artery. A 2-cm segment of the peroneal artery is sharply dissected. Crossing venae comitantes are ligated and divided. Attention is then directed to the groin.

Figure 2: Exposure of the Great Saphenous Vein

A vertical curvilinear skin incision is started overlying the right common femoral artery. The incision is extended down the upper medial thigh along the preoperatively mapped great saphenous vein. The great saphenous vein is identified and traced towards the saphenofemoral junction. The saphenofemoral junction and an adjacent 5-cm segment of the saphenous vein are circumferentially dissected. Venous branches originating from this segment are isolated and divided. The anterior aspect of the saphenous vein is then exposed from the saphenofemoral junction to the lower leg through one continuous incision. If the vein is very small and prone to spasm, the vein is exposed for short segments at a time.

Figure 1

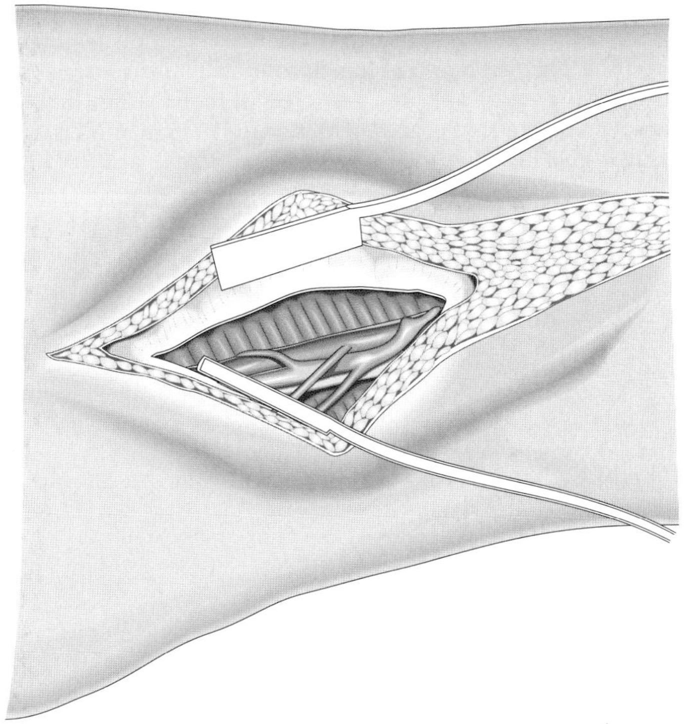

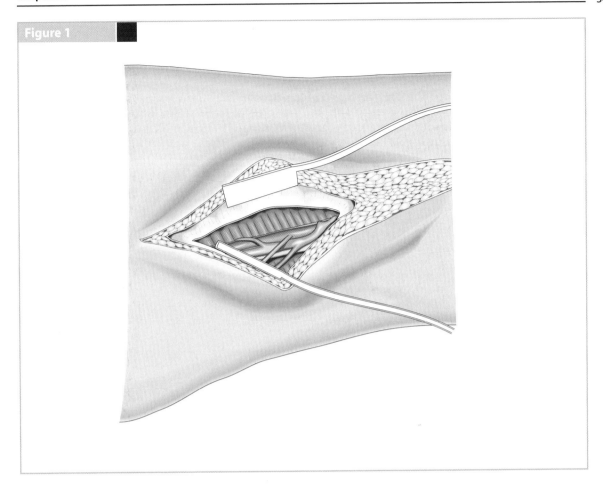

Figure 2

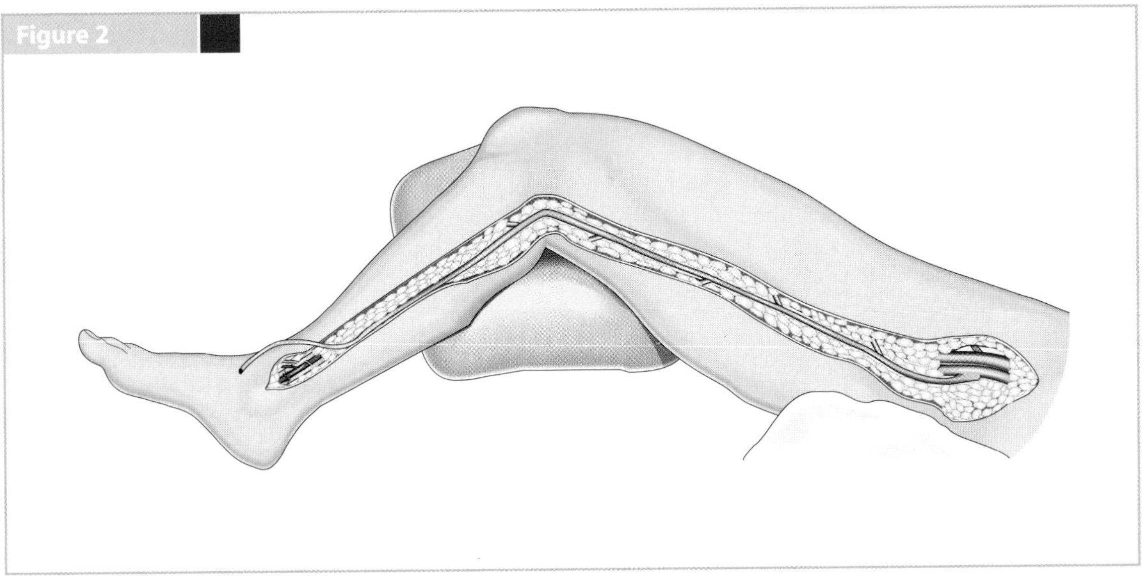

Figure 3: Exposure of the Donor Vessel

The subcutaneous tissues overlying the femoral pulse are incised with the electrocautery. The common femoral artery is exposed and sharply dissected circumferentially. The encountered lymphatics are ligated and divided. The dissection is extended proximally to the inguinal ligament and distally to include the superficial femoral and profunda femoris arteries. The common femoral, superficial femoral and profunda femoris arteries are encircled with Silastic vessel loops. Minor branches of the common femoral artery are identified and spared.

Figure 4: Construction of the Proximal Anastomosis

A 5000 units of Heparin (75 units/kg) is given intravenously. A side biting clamp is applied on the common femoral vein and the saphenous vein is transected incorporating the saphenofemoral junction and a 1-mm rim of the femoral vein. This allows for a generous proximal anastomosis. The femoral venotomy is then closed with a running 5-0 Prolene suture. The saphenofemoral valve is excised under direct vision using Potts scissors. The common femoral artery, profunda, and superficial femoral artery are clamped. A longitudinal arteriotomy in the common femoral artery is performed and extended with Potts scissors for 1 cm. The proximal anastomosis is constructed between the hood of the saphenofemoral junction and the femoral arteriotomy with a running 5-0 Prolene suture. Prior to completing the suture line, backbleeding, forward flushing and irrigation of the anastomosis with heparinized solution is performed. The anastomosis is then completed and checked for hemostasis.

Figure 3

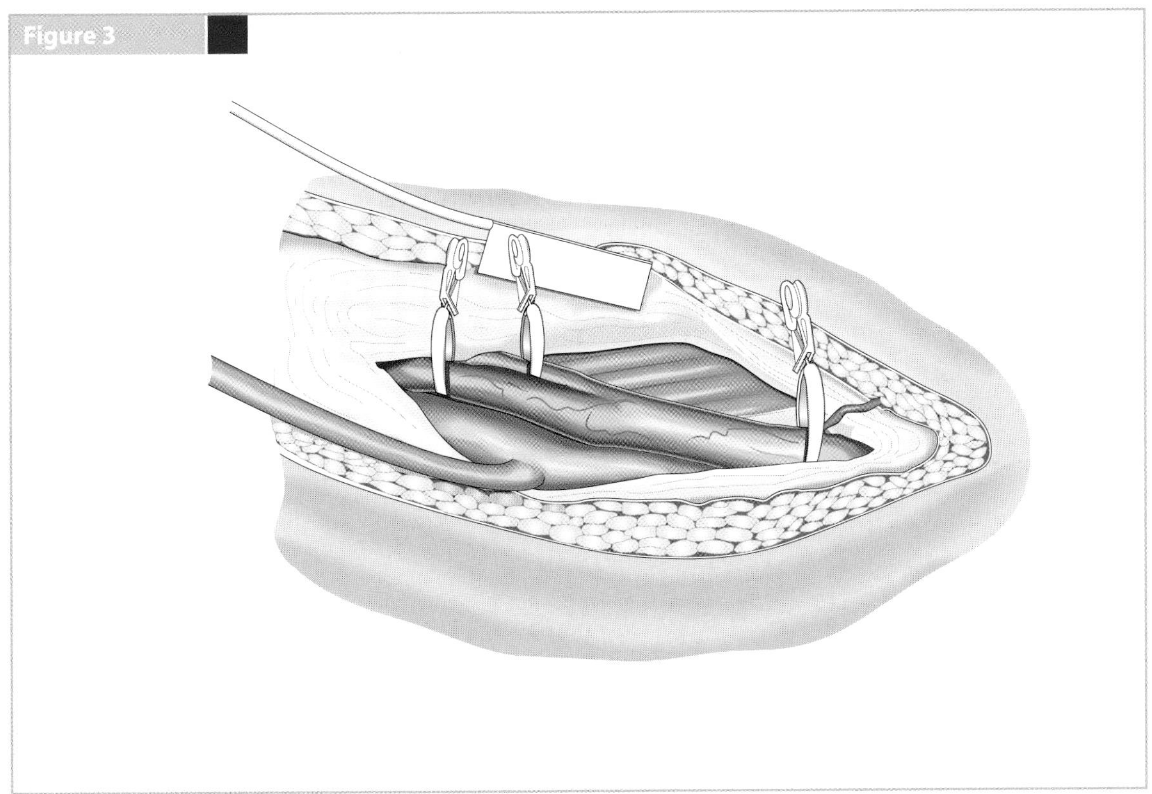

Figure 4

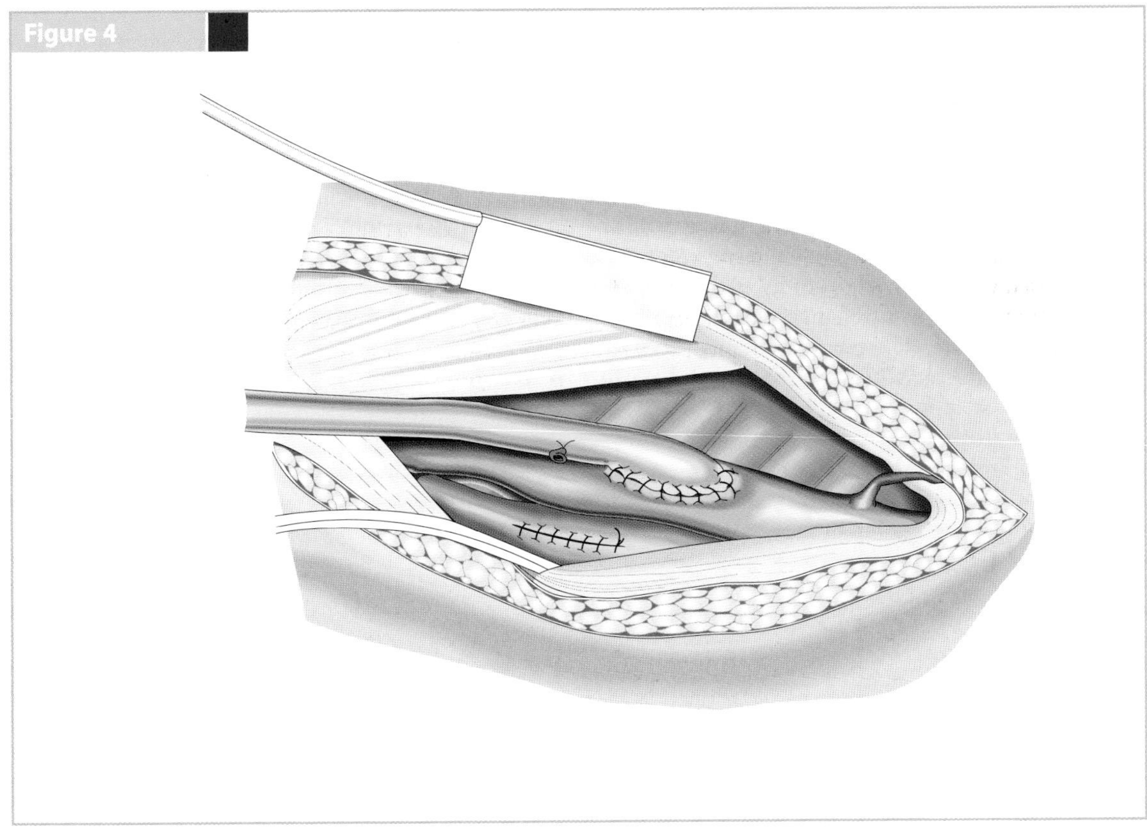

Figure 5: Valvulotomy

With the vein arterialized, the skin overlying the vein is incised and the vein sequentially exposed. The remaining valves are then disrupted using a retrograde valvulotome introduced through side branches and the distal end of the saphenous vein. Vein branches identified during dissection and by Doppler examination are ligated. The flow through the vein end is checked to be pulsatile. The distal end of the vein is controlled with a Yasargil/bulldog clamp.

Figure 6: Construction of the Distal Anastomosis

Trauma to the target vessel during the construction of the distal anastomosis is to be minimized. To minimize the injury, the target vessel can be controlled in various manners. One option is to use a sterile tourniquet. Alternatively the vessel can be controlled from within by using internal occluders. The tourniquet is ideal with calcified vessels and when the vessels are deep.

A tourniquet is placed above the knee and an Esmarch rubber bandage is applied to the foot and wrapped proximally to exsanguinate the leg. Following leg exsanguination, the tourniquet is inflated to 250–350 mmHg. A 1-cm arteriotomy is then created in the anterior wall of the change to tibial/peroneal artery. The vein is transected at the appropriate length. The transected end is incised along its posterior aspect spatulating the vein. The distal anastomosis to the peroneal artery is constructed with a running 7-0 Prolene suture. Prior to tying the suture line, the tourniquet is deflated. Backbleeding, forward flushing and irrigation of the anastomosis with heparinized solution is performed. The sutures are tied and checked for hemostasis. A 20G angiocatheter is then introduced into a side branch in the vein near the proximal anastomosis and an intraoperative arteriogram is performed to evaluate the anastomosis and check for any retained valves, filling defects or kinks. The angiocatheter is later removed and its puncture site repaired with a 6-0 Prolene suture. The suture lines and the wounds are then rechecked for hemostasis. The presence of good Doppler signal in the foot at the level of the dorsalis pedis and posterior tibial arteries and a good augmentation of the signal with compressing and releasing the vein graft is demonstrated.

■ **Wound Closure.** The wounds are all irrigated with antibiotic solution. The subcutaneous tissue in the groin wound is closed in two layers of 3-0 Vicryl suture. The fascia overlying the soleus muscle is partially closed with 3-0 Vicryl suture. The skin is closed with staples.

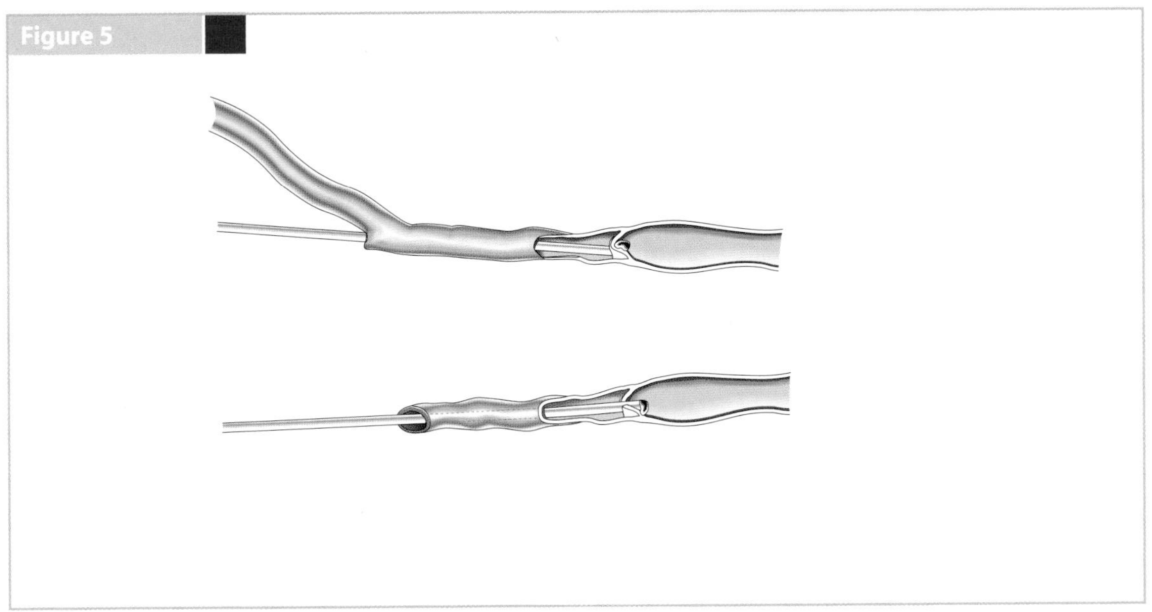

Figure 5

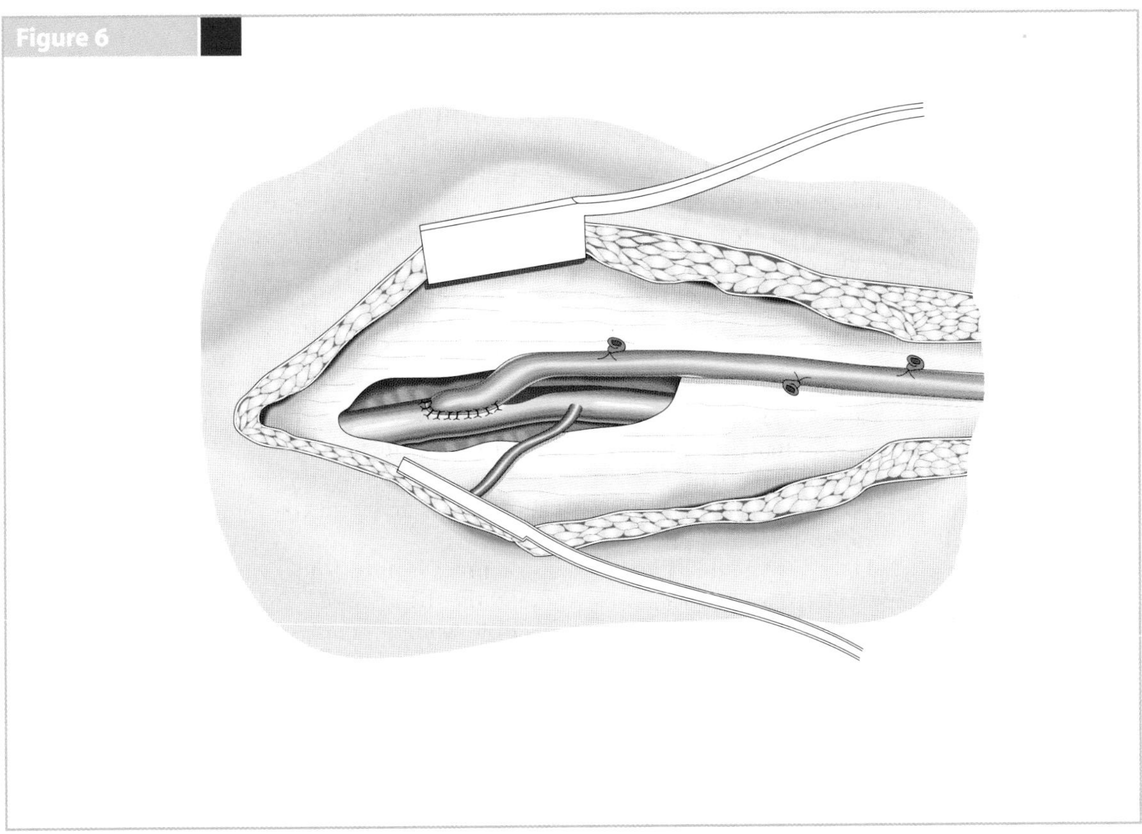

Figure 6

CONCLUSION

The primary patency rate of in situ femoroinfrapopliteal bypasses is reported to range from 85–90% at 1 year to 65% at 5 years. Secondary patency rates of 95% at 1 year and 80–90% at 5 years have been reported. Postoperative surveillance is essential to identify failing bypasses that can be salvaged prior to occlusion. Our surveillance protocol consists of physical examination, ankle brachial index and color duplex surveillance at 1 month postoperatively then every 3 months in the 1st year, every 6 months in the 2nd year and yearly thereafter. All patients should be placed on antiplatelet therapy. Routine anticoagulation with coumadin has not been proven to be advantageous and is recommended only in patients with known or suspected hypercoagulable states.

CHAPTER 30

Femoral to Anterior Tibial Artery Bypass with Non-reversed Great Saphenous Vein

Jamal J. Hoballah, Timothy F. Kresowik

INTRODUCTION

A non-reversed great saphenous vein bypass has several advantages. Such a bypass allows for a good size match between the vein and the target infrapopliteal artery. The valvulotomy may be easier to perform as the vein is free in the surgeon's hands rather than still attached to the leg. It also allows for tunneling the bypass through various routes decreasing its vulnerability should a wound complication develop. Furthermore, it allows for flexibility in using different inflow sources especially when the usable vein length is limited and a more distal inflow source is necessary for the vein to reach the target vessel. Its potential disadvantages include vein ischemia during harvesting and trauma to the vein and endothelium during harvesting and valvulotomy.

■ **Patient Positioning.** The patient is placed supine on the operating table. The arms are tucked or placed at 80°. Normal bony prominences are padded. The appropriate lines are placed, and regional/general anesthesia is induced. A Foley catheter is placed under sterile technique. The patient's lower abdomen and both lower extremities are circumferentially prepped and draped in the usual sterile fashion. Preoperative antibiotics are administered prior to skin incision.

Figure 1: Exposure of the Target Vessel

A 10–12 cm vertical skin incision is performed 2 cm posterior and parallel to the tibia. The skin incision is deepened through the subcutaneous tissue until the fascia is identified. The fascia is incised exposing the tibialis anterior and extensor digitorum muscles. Gentle blunt dissection between these two muscles is performed and a self retaining retractor is placed deeper in the wound exposing the anterior tibial artery and veins. A 2-cm segment of the anterior tibial artery is sharply dissected. Crossing venae comitantes are ligated and divided.

■ **Exposure of the Donor Artery.** A vertical skin incision overlying the right common femoral artery is made extending down the upper medial thigh along the preoperatively mapped great saphenous vein. The incision is deepened through the subcutaneous tissues with electrocautery. The encountered lymphatics are ligated and divided. The common femoral artery is exposed and sharply dissected circumferentially. The dissection is extended distally to include the superficial femoral and profunda femoris arteries. The common femoral, superficial femoral and profunda femoris arteries were encircled with Silastic vessel loops. Crossing veins over the profunda femoris artery are ligated and divided. The distal profunda branches are isolated.

■ **Vein Exposure and Harvest.** The great saphenous vein is identified in the groin or lower leg. The vein is exposed from the saphenofemoral junction to the lower leg through one continuous incision or through multiple incisions separated by skin bridges. Dextran-heparin-papaverine solution is infused into the saphenous vein through a blunt needle that is placed in a side branch in the most distal aspect of the vein. The saphenous vein is harvested and its tributaries ligated with 3-0 silk ties. The vein can also be harvested using endoscopic techniques. We tend to limit endoscopic harvesting to the above knee segment of the vein and to avoid it when dealing with small diameter veins.

Figure 1

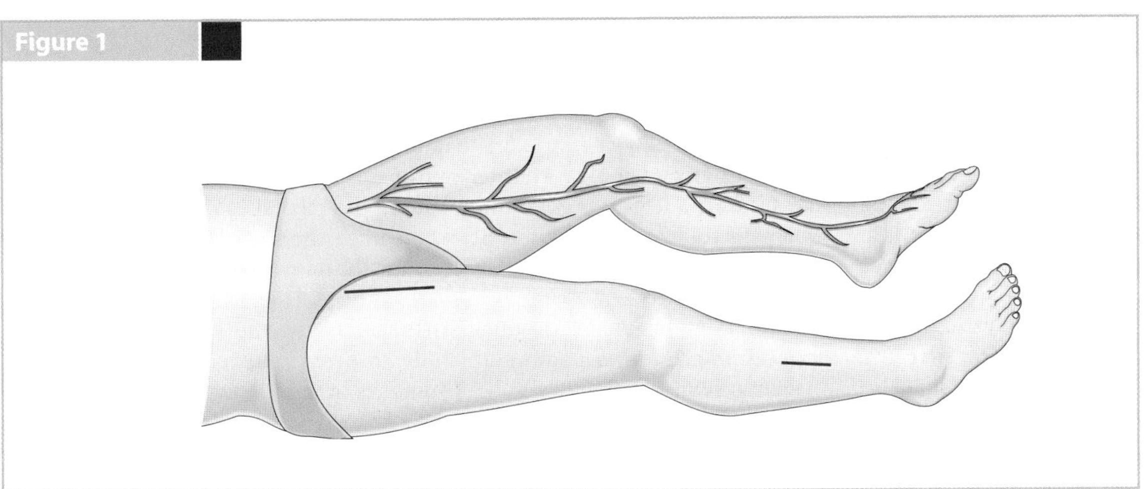

Figure 2A–C: Tunneling

A tunnel is created using a Kelly-Wick or a Gore-Tex tunneler. Our preference is to tunnel subcutaneously crossing from medial to lateral in the thigh and continuing laterally to the target vessel in the leg. Bypasses originating distal to the femoral bifurcation, i.e., from the profunda femoris artery, are first tunneled posterior to the sartorius muscle and then exiting into the subcutaneous layer in the thigh to avoid acute angulation by the sartorius muscle. Alternatively, the tunnel can be subcutaneous along the medial aspect of the thigh and knee and crossed from medial to lateral below the knee anterior to the tibia. Another option is to create a subcutaneous/subfascial tunnel along the medial aspect of the thigh and knee. Below the knee, the tunnel crosses from medial to lateral through the interosseous membrane. Crossing through the interosseous membrane requires additional dissection below the knee and should be done carefully to avoid inadvertent bleeding from muscular branches in the tunnel.

Figure 2A

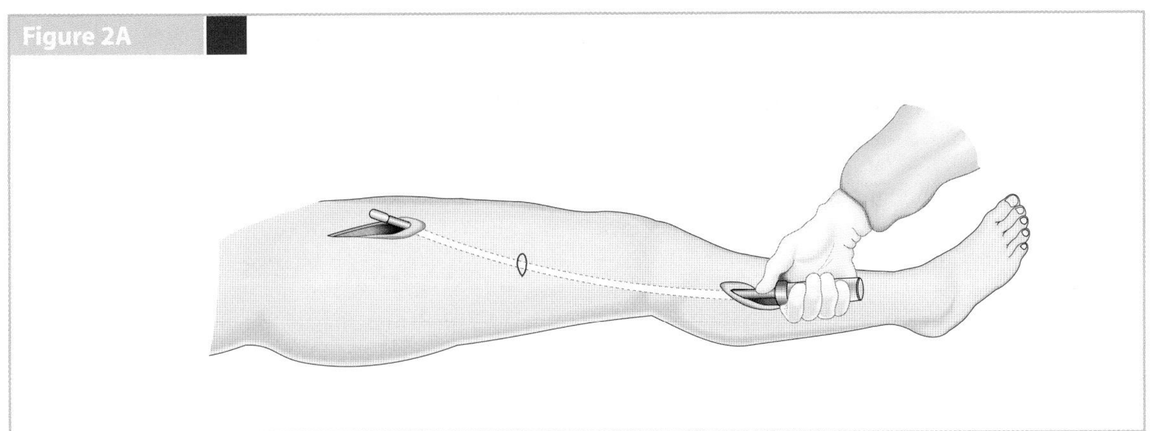

Figure 2B

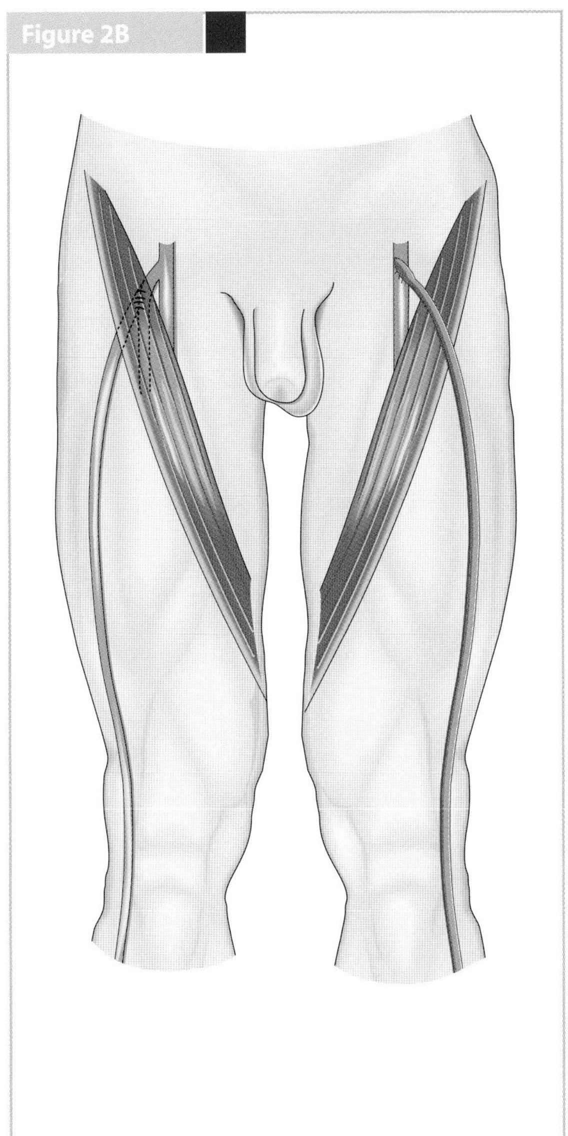

Figure 2C

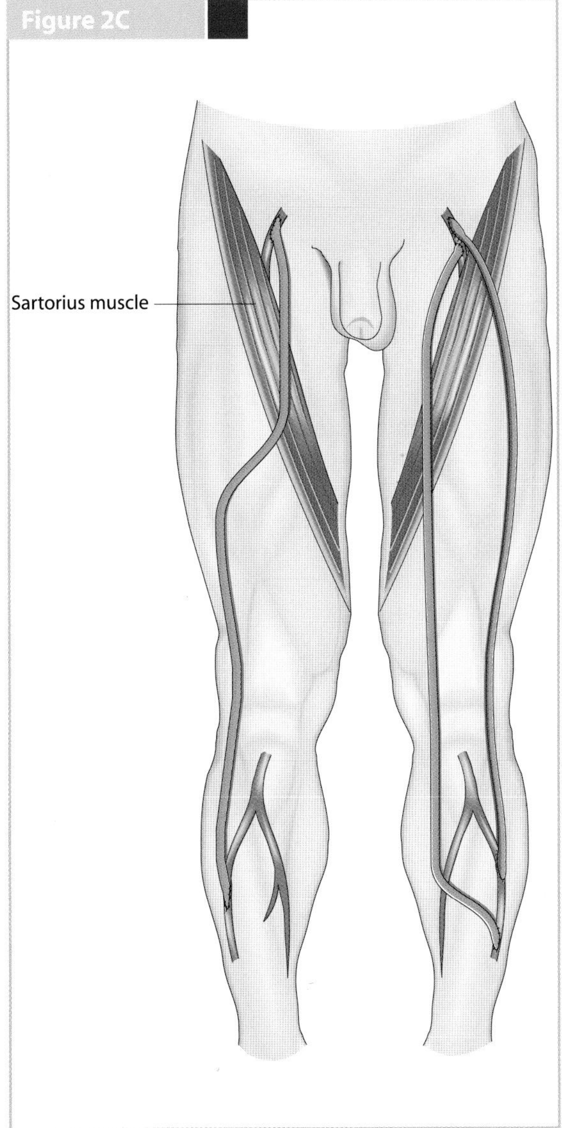

Figure 3: Proximal Anastomosis

Heparin is given intravenously at 75 units/kg. A side biting clamp is applied on the common femoral vein and the saphenous vein is transected incorporating the saphenofemoral junction and a 1-mm rim of the femoral vein. The femoral venotomy is closed with a running 5-0 Prolene suture. The saphenofemoral valve is then excised under direct vision using Potts scissors. The profunda femoral artery is clamped. A longitudinal arteriotomy in the profunda femoris artery is performed and extended with Potts scissors for 1 cm. The proximal anastomosis is constructed between the hood of the saphenofemoral junction and the femoral arteriotomy with a running 6-0 Prolene suture. Prior to completing the suture line, backbleeding, forward flushing and irrigation of the anastomosis with heparinized solution is performed. The anastomosis is then completed and checked for hemostasis. The remaining valves are then lysed using a retrograde valvulotome introduced through side branches and the distal end of the saphenous vein. The flow through the vein is checked to be pulsatile. The end of the vein is ligated with a 2-0 silk tie. The vein is rechecked for hemostasis. The vein is then passed through the tunnel avoiding any twists.

Figure 4A, B: Distal Anastomosis

A tourniquet is placed above the knee and an Esmarch rubber bandage is applied to the foot and wrapped proximally to exsanguinate the leg. The tourniquet is then inflated to 250–350 mmHg. A 1-cm arteriotomy is created in the anterior wall of the anterior tibial artery. Alternatively a 1-cm arteriotomy is created in the anterior wall of the anterior tibial artery and an appropriate size internal occluder (2.0, 2.25, 2.50 mm) is introduced into the lumen. Proximal and distal control of the anterior tibial artery with vessel loops, vascular clamps or bulldog clamps is avoided to minimize severe spasm and trauma to the artery at the clamp site.

The vein is transected at the appropriate length. The transected end is incised along its posterior aspect spatulating the vein. The distal anastomosis to the anterior tibial artery is constructed with a running 7-0 Prolene suture. Prior to completing the suture line, backbleeding, forward flushing and irrigation of the anastomosis with heparinized solution is performed. The anastomosis is then completed and checked for hemostasis.

A 20G angiocatheter is then introduced into a side branch in the vein near the proximal anastomosis and an intraoperative arteriogram is performed. The angiogram is used to confirm a patent anastomosis with no evidence of any retained valves, filling defects or kinks. The angiocatheter is removed and its puncture site repaired with a 6-0 Prolene suture. The suture lines and the wounds were then rechecked for hemostasis. A Doppler signal in the foot at the dorsalis pedis with a good augmentation of the signal with compressing and releasing the vein graft are demonstrated.

■ **Wound Closure.** The wounds are all irrigated with antibiotic solution. The subcutaneous tissue in the groin wound is closed in two layers of 3-0 Vicryl suture. The fascia overlying the anterior tibial muscle and extensor hallucis muscles is partially closed with 3-0 Vicryl suture. The skin is closed with staples.

Figure 3

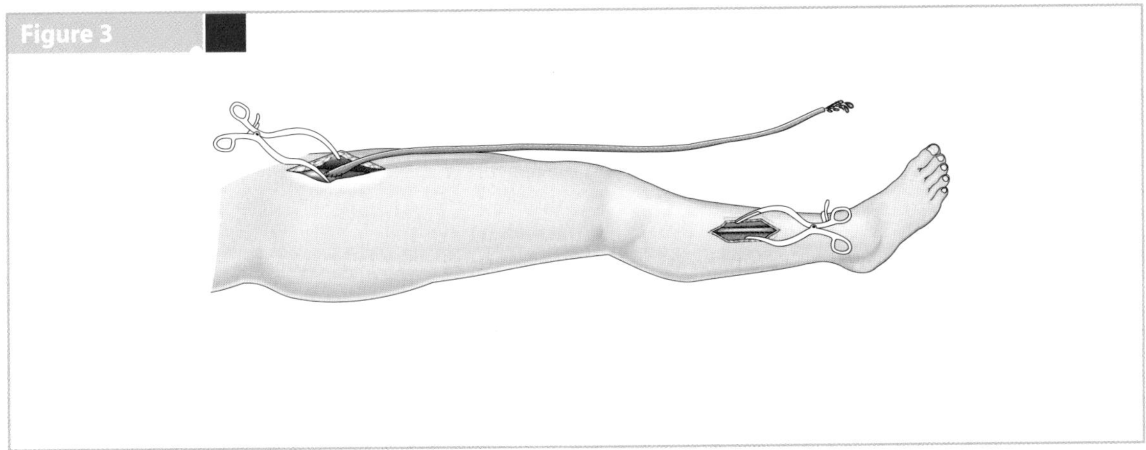

Figure 4A

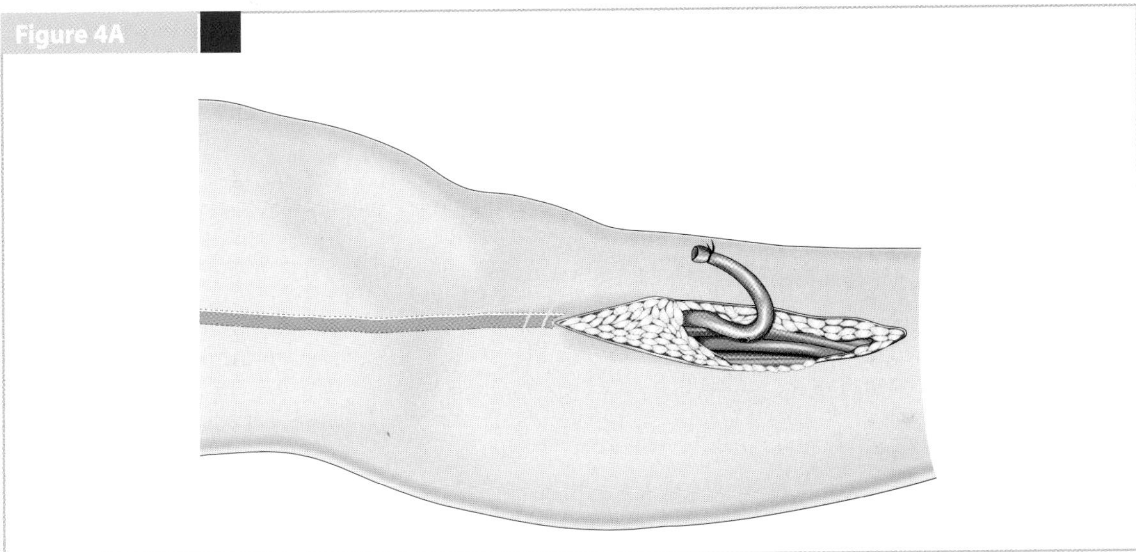

Figure 4B

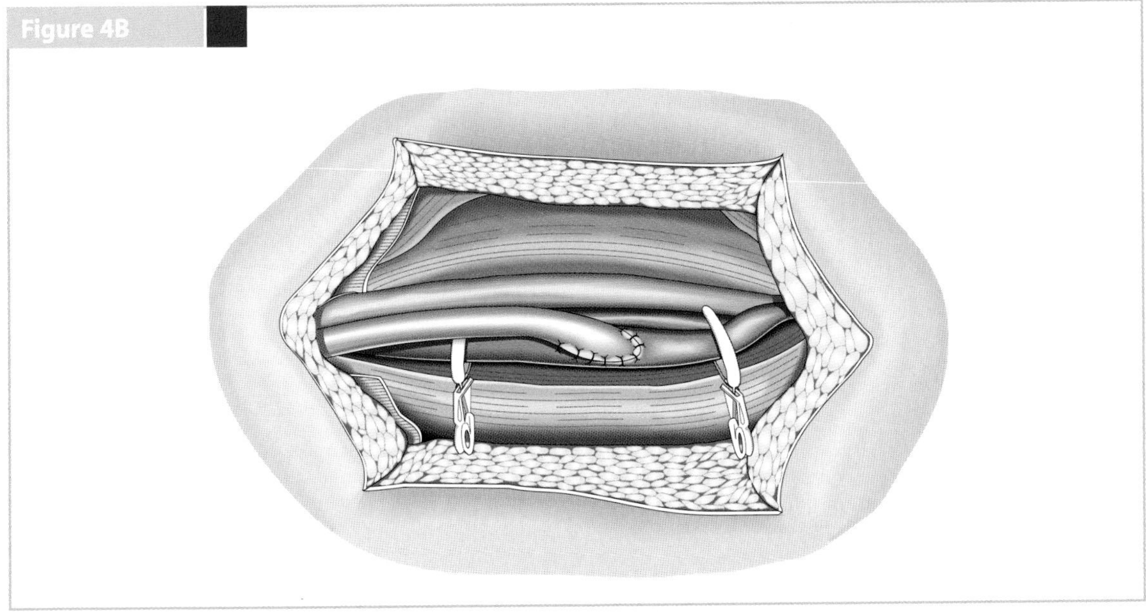

CONCLUSION

Non-reversed vein passes is a useful and simple technique that allows a good vein to artery match and flexibility in tunneling and revascularization.

For a description of the common femoral to peroneal artery bypass with an adjunctive vein collar/AV fistula, refer to Chap. 31 by Calligaro and Dougherty.

SELECTED BIBLIOGRAPHY

Ascer E, Veith F, Gupta S (1985) Bypasses to plantar arteries and other tibial branches: An extended approach to limb salvage. J Vasc Surg 8:434

Bridges R, Gewertz BL (1980) Lateral incision for exposure of femoral vessels. Surg Gynecol Obstet 150:733

Danese CA, Singer A (1968) Lateral approach to the trifurcation popliteal artery. Surgery 63:588–590

Dardik H, Dardik I, Veith FJ (1974) Exposure of the tibioperoneal arteries by a single lateral approach. Surgery 75:377–382

Dardik H, Elias S, Miller N et al. (1985) Medial approach to the anterior tibial artery. J Vasc Surg 2:743

Dardik H, Ibrahim IM, Dardik II (1979) The role of the peroneal artery for limb salvage. Ann Surg 189:189–198

Hoballah JJ, Chalmers RT, Sharp WJ et al. (1996) Lateral approach to the popliteal and crural vessels for limb salvage. Cardiovasc Surg 4:165–168

Imparato AM, Kim GE, Chu DS (1973) Surgical exposure for reconstruction of the proximal part of the tibial artery. Surg Gynecol Obstet 136:453–455

Minken SL, May AG (1969) Use of the peroneal artery for revascularization of the lower extremity. Arch Surg 99:594–597

Naraysingh V, Karmody AM, Leather RP, Corson JD (1984) Lateral approach to the profunda femoris artery. Am J Surg 147:813–814

Nunez AA, Veith FJ, Collier P, Ascer E, Flores SW, Gupta SK (1988) Direct approaches to the distal portions of the deep femoral artery for limb salvage. J Vasc Surg 8:576–581

Padberg FT Jr (1998) Lateral approach to the popliteal artery. Ann Vasc Surg 2:397–401

Usatoff V, Grigg M (1997) Letter to the editor. A lateral approach to the below-knee popliteal artery without resection of the fibula. J Vasc Surg 26:168–170

Veith FJ, Ascer E, Gupta SK, Wengerter KR (1987) Lateral approach to the popliteal artery. J Vasc Surg 6:119–123

CHAPTER 31

Femoro-peroneal PTFE Bypass with Adjunctive AV Fistula/Patch

Keith D. Calligaro, Matthew J. Dougherty

INTRODUCTION

Severe lower extremity arterial insufficiency is manifested by rest pain, ischemic ulceration or gangrene. Patients with these problems are faced with a major amputation if revascularization is unsuccessful or not possible. Although autogenous vein provides better patency rates than prosthetic grafts, vein is not always available.

Prosthetic bypass grafts to the above-knee popliteal artery yield an acceptable (approximately 50%) 4-year primary patency rate (Veith et al. 1986). However, prosthetic graft bypass to infrapopliteal vessels, such as the tibial or peroneal arteries, yields a dismal 10% primary patency rate after 4 years when no other medical or surgical adjuncts are used (Veith et al. 1986). Autogenous vein grafts yield dramatically better long-term patency and other adjuncts are usually not necessary. Various procedures have been promoted to improve long-term success for prosthetic bypass grafts to infrapopliteal arteries. As low blood flow velocity (due to resistant outflow beds) through thrombogenic graft material may cause graft thrombosis, increasing graft flow is one strategy. Construction of an arteriovenous (AV) fistula at the distal anastomosis results in higher flow rates in the graft. Intimal hyperplasia at the distal anastomosis is another cause of graft failure. Placement of a vein patch or cuff at the distal anastomosis may lessen compliance mismatch and result in less intimal hyperplasia, or may move the zone of intimal hyperplasia away from the outflow track (Ascer et al. 1996). Both of these techniques have been reported to enhance patency of these disadvantaged grafts.

Ascher has proposed that a combination of these two techniques may offer advantages of both methods and also be technically easier: a peroneal or tibial vein is sutured end to side to the crural artery and a prosthetic graft is then sutured end to side to the vein. Taylor has devised a vein patch that lies on the distal part of the prosthetic graft and the artery (Taylor et al. 1992). We will outline the technical aspects of performing an Ascher AV fistula and a Taylor vein patch at the distal anastomosis of a prosthetic graft anastomosed to the peroneal artery.

Complications of lower extremity arterial bypasses include graft thrombosis, infection, amputation, bleeding, local nerve injury, and cardiac and pulmonary complications.

PROCEDURE

An epidural catheter is placed for anesthesia and postoperative analgesia and a radial artery catheter is placed for blood sampling and blood pressure monitoring. Intravenous antibiotics are administered 30 min prior to incision. The patient is positioned supine.

The inflow artery (common or superficial femoral or popliteal) is dissected through an appropriate incision. When the peroneal artery proximal to the midpoint of the tibia is the site for distal anastomosis, a medial approach to the artery is used. The soleus muscle is divided at its tibial insertion and the posterior tibial artery is identified. The dissection continues along the fascia anterior and lateral to the posterior tibial artery, until the peroneal artery is identified. The prosthetic graft is tunneled medially in the subcutaneous plane to the peroneal artery, unless the popliteal fossa has been exposed in which case the graft is tunneled anatomically between the heads of the gastrocnemius muscle and in the subsartorial plane.

When the distal anastomotic site is the distal half of the peroneal artery, we prefer a lateral approach, resecting approximately 3 cm of the fibula. The distal 5 cm of the fibula must be left intact or the ankle joint may become unstable. The prosthetic graft is tunneled subcutaneously in the thigh, to just lateral to the patella and anterior to the fibular head, and to the distal peroneal artery.

The patient is anticoagulated with 100 units heparin/kg intravenously and activated clotting times are maintained above 200 s. The inflow artery is clamped and the end-to-side proximal anastomosis is constructed.

Figure 1A, B

Venous tributaries anterior to the peroneal artery are divided and ligated with fine silk ties. The appropriate arterial site for distal arterial anastomosis is exposed. If the vessel is calcified, the leg is exsanguinated with an Esmarch bandage and a calf or thigh tourniquet inflated to 350 mmHg is utilized in lieu of vessel loops or clamps. This technique also obviates extensive arterial dissection. The adjacent peroneal vein is dissected free for fistula construction, while saphenous or arm vein is harvested for vein patch. The distal peroneal vein is ligated. If venous backbleeding occurs it is controlled with a small bulldog clamp. The vein is spatulated approximately 10 mm. Figure 1A shows the preferred site of transection of the adjacent vein relative to the arteriotomy, and Fig. 1B shows the vein prepared for end-to-site anastomosis to the infrapopliteal artery.

Figure 1A

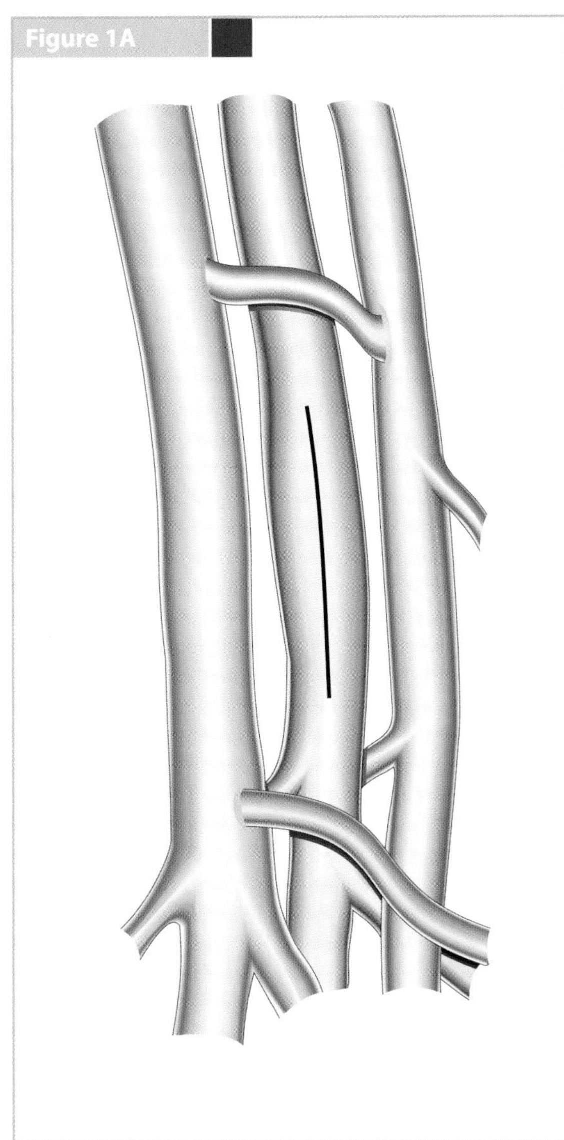

Figure 1B

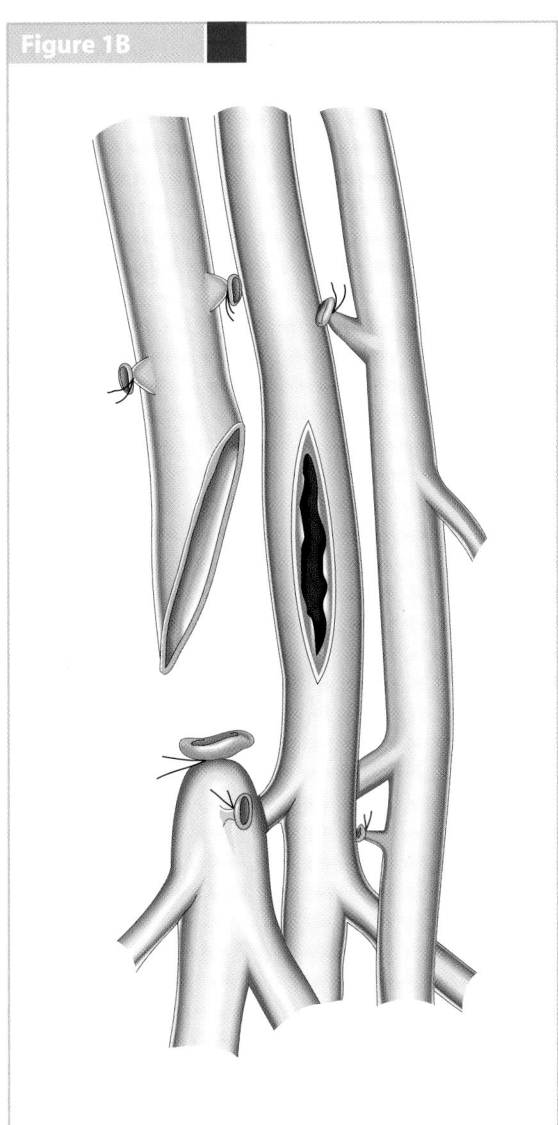

Figure 2A, B

A 10-mm arterotomy is made on the peroneal artery. The spatulated peroneal vein is sutured to the anterior aspect of the artery with a fine-running monofilament suture. The vein is thin-walled and fragile and gentle; meticulous technique is critical. After the vein-to-artery anastomosis is completed, a venotomy is made on the hood of the vein extended proximally for about 10 mm, centered over the heel of the venoarteriostomy.

Figure 2A

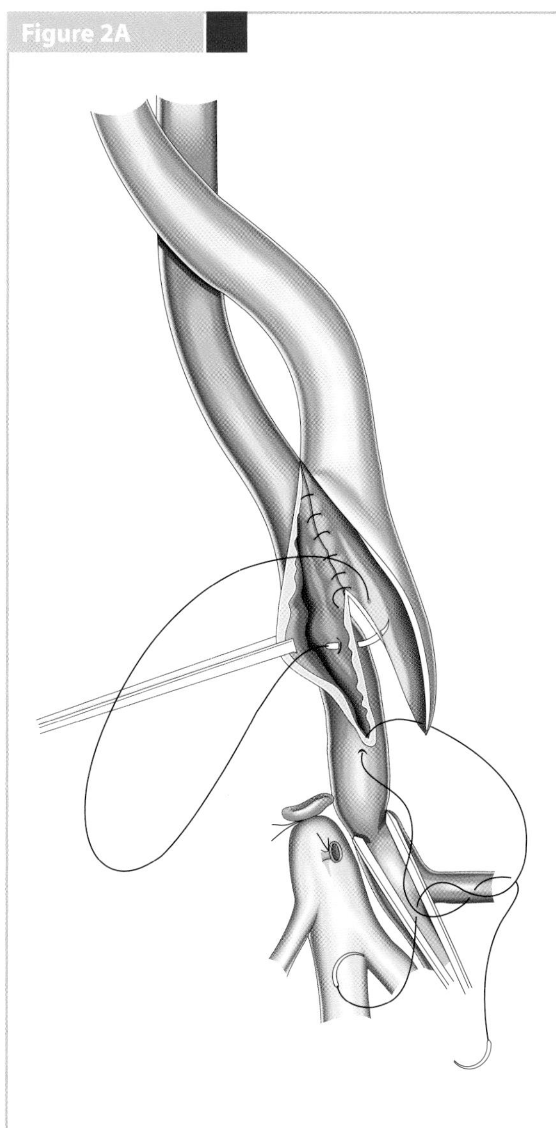

Figure 2B

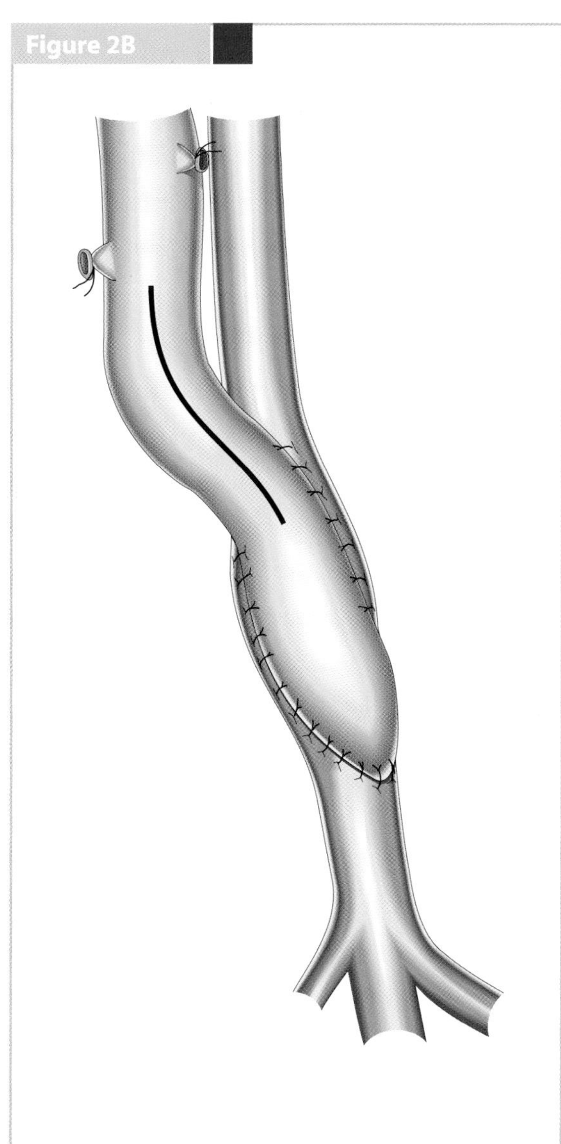

Figure 3A, B

After the venotomy is made, the prosthetic graft is spatulated 10 mm and anastomosed with fine monofilament suture. Clamps or vessel loops on the peroneal vein are first removed, or the tourniquet is deflated.

Figure 3A

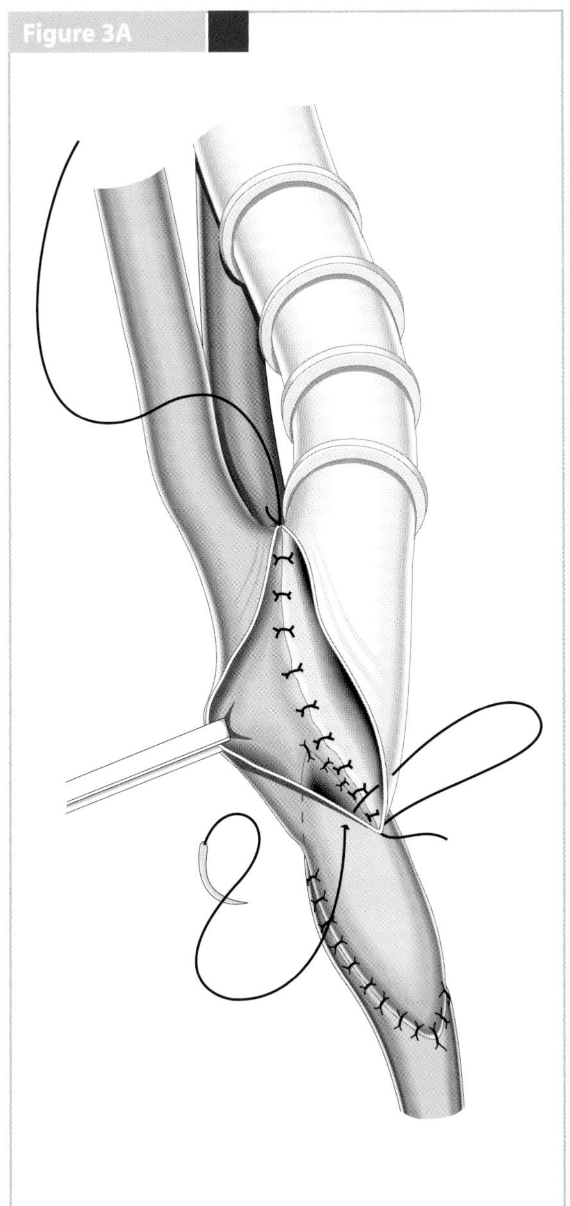

Figure 3B

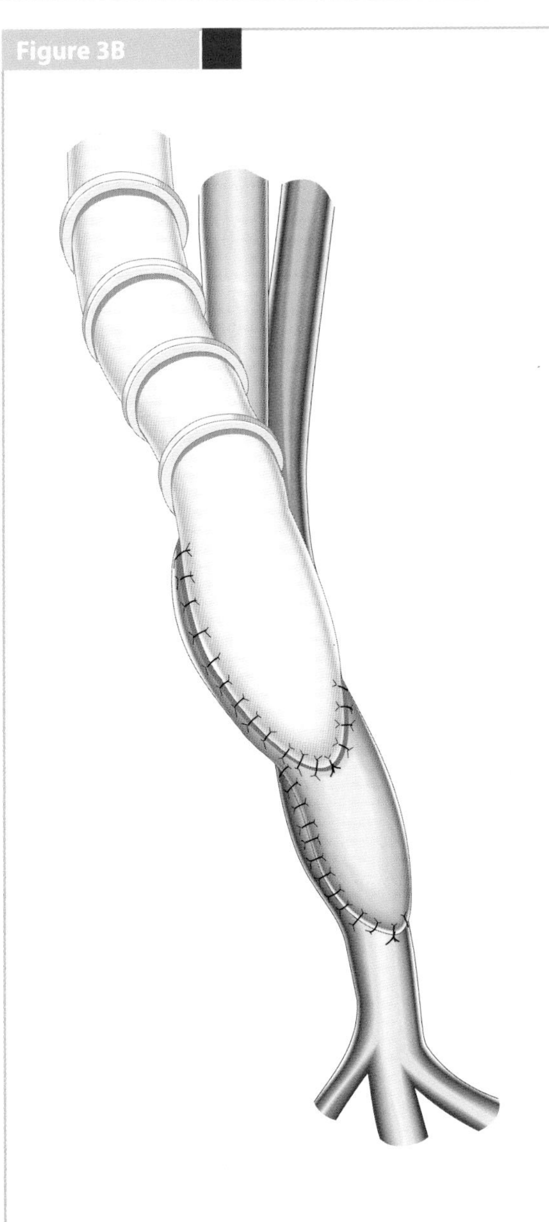

Figure 4A, B

The prosthetic graft lies anterior to the peroneal vein, which is anterior to the peroneal artery. In this manner, an AV fistula has been constructed to enhance flow through the graft via the fistula, and the vein acts as a cuff to potentially diminish development of intimal hyperplasia.

If the outflow proximal peroneal vein is large, the potential exists for arterial "steal" from the distal arterial tree. Significant steal may result in persistent limb ischemia despite a patent graft. One method to prevent steal is to "band" the proximal outflow peroneal vein to limit flow through the fistula. If there is any question of adequacy of pedal perfusion, arterial pressure is measured at the hood of the distal anastomosis. A pressure of 100 mmHg is usually sufficient to perfuse the foot; if lower, the vein fistula is narrowed with Weck clips applied tangentially until the target pressure is achieved.

In Fig. 4, the completed bypass demonstrates the final configuration of distal AVF/VI without banding of venous outflow (**A**) and with banding (**B**).

Figure 5

If a Taylor vein patch is to be constructed, an appropriate length of suitable saphenous or arm vein is harvested. A 30-mm arteriotomy is made. The prosthetic graft is fashioned by spatulating it over 30 mm, then excising the distal half. The hood of the graft is then incised 15 mm. The prosthetic graft is sutured to the proximal half of the peroneal artery arteriotomy. The vein patch is sutured to the distal peroneal artery arteriotomy and the prosthetic graft with a running monofilament suture.

In Fig. 5, the critical distal interrupted sutures between the vein patch and artery are all inserted under direct vision before any are tied.

Figure 6

The Taylor vein patch extends over 15 mm of the prosthetic graft and 15 mm of the peroneal artery. Adequate vein caliber is critical to avoid kinking.

A completion arteriography is performed using 20 cc of contrast injected through a 21-gauge needle into the hood of the graft. With the Ascher fistula, inflow occlusion is not used as contrast will preferentially opacify the vein at low pressures, but for the Taylor patch inflow occlusion may improve imaging. The wounds are irrigated with antibiotic solution and closed with absorbable suture to the subcutaneous fascia. Skin is closed with clips or nylon sutures.

In Fig. 6, the correct appearance of the completed vein patch is tapered smoothly to enable a gradual reduction in diameter.

Figure 4A

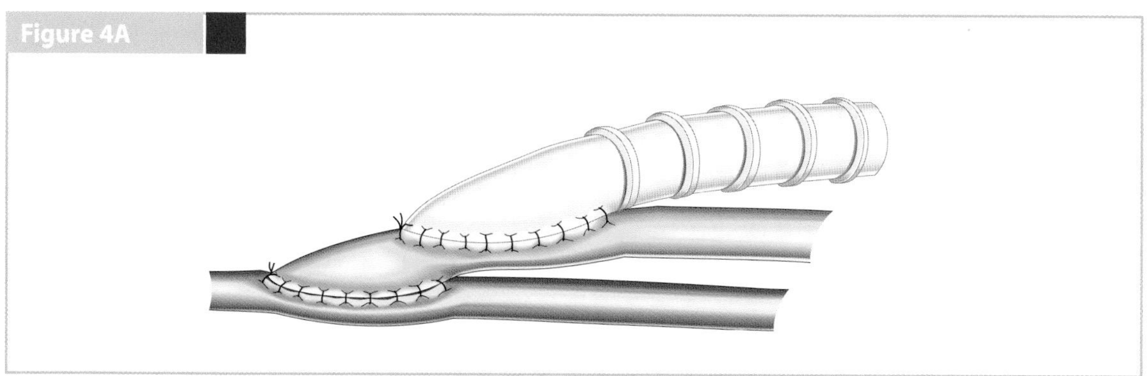

Figure 4B

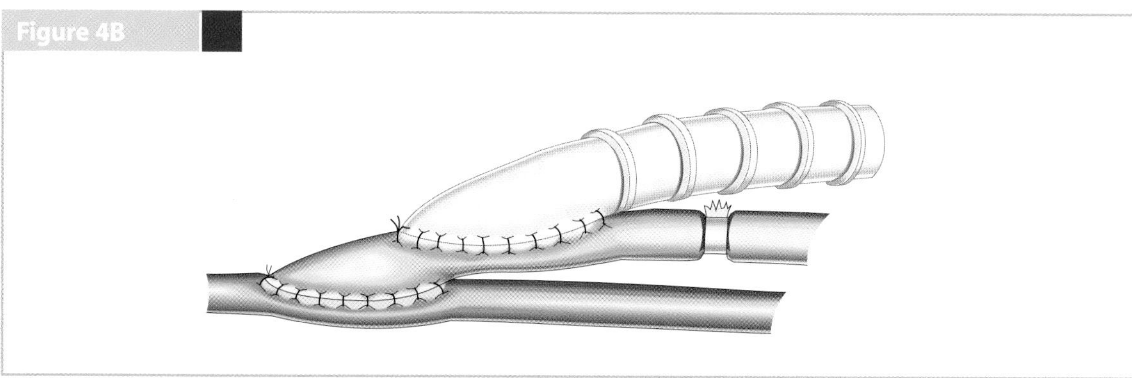

Figure 5

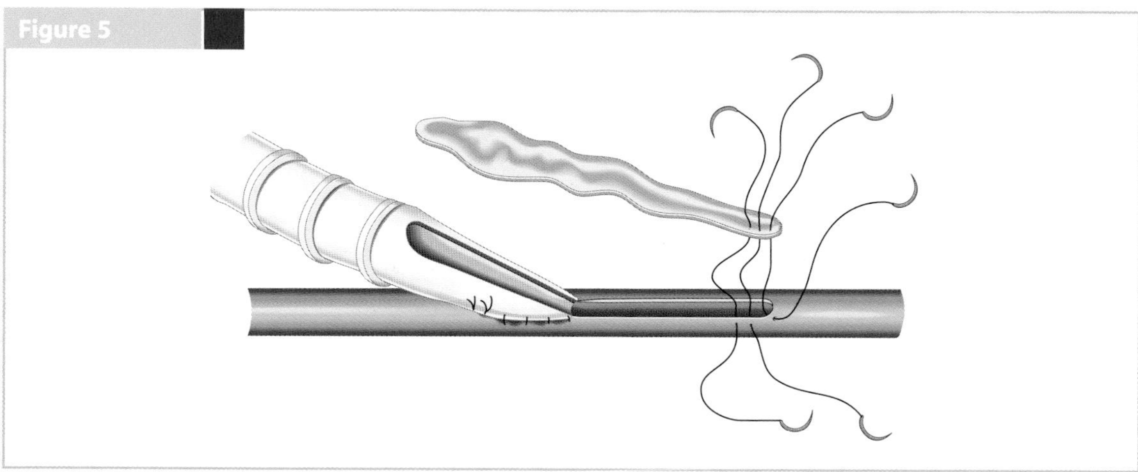

Figure 6

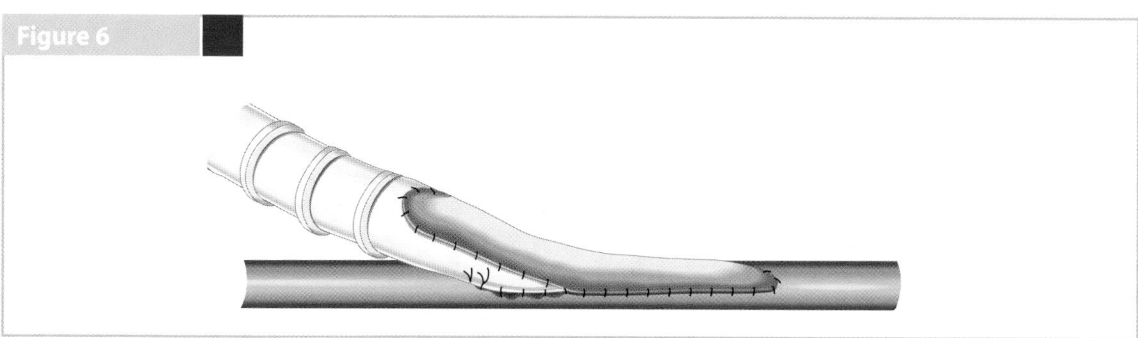

CONCLUSION

Construction of an adjunctive Ascher AV fistula or Taylor vein patch at the distal anastomosis of prosthetic grafts to the peroneal artery may improve long-term patency rates of these grafts.

REFERENCES

Ascer E, Gennaro M, Pollina RM et al. (1996) Complementary distal arteriovenous fistula and deep vein interposition: A five-year experience with a new technique to improve infrapopliteal prosthetic bypass patency. J Vasc Surg 24:134–143

Taylor RS, Loh A, McFarland RJ et al. (1992) Improved technique for polytetrafluoroethylene bypass grafting: long-term results using anastomotic vein patches. Br J Surg 79:348–354

Veith FJ, Gupta SK, Ascer E et al. (1986) Six-year prospective multicenter randomized comparison of autologous saphenous vein and expanded and polytetrafluoroethylene grafts in infrainguinal arterial reconstructions. J Vasc Surg 3:104–114

Part VI Vascular Access

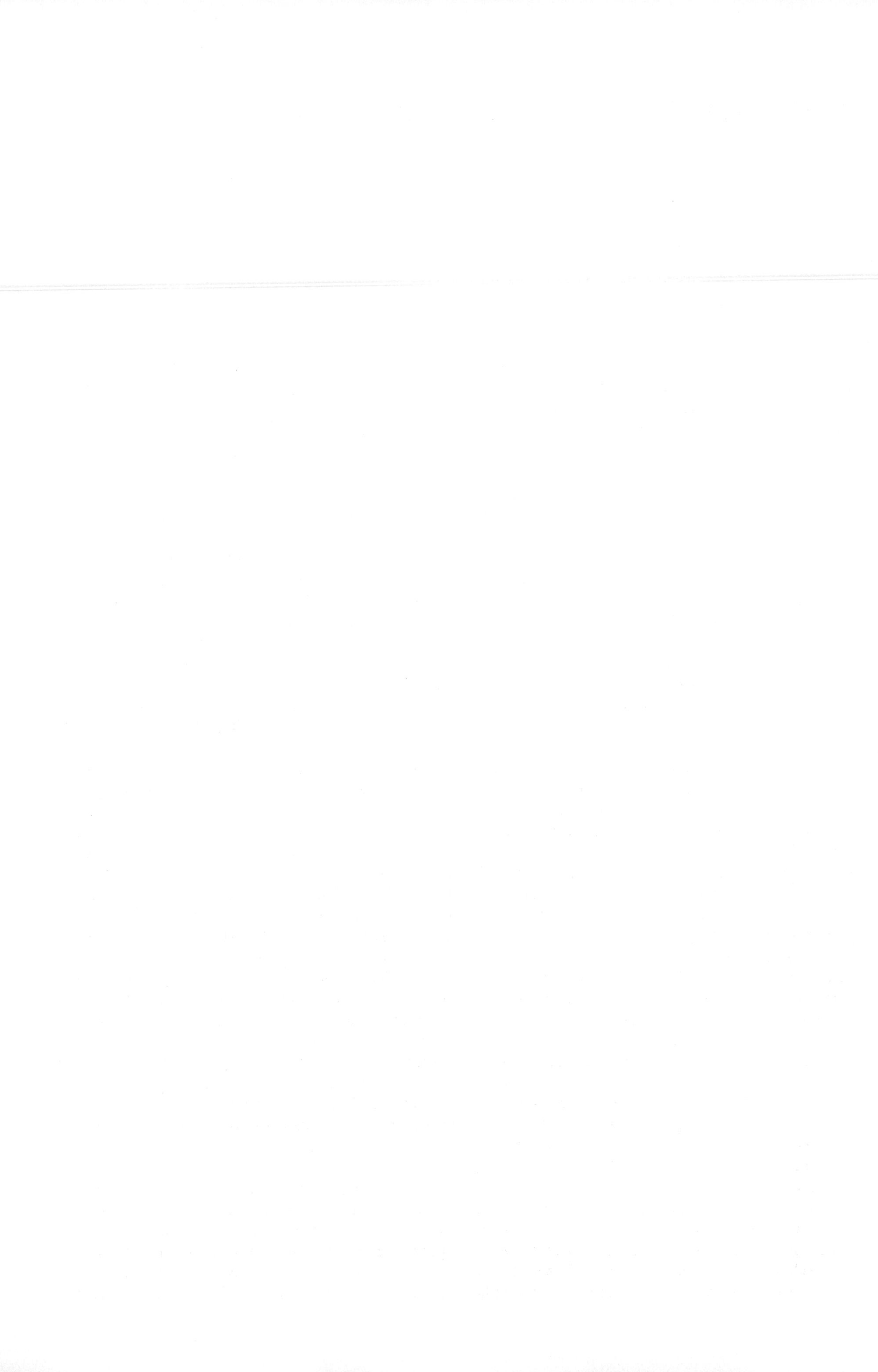

CHAPTER 32

Vascular Access

Paul Srodon, John Lumley

INTRODUCTION

The prime indication for long-term vascular access is hemodialysis for end-stage renal disease (ESRD). Transplantation is the preferred option for these patients, but dialysis is needed while awaiting an appropriate kidney, and some patients are unsuitable for transplantation.

Hemodialysis requires reliable repetitive access to the circulation that can provide flow of up to 400 ml/min. Access techniques have evolved over the last 50 years. Repeatable access first became possible with the introduction of the Quinton-Scribner arteriovenous shunt in 1960, but this external fistula gave way to the Brescia-Cimino fistula in 1966. Central venous catheters (CVCs) have been available for more than 30 years and provide immediate temporary, and sometimes permanent, access, but if used too early and for too long, they may result in stenosis and occlusion of major veins that would complicaate or prevent the formation of distal forms of access.

Patients with ESRD often have significant co-morbidity, and an increasing number of elderly patients are dialyzed. Co-morbid factors influencing the choice and success of access include: diabetes; cardiovascular problems – hypertension, hyperlipidemia, smoking, anemia, arrhythmias, and left ventricular failure. These may lead to poor tolerance of rapid fluid shifts, which may occur in dialysis. Uremia may be accompanied by proteinuria, phosphate retention, metabolic and keto-acidosis, increased ammonia production, defective drug metabolism and clearance, central nervous system depression, autonomic and peripheral nerve palsies, and visual impairment. Thrombogenic factors include platelet dysfunction and prescribed anticoagulants for arrhythmia and possible prosthetic valve disease; and there may be concomitant disorders from diabetes and homocystinuria. If continuous ambulatory peritoneal dialysis (CAPD) is being considered, previous abdominal surgery, hernias and obesity may be contraindications.

Social influences on the choice of dialysis include employment, social support, and the proximity of the dialysis unit, and the type of transport available.

The mode of presentation has a marked influence on the choice of access, as immediate dialysis may be needed. However, referral and assessment in a dedicated access clinic allow mental and physical preparation of the patient, including involvement in the choice of dialysis technique. Planning ahead can also allow the establishment of a permanent fistula a few months ahead of requirement, allowing this to mature and avoiding the need for CVC temporary lines; the whole amounting to specific tailoring to the individual patient for counseling and arriving at an informed decision.

The number of sites available for venous access is limited and it is, therefore, essential to optimize their use, starting as far distally in the upper limbs as vessels will allow. The first fistula can dictate subsequent lifelong management of the patient undergoing dialysis and must, therefore, be undertaken by the most skilled surgeon available. Radiocephalic fistulae satisfy the distal criteria and also carry the lowest long-term morbidity. However, initially, and possibly long-term, they do not necessarily deliver high enough flow rates for adequate dialysis, and for this reason, since the availability of synthetic grafts, primary grafting is the procedure of choice in some units, particularly in the United States where the overall incidence is 68% and up to 80% in selected units. This led to the National Kidney Foundation/Kidney Disease Outcome Quality Initiative (KDOQI) guidelines recommending that primary A-V fisculae should be constructed in at least 50% of all new renal failure patients electing to receive long term hemodialysis. Veins should be mapped and all previous surgery, injection sites and traumatized area must be identified through the history, scars and other evidence of injury. Veins may be difficult to find and, subsequently, to needle in a fatty arm, or if the arm is edematous; previous CVC catheters may have damaged the subclavian vein, and the existence of a pacemaker is a contraindication to the use of a limb, if there are alternatives.

The lengths of vein must accommodate two needles with enough separation to avoid recirculation, and their position must allow comfortable positioning of the arm during many hours of dialysis. The application of an upper arm venous cuff facilitates palpation, assessment of distensibility (often reduced in the diabetic patient), and the distribution and continuity within the superficial venous system. Assessment of continuity is aided by tapping the vein distally, and feeling for the proximal venous impulse. Arterial inflow is assessed by palpation of all limb pulses and the measurement of blood pressure, while looking for signs of distal ischemia, such as loss of subcutaneous fat, tapering of digits, thin skin and superficial ulceration. Allen's test assesses ulnar flow, and possible consequences of a radiocephalic steal: the radial and ulnar arteries are compressed at the wrist, after the patient has forcefully made a fist to empty blood from the hand. The hand is opened up, and the radial artery released, to assess recirculation; the process is repeated, releasing the ulnar artery. If there is clinical suspicion of abnormal anatomy or stenotic disease, Duplex ultrasound or angiography may be necessary. Both arms are examined, and the neck and upper chest, for collateral veins, suggestive of deep venous problems; also assessment of the lower limb vasculature for immediate or possible later use. A fistula in the nondominant arm is less likely to be traumatized, allows better everyday function, and is also easier for a patient to self-needle. The choice, however, is dictated by the quality of the existing vasculature.

Once the limb has been chosen, the patient must be aware that it must no longer be used for taking blood pressure, for venous access, or for insertion of any lines. This awareness may be heightened by removing any watch or bracelets from the limb.

Duplex ultrasound of the arterial tree may identify upper limb atherosclerotic disease, and abnormalities such as reversed flow, steal and pseudoaneurysms. It is also used to map the site, continuity and diameter of the superficial veins, comparing both upper and lower limbs, previous surgery being noted in the latter. In the upper limbs 70% of the blood flows in the superficial veins, this being the reverse of the lower limb. Mapping identifies anomalous anatomy, missing or stenotic segments of vein, intimomedial thickness, intimal hyperplasia and valve leaflets. The technique also allows the identification of perivascular abnormalities, such as hematoma and infection. Flow may be measured in the straight length of established fistula, or vein, or prosthetic graft. Flows of <300 ml/min may require radiological investigation. When assessing the subclavian vein, spontaneous phasic flow, in time with respiration should be present, together with cessation of flow with a Valsalva maneuver, and augmentation with distal compression of the limb. Subclavian stenosis usually occurs between the clavicle and first rib, and this vessel and the internal jugular veins are well visualized by ultrasound. However, the clavicle and sternum often inhibit good visualization of the innominate veins and the superior vena cava. Ultrasound is a valuable means of follow-up of fistulae and grafts, particularly once an abnormality has been detected.

Figure 1: Radiocephalic Fistula (Brescia-Cimino)

Suitability for radiocephalic fistula is confirmed by preoperative assessment: Allen's test must demonstrate that both radial and ulnar arteries are patent, and a tourniquet applied to the upper arm must show filling of the cephalic vein. If there is suspicion that the cephalic vein may be damaged or occluded, or of upper limb arterial insufficiency, these vessels should be assessed by Duplex ultrasound. Venography is required if there has been previous ipsilateral subclavian vascular access; when subclavian vein stenosis is present, radiologically guided balloon dilatation and stenting may be possible. If these precautions are not observed, early failure of the fistula may result.

The preferred site for the fistula is 3 cm proximal to the wrist, in the nondominant arm; although some surgeons prefer a more distal anastomosis in the anatomical 'snuffbox'. The radial artery and the cephalic vein, with its branches, are marked (Fig. 1). The procedure may be performed using local, regional or general anesthesia. Regional block may assist surgery by producing vasodilatation. The patient lies supine, with the chosen arm resting on an armboard in abduction. The arm is prepared from the fingers to the elbow. The upper arm is covered with a small drape encircling the elbow, and the hand with a small drape encircling the wrist. The arm is then placed on drapes covering the arm-board, with the markings uppermost; large drapes are used to cover the remaining areas.

Figure 1

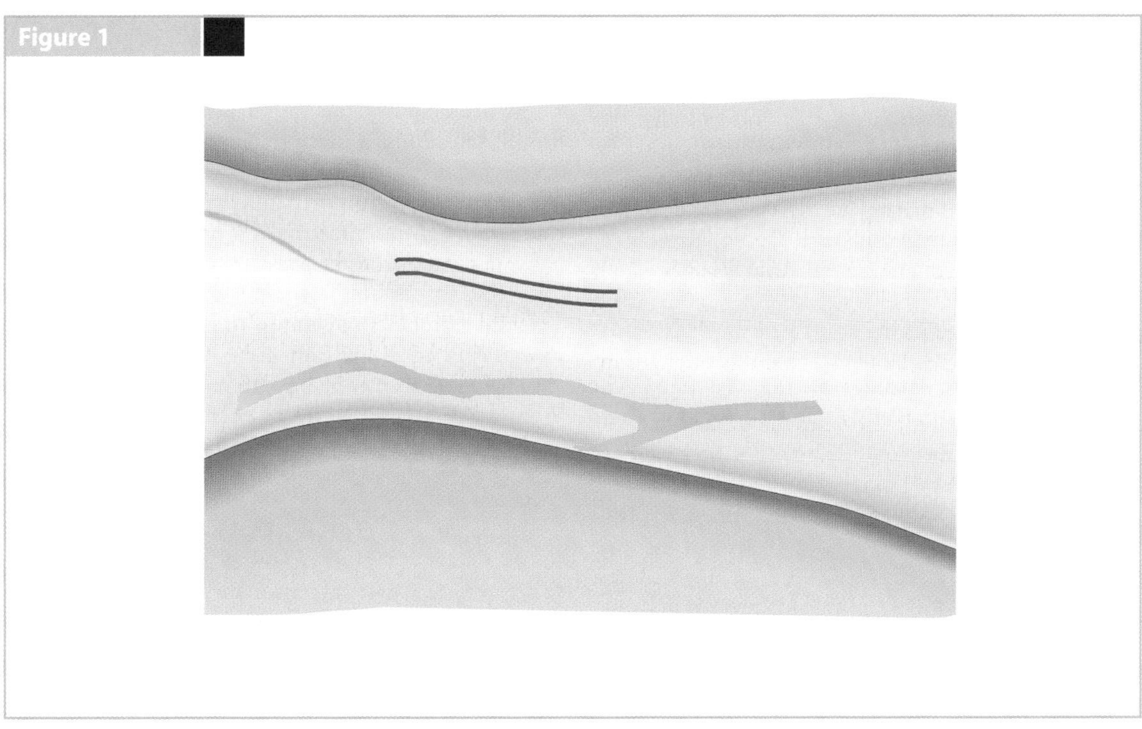

32

Figure 2

A 5-cm axial skin incision is made between the radial artery and cephalic vein, extending proximally from the level of the wrist. A smaller transverse incision may be used where the artery and vein lie together. The cephalic vein is mobilized from the subcutaneous tissue along the length of the incision, preserving the radial nerve. The deep fascia is divided along the length of the incision, and the radial artery mobilized. Small branches of the radial artery may be ligated in continuity with 4/0 silk, and divided. The vessels must be sufficiently mobilized to allow them to be drawn together for anastomosis without tension. The deep fascia is divided to such an extent that the vessels are not compressed by its edge.

Figure 2 shows the radial artery, that has been mobilized along a similar length. The deep fascia overlying it is divided in line with the vessel and will also require division proximally and distally beyond the length of mobilization to ensure that the uncut edge does not produce pressure or angulation. Small branches can be diathermied well away from the vessel with a bipolar coagulator, or the distal end can be coagulated after division. At a later stage a branch can be cut across at its base to commence the arteriotomy.

Figure 3

Bulldog clamps are applied to each end of the mobilized radial artery, and to the distal cephalic vein; valves should prevent backbleeding from the proximal vein. Alternatively the vessels may be controlled and occluded by encircling each end with double-loops of fine Silastic vascular slings. Heparin 50 units/kg may be given intravenously prior to occluding the vessels. At about 1 cm from the midpoint of the exposed portion of artery, a hollow needle is passed through its wall, advanced up to 1 cm distally along the lumen, and passed back out again. The upturned tip of a number 11 scalpel blade is engaged in the hollow needle-point, and these are drawn back together to create an arteriotomy. This can be extended to 1.5 cm in length with angled Pott's scissors if required. A similar technique is used to create an adjacent venotomy. The arteriotomy is typically made laterally, and the venotomy medially, so that the vessels have a natural lie when anastomosed.

The vein is flushed with heparinized saline: this often demonstrates a patent valve in the distal portion.

In Fig. 3, attention is directed at the vein and a similar technique is being used for the venotomy. The needle has been introduced on the medial aspect of the vein. The point has been advanced through the lumen, and extruded on the medial aspect distally. The point of a No. 11 blade is engaged in the hollow of the needle, ready for advancement and division of the intervening vein wall.

Figure 2

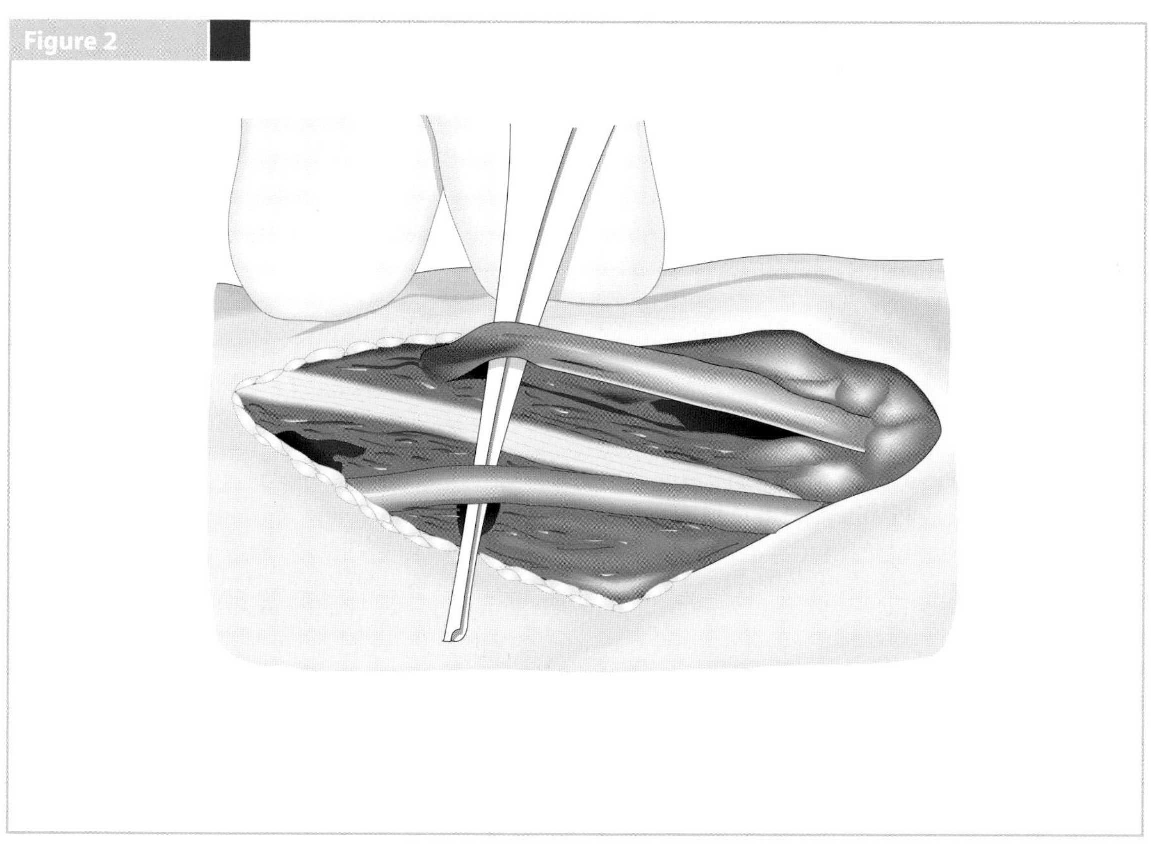

Figure 3

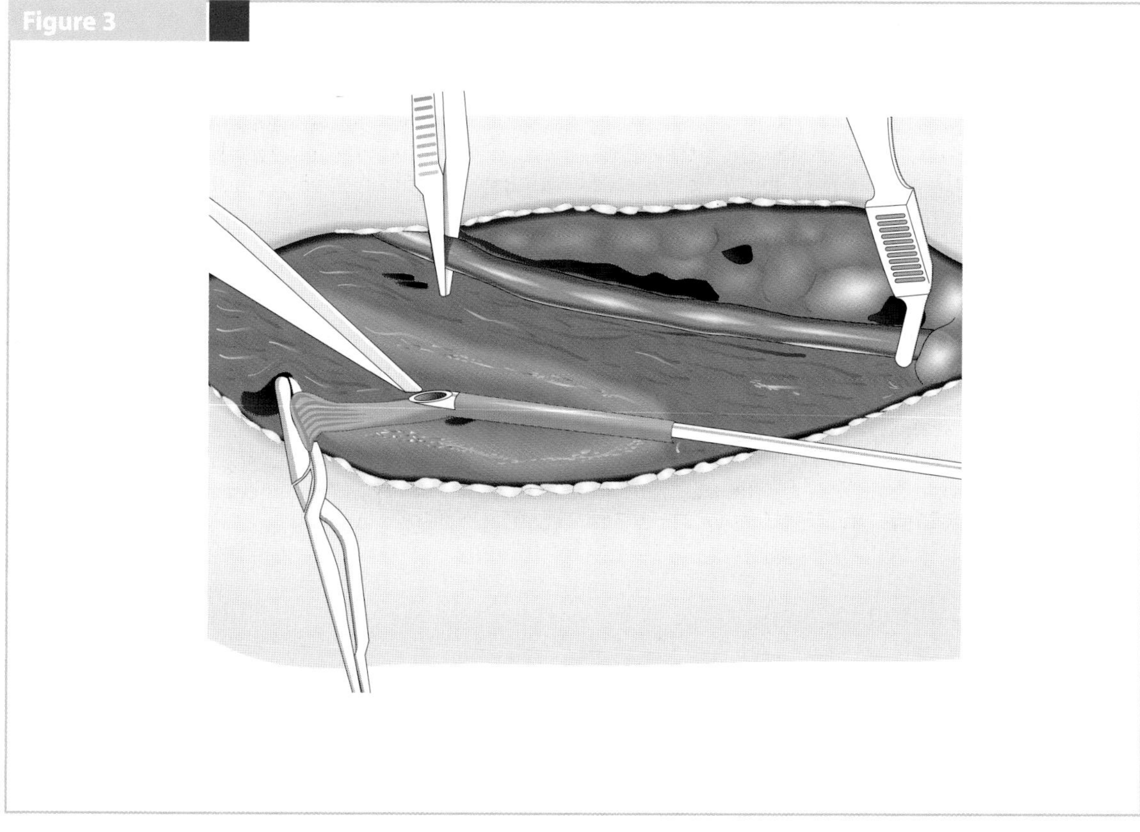

Figure 4

The side-to-side anastomosis is fashioned between stay sutures placed between the ends of the arteriotomy and venotomy. The anterior suture line is completed first, and the proximal suture tied to the distal stay. The anastomosis is rotated 180°, in whichever direction it most freely moves, by passing the stays beneath one of the vessels. The posterior wall of the anastomosis is then fashioned – just prior to completion, a probe is passed to check the adequacy of the lumen, and all vessels are flushed with heparinized saline. The anastomosis is completed, tying to the proximal stay, and tested by removing the distal venous clamp. The anastomosis is covered with a swab, and the clamps removed – the swab should be kept in place for 5 min to allow the suture holes to seal.

If an end-to-side anastomosis is preferred, the distal cephalic vein is ligated in continuity with 4/0 silk, and divided. The proximal vein end is prepared, and the anastomosis fashioned, as in a distal arterial vein-bypass procedure.

The vein is examined for constricting adventitial bands – which must be divided, and for compression at the divided edge of the deep fascia – which must be adequately incised. There must be pulsation in each arterial limb, and a thrill in the proximal venous limb – if not, the fistula must be reexplored via an incision along the vein, between the two suture lines. A probe may be gently passed into each vessel, and a 4Ch Fogarty catheter may be required to remove thrombus. The venotomy is closed with a continuous 6/0 Prolene suture. An intraoperative Doppler probe may be used to confirm good quality flow waveforms in each vessel.

Subcutaneous tissues may be closed with continuous or interrupted 3/0 Vicryl sutures, and the skin with continuous intradermal 3/0 Monocryl.

The wound is covered with a light dry dressing, or small occlusive dressing. The area is then protected with a Gamgee pad, lightly taped on the opposite side – but not circumferentially. As the patient recovers, the arm is nursed slightly raised on pillows. Hourly observation is undertaken for 12 h: to confirm the presence of a thrill and bruit in the cephalic vein immediately distal to the anastomosis; to identify anastomotic bleeding, as overt hemorrhage or wound hematoma; and identify ischemia of the hand. In all such cases, reexploration is required.

Figure 4

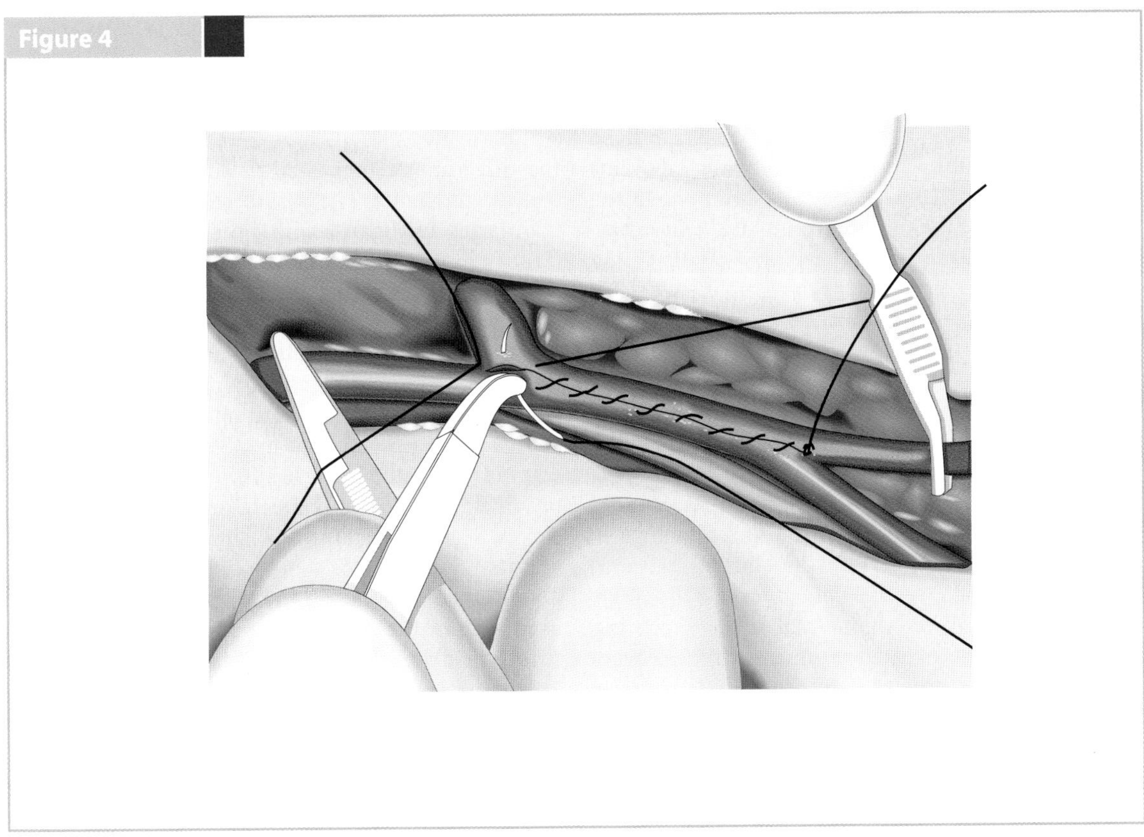

Figures 5, 6: Cubital Fossa Fistula and Basilic Vein Transposition

If preoperative assessment, or preference, is against formation of a radiocephalic fistula, access may be created in the cubital fossa. The cephalic vein, antecubital vein or basilic vein is anastomosed to the brachial artery. If the upper arm uphalic vein is patent by duplex ultrasound, a brachio cephalic fistula at the cubital fossa will provide the simplest access. If the basilic vein is used, it must be transposed superficially, as it lies too deep to allow easy puncture for dialysis.

The patient is assessed, anesthetized, and positioned in a similar manner to that for a radiocephalic fistula; except that Allen's test is unnecessary. Markings should indicate the brachial artery, and the cephalic, median cubital or basilic veins. The arm is prepared from the fingers to the shoulder region, including the axilla. A drape encircles the shoulder, and the hand is covered with a small drape encircling the wrist. The arm is placed supine, on drapes covering the arm-board, and large drapes are used to cover the remaining areas.

If the cephalic or median cubital veins are to be used, a transverse skin incision is made over the cubital fossa, and these veins are mobilized from the subcutaneous tissues. The antecubital vein is ligated with 3/0 silk close to the basilic vein, and divided. Flushing with heparinized saline may reveal valves preventing flow towards the cephalic vein – a dilator is passed to rupture these valves. If the cephalic vein is to be used, it is ligated and divided just proximal to the origin of the antecubital vein, so that the distal cephalic vein still drains to the basilic.

For basilic vein transposition, an oblique antecubital incision through skin, subcutaneous tissue and deep fascia is used to expose the median cubital and basilic veins, adjacent to the brachial artery. In this case, two further axial incisions are made along the upper arm, and a transverse incision in the axilla. Alternatively, a single long axial incision is used in the direction of the basilic vein, from the cubital fossa to the axilla. The basilic vein is mobilized, and tributaries are ligated with 3/0 silk and divided – a large tributary enters the vein at the junction of the middle and upper thirds of the upper arm. Finger dissection and forceps on a curved tunneler can be used to fashion a subcutaneous tunnel, from the deep aspect of the axilla to the antecubital incision. A small swab drawn into the tunnel ensures that it is adequate, and encourages hemostasis. The distal basilic vein is ligated with 3/0 silk, and divided. The free proximal basilic vein is drawn out of the axillary incision, laid in its natural orientation over the arm, and its upper surface marked with methylene blue. Long forceps passed via the antecubital incision are used to draw the vein into the superficial tunnel, ensuring that the marked surface remains uppermost. Valves prevent backbleeding, but a small bulldog clamp may be used to hold the vein in its correct orientation.

Figure 5 shows the toweling complete and the incisions marked. These include a transverse incision in the apex of the axilla, two longitudinal incisions in the upper arm, and an oblique incision along the course of an antecubital vein. The additional lines on either side of the latter indicate the position of the brachial artery. If a length of basilic vein is required from the medial aspect of the upper forearm, an additional incision is made. Figure 6 shows division of the vein distally and exterioration, with the addition of orientation marks. A subcutanous tunnel has been fashioned along the upper arm by blunt digital disection. A swab has been drawn into the tunnel to ensure there are no constuction residural bands and to provent hemostosis.

Figure 5

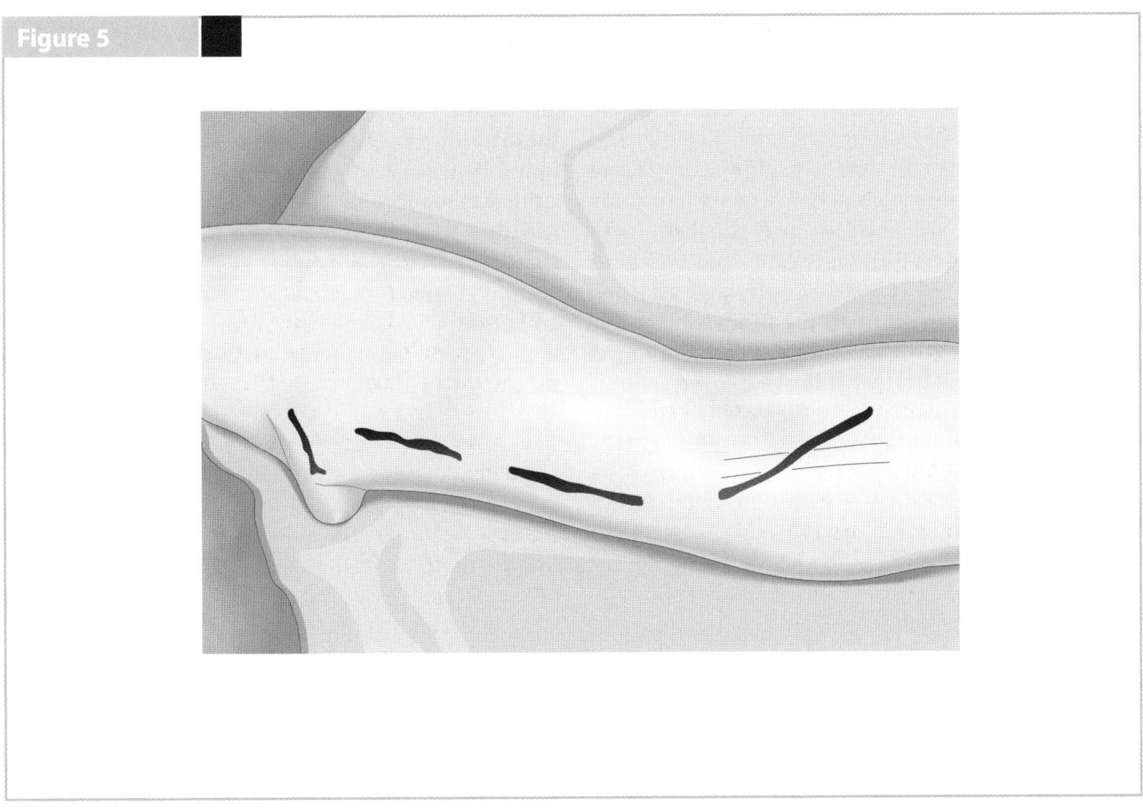

Figure 6

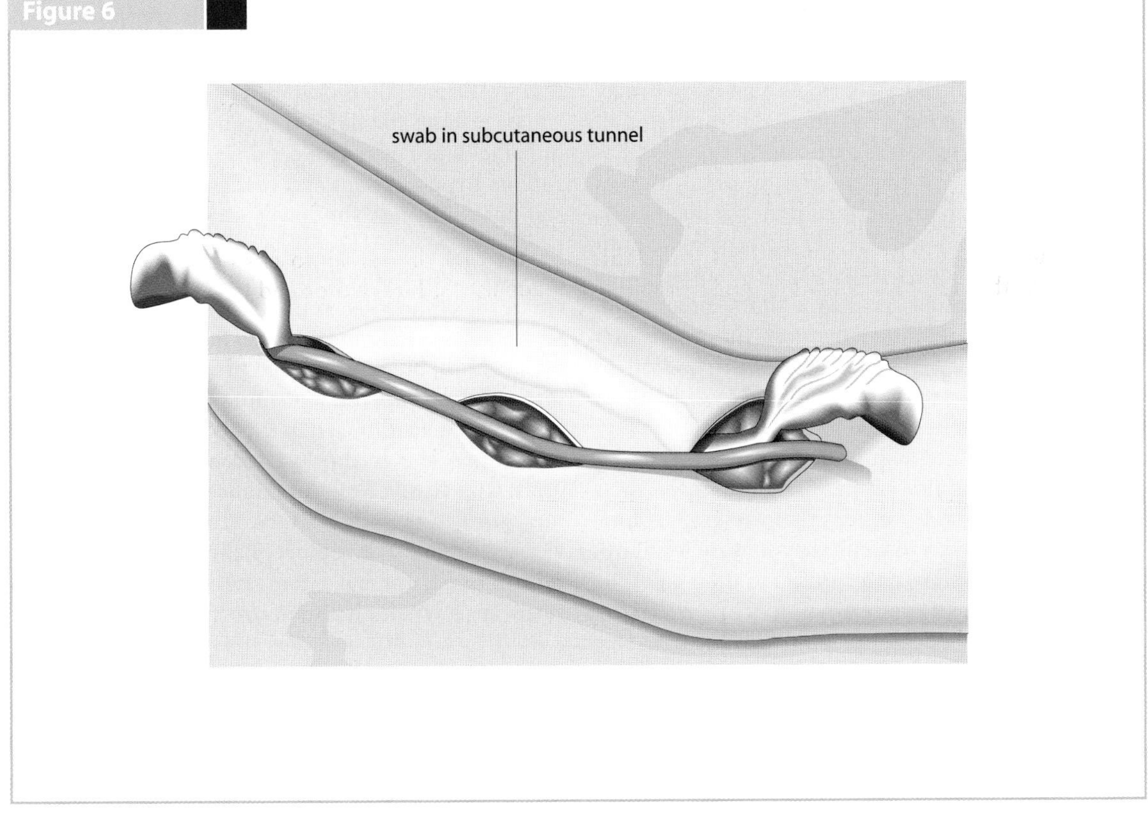

Figure 7: First Side of Anastomosis Completed

The brachial artery is exposed in the cubital fossa, incising the deep fascia longitudinally. The bicipital aponeurosis, and small veins crossing the artery, are divided. The artery is clamped, a 1-cm arteriotomy fashioned, and the vessels are flushed with heparinized saline, in a similar manner to that for a radiocephalic fistula. The basilic vein, still attached proximally, is drawn through the tunnel, using the markings to prevent rotation, to the incision in the cubital fossa. The distal end of the vein is incised axially on the side nearest the brachial artery, to match the arteriotomy. An end-to-side anastomosis is fashioned between stay sutures using 6/0 Prolene, in a similar manner to that described for the radiocephalic fistula. After completion and hemostasis, any constricting adventitial bands across the vein are divided, and presence of a thrill is confirmed in both distal and proximal basilic vein. Closure and postoperative management are similar to that for radiocephalic fistula.

Figure 8: Synthetic Graft Fistulae

Grafts have been used for salvage access for over a quarter of a century. In recent years, however, they have been more widely accepted as a primary procedure. The graft fistula overcomes the problems of inadequate forearm veins, particularly those of diabetic patients; these being the commonest group of patients presenting for dialysis in the United States. A 6-mm non-reinforced PTFE is the prosthetic graft of choice. It provides a large, uniform surface area that is easy to needle and has a short maturation. Saphenous vein grafts may be used, but harvesting requires an additional procedure and a period of maturation is necessary. They are more difficult to unblock, and are not proven to be of greater longevity than their synthetic equivalents.

Surgical technique is similar to that for lower limb synthetic bypass grafts, except that the graft is tunneled subcutaneously to facilitate puncture for dialysis. The vessels used vary according to their suitability and availability. Common patterns are: radial artery to cubital fossa veins, brachial artery to axillary vein, axillary artery to contralateral axillary vein, and femoral artery to femoral vein.

Lower limb fistulae are inconvenient, and have a high incidence of complications – particularly 'steal', venous hypertension, and cardiac failure from substantial shunting. The lower limb is therefore only used once all other access sites have been exhausted. An alternative to the lower limb synthetic fistula is to create a saphenous vein loop. The marked long saphenous vein is mobilized to knee level, as in a vein bypass graft, but left attached proximally. It is drawn into a curved subcutaneous tunnel over the anterior thigh, and anastomosed to the femoral artery.

Figure 8 shows the anastomoses of a synthetic graft, with fistula flow commenced. The distal anastomosis is to the ulnar artery. Proximally, veins previously used for a radiocephalic fistula have been reconfigured for an ulnar-antecubital graft. The Gore-Tex graft lies within a subcutaneous tunnel.

Figure 7

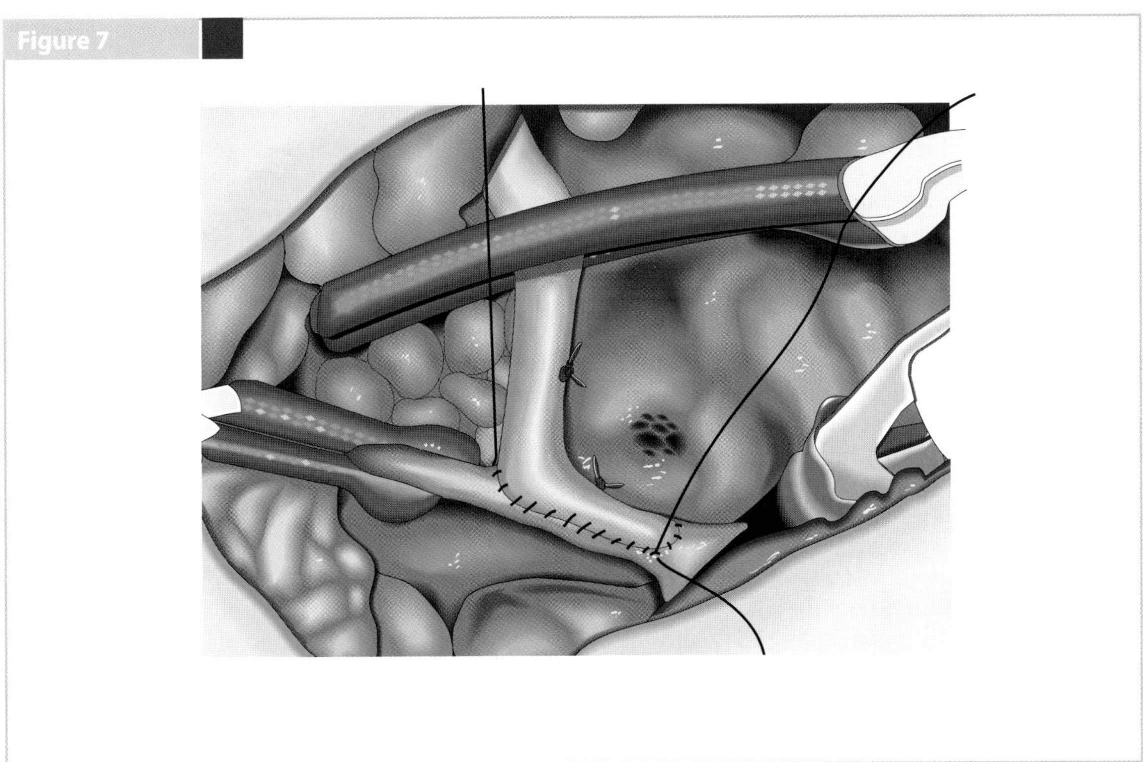

Figure 8

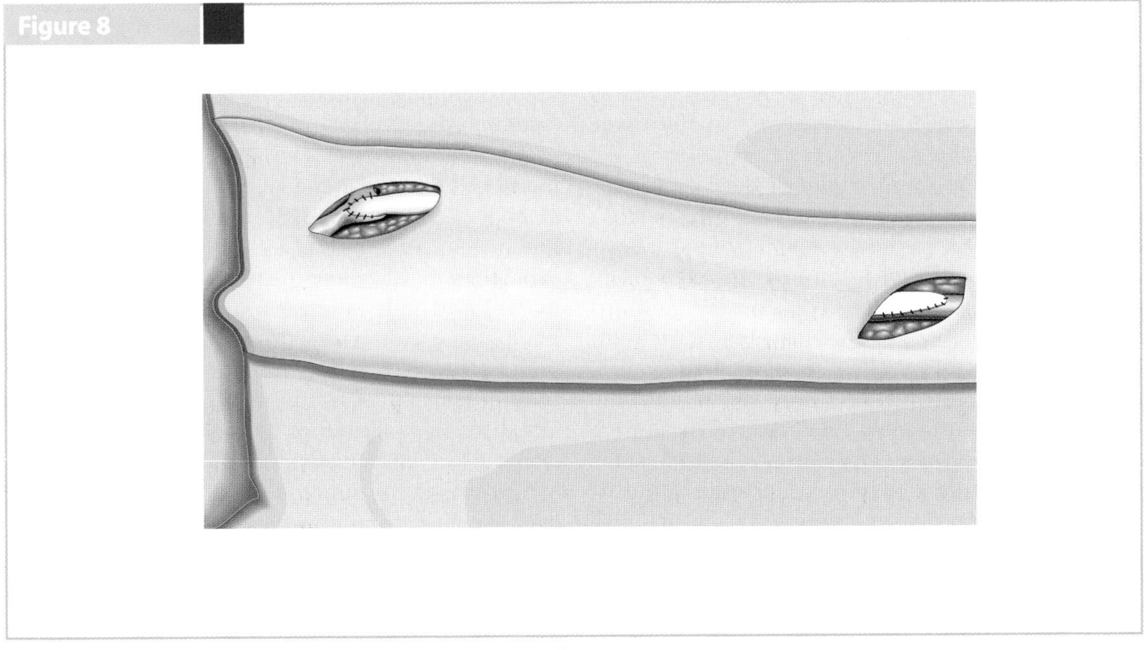

Figure 9: Hickman Line and Permacath

Synthetic lines for central venous administration of drugs (Hickman line), or for dialysis (Permacath) can be placed via a percutaneous or open surgical technique. Subclavian or jugular routes may be used, but there are preferential locations for each type. A Hickman line is best located in the right subclavian vein, as this is technically simplest, and lends itself well to a local anesthetic technique. Single lumen lines are less likely to suffer complications – a double lumen line should only be used where oncologists require simultaneous central infusions. A Permacath is best located in the right internal jugular vein; as when placed in the subclavian vein, these long-term catheters may cause venous stenosis, which results in the failure of any subsequent arm fistula. The right internal jugular vein offers a shorter, more direct route to the right atrium, than the left.

The patient is positioned supine. The right side of the neck and chest wall are prepared from the ear lobe to the costal margin, and out to the shoulder. Drapes are placed: over the right arm; over the left side of the chest; from the tip of the shoulder across the posterior triangle of the neck, to the right ear lobe; and from just below the nipple, to cover the lower body (Fig. 9). Air is expelled from the Hickman line by flushing all ports with saline. A local anesthetic mixture of 10 ml 1% xylocaine with 1:200,000 adrenaline and 10 ml 0.5% bupivacaine is used: 2 ml is injected subcutaneously at the tissue depression palpable just below the junction of the middle and lateral thirds of the clavicle; 1 ml is injected more deeply under the clavicle at this point – after drawing back on the syringe to avoid intravascular injection; and 2 ml is injected subcutaneously at the lateral border of the sternum, over the third intercostal space – the surface marking of the right atrium. The injecting needles are left in place to identify these points. A spinal needle is used to inject the remaining local anesthetic subcutaneously, along a line between the two points. The local anesthesia is supplemented with sedation, administered by an anesthetist with appropriate monitoring and maintenance of the airway.

The operating table is tilted head down to fill the veins. The guidewire needle is attached to a 5-ml syringe; free action of the syringe plunger is confirmed, and all air is expelled. An assistant reaches beneath the drapes, and pulls the patient's right arm caudally, to draw the shoulder out of the way. The needle is advanced through the skin at the junction of the middle and lateral thirds of the clavicle, in a horizontal plane, aiming toward the sternal notch. The syringe plunger is drawn back under gentle pressure throughout. If the advancing needle is arrested by the clavicle, it is withdrawn a little, then advanced again with a slight downward angle – it is safest to underestimate the degree of inclination, and come to rest against the clavicle, as too steep an angle results in a pneumothorax. When the subclavian vein is punctured, dark venous blood quickly fills the syringe – at this point the needle must be held perfectly still, and the syringe removed. Dark venous blood slowly drips out of the needle. Accidental puncture of the subclavian artery rapidly fills the syringe with bright red blood, and strong pulsatile bright red bleeding is observed on disconnection. The needle should then be removed, and pressure applied with swabs above and below the clavicle for 4 min, before reattempting venous puncture. If there is any doubt, a sample of this blood may be sent for gas analysis.

The guidewire is advanced through the needle, down to the right atrium, under X-ray screening – when just at the right atrium the guidewire tip is seen to move with the cardiac action. The guidewire needle is removed – the guidewire must not be drawn back with the needle in place, as this may strip off a layer of wire, and prevent subsequent removal of the guidewire. The exposed guidewire length is measured, and used to calculate the surface-atrial distance – commonly supplied guidewires are 50 cm long.

The operating table is leveled, and 1-cm transverse incisions are made at the guidewire entry point, and at the lowermost point of the anesthetized track. The line introducer is passed diagonally upwards to the subclavian incision, and the Hickman line is attached to the lower end, and drawn through the track. The implantable cuff is drawn through the track, and then back until it is caught by the subcutaneous tissues, at about 5 cm from the lower tunnel opening. The distal line is trimmed to the length of the calculated surface-atrial distance.

The plastic introducer-sheath is carefully passed over the guidewire, and the guidewire is removed. The Hickman line is pushed through this sheath, as far as is possible. The introducer-sheath is then split, and withdrawn – whilst maintaining constant finger-pressure at the entry point, to avoid accidentally withdrawing the Hickman line. The remaining protruding kink in the Hickman line is pushed down with forceps. A 10-ml syringe of heparinized saline is used to check the patency of each lumen – by first drawing back a little, and then flushing. The final

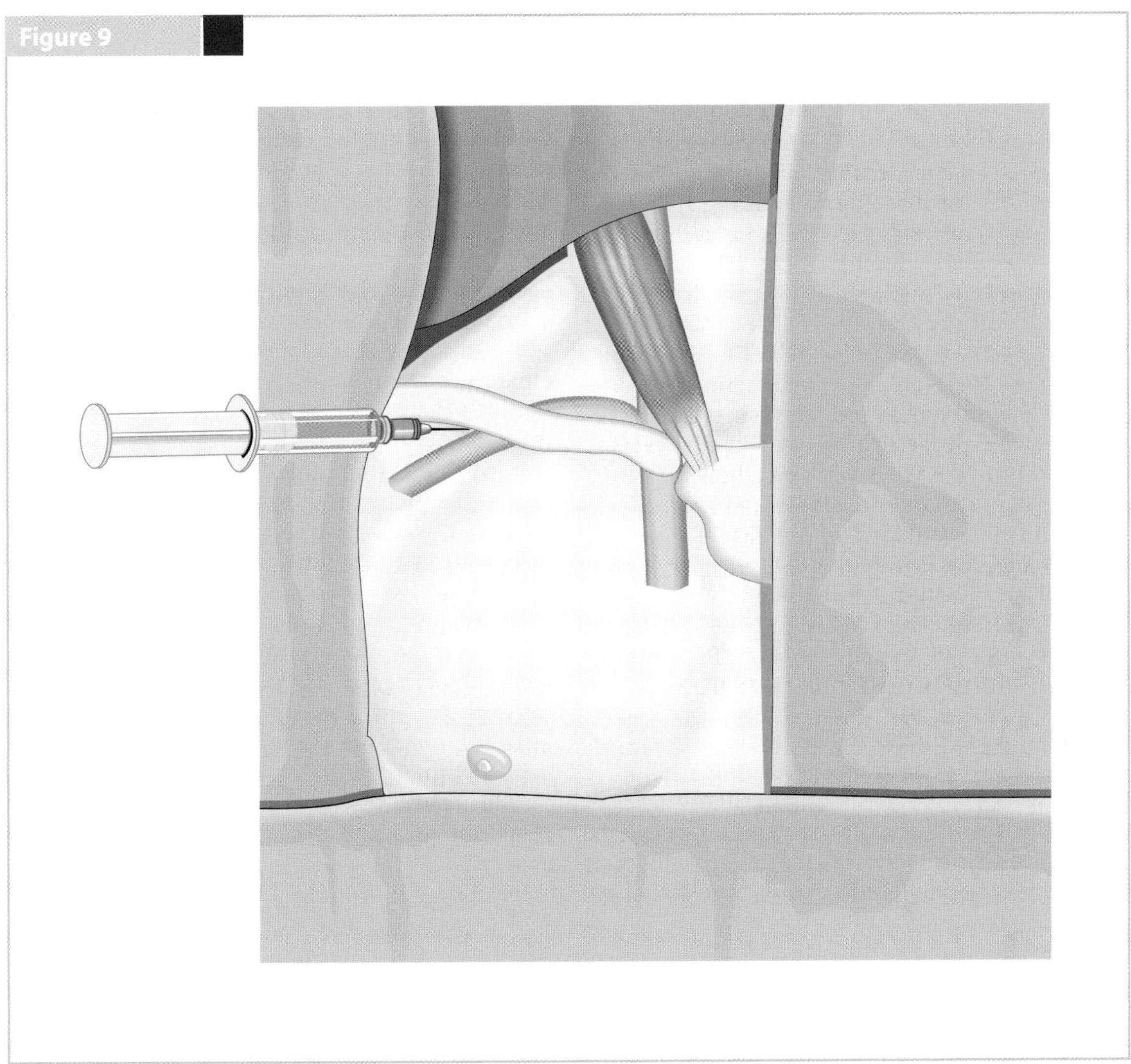
Figure 9

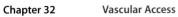

Figure 9: Hickman Line and Permacath (continued)

position of the line is confirmed by X-ray screening – the tip should lie just in the right atrium. The subclavian incision is closed with a single 4/0 nylon suture, and the line is secured at the tunnel entry with a 'roman-sandal' style 2/0 silk suture. Extreme care must be taken not to puncture the line with the suture or forceps.

For a Permacath, or a Hickman line, when a jugular location is preferred, the guidewire needle is introduced in a similar manner between the sternal and clavicular heads of the sternomastoid muscle. An ultrasound device may be used to locate the jugular vein; this can be made more prominent by asking the patient to perform a Valsalva maneuver. The tunnel is made directly upward to this point, but the remainder of the procedure is identical.

When a patient has had multiple previous Hickman lines, or where the facility for percutaneous insertion is not available, an 'open' approach may be used. The procedure uses identical preparation and position to that described above, and may be performed with the patient under general or local anesthesia. A 2.5-cm transverse incision is made over the divergence of the sternal and clavicular heads of the sternomastoid muscle, and extended through the subcutaneous tissue and platysma. A small, blunt artery clip is used to dissect deeply, by gently opening it in a longitudinal plane, gradually working down each side of the jugular vein. A small angle artery clip is used in a similar manner to free the underside of the vein, and separate it from the vagus nerve. Great care must be taken, as a posterior tear in the vein is difficult to deal with. In the event of a venous tear, bleeding should be immediately controlled by pressure, the area swabbed dry, and packed with a small swab for 4 min. Small tears self-seal, but others may require repair with 6/0 Prolene.

Two Silastic slings are passed under the mobilized vein, and gently tensioned by clips on their ends, and allowed to hang over the upper and lower wound edges. The tunnel is created, and the line passed through it, as described above. In this case it is necessary to estimate the internal length of the line, and trim it accordingly. A 6/0 Prolene pursestring suture is placed in the vein, and an upturned number 11 blade is used to make a small longitudinal 'stab' venotomy in its center. Gentle tension on the sloops controls bleeding. Forceps are used to pass the line distally through the venotomy. The position of the line is adjusted under X-ray control, and the pursestring is gently tightened and tied. The procedure is completed in a similar manner to that for a percutaneous line.

CONCLUSION

Once established, an arteriovenous fistula gradually 'matures' as the vein dilates, and flow increases. It takes 4 months for a radiocephalic fistula to have sufficient flow to allow access for dialysis. Premature use may result in inadequate dialysis, from recirculation in a low flow fistula; or more importantly thrombosis of the fistula, from damage to the poorly developed vein. Synthetic fistulae may be used for access almost immediately, as soon as the local effects of the surgery have settled.

The radiocephalic fistula is preferred because it leaves most opportunity for subsequent access at more proximal levels, and adds to the duration of dialysis available to the patient. Technical success in appropriately selected patients may be up to 93% (Burkhart and Cikrit 1997); but many radiocephalic fistulae do not mature sufficiently for dialysis, or fail within the 1st year. Primary patency at 1 year may be as low as 54%, and at 5 years 36% (Dixon et al. 2002). Veins of less than 2 mm diameter are best avoided. Flow only reaches its peak when the vessel is more than 75% the diameter of the feeding artery. Debate continues as to the preference of side-to-side or end-to-side anastomoses. The former provides additional vessels, but is also more conspicuous due to the dilated veins of the dorsum of the hand.

The brachiocephalic fistula produces a higher initial flow rate, but a shorter length of needlable vein and a higher incidence of steal. The anastomotic opening should be less than 5–7 mm, an end-to-side anastomosis is fashioned to reduce the incidence of distal venous hypertension. The cephalic vein is usually chosen as the basilic is more deeply placed and difficult to needle; also the needles are less favorably positioned for patient comfort during dialysis. The alternative of superficial transposition of the basilic vein is more complex surgically, but may produce satisfactory fistula access and flow. Patency of fistulae at the cubital level is between 55% and 90% at 1 year.

Synthetic graft-fistulae have a longevity of 11/2–5 years, and a maximum 7 years. The graft may be placed longitudinally along the forearm, from the radial artery to the cubital vein, but the brachial artery is the preferred donor vessel, the prosthetic loop lying in the forearm or, with more proximal take-offs, the upper arm. Careful fashioning of a tightly applied tunnel supports the graft and allows early needling; successful 24–70 h needling has been reported without graft problems when acute dialysis was needed, the graft being placed under slight tension. Platelet aggregation and intimal hyperplasia are common findings at the venous anastomosis in PTFE grafts, and long-term monitoring is essential. Thrombosis and infection occur in 45% of patients within 2 years.

A dedicated vascular access team has a key role in the monitoring and documentation of fistula progress. Duplex surveillance of fistulae and early surgical or radiological intervention for stenosis of the vein may improve secondary patency by up to 10% (Berman and Gentile 2002).

REFERENCES

Berman SS, Gentile AT (2002) Impact of secondary procedures in autologous arteriovenous fistula maturation and maintenance. J Vasc Surg 36:367–368

Burkhart HM, Cikrit DF (1997) Arteriovenous fistulae for hemodialysis. Semin Vasc Surg 10:162–165

Dixon BS, Novak L, Fangman J (2002) Haemodialysis vascular access survival: upper arm native arteriovenous fistula. Am J Kidney Dis 39:92–101

Part VII Amputations

CHAPTER 33 Amputations

Kingsley P. Robinson, John Lumley

INTRODUCTION

Amputation is one of the most ancient operations and its principles were well documented by Hippocrates and his successors. In the dark ages, amputation stumps were treated with boiling oil to obtain hemostasis as knowledge of the ligature was lost to this era. Re-discovery of the ligature is usually attributed to Ambroise Paré; the extensive number of lower limb amputations in warfare and the skill of the army surgeons of the 18th and 19th centuries are legendary.

In the Western world, the past 40 years have seen a marked transformation in the indications for lower limb amputation, from those of trauma and infection to that of arteriosclerosis, the latter now making up over 90% of elderly patients attending limb fitting centers.

Vascular patients coming to amputation are frequently old and may also be suffering the cardiac and cerebrovascular consequences of their disease. Hypertension and diabetes frequently coexist. The patients are almost always smokers and respiratory problems are common, while the limb disease may have associated infection, and knee and hip contractures. To combat these various problems, a skilled team of surgeons, nurses, physiotherapists, occupational therapists and social workers is required and, if possible, at least a few preoperative days allowed for full assessment of the patient and his or her home environment.

Vascular surgeons and their teams must be well versed in amputation techniques and ensure that their patients are expertly managed, as the disability produced by failing to attend to this aspect of vascular disease can outweigh the benefits gained elsewhere.

A full explanation must be given to the patient for the need for the amputation and its consequences. The patient's acceptance is vital to subsequent management, although existing disability and the often long-term acquaintance with the surgeon means that this is rarely a problem. Similar discussions must be held with the patient's spouse and other relatives and carers to assess the degree of home support available.

Adequate pain relief must be given, and infection and diabetic problems controlled. Pressure areas must be meticulously treated as pain may restrict the patient's movements and endanger the skin of the buttocks and other leg. Preoperative physiotherapy is directed at respiratory problems and the assessment of the severity of any contractures, the patient's balance and the strength of their upper limbs. These factors and the presence and condition of the other leg influence future mobility.

It may be decided that the patient would be best suited to a wheelchair existence, and in this case a full home assessment is necessary. This includes consideration of the number of steps and stairs, the need for ramps, the width of doors and corridors, the need for rails, the flooring, the height of sinks, baths, toilets, cooking facilities, cupboards and light switches, and available transport.

When a postoperative prosthesis is proposed, a preparatory fitting is of value. Specialist procedures such as the application of an instant prosthesis bring the surgeon and prosthetist into regular contact. The surgeon must maintain close liaison with the prosthetist regardless of any physical separation of their respective institutions. In this way, they will remain aware of all new developments that could add to the comfort and progress of their patients.

The selection of a lower limb amputation site is influenced by many factors. In general as much length should be preserved as possible, aiming for maximum restoration of function. There is no adequate substitute for the patient's own knee, and a long length of limb improves leverage in a patient in bed or a wheelchair. However, there is nothing to be gained by preserving fixed useless lengths of limb or unhealed painful and potentially dangerous areas. Hip contraction of up to 10% can usually be catered for in a prosthesis, and occasionally knee flexures of up to 30%. In predicting likely healing, the state of the skin, the subcutaneous tissues and any surrounding infection are of major importance. Many indices of pressure, blood flow and tissue oxygenation are available, but difficult to interpret. If healing is in doubt it is worth trying a below-knee rather than an above-knee amputation, as healing is usually in the region of 70% and this increases with the experience of the surgeon. Bleeding and the state of the deep tissues can be assessed at operation.

The chances of walking with a below-knee amputation are at least double that of an above-knee amputation, but this also reflects case selection, as does a lower operative mortality. However, a second operation also has the affect of more than doubling the mortality. In an old and frail patient, with a short life expectancy, and who would be unlikely to withstand the second operation or carry the weight of a prosthesis, it is wiser to accept a wheelchair existence and an early hospital discharge by proceeding directly to an above-knee amputation.

The general morale of all patients must be carefully assessed and it must be remembered that 50% of the patients surviving a lower limb amputation for 5 years require amputation of the second limb.

OPERATIVE TECHNIQUE

The technique used in amputation surgery should equate to the skills needed for its vascular counterpart. Tissue should be handled with care and specific attention given to hemostasis and the precise apposition of cut skin edges. Speed is not usually a major prerequisite although it must be considered in elderly sick patients. Consideration must also be given to the control of diabetes and hypertension. Prophylactic antibiotics should be given to combat the risk of gas gangrene and additional culture specific antibiotics to treat overt infection. Major amputations are most conveniently carried out with the patient under general anesthesia but regional techniques may be applicable. Epidural/spinal anesthesia may also be continued as epidural analgesia, to control postoperative pain and to facilitate early mobilization.

Skin flaps should be measured and marked, with a waterproof marker; a piece of tape placed around the circumference at the amputation site can be folded in two to mark the equal anterior and posterior flaps. Deep fascia and muscles are usually divided at the same level as the skin. Bones are divided more proximally to allow muscle cover of the cut ends. Large vessels should be identified and tied individually; bleeding muscle may require underrunning sutures to control hemorrhage. Nerves are pulled down and cut transversely with a knife as far proximally as possible, to allow retraction from the wound edge, thus reducing subsequent neuroma formation. A large major nerve containing a vessel, such as the sciatic, may be ligated; this does not increase postoperative neuroma formation; phantom pains are unusual in patients with chronic vascular disease.

Bones are divided with an electric, flat bladed or a Gigli saw to provide a smooth cut surface; sharp edges are filed away. Bone cutters and nibblers are best avoided as they can fracture the ends and leave sharp edges. Periosteum, with its muscle attachments, is raised from distally to the line of the bone division, so that it can be used later to cover the bone end and help to secure sutures. Bone dust should be washed away and bone wax may be used to control troublesome bleeding from the marrow (but sparingly, as it can produce a foreign body response and sinus formation). Muscle is usually joined over the bone ends, retaining its length and power of leverage. This closure is referred to as myoplasty; myodesis, in which holes are drilled through the bone and the muscle bundles tied to it, promotes retention of their action. Drains can be avoided if hemostasis is good and infection is absent. This also avoids the necessity of disturbing any dressing for their removal after 2–3 days. When they are used, they should be fixed outside the dressing to allow removal without disturbing the dressing – this requires great care not to pull them out during closure. Skin strips can replace sutures, although ischemic changes are rarely referable to the latter.

Attention to amputation dressings is of vital importance, as they can compromise the viability of the skin flaps. They should not be applied under tension, and direct application of elasticated bandages must be avoided. Loose weave two-way stretch bandage can be applied over wool, but heavy and one-way stretch varieties should be avoided. In the absence of pain and fever, a well-applied dressing is best left for 2 weeks at which time it is taken down, the sutures examined and, if satisfactory, stump bandaging commenced. Sutures are retained for 2–3 weeks.

Prophylaxis against deep venous thrombosis using low molecular weight heparin is advised until the patient is fully mobile. Skin care and chest physiotherapy are started immediately postoperatively. Stumps should not be raised on pillows, as this can promote hip and knee flexion contractures; epidural analgesia should be considered to facilitate hip flexion and quadriceps exercises after 24 h, followed by progressive mobilization in bed. After 2–3 days, the patient may progress to parallel bars and walking with crutches.

A pneumatic pylon can be applied to an asymptomatic stump after 3–4 days, but is safer left until 10 days; the first prosthetic fitting is done once the wound has healed. It is essential for the patient to receive skilled prosthetic management, particular care being required of a recent wound. Early fitting, the most advantageous being in theater at the completion of the amputation, is practiced in some centers; success requires a skilled team to monitor progress and recognize any complications.

Amputations for vascular problems are more liable to break down than those undertaken in younger patients for trauma. Patellar-tendon bearing prostheses require particular care, appropriate weight distribution being necessary to prevent irreversible damage of a new amputation stump.

During rehabilitation, attention is given to the development of the muscles of the other leg, the trunk and upper limbs. Healing may be delayed in a third of below-knee vascular amputations, and early excision of obvious major ischemic areas and hematoma is advised, as is debridement to accelerate healing and early discharge from hospital.

Figures 1, 2: Toe Amputation

When amputating a toe in a patient with peripheral vascular disease, toe blood pressure should be at least 40 mmHg. As much length should be preserved as possible. A circumferential incision should be made around the toe, avoiding fish-mouth incisions as these may further interfere with flap blood supply. Extension of incisions onto the dorsum of the foot must also be avoided whenever possible. Bones are divided through the neck or the body of the phalanx, nibbling away bone to allow tension free anteroposterior closure of the skin; cartilage is best avoided at the end of the stump. Anteroposterior skin closure may be with sutures or skin tapes to provide apposition without tension.

In the case of the great toe, whenever possible the metatarsophalangeal joint should be preserved as this improves stability when walking. When the underlying lesion is vasculitis, diabetic neuropathy, trauma or the patient has undergone revascularization, the blood supply of the flap is less critical and the amputation follows the line of infection or necrosis.

Figure 1 shows circumferential incision excising the gangrenous tip. The tendons have been pulled down, cut as short as possible and allowed to retract. The bone has been divided through the neck of the proximal phalanx, a nibbler is being used to remove the head of this bone. Cartilage is best avoided at the base of these amputations.

Figure 2 shows anteroposterior closure of the wound with skin tapes. Interrupted nylon sutures are equally effective, but tapes are preferred if there is any ischemia of the skin edges.

Figure 3: Ray Amputation

When infection passes along one of the tendon sheaths into the sole or involves the bone of a metatarsal ray, ray excision is appropriate, as healing is possible by secondary intention. Such an amputation is inappropriate in the ischemic foot. Careful attention must be given to foot supports and footwear, as with all neuropathic feet the patients must be taught to inspect the foot directly and with a mirror each day for areas of redness and ulceration. If the patient's eyesight does not allow this, it must be carried out by another party. Focal infection of the head of a metatarsal may be excised through a small dorsal incision, and any penetrating ulcers on the sole excised, allowing through and through drainage without a full ray incision.

Figure 3 shows ray excision of the second and third toes; healing is aided by the application of a split skin graft. Skin may be taken at the time of the ray excision and laid on after 3 or 4 days, as in this patient, although if infection has been totally excised, and there is no residual inflammation, skin may be laid on as a primary procedure.

Figure 1

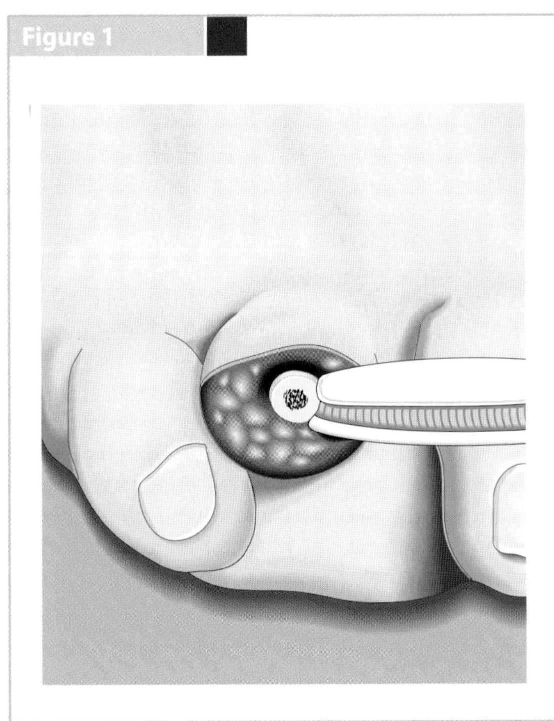

Figure 2

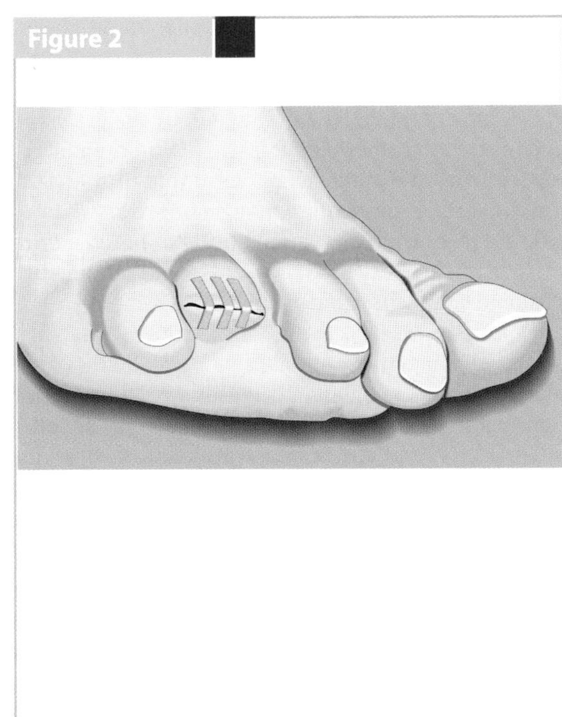

Figure 3

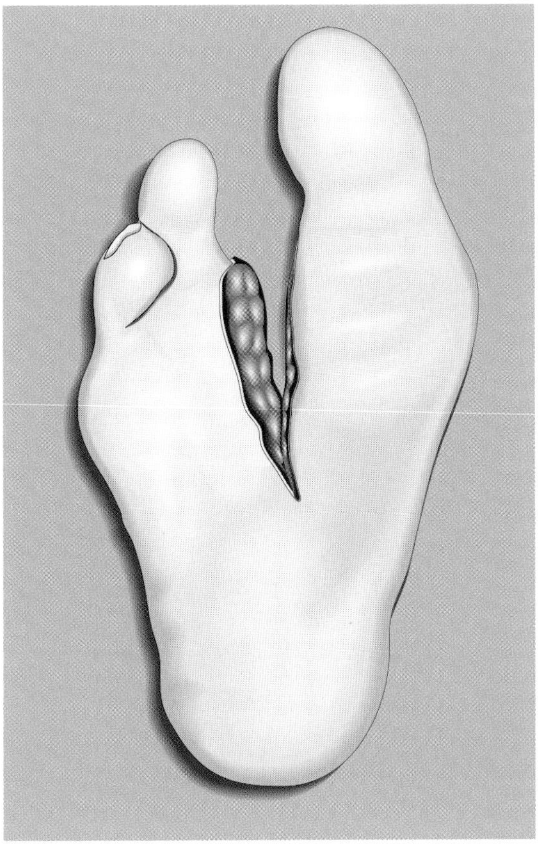

Figures 4–8: Transmetatarsal Amputation

When infection involves all the toes, or the great toe and most of the other toes, it is usually more satisfactory to proceed to transmetatarsal amputation. Again proximal revascularization may be necessary to provide an adequate blood supply for healing. The dorsal incision is at the level of the neck of the metatarsals, and the plantar flap at the base of the toes. An electric or Gigli saw is used to divide the metatarsals, usually through the proximal shaft, care being taken to protect the skin flaps during this procedure. All non-viable tissue and infected tendons and sheaths must be removed. If residual infection is present, delayed closure may be necessary. The plantar flap is approximated to the dorsal and may need fashioning and debulking to allow accurate apposition. Precautions with dressings are as previously described.

When there is no marked ischemia, a guillotine procedure may be undertaken with primary skin grafting, or a transtarsal or Syme's amputation considered.

Figure 4 shows the dorsal flap being incised on to the necks of the metatarsals. In Fig. 5 the plantar flap is incised. The plantar fat pad and fascia are retained on the flap, and the incision passed deeply on to the heads of the metatarsals and then followed along the metatarsals to an appropriate level, usually the midshaft. Figure 6 shows a Gigli saw being used to divide the metatarsals through their shafts. Care must be taken to protect the skin flaps during this procedure. In Fig. 7 the amputation is completed and all non-viable tissue excised, while in Fig. 8 the plantar flap has been approximated to the dorsal, and is being retained by skin tapes. There is still some lateral bulging of the subcutaneous tissues, which will require an extra tape or suture. The plantar flap is slightly narrow in this patient, because of the line of ischemic demarcation.

Figure 4

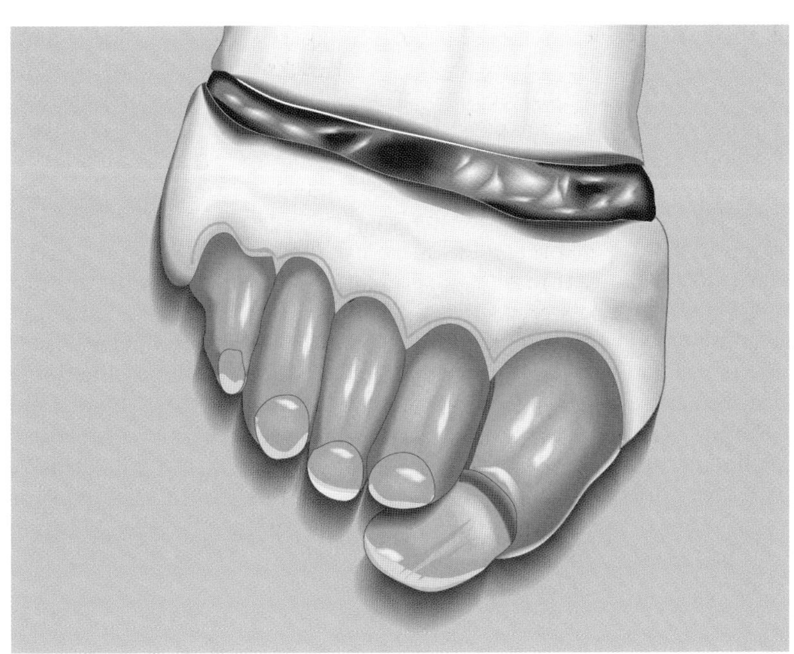

Figure 5

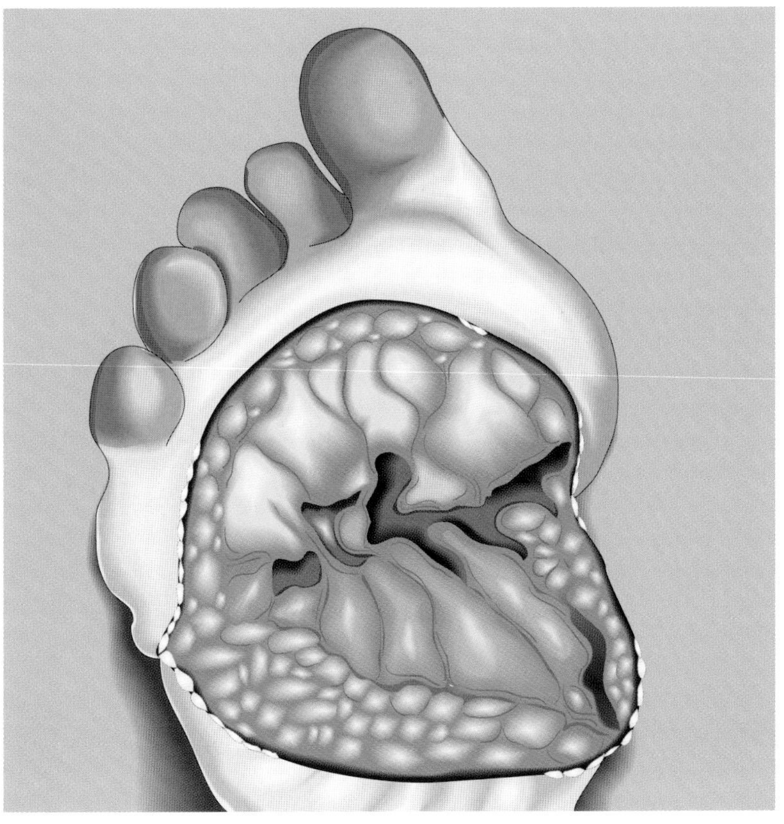

Figure 6–8

Figure 6

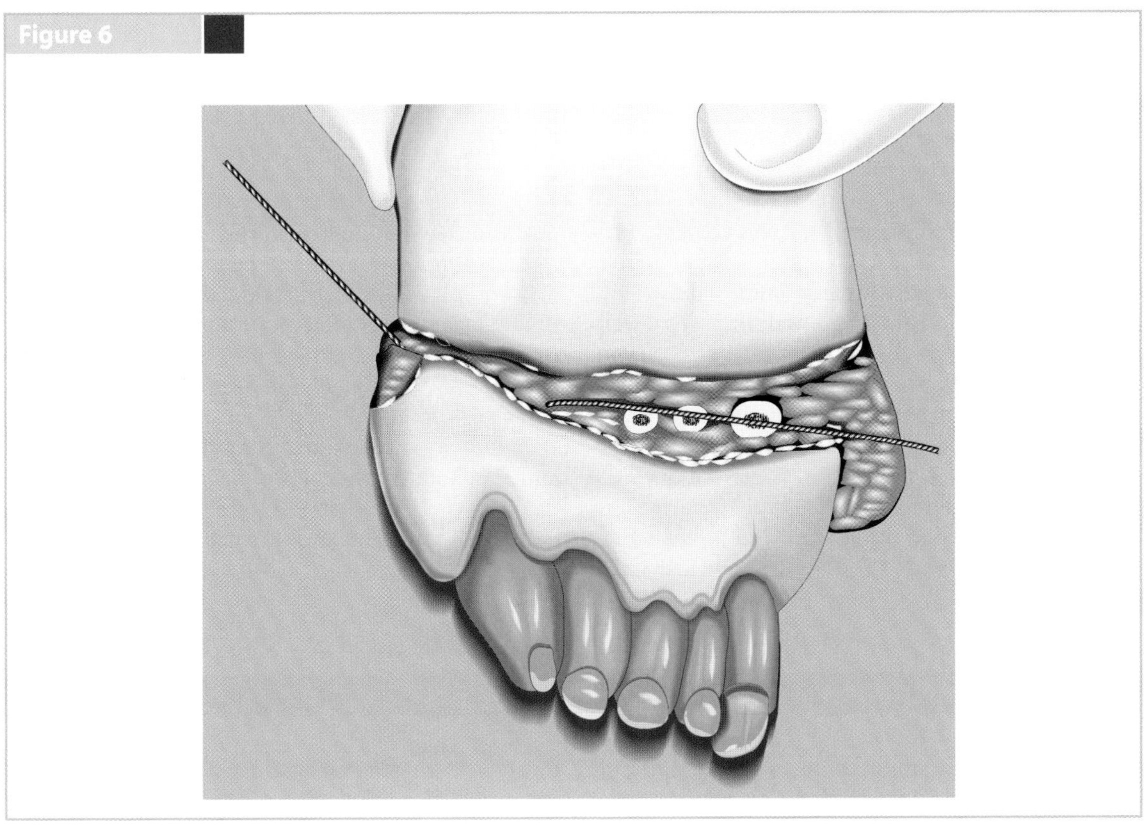

Figure 7

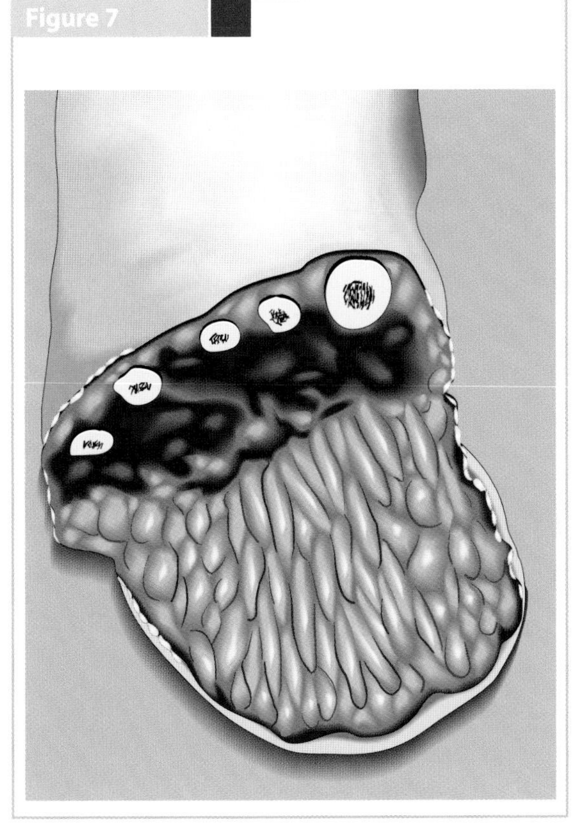

Figure 8

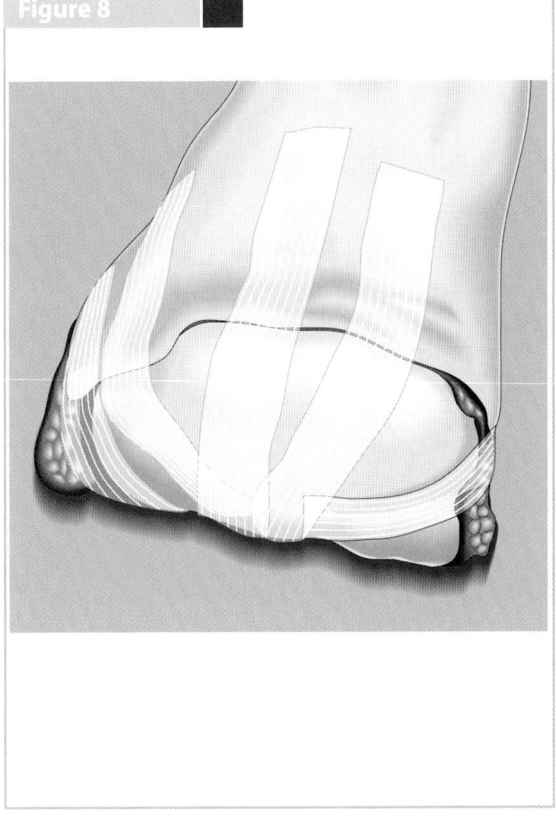

Figures 9–11: Syme's Amputation

A Syme's amputation retains the lower leg, which is of advantage in leverage and stability when in bed. Syme's amputation originally described an ankle disarticulation, but was later applied to removal of the articular surface and malleoli for end bearing. Providing a suitable prosthesis is difficult. Weight is concentrated on a narrow area, and stability and mobility may be no better than walking with a well-fitted below knee prosthesis.

A long plantar flap is required and this may not be possible in a vascular patient. After marking and incising the skin flaps, the extensor tendons are divided at the same level, the section is carried onto the ankle joint and the foot dislocated posteriorly. This exposes the lower end of the tibia and fibula, which are divided transversely through the bone just above the joint, removing the malleoli but leaving the maximal length of the tibia. Sharp dissection is used to remove the bones of the foot, staying close to the periosteum. A preferable modification retains the posterior few millimeters of the calcaneum, with the Achilles tendon attached, to be turned anterosuperiorly and placed over the transected lower end of the tibia. The anterior tendons are sutured to the plantar fascia followed by skin closure. In vascular patients healing can be slow. Figure 9 shows skin flaps for a Syme's amputation.

Figure 10 shows transverse division of the tibia and fibula above their lower articular surfaces, and through the calcaneum. Figure 11 shows the final boney configuration and skin closure.

BELOW KNEE AMPUTATION

Original below knee amputations used equal anterior and posterior flaps, preserving about half the tibia. Subsequent developments have come from both vascular surgeons and prosthetists. The former noted the adequate blood supply to the superficial calf muscles, even in severe ischemia, and the prosthetists emphasized the value of the short patellar-tendon bearing prosthesis, rather than long below knee leverage.

Figure 9

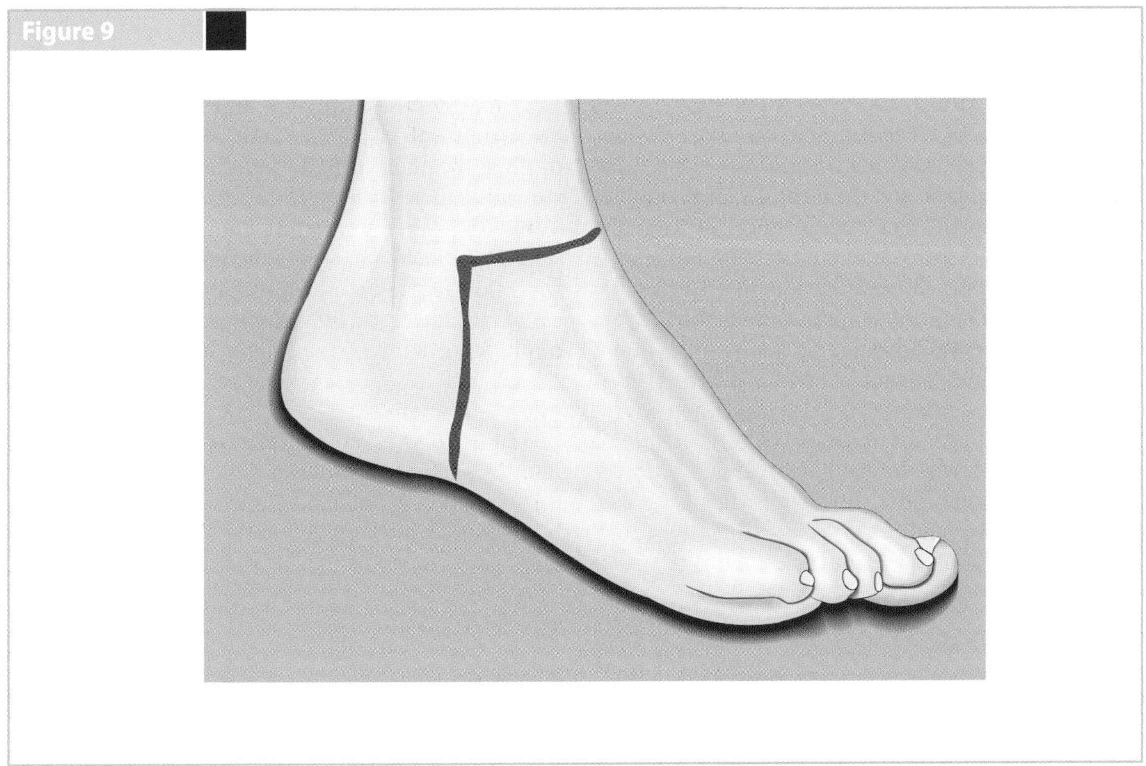

Figure 10

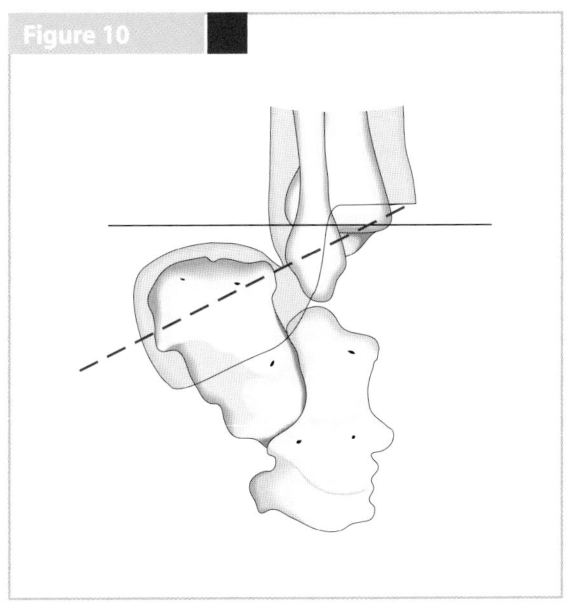

Figure 11

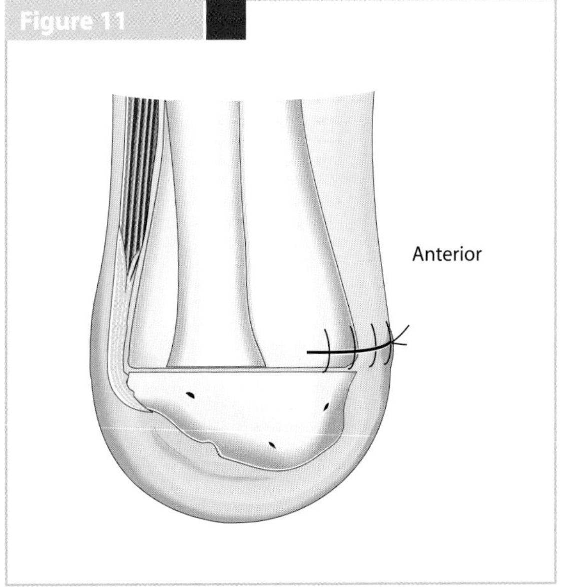

Figure 12

The long posterior flap, as advocated by Burgess, has become a much-used procedure in vascular patients. A double layer of wool is placed around the thigh beneath a tourniquet, and the ischemic limb double-wrapped and sealed. Skin preparation is from the upper thigh to the ankle. Accurate skin marking is necessary, as with all amputation procedures. Of prime importance is the length of the bone section, the skin flaps being fashioned to ensure subsequent tension free bone coverage. The anterior flap is 12.5 cm from the joint line. For a patellar tendon bearing prosthesis, 12 cm is the preferred upper limit of tibial length, but the prosthesis can be applied to stumps as short as 5 cm from the joint line.

Figure 12 shows toweling completed. The foot is sealed and its bandage tied, without towel clips. The leg is exposed; towel allows mobility and a cut-off: an assistant is able to lift the thigh without exposing unprepared skin.

Figure 13

The width of the anterior flap is a third of the circumference and a gentle curve is fashioned between them on each side. The anterior skin flap is incised onto the bone, transecting the anterior muscles onto the interosseous membrane. Anterior tibial vessels are ligated (the artery is often already occluded). The periosteum is divided at the level of the skin incision and raised, with its attached muscles, to the level of bony division.

In Fig. 13 attention is given to the tibial division. The periosteum has been divided at the same level as the muscle transection and stripped proximally with a rougine, so that the bony division is approximately 2.5 cm proximal to the muscles. The periosteum is preserved so that it can be used to take stitches in the subsequent closure.

Figure 12

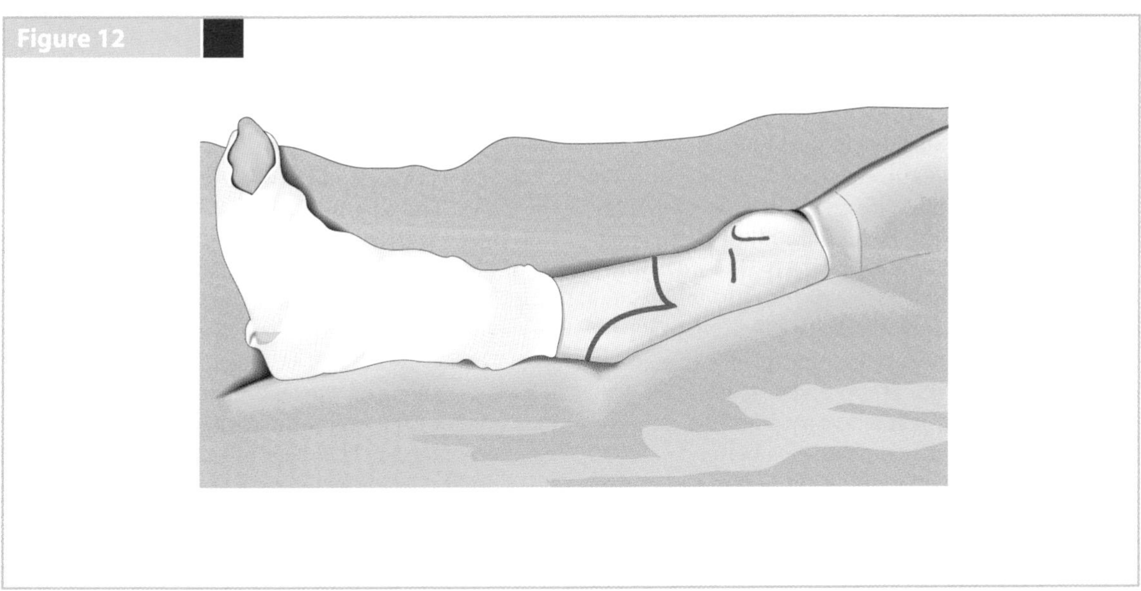

Figure 13

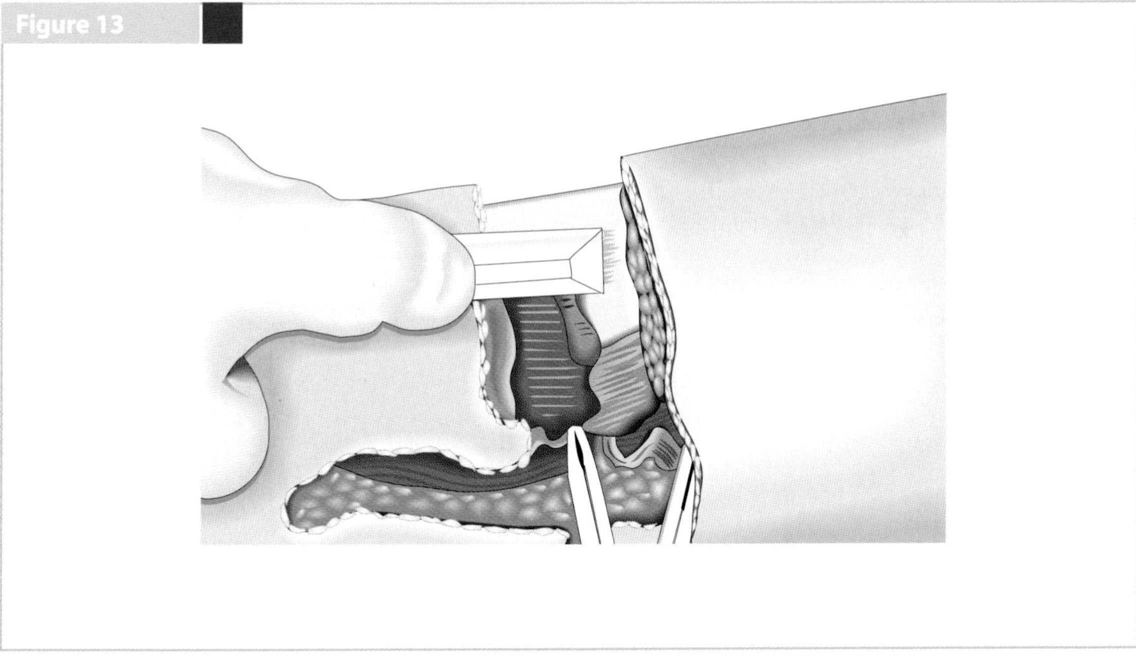

Figures 14–16

The anterior bevel on the tibia is conveniently first sawn at 45° through a third of the bone diameter and the bone then divided transversely, in line with the depth of the first cut. With an electric saw, however, it is usually possible to fashion the bone with a single cut. The fibula is divided effectively with a Gigli saw 1 cm proximal to the tibia. If osteoplasty is being considered, a piece of fibula is removed from the amputated limb and used to produce a bridge between the two bones. Sharp edges of tibia are filed free and the filings washed away from the amputation site. Meticulous hemostasis is obtained.

Figure 14 shows an oblique cut being made to remove the anterior sharp border when dividing the tibia. In this picture, retractors are being used to keep the skin clear of the bony transection, and the first saw cut is being made obliquely downwards through approximately a third of the cross-section at an angle of 45°.

In Fig. 15 the second saw cut is at right angles to the bone. The saw masks the initial oblique cut in this view.

In Fig. 16 the bony division is completed and the amputation completed. The gastrocnemius muscle has been divided at the same level as the posterior flap. The soleus muscle has been transected obliquely; it is seen lying on the tendon of the gastrocnemius and much of the bulk of its contribution to the calf has been excised. The deep muscles of the calf have been divided transversely at a level just distal to the bone, similar to the anterior group.

In this picture tension is being applied to the tibial nerve, which is being divided with a scalpel and will then retract away from the wound.

Figure 14

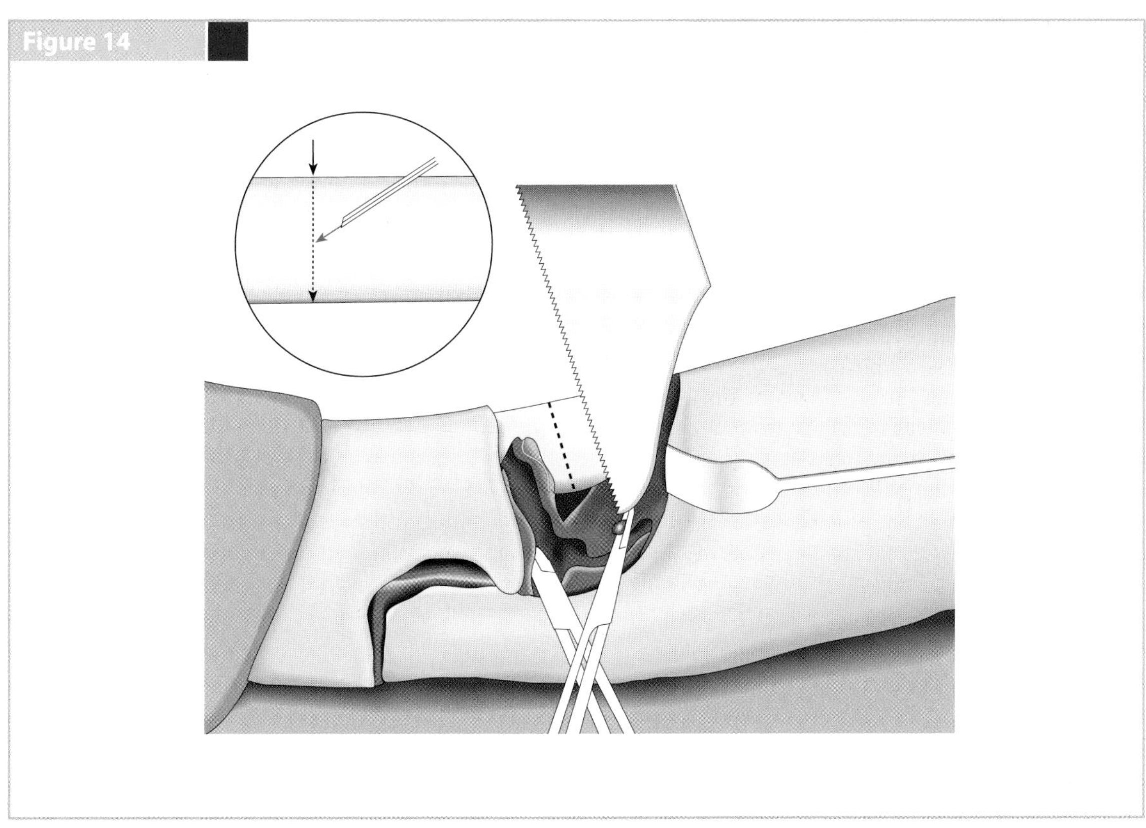

Figure 15

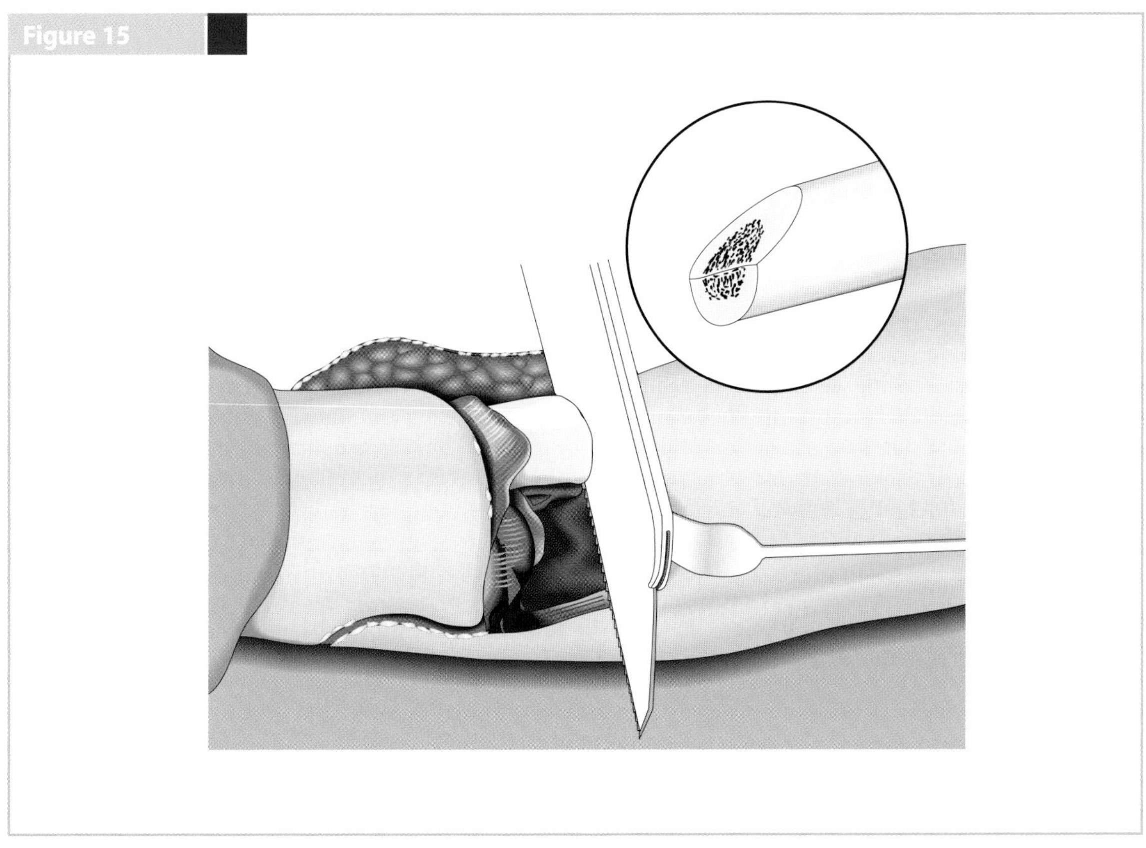

Figure 16

Figures 17, 18

The posterior flap is extended onto and through the deep fascia; gastrocnemius is divided at the same level. The soleus muscle is transected obliquely, or completely removed, as this reduces much of the bulk of the calf and facilitates closure. The deep muscles of the calf are divided at the level of the tibial division, posterior tibial and peroneal vessels are ligated, and hemostasis obtained of the soleal veins (often by underrunning sutures). Tibial and common peroneal nerves are pulled down, divided proximally and allowed to retract.

The skin edges are approximated, to assess whether this can be undertaken without any tension or whether further debulking of muscle is required. Great care must be taken with any skin fashioning never to cut across a skin base. A suction drain may be inserted if there is residual oozing. The drain may be left unstitched for ease of removal at a later stage but must be taped, and great care taken that it is not dislodged during subsequent closure.

In Fig. 17 once the amputation is completed and hemostasis obtained, attention is given to the ease of closure. In this picture the sharp rim of the divided tibia is being filed down. Attention is also given to the bulk and shape of the muscles, which will be closed anteroposteriorly. It may be necessary to remove more of the soleus from the deep surface of the gastrocnemius and attention is given to the shape of the skin flaps. The edges of the posterior flap can be reduced but great care must be taken never to cut across its base.

Figure 18 illustrates the completed amputation showing the anterior crural and deep posterior calf muscles transected at the level of the bone. The gastrocnemius muscle is preserved, but the bulk of the soleus has been excised to reduce bulk while still retaining the important collateral vessels through the gastrocnemius and between the bellies of these two muscles. The skin is being pulled proximally to show the transection of the bone, with the anterior tibial spine cut obliquely and the edges filed. Sawdust and bone filings have been washed away to avoid any areas of subsequent calcification in the superficial tissues. The periosteal rim is seen around the bone. The fibula in this case has been divided at a more proximal level.

Figure 16

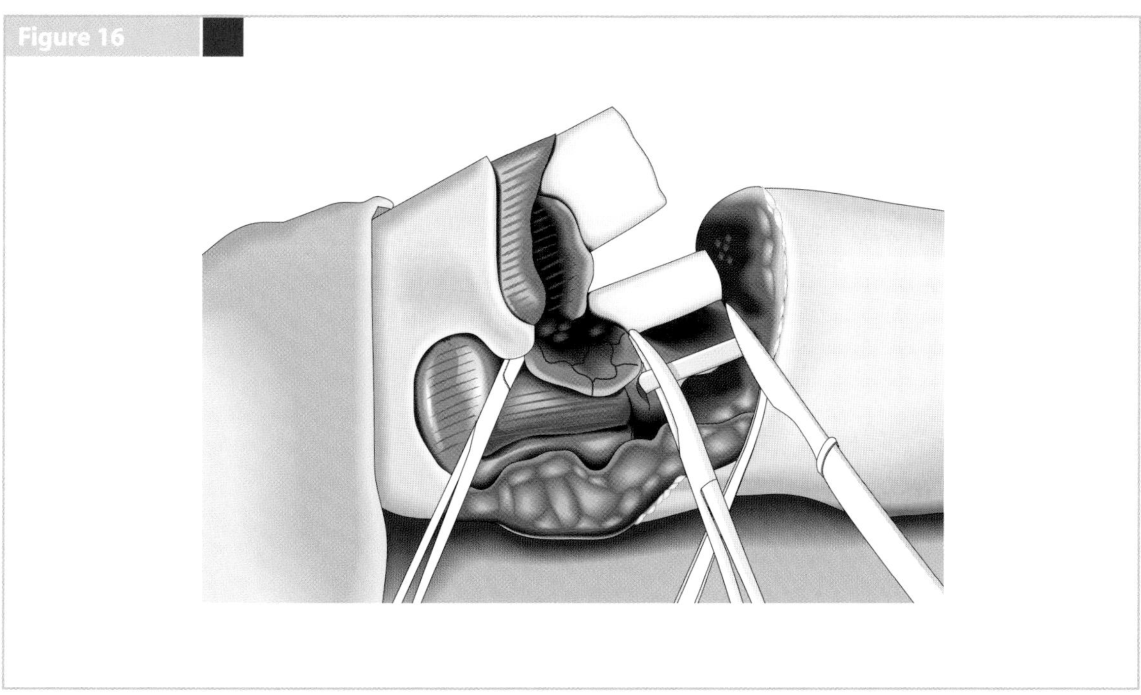

Figure 17

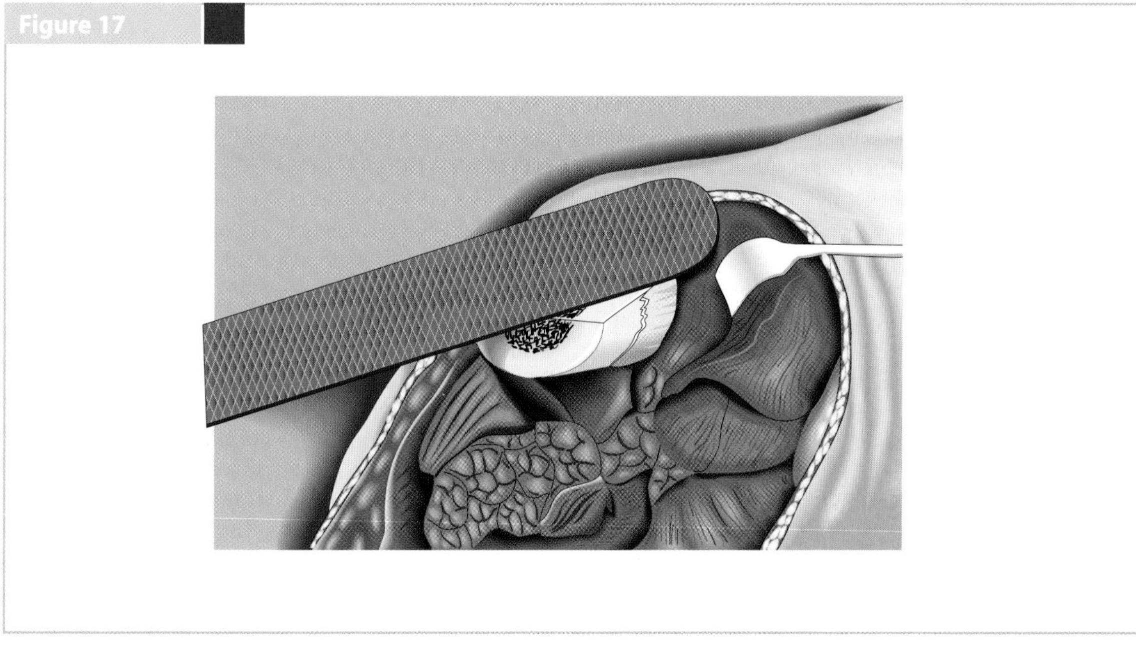

Figure 18

Figures 19–21

The gastrocnemius is sutured to the anterior crural muscles, periosteum and the interosseous membrane, with interrupted mattress sutures. Suturing the anterior and posterior layers of the deep fascia completes deep closure. No subcutaneous layer is required but meticulous apposition of the skin is necessary with suture or skin tapes.

Figure 19 shows the anteroposterior closure. A few stitches have already been placed in the soleus, tacking it to the periosteum on the front of the tibia, and now the fascia on the deep surface of the gastrocnemius is being sutured to the deep surface of the anterior crural muscles and the interosseous membrane. Interrupted mattress sutures of an 0 absorbable suture are being applied.

In Fig. 20 the muscle closure proceeds more superficially. In this picture the deep fascia over the calf is being sutured to the deep fascia over the anterior crural muscles.

Figure 21 shows the closure completed; the deep fascia has been sutured anteroposteriorly. No subcutaneous layer has been used in this patient, but interrupted mattress and plain sutures of monofilament nylon have been applied to the skin. Skin tapes may be used. No stay suture has been applied to the drain, which can therefore be removed in the early postoperative period without taking the dressings down. When this technique is used, however, care must be taken not to pull the drain out when applying the dressing.

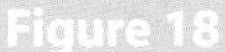
Figure 18

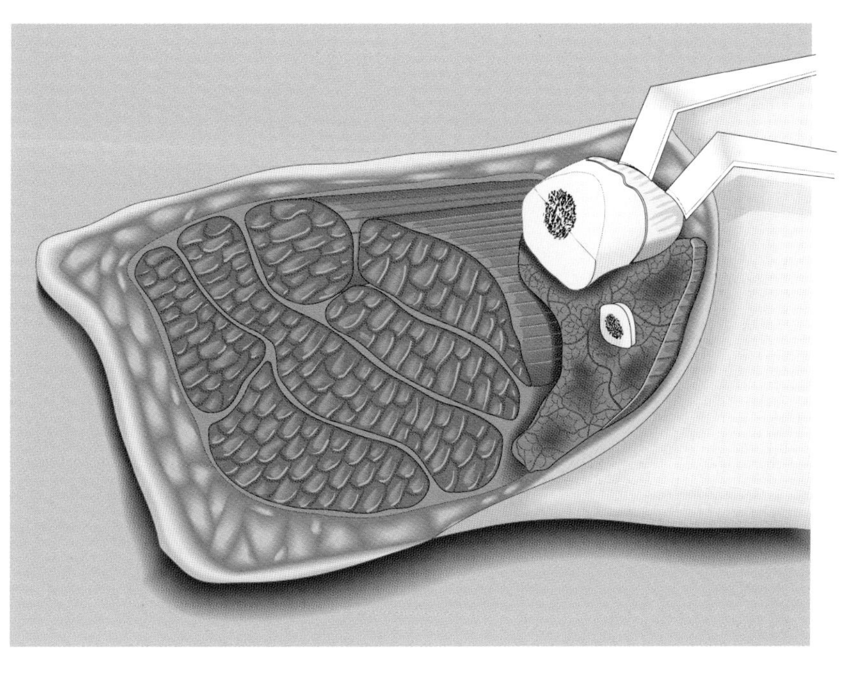

Figure 19

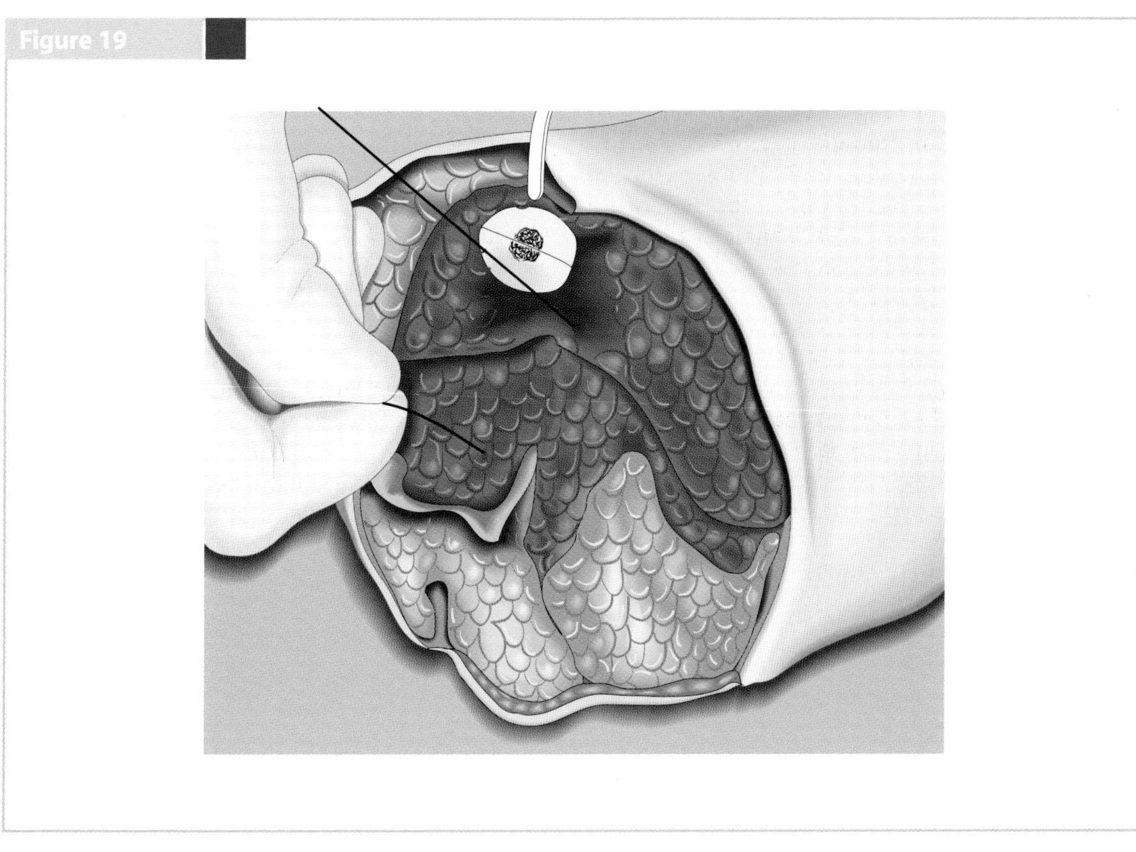

Figure 20, 21

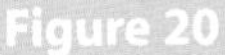

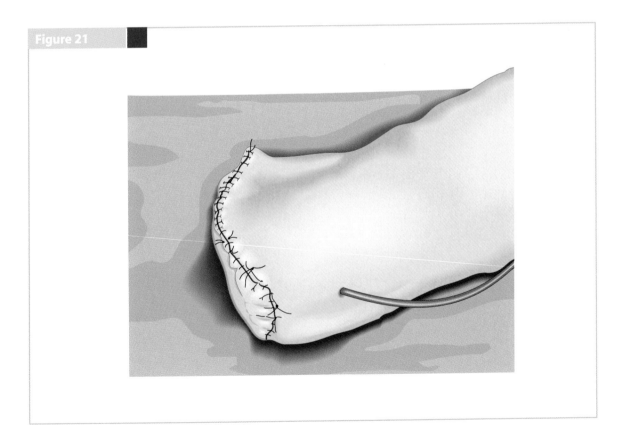

Figure 20

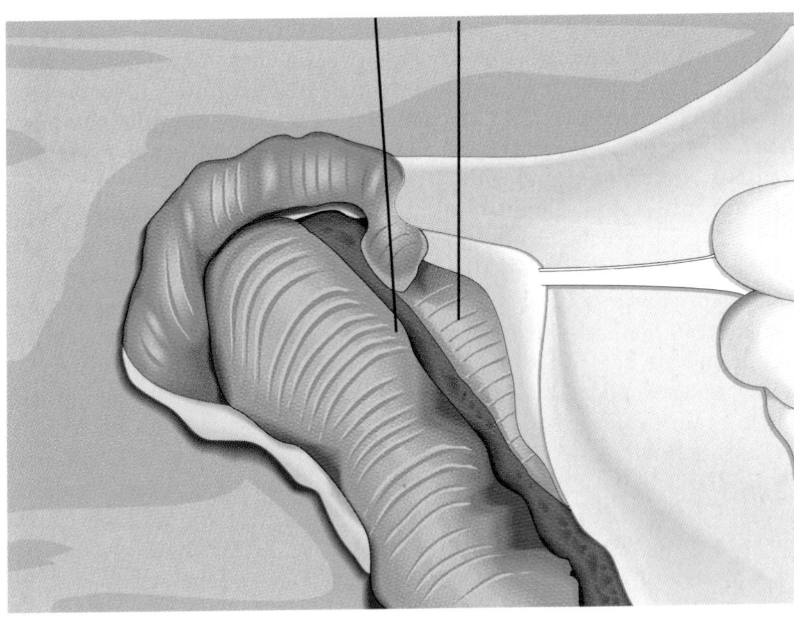

Figure 21

Figures 22–24

The dressing is applied (Fig. 22) with a generous application of wool (Fig. 23), and light two-way stretch bandage, followed by a second layer of wool and bandaging, to ensure uniform support without compromising the residual circulation. Figure 24 shows the completed stump bandaging. Bandaging is of particular importance in ischemic amputations, as excessive pressure may prejudice the viability of skin flaps. A loosely applied dressing may allow edema of the operation site, accentuated by any constriction at the level of the knee joint. Similarly, removal of the dressing on the 4th and 5th day will allow sudden edema of the stump, and reapplication of the dressing at this time can again cause constriction at the level of the knee, and endangers the viability of the flaps. Generally, the dressing, if well applied, can be left for 10 or 12 days. The drain can be pulled out on the 4th or 5th day without interfering with the dressing. Skin sutures are removed at 14–20 days. Burgess advocated the application of a plaster of Paris backslab or complete plaster over the dressing, leaving it undisturbed for 3 weeks.

In the absence of progressive pain or unexplained pyrexia, dressings should be left until healing is anticipated. A number of further alternatives have been advocated, for example exposure of the stump within an intermittent positive pressure device. A simple alternative is to place a thin single dressing over the wound with no bandaging. Although this allows initial edema, there is no risk of compromising the blood supply at the knee level, and the progress of the stump can be monitored more closely. This technique provides a safe alternative for the inexperienced as well as the experienced surgeon. Attention must be given to maintaining an extended knee joint, and early gentle active movement is encouraged. The single amputee who is physically capable should walk early on crutches. Use of the knee in a pneumatic device for walking can be considered after 10 days, when there are no signs of infection or ischemia, and the wound looks stable.

Figure 22

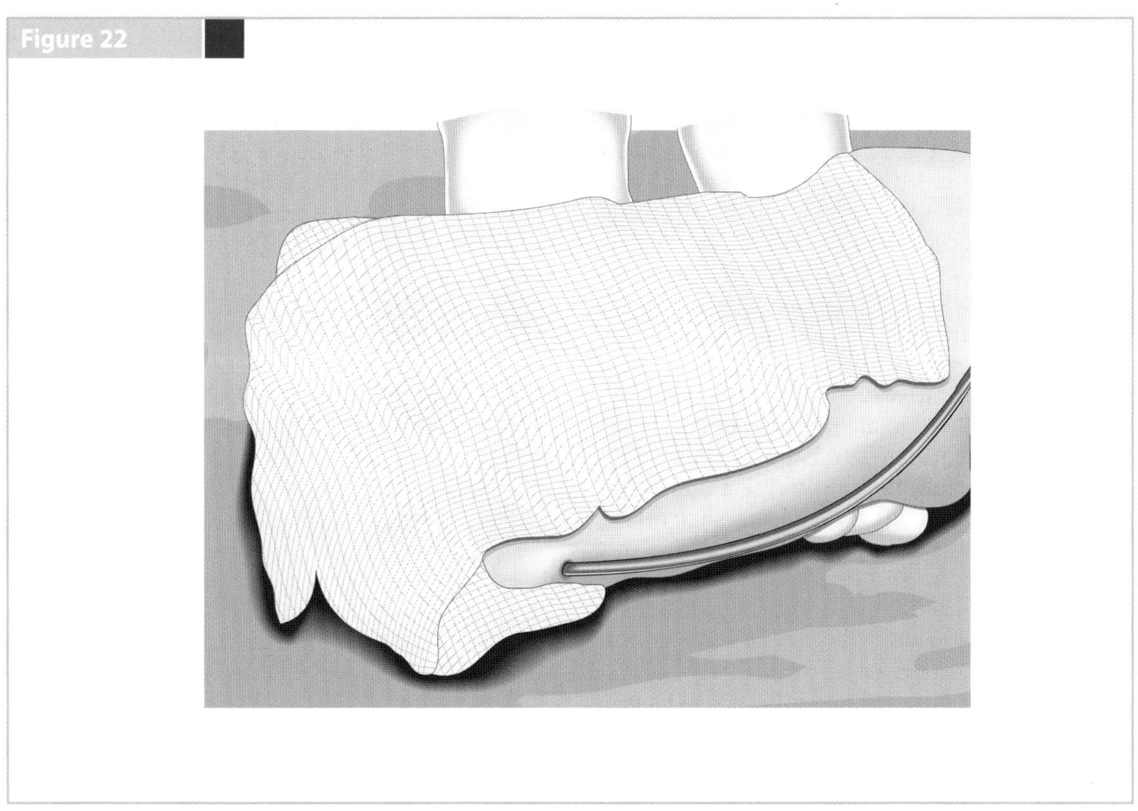

Figure 23

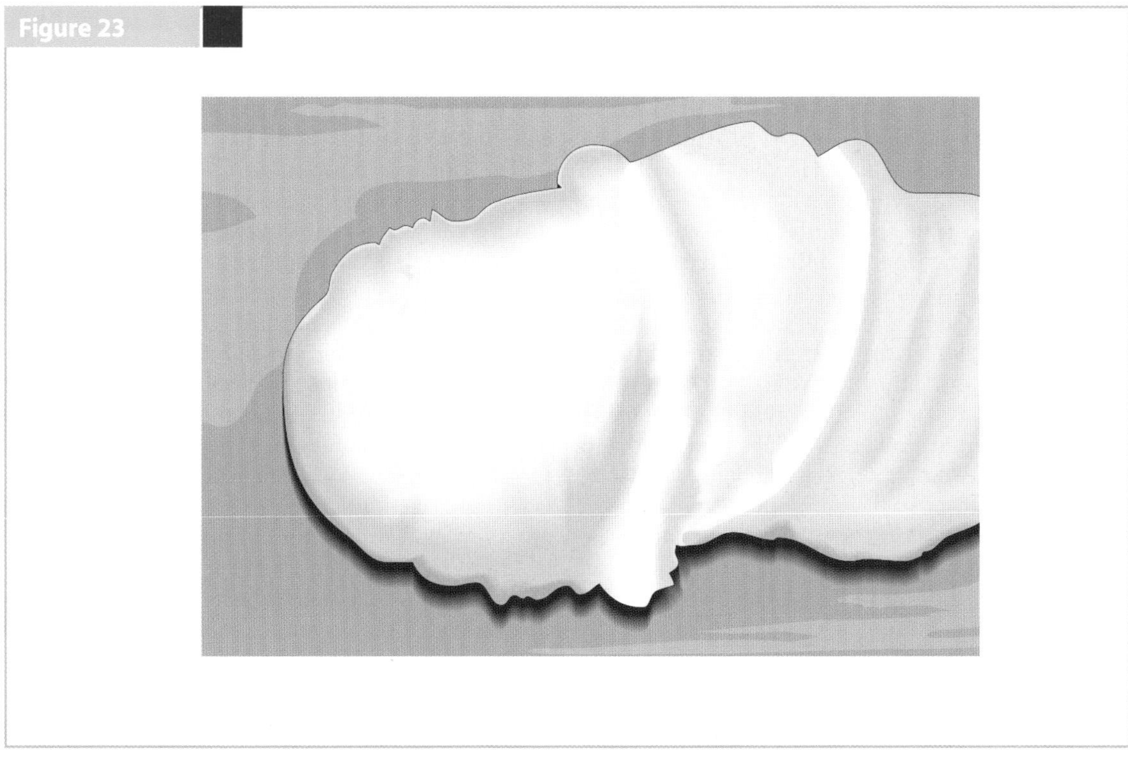

Figure 24

Figure 25: Skew Sagittal Flap Myoplastic Transtibial Amputation

The skin incision is marked between 10 and 14 cm below the articular surface of the tibia (determined by the patient's build and placed proximal to the maximum diameter of the calf muscle). With this reference line, the equal semicircular flaps are formed, skewed from the sagittal plane by 40°. This is achieved by marking the anterior intersection 2–2.5 cm lateral to the subcutaneous anterior border of the tibia. By halving a piece of tape passed around the circumference at the reference level, diametrically opposite the intersections are marked on the posteromedial aspect of the leg. With the same tape quartered, the mid-point of the flaps is marked and the same quarter circumference length used to determine the length of each semicircle. Flaps are now drawn free hand, making sure the anterior part of the flap is not compromised by a wide radius curve, as this portion of the suture line comes to overlie the more prominent anterior aspect of the tibial stump.

An upward extension of the anterior incision over the anterior tibial compartment for 2 cm gives adequate access to both this and the peroneal compartments. The skin flaps include the subcutaneous fat, the deep fascia and the periosteum, ensuring no separation as the flaps are lifted to expose the musculature. The long and short saphenous veins are ligated, avoiding the saphenous and sural nerves. The periosteum is raised from the tibia to be included in the deep surface of the flap.

The extensor muscles are divided transversely, after separately dividing the anterior tibial nerve and ligating the anterior tibial vessels. The dissection is extended laterally to divide the peroneal muscles and identify the common peroneal nerve, dividing it under tension as high as possible. The exposed interosseous membrane is incised and the periosteum is elevated around the tibia and fibula to the level of the bony section. The curved tibial division is best undertaken with a cantilever power saw (Stryker), and the fibula divided 5–10 mm proximal to this level. Copious irrigation is required to remove bone dust and prevent heating of the cut surfaces. A bone hook inserted into the distal fragment of the tibia can be lifted to expose the tibialis posterior muscle. When this is divided the peroneal and posterior tibial vessels can be seen, together with the tibial nerve.

Figure 25 shows the patient prior to skin preparation on the operating table with a tourniquet in place and the skin marked indicating the displacement of the anterior intersection of the skin flaps from the tibial crest.

Figure 24

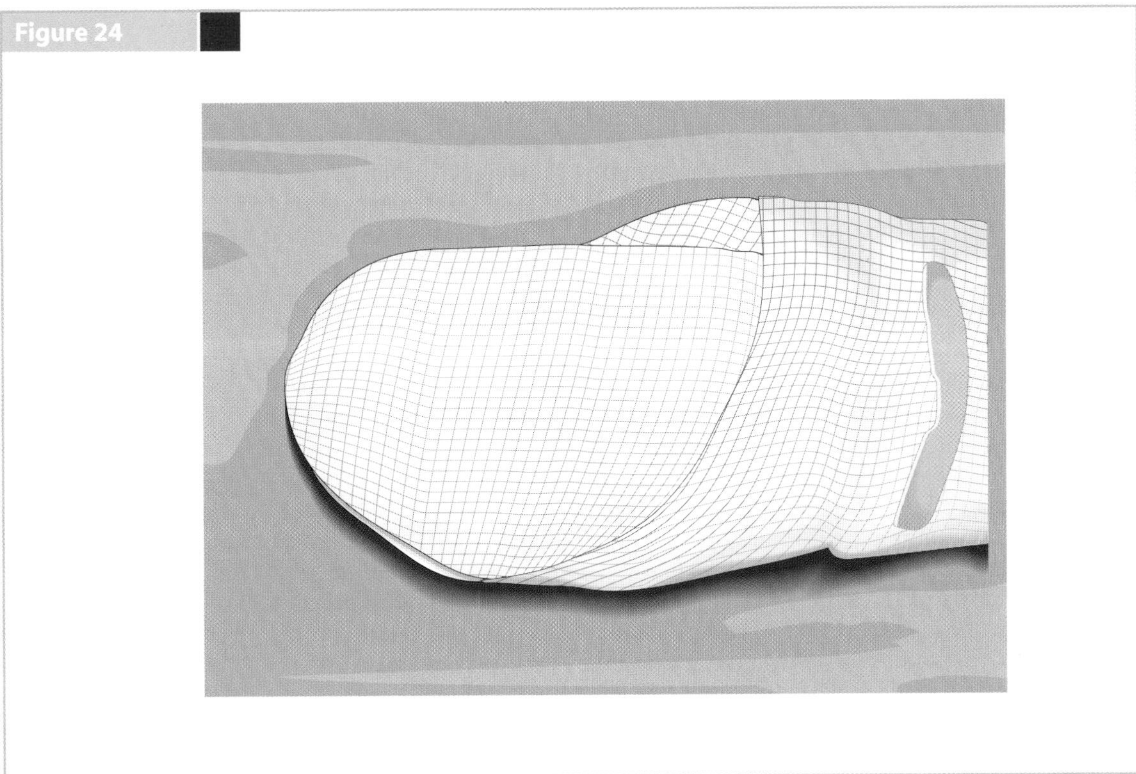

Figure 25

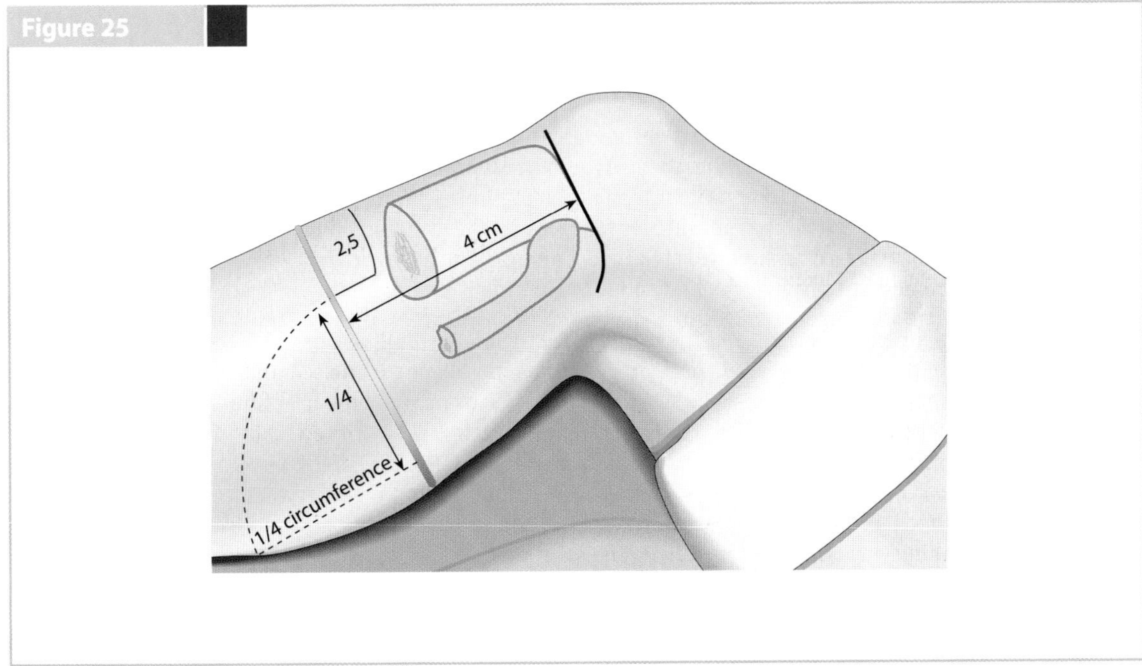

Figures 26, 27

At this stage a plane can be developed superficial to these structures to expose the gastrocnemius and soleus muscles well down the leg, enabling them to be divided transversely. Sufficient length of tissue is preserved to fold over the bone ends and create a myoplasty. Once the gastrocnemius mass is divided, the specimen is removed and the vessels dissected clear of the posterior tibial nerve for ligation; the nerve is divided high under traction. The gastrocnemius muscle is displayed by traction with two tissue forceps and a long incline is cut with a large scalpel or amputation knife, preserving the soleal compartment. The muscle flap must also be narrowed by resection of tissue from the medial and lateral sides of the flap so that when it is rotated anteriorly, it does not produce any widening of the stump.

The sculpturing of the mass is a key element in producing an ideal shape to the finished stump. Many soleal sinuses and veins with small arteries require underrunning with stitches to obtain effective hemostasis. Attention must be paid to the tibia and fibula bone ends, which must be shaped to a smooth and rounded profile. This can be achieved with a rasp and bone files. On completion of bony sculpturing, the tourniquet is released and hemostasis ensured before insertion of a suction drain. Muscle flaps are rotated anteriorly and trimmed to make a compact junction with the anterior tibial fascia and tibial periosteum.

Skin flaps are accurately cut to the marked design, without tension and with minimal redundancy. By inserting central and halfway marker stitches, the flaps can be sutured with vertical mattress sutures to incorporate the deep aspects of the superficial fascia; 3/0 nylon is recommended to provide the best blood supply to the skin edge with an 8–10 mm stitch spacing to avoid excessive sutures. Stitches can be alternated with 5-mm adhesive strips. Intradermal sutures are not recommended, as they tend to produce superficial skin necrosis. The oblique skewed scar does not cross the bone end of either the tibia or fibula, and is strong enough to withstand early activity.

At the conclusion of the operation, the amputation stump should be slender with parallel or tapered sides, a rounded end, and an adequate but not excessive soft tissue covering of the bone ends. A minimum dressing is applied, and cotton gauze fluffed and held in place with a soft mesh bandage to avoid areas of high pressure.

The patient is instructed when conscious to extend the knee and avoid knee flexion while undertaking quadriceps exercise from the earliest stage. Hip and knee extension are emphasized and a pillow is not allowed under the residual limb. Knee extension exercise can be commenced on the day of operation and general body exercise the following day. The patient is taught to transfer into a wheelchair and instructed in the use of a stump board to prevent the stump becoming flexed and dependent. By the third day, the patient can use the pneumatic walking aid inflated to 40 mm of mercury to meet standing with ground contact between parallel bars under supervision. In the most favorable cases, a patellar-tendon-bearing socket has been provided on the 10th postoperative day. With uneventful wound healing, a definitive prosthesis can be used between the 14th and 21st postoperative day and without any complication factors, early discharge is achieved within 20 days of the operation.

Figure 26 shows the transtibial skew flap amputation at the conclusion of the dissection; the gastrocnemius soleal myoplasty is displayed, and the bone shaping is complete. In Fig. 27 the anterior folding of the myoplasty is shown completed prior to the skin closure and drain insertion.

Figure 26

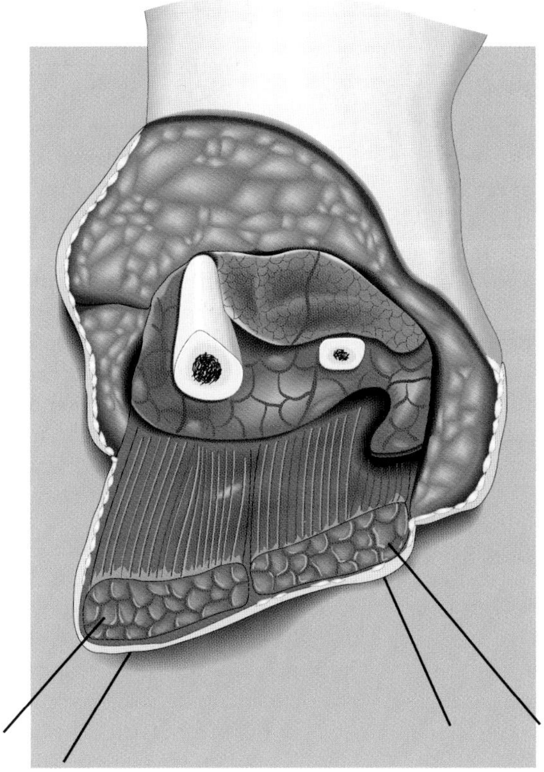

Figure 27

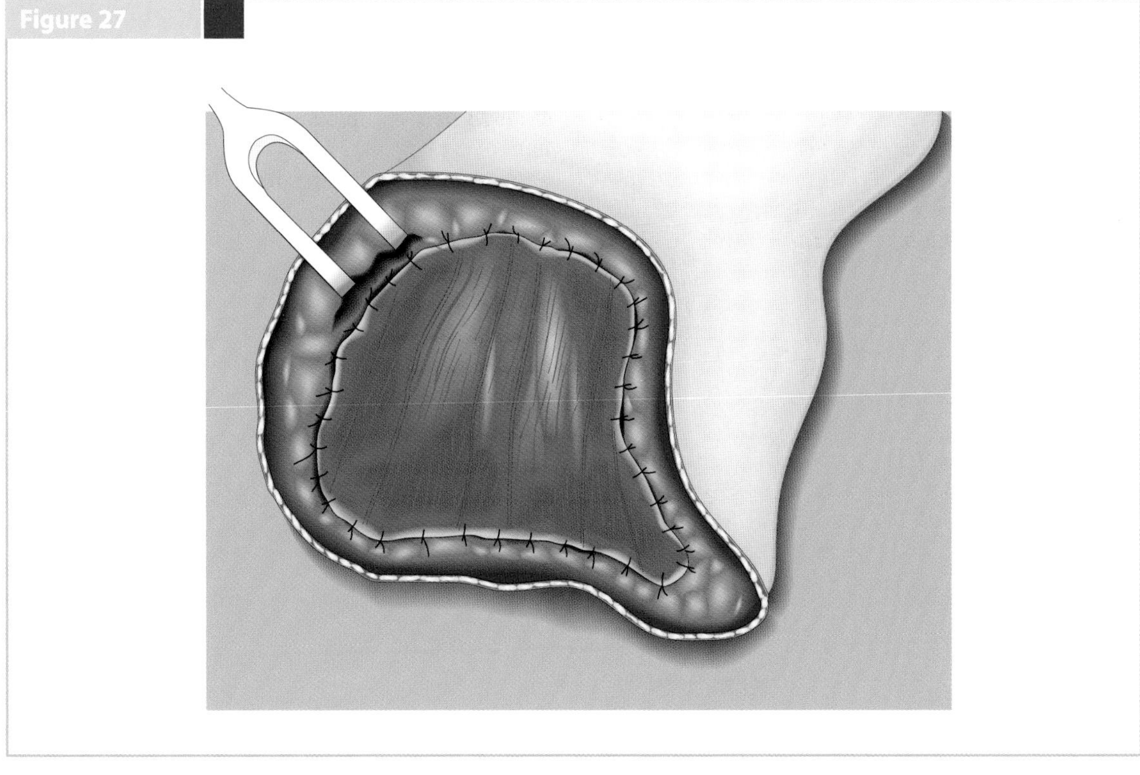

Figures 28, 29: Through-Knee Amputation

A through-knee amputation can provide an end-bearing stump. It is not favored by prosthetists, as it requires an external knee joint, and this is cosmetically unattractive. It also extends anteriorly and requires more space, as when sitting in a bus or an aircraft. Skin healing is also poor at the knee level in ischemic patients, although mediolateral rather than anteroposterior flaps improve this situation. Skin healing can be improved by dividing the bone through the distal femur, either at the level of the intercondylar notch, or at 6 cm for the Gritti-Stokes amputation. The Gritti-Stokes procedure removes the back of the patella to fix it to the divided femur; although favored in some centers, the uncertainty of this union and the subsequent non-weight bearing stump have no advantages over the standard above-knee procedure.

Sagittal skin flaps are preferred, semicircular flaps extending from the attachment of the patellar tendon on the tibia anteriorly, to the middle of the popliteal crease posteriorly. The patellar tendon is divided from its tibial attachment. In the transcondylar amputation, the patella is removed by sharp dissection close to the anterior periosteum, if possible preserving the continuity of the anterior tendinous covering. Hamstring tendons are divided at their tibial and fibular attachments. Gastrocnemius is divided from its femoral attachments by sharp dissection. The popliteal vessels and saphenous and other veins are ligated, and the tibial and common peroneal nerves divided under tension.

The patellar tendon is sutured to the cruciate ligaments and the hamstring tendons, these coming to lie within the intercondylar notch. Careful apposition of the deep fascia and skin complete the procedure. Caution is taken with bandaging as with below-knee procedures.

Figure 28

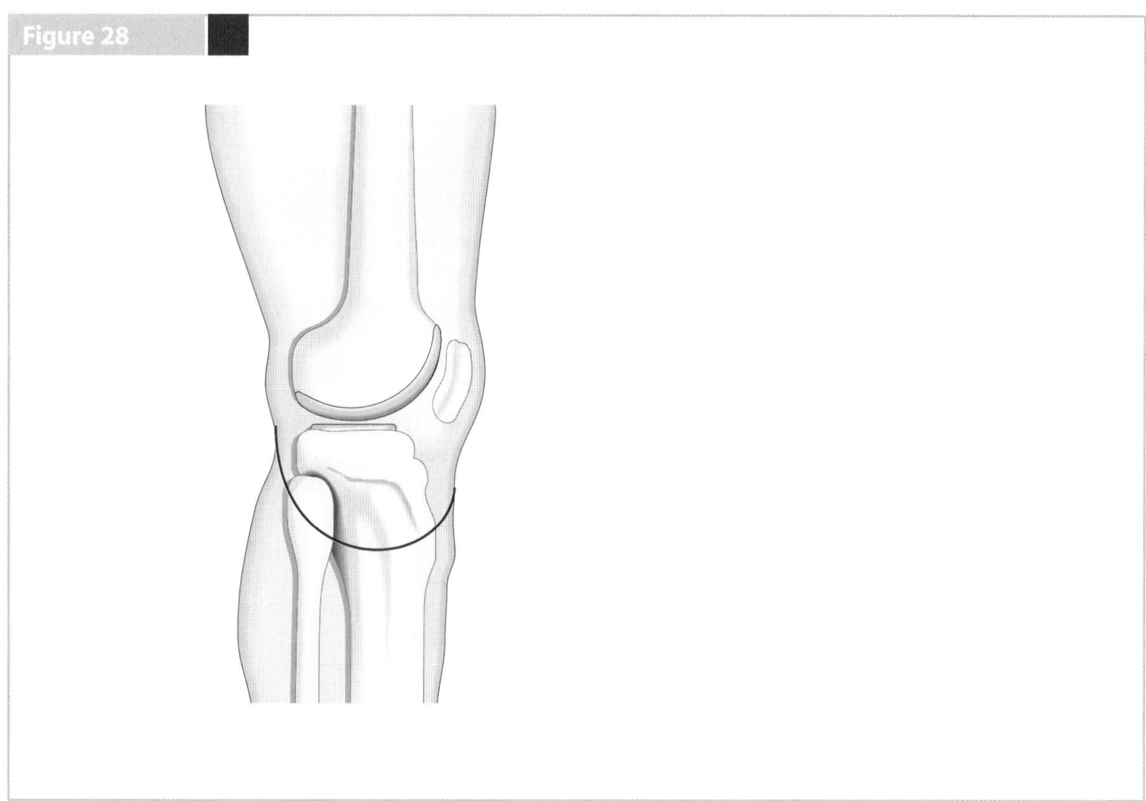

Figure 29

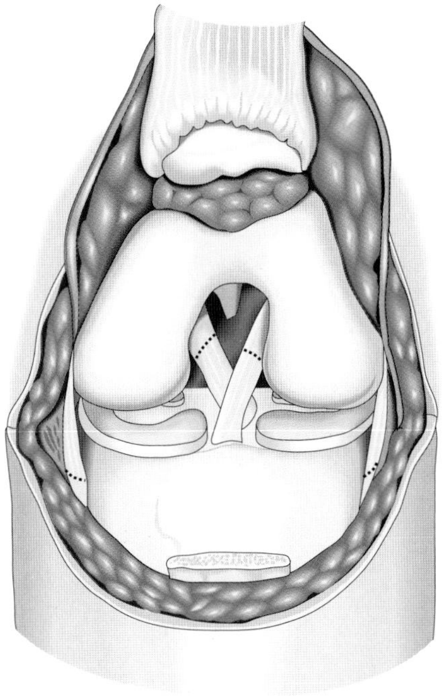

Figure 30: Above-Knee Amputation

Above-knee amputations have a much higher primary healing rate than below-knee in the severely atherosclerotic patient. However, these patients have a higher mortality, as they are often frail, and have associated cardiovascular and cerebrovascular problems, as well as chronic respiratory and sometimes neoplastic disease. The level of bone section is related to the size of the knee mechanism required for an above-knee prosthesis; usually 15 cm clearance above the knee joint is required. Within these limitations, and the dictate of the underlying disease, as much length of bone as possible should be preserved, with particular respect to the adductor group of muscles, which are essential to prevent a prosthesis from slipping laterally.

In vascular patients, flaps are usually equal, even if they become mediolateral or obliquely placed because of previous incisions in the thigh. The underlying fascia is divided in line with the skin flaps; the muscles are divided at a similar level, this being at least 5 cm distal to the proposed bony division. The periosteum is divided at the level of the muscular division and then raised proximally with a rougine to the level of the bony division. Bone is divided with a saw and sharp edges filed away.

Figure 31

Muscles are approximated in layers over the bony end. The periosteum is first closed anteroposteriorly. The adductors are then sutured to the iliotibial tract, with interrupted mattress sutures, and finally the bulk of the quadriceps tendon is sutured anteroposteriorly to the hamstring muscle bellies. The deep fascia provides good subcutaneous approximation of the flaps and interrupted sutures are applied to the skin. A suction drain is placed in one of the deeper layers and brought out laterally. It may be left unsutured as previously described.

Disease sometimes dictates an amputation at a higher level. Bandaging is more difficult in this situation. The conical nature of the upper thigh makes it difficult to apply an even pressure over the stump and there is a tendency for the dressing to slip off. Care must be taken, however, to avoid any proximal constriction and a single light dressing and exposure may be the most appropriate management. If a dressing is applied, some form of "braces" strapping to the bandaging is advisable to maintain a longitudinal pull and hip spica bandaging. As with other amputations, careful monitoring and physiotherapy in the immediate and later postoperative period are essential to ensure that flexion contractures do not occur. The hip must not be flexed on any support but must rest on the bed during the immediate postoperative period; gentle passive extension is started from the first postoperative day.

Figure 30

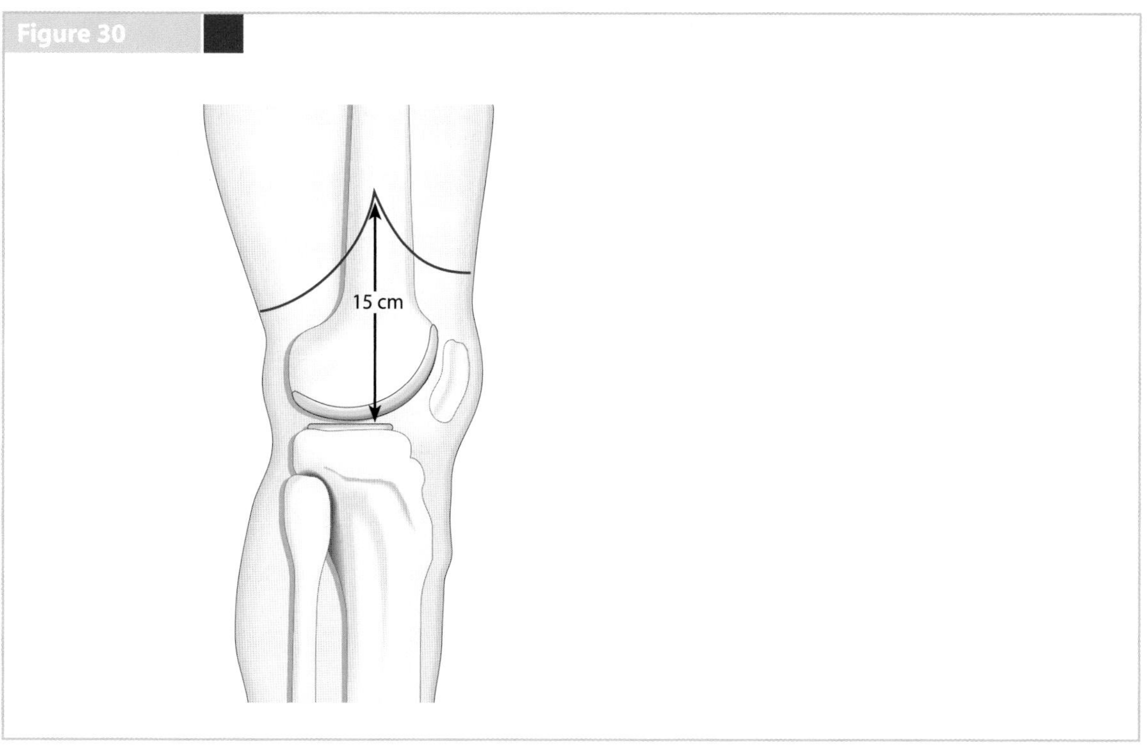

Figure 31

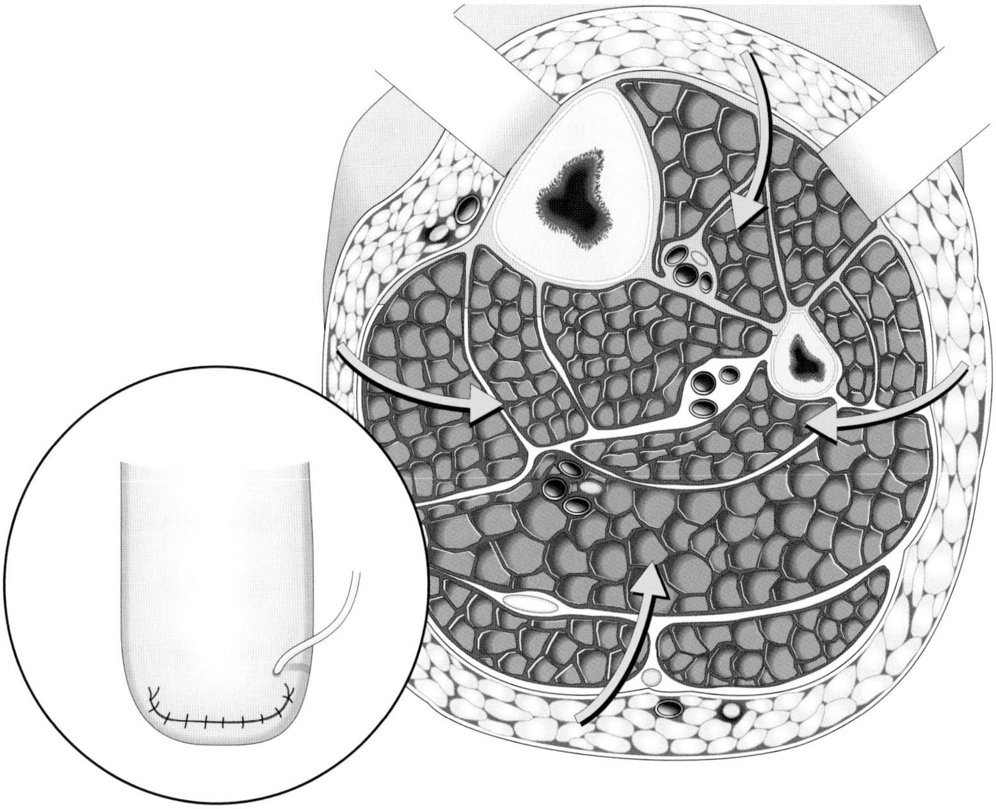

Part VIII Venous

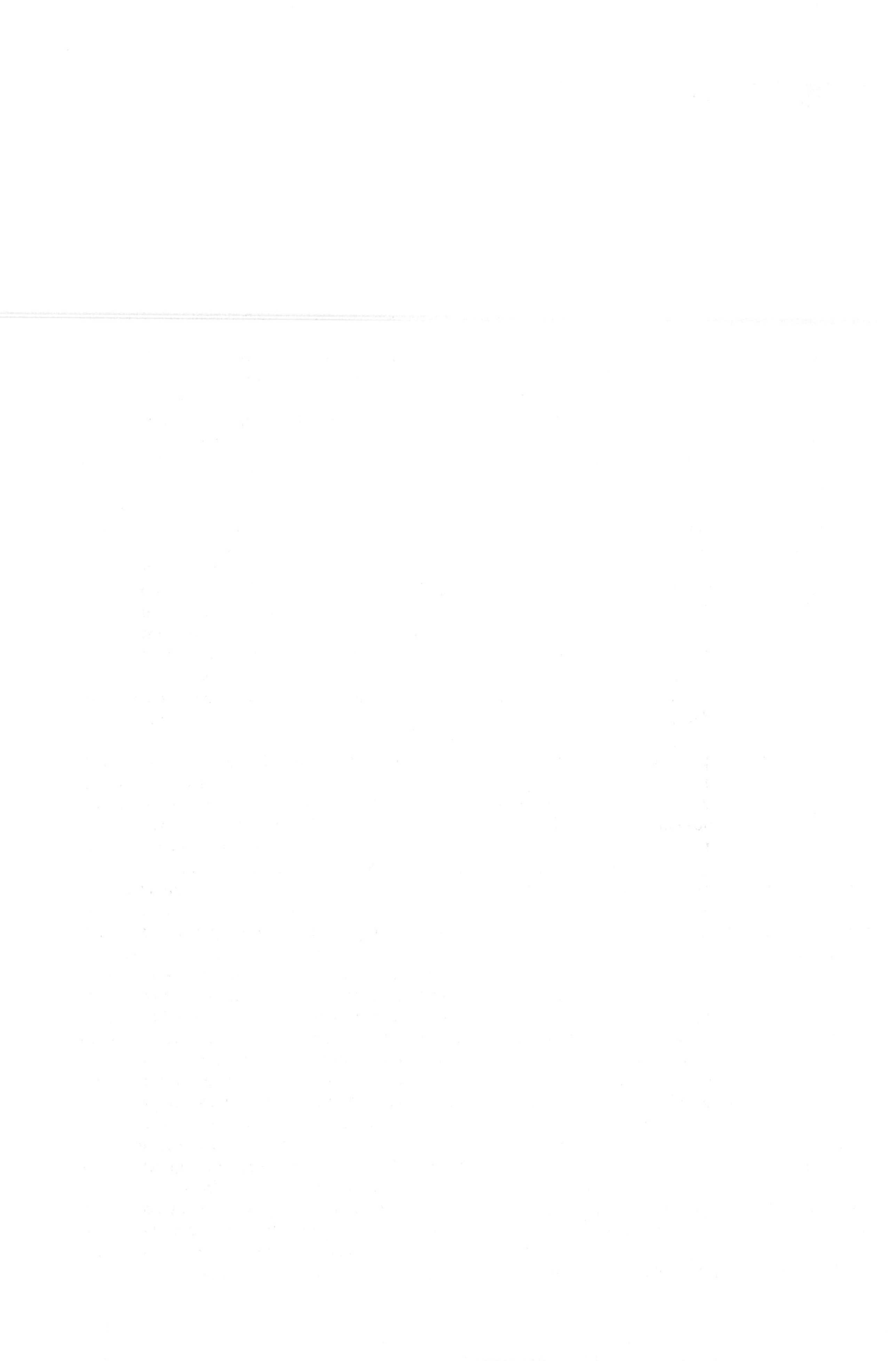

CHAPTER 34

Surgery of the Veins

Colin D. Bicknell, Nicholas J.W. Cheshire

INTRODUCTION

Venous disease of various forms affects 30% of the 35–70 year old population in the United Kingdom (Franks et al. 1992). The vast majority of venous surgery is for superficial varicosities; operative treatment of other venous disease is relatively uncommon, but remains an important lesson for the vascular surgeon.

Varicose veins are dilated, tortuous vessels of the leg arising as a direct result of superficial venous reflux. The disease is most commonly primary, associated with a familial disposition, but may rarely be secondary to pelvic disease such as benign masses (e.g., fibroids) or carcinoma which obstruct venous outflow of the lower limbs.

Clinical examination of varicose veins should identify the distribution of varicosities and determine the sites of venous incompetence. Varicosities of the medial thigh and leg, a cough impulse over the sapheno-femoral junction, downward transmission of impulses when tapping the long saphenous vein and control of varicosities with a tourniquet applied to the upper thigh (Trendelenburg's test) all indicate reflux from the sapheno-femoral junction leading to varicosities of the long saphenous vein. Short saphenous vein reflux may present with varicosities over the posterior and lateral leg and control of varicosities only with a tourniquet applied below the knee. Perthes' test is performed by applying a tourniquet just below the knee and requesting the patient to walk or mark time. Venous claudication during this manoeuvre implies deep venous obstruction.

The hand-held Doppler can be used effectively in clinic to detect reflux, by insonating the sapheno-femoral and sapheno-popliteal junctions. Blood is encouraged into the deep system by firmly squeezing the calf. Release of the calf allows the examiner to listen to reflux of blood into the superficial veins at each site.

The medical treatment of uncomplicated varicose veins producing symptoms such as aching and minor skin changes is dependent on increasing venous return from the lower extremities. Advice to exercise regularly, avoid standing for long periods and raising the feet is useful but can be difficult to enforce in a working population. Above knee compression stockings (Class II) worn continuously when upright will aid venous return and relieve minor symptoms.

Venous insufficiency complicated by ulcers requires regular appropriate dressings and, in the absence of arterial insufficiency, compression bandaging.

Compression sclerotherapy can be used to treat fine subcutaneous venules, which are cosmetically unsightly. A needle is inserted into the veins under magnification and a mild sclerosant (such as sodium tetradecyl sulfate) is injected directly into the vein. The leg is then firmly bandaged for an extended period of time to compress the sclerosed veins. Sclerosant is now rarely used in larger varicosities due to the high recurrence rate after this procedure.

Varicose vein surgery is undertaken for superficial venous insufficiency in the absence of deep venous obstruction for a wide range of symptoms including leg aching, skin changes, venous eczema, thrombophlebitis and recurrent bleeding. Surgery for cosmetic reasons alone is a common practice but may be difficult to justify in an ever resource conscious Health Service. Surgery for varicose veins is also indicated to promote ulcer healing.

Preoperative investigation of lower limb varicosities relies on duplex Doppler ultrasound examination. Sapheno-femoral, sapheno-popliteal and deep venous reflux can be observed. Perforating branches can also be mapped and the full pattern of reflux is used to plan the operative procedure. Sapheno-femoral junction ligation, long saphenous vein stripping and multiple avulsions is the commonest of venous procedures. Short saphenous vein ligation and avulsion of smaller veins is a less common procedure but must be correctly performed to avoid recurrence.

Subfascial endoscopic perforating vein surgery (SEPS) is a relatively new technique to complement the established venous procedures. Significant perforating veins are mapped out using duplex examination, and the perforating vein is visualized during the operation using an endoscope placed underneath the deep fascial layer of the leg. Ligation with clips can be performed under direct vision.

Figure 1: Sapheno-femoral Junction Ligation and Long Saphenous Vein Stripping

Preoperatively visible and palpable varicosities are marked using permanent ink with tramlines either side of the vein. Marking the vein directly causes tattooing of the skin if the marked area is incised and should be avoided. This essential part of the operation is performed with the patient standing on a stable, cloth covered platform, in a well-lit environment. After a few minutes the veins become filled so they are easily identified. A palpable saphena varix is also marked to facilitate identification of the sapheno-femoral junction.

The operation is performed with the patient under general anaesthetic. The patient is positioned in the supine position. The leg is held above the table by the foot by a member of the theatre team and the skin is prepared from the ankle of the affected limb to the level of the umbilicus, preparing the lower quadrant of the abdomen. The groin area is prepared last of all. The leg is placed with the hip externally rotated and abducted with the knee slightly flexed onto a sterile drape.

Sterile drapes cover the contralateral limb, and the remainder of the patient and the foot are shut off with a separate small sterile drape, which is securely fastened. The groin is isolated from the wound with a drape folded into a small long oblong and placed vertically to cover the genitals.

In the supine patient the sapheno-femoral junction lies two fingers laterally and two fingers inferiorly from the pubic tubercle. An oblique incision, centred over the surface marking of the sapheno-femoral junction, is made into the skin within a skin crease of the groin.

Figure 2

The incision is deepened through the superficial fat layer. The fibrous part of the superficial fascia at this level can be identified as a thin layer, which is incised in the same direction as the skin incision. The underlying adipose tissue typically bulges out of this break in the fascia.

The dissection is continued through the fat using small (e.g., Langenbach) retractors to identify the vein. A vertical sweep with a small swab can also be utilized to clear the tissue from the long saphenous vein, which is easily found using this technique.

Figure 1

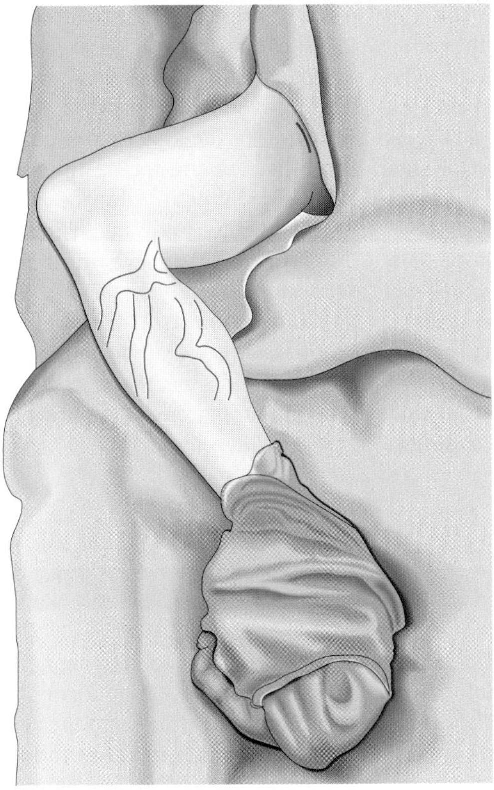

Figure 2

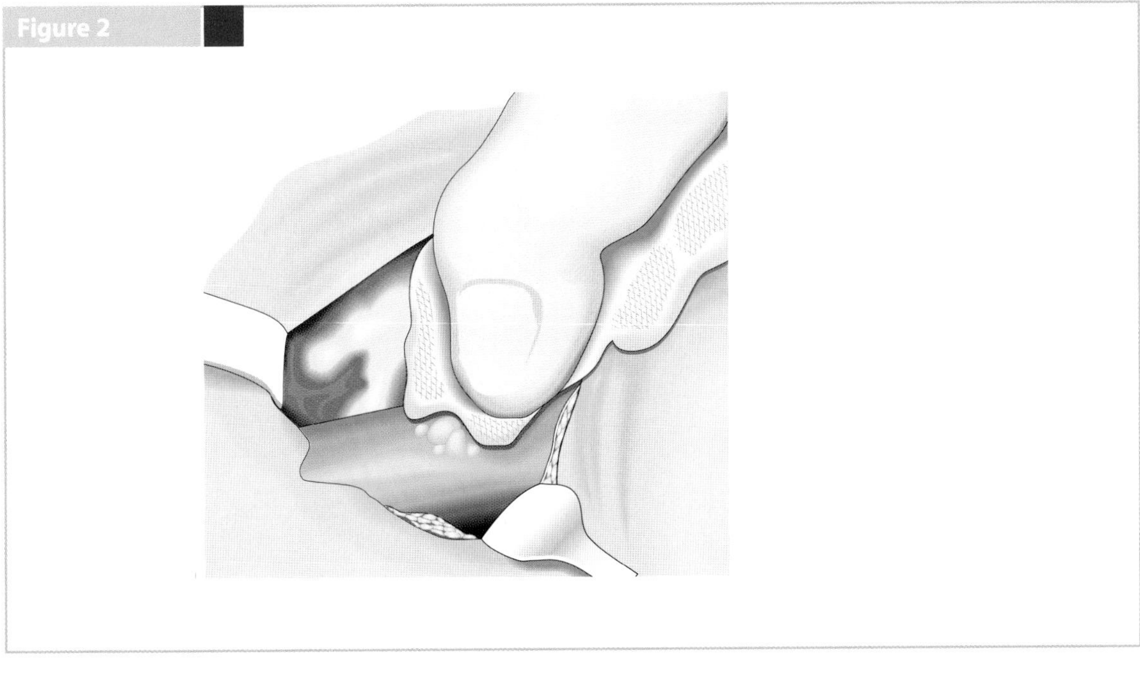

Figure 3

Once the long saphenous vein is located and the overlying tissue has been cleared the long saphenous vein is dissected free of the surrounding tissue. The dissection should be performed near to the vein wall as this plane is relatively avascular and allows excellent definition of structures. The wound is held open during this stage by a self-retaining (Travers) retractor.

Six named tributaries of the long saphenous vein in close proximity to the junction can be identified. The superficial and deep external pudendal veins, a circumflex iliac vein, an external inferior epigastric vein, a posteromedial branch and an anterolateral branch of the long saphenous vein should be dissected. Commonly pairs of veins share a common trunk, joining together a variable distance away from the sapheno-femoral junction. Often the superficial external pudendal artery is encountered and may be ligated to allow an improved access to the junction. Branches of the long saphenous vein are not divided until the sapheno-femoral junction is clearly identified as a T-junction between the femoral vein running vertically underneath the cribiform fascia and the long saphenous vein that emerges from the saphenous opening.

There is no need to dissect the femoral vein above and below the sapheno-femoral junction as long as the junction is clearly identified and no branches of the long saphenous vein remain.

Figure 4

All tributaries of the long saphenous vein are clipped, divided and ligated separately, after the junction has been clearly identified. Application of Ligaclips is an alternative and acceptable method of securing these branches. Tributaries that join into a common trunk prior to joining the long saphenous vein are ligated separately as these may form a potential site for recurrence with reflux from the venous drainage of the abdominal wall and pelvis to the superficial venous system of the thigh.

Figure 3

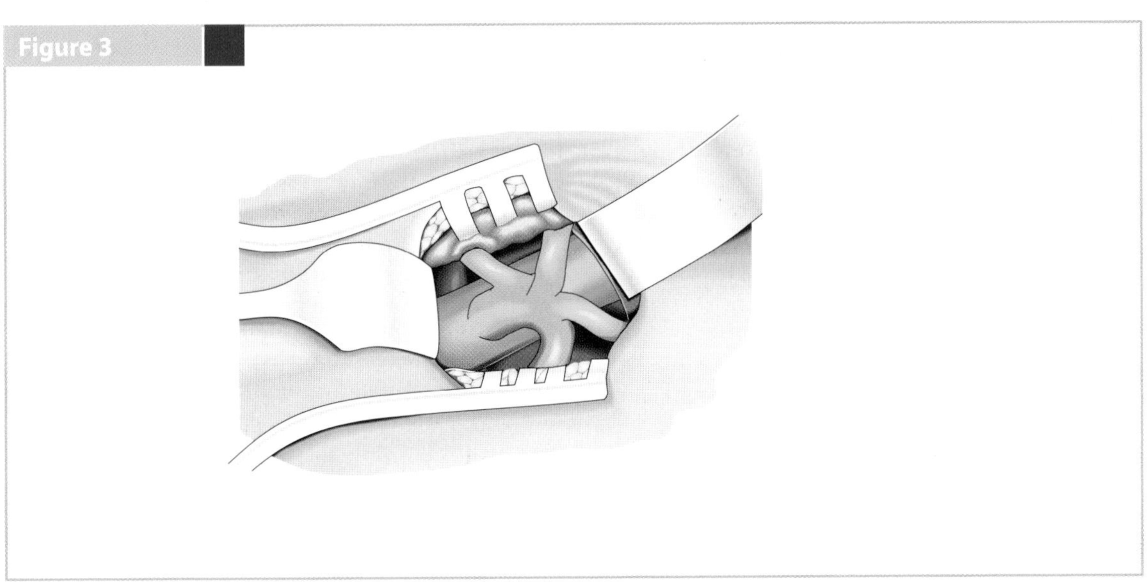

Figure 4

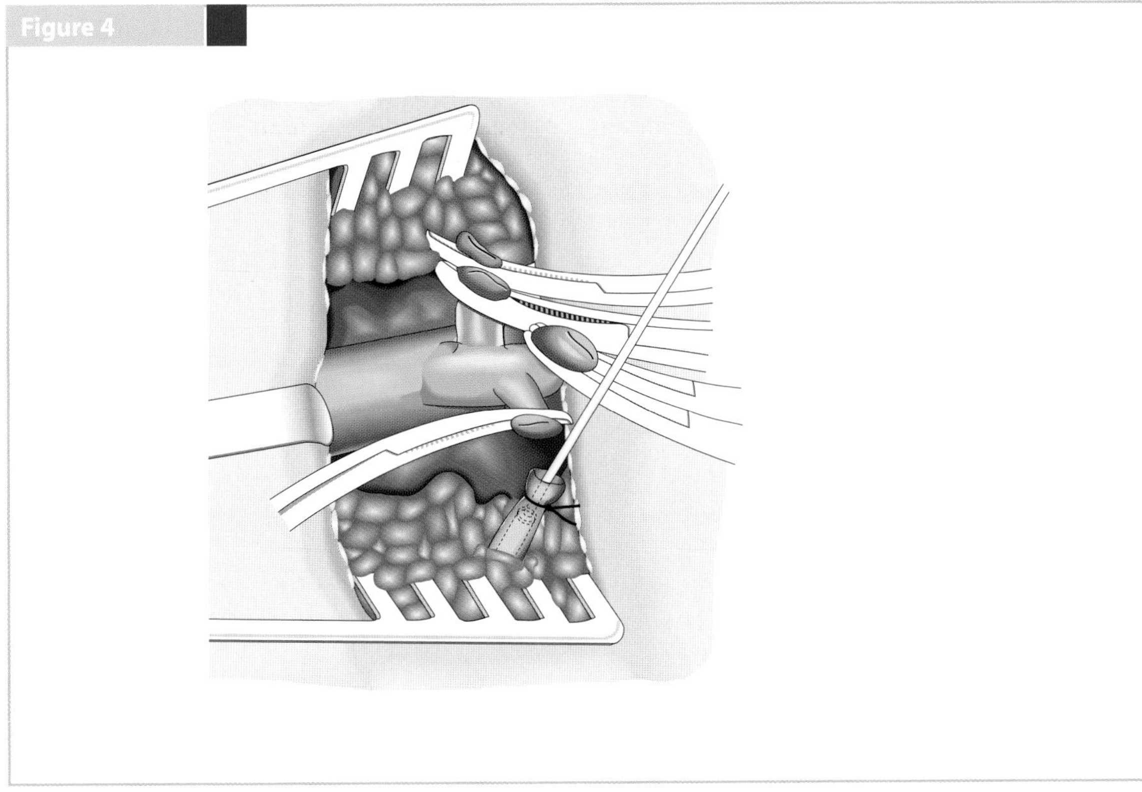

Figure 5

Two clips are applied to the long saphenous vein flush to the junction. The long saphenous vein is divided between the two clips and the long saphenous vein is suture ligated for security. The ligation should be flush with the femoral vein. Care must be taken not to cause narrowing of the vein or leave a blind ending sac.

Figure 6

A haemostat is placed on the superior free end of the long saphenous vein and the vein is freed from the surrounding tissue in the upper thigh with gentle finger dissection, ligating any further branches that are encountered. Often the anterolateral and the posteromedial branch of the long saphenous vein join in the upper thigh rather than around the junction and are identified and ligated in this way. If these are not dealt with appropriately they may bleed excessively after stripping. Bandaging of the upper thigh may not sufficiently compress these veins and they can lead to groin hematoma.

Figure 5

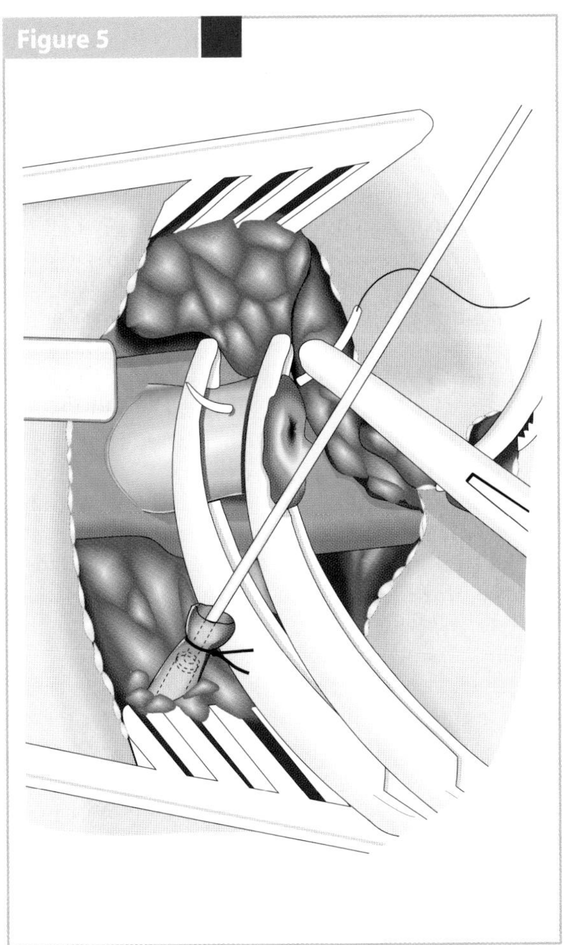

Figure 6

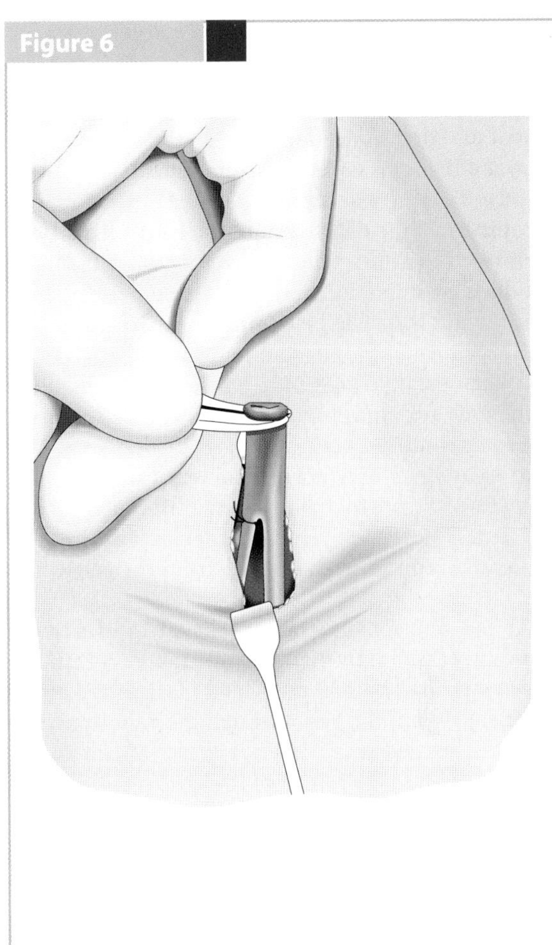

Figure 7

Stripping of the long saphenous vein in the thigh removes the communication between tributaries of the vein and the long saphenous vein. This is ideally set up after ligating the sapheno-femoral junction, but stripping may be delayed until avulsions have been performed to avoid excessive haemorrhage from the site during completion of the operation before bandages are applied. The procedure is explained in this section for ease of understanding.

A haemostat, using gentle tension, holds the long saphenous vein and a double length silk tie is loosely placed around the vein. A single, loose throw of a knot is used only. A horizontal venotomy is made using fine scissors to divide half the circumference of the vein. Holding the vein under tension during this procedure reduces haemorrhage from the venotomy site.

As the vein remains under tension the stripping device is passed into the lumen of the vein through the venotomy. The stripping device is directed at the posterior wall of the vein through the venotomy site and then turned in an inferior direction threading the stripper into the lumen of the vein.

Figure 8

The stripper is passed inferiorly in the lumen of the long saphenous vein to just below the level of the knee joint. Gentle pressure only is required to advance the instrument within the vein. If the stripper is impeded in its progress it is withdrawn slightly, rotated and another attempt is made to pass the stripper through the correct channel. This process can be aided by directed pressure over the tip of the stripper to push the tip into an alternative tributary.

The tip is located immediately below the knee by palpating the skin over the stripper head. Any attempt at stripping the vein further inferiorly carries a significant risk of saphenous nerve damage and should not be routinely performed. Damage to this nerve leaves the patient with anaesthesia over the medial portion of the leg, or in some cases hyperesthesia, which can have a severe impact on patient lifestyle following the operation. Damage to this nerve is a frequent cause for litigation.

A small vertical incision is made directly over the tip of the stripper, just long enough to admit the tip of the stripper. The vein is located at this level using a vein hook (see avulsion technique), and clamped below the tip of the stripper. A venotomy is made to allow passage of the stripper out of the vein.

The stripper is advanced until the end is at the venotomy site at the superior section of the long saphenous vein. The loose silk tie is fastened securely at the superior end around vein and stripper.

A large head can be attached to the vein stripper, which encases the vein when it is pulled through the thigh. However, a secure tie around the vein and stripping device will invert the vein as it is pulled through with minimal surrounding tissue trauma and a smaller scar below the knee (Durkin et al. 1999). This technique is described as perforate invagination (PIN) stripping of the long saphenous vein and can be performed with a reusable conventional PIN stripper or with disposable plastic stripping devices.

Figure 7

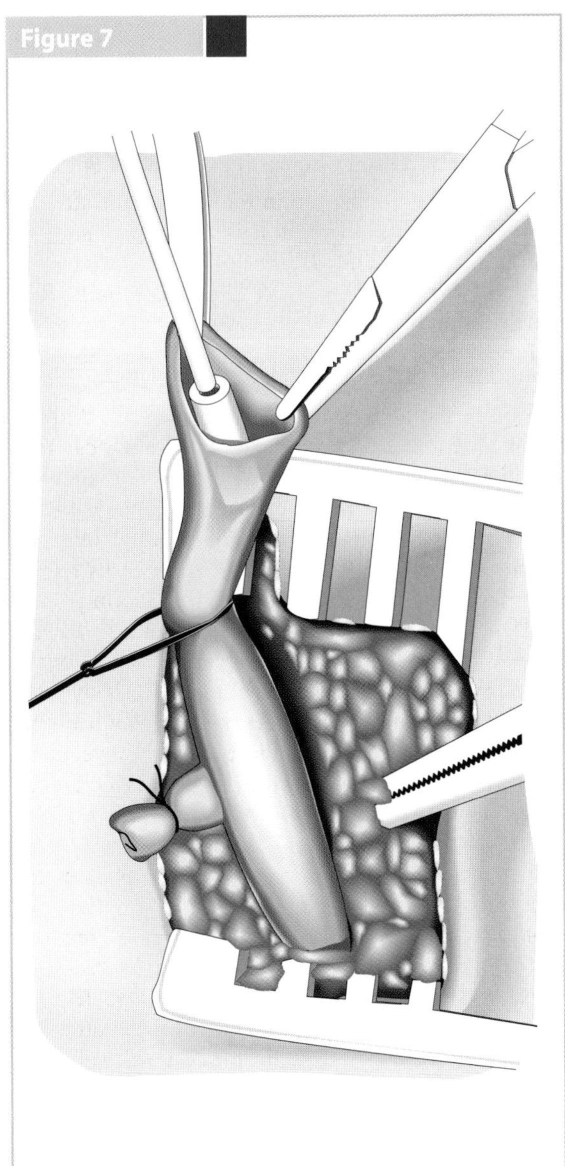

Figure 8

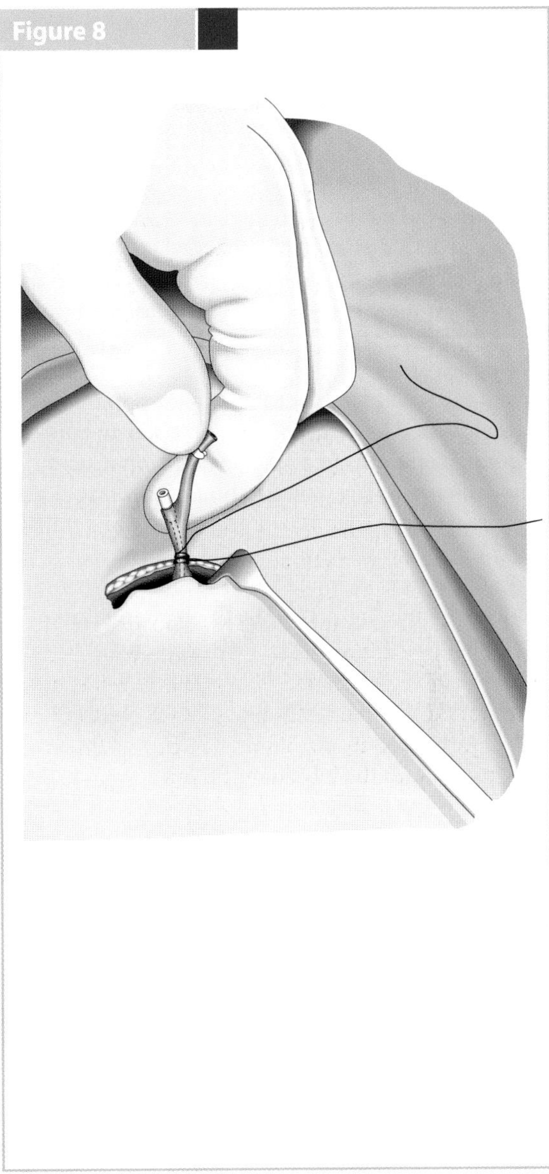

Figure 9

An assistant holds the long silk tie as stripping is performed. The vein is stripped by applying controlled traction to the lower end of the stripper, pulling in an inferior direction. The vein is inverted as the stripper is pulled down to knee level and tributaries are avulsed. Once the vein is stripped the long silk tie is used to remove the vein and stripping device from the groin wound. This method of stripping allows the incision at the knee to remain small and cosmetically acceptable. If the surgeon is satisfied he/she has removed the whole length of the vein the apparatus can be removed. The silk tie may be used to pull the stripping apparatus in a reverse direction if stripping is not adequate. The continuation of the long saphenous vein into the leg is ligated or carefully removed with multiple avulsions.

As the vein is stripped some surgeons use a tourniquet, which is applied to the thigh after exsanguinating blood from the leg. This prevents excessive bleeding from veins that have been avulsed in the thigh following stripping and during avulsions of veins in the leg.

Figure 10

The tunnel formed by the stripping apparatus may become filled quickly with blood from avulsed veins in the thigh. A thigh hematoma can take weeks to resolve, causing pain and delay in return to normal activity. Sweeping the skin from distal to proximal, expressing the blood from the groin wound, can clear the tunnel. An alternative method is to roll a swab along the length of the thigh.

Adequate hemostasis is achieved at the groin wound with diathermy. The fibrous part of the superficial fascia is closed using an absorbable polyglactin (Vicryl) suture and the overlying skin is closed. The use of a subcuticular monofilament (e.g., polypropylene) suture gives good cosmetic results. A long acting local anaesthetic agent is injected into the wound to provide short-term pain relief and early mobilization.

The distal incision for removal of the stripper is closed using interrupted monofilament sutures. Multiple avulsions are performed as described later in this chapter and dressings and bandages are applied to the leg and upper thigh.

Figure 9

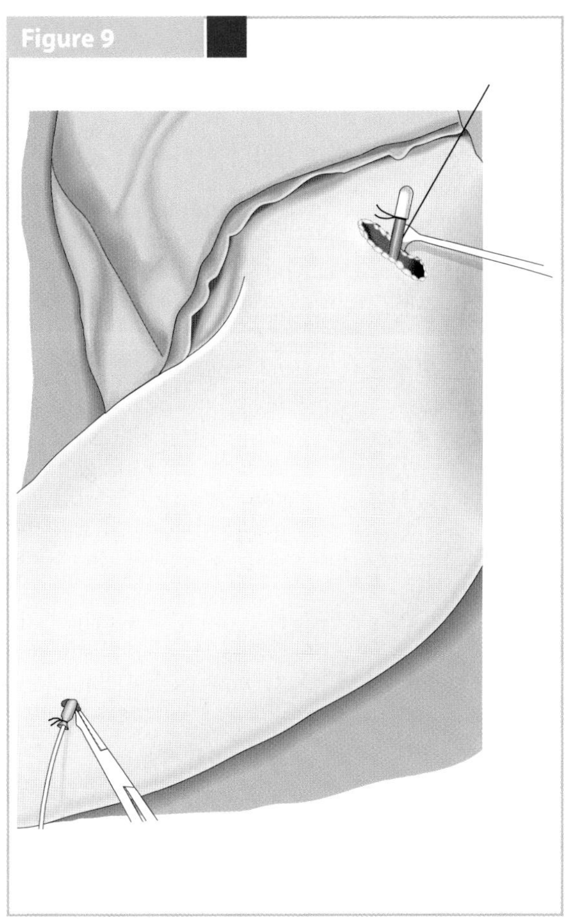

Figure 10

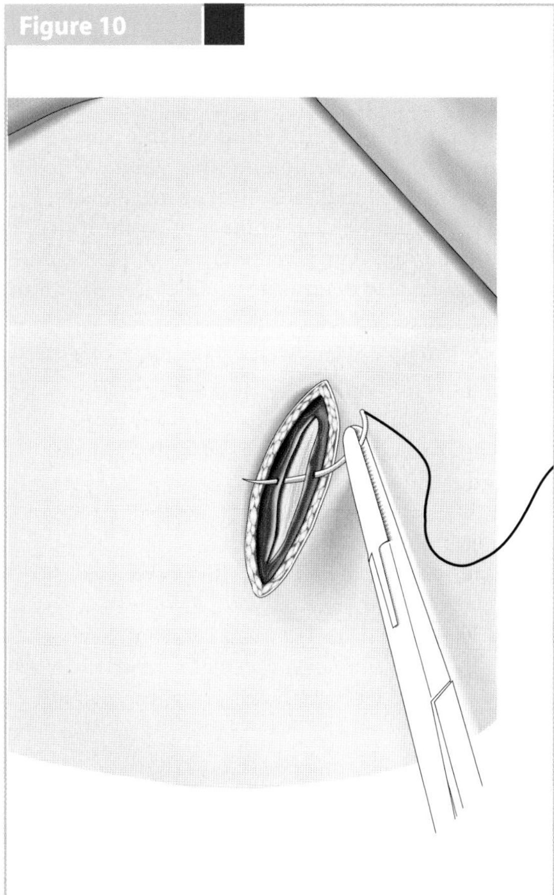

Figure 11: Short Saphenous Vein Ligation

Preoperative duplex Doppler ultrasound examination is required to identify the variable site of the sapheno-popliteal junction in the popliteal fossa. There are various methods of marking the site, but the surgeon must be clear of the level of the junction from the marking in permanent ink. Duplex examination should also determine whether there is reflux of large gastrocnemial veins around the sapheno-popliteal junction and the presence of a Giacomini vein. This process is essential and short saphenous surgery should not be attempted without prior duplex examination.

With the patient in the standing position the courses of the major varicosities of the leg are marked, using a permanent marker, with tramlines either side of the vein as described in the previous section.

Figure 11

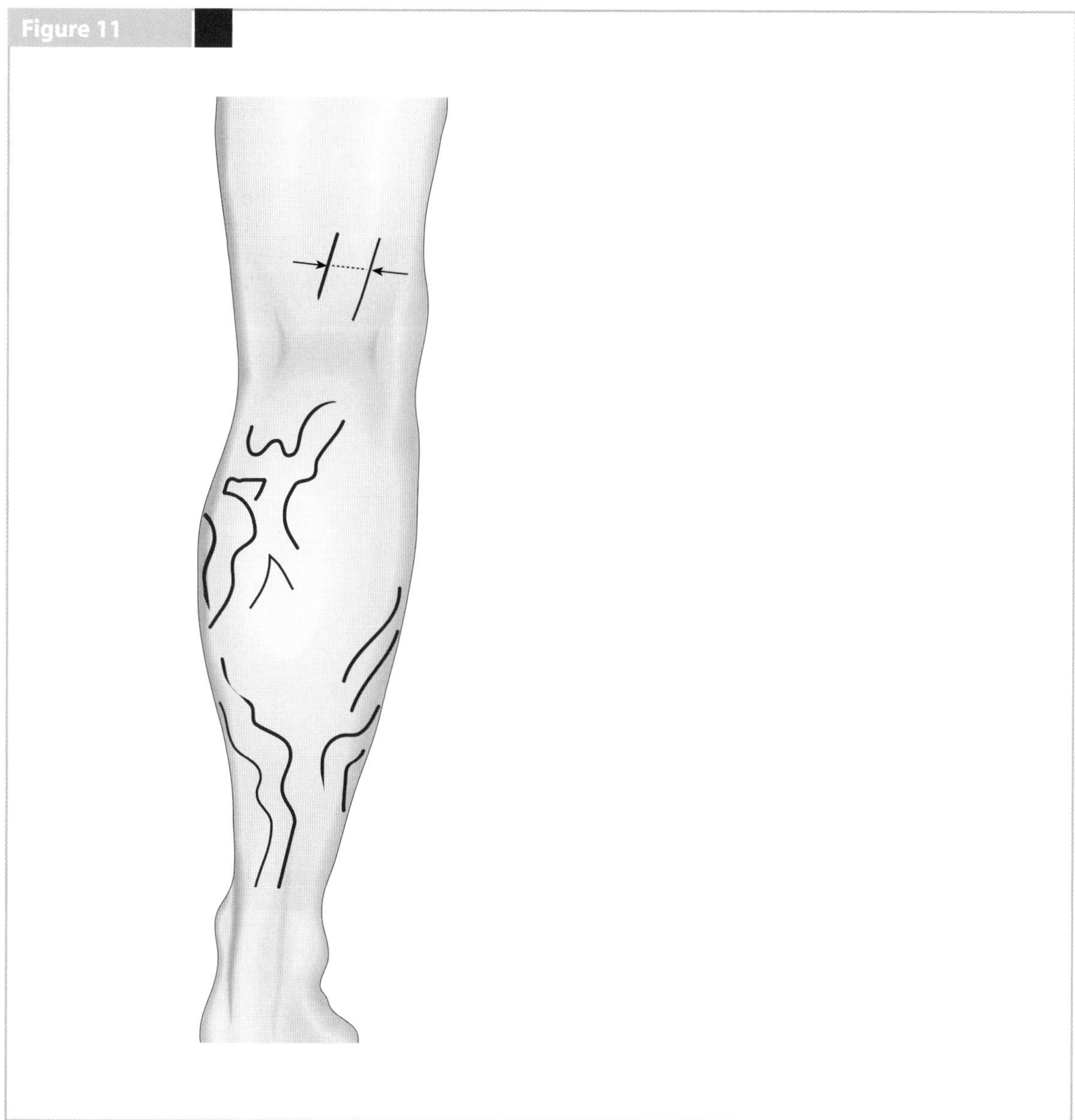

Figure 12

The operation is performed with the patient under general anaesthetic. The patient is positioned on the operating table either on the opposite side to that of surgery, with the leg for operation uppermost, or in the prone position. Both provide an adequate operating position, but the prone position is more difficult to achieve. Care must be taken in both instances to maintain airway devices and attached devices when positioning the patient. Positioning must be undertaken in a controlled fashion and under the direct supervision of the operating surgeon and anaesthetist. The patient is stabilized on the side with the use of sandbags and tape around the upper body.

The skin of the lower limb is prepared from the ankle to upper thigh whilst an unscrubbed member of the team holds the foot. Towels are placed to cover the upper and mid thigh, the contralateral limb and the rest of the patient. The foot is shut off with a separate small drape and securely fixed.

The skin incision is made transversely in the skin overlying the popliteal fossa, at the level of the sapheno-popliteal junction indicated by duplex assessment.

Figure 13

The incision is deepened through the subcutaneous fat to the deep fascia overlying the popliteal fossa and this subcutaneous tissue is cleared from the fascia using a firm sweeping motion with a small swab. The deep fascia at this level is seen as a glistening sheet of fibrous tissue.

The deep fascia is incised longitudinally to allow the vein to be followed along its course in the popliteal fossa to the sapheno-popliteal junction.

Figure 14

The dissection is continued within the popliteal fossa to locate the short saphenous vein. The tissue surrounding this vein is carefully cleared. Dissection should be carried out close to the vein wall, as this plane is relatively avascular. As long as the preoperative Duplex examination has confidently excluded severe reflux within the gastrocnemial veins there is no need to follow the short saphenous vein superiorly to identify the sapheno-popliteal junction. This avoids deep dissection in the popliteal fossa, avoids nerve damage, and division of functioning gastrocnemial veins may cause venous outflow obstruction from the calf muscles and venous claudication. Branches of the short saphenous vein are ligated separately and the short saphenous vein is divided between two haemostats, taking care not to damage the sural nerve. The superior trunk of the short saphenous vein is suture ligated to ensure security of the ligature in the postoperative period.

Occasionally, the Giacomini vein is located, passing from the short saphenous vein superiorly. It eventually meets with the long saphenous vein to provide a connection between long and short saphenous systems. It is an important site of recurrence and must be ligated separately.

Figure 12

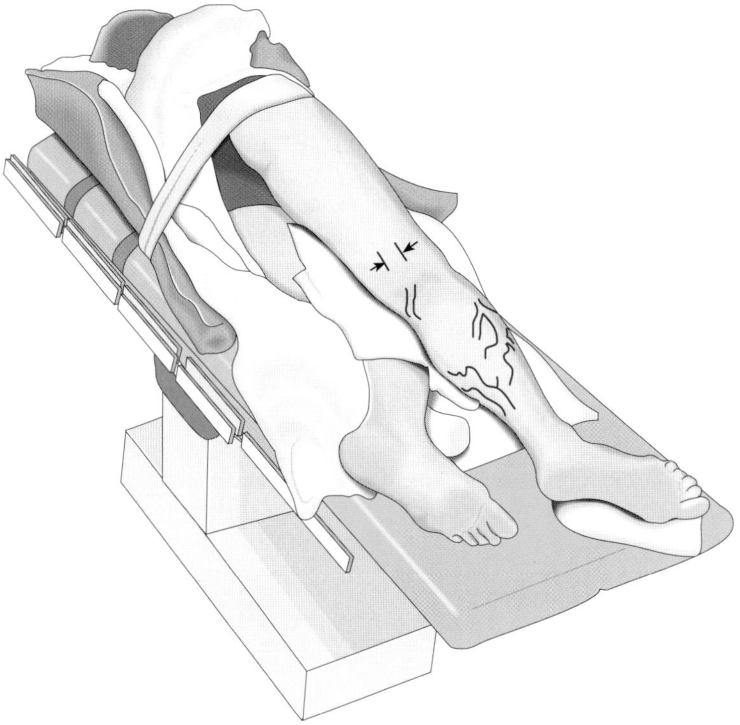

Figure 13

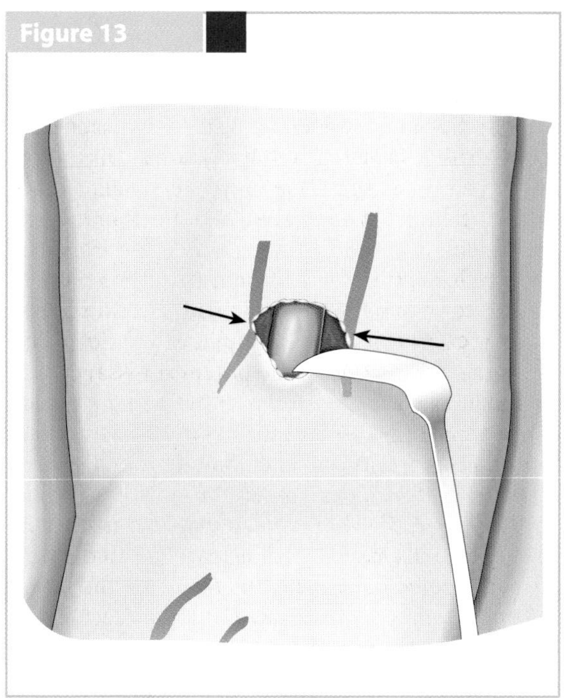

Figure 14

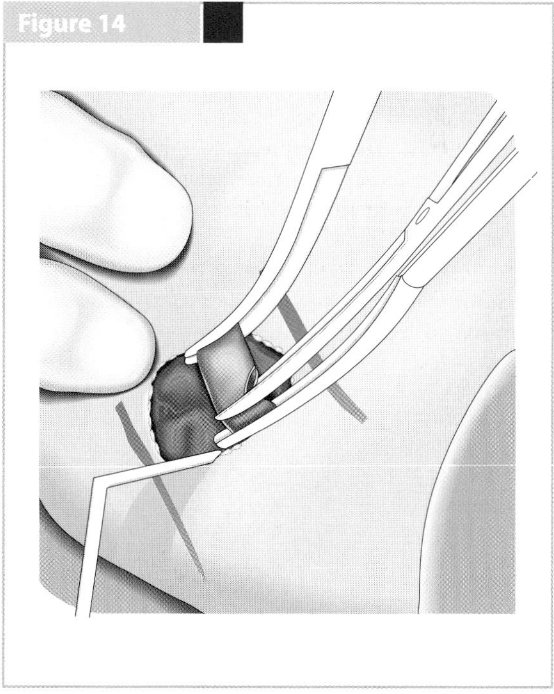

Figure 15

Stripping of the short saphenous vein is a debated issue as it carries a significant risk of associated sural nerve damage. A preferred approach to stripping of the vein is serial avulsions of the short saphenous vein.

Using the index finger, the superior part of the short saphenous vein is mobilized from its attachments as far as possible in an inferior direction in the leg. A vertical stab incision is made in the skin over the point to which the vein has been mobilized and a vein hook is used to avulse the vein through the stab incision. Confirmation that this is a continuation of the short saphenous vein is made as the skin is tented up between the short saphenous vein in the popliteal fossa and the avulsed vein. At this point if the accompanying nerve is visualized it can be carefully freed from the vein. The superior section of vein can be extracted from this small incision.

Serial avulsions can be repeated along the course of the short saphenous vein, which has been marked preoperatively. Multiple avulsions are then used to remove the varicose tributaries of this vein. The technique for this is described in this chapter.

A drain is not usually required in the popliteal fossa. Secure haemostasis is ensured with careful diathermy and ligation of larger vessels and vessels closely associated with nerves.

The deep fascia is closed longitudinally with an absorbable polyglactin (Vicryl) suture. The skin of the flexor surface of a joint should be closed with patient comfort in mind, and a subcuticular suture is a suitable choice. A dressing is applied over the wound.

Avulsion sites (see Figs. 19, 20) are closed appropriately and the leg is dressed and bandaged as detailed in the section dealing with avulsion of veins and dressing of the leg.

Figure 15

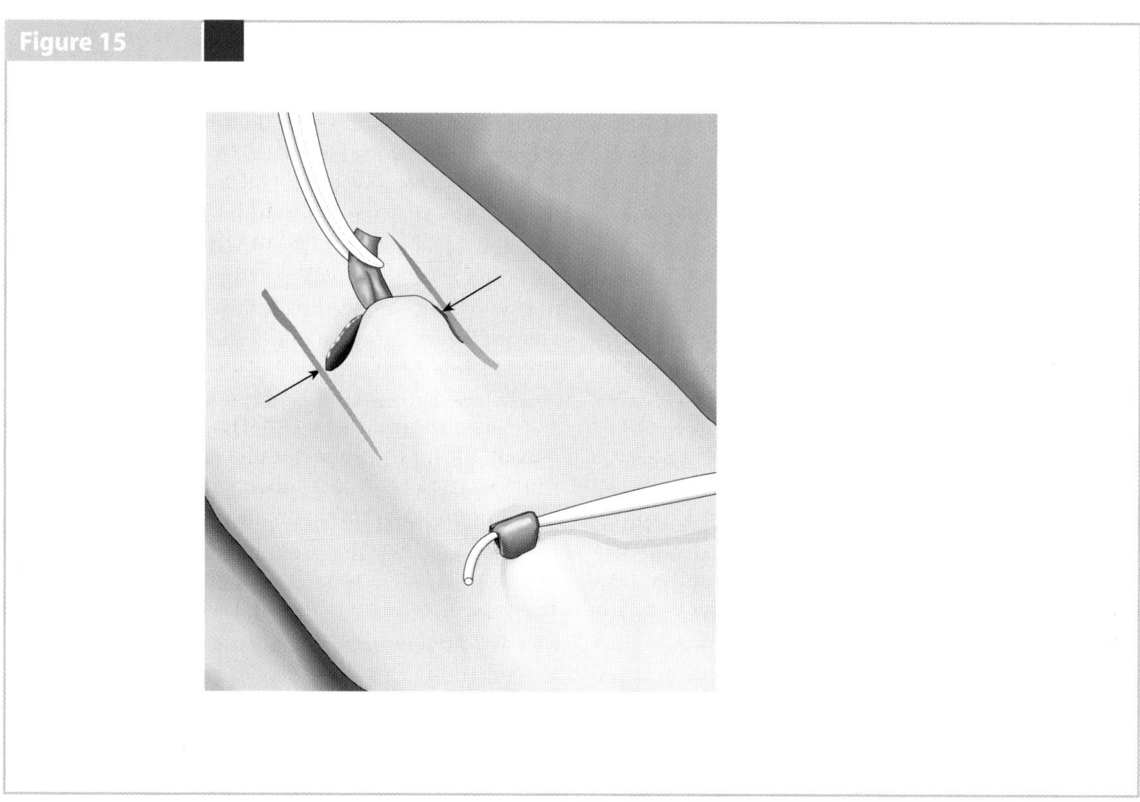

Figure 16: Subfascial Endoscopic Perforator Surgery (SEPS)

This is a technique for dividing calf perforating veins without the need for extensive incisions in already diseased skin. The technique can be used in association with other superficial venous surgery (common in mainland Europe) or as a stand-alone procedure and may be indicated in the management of venous ulcers and severe lipodermatosclerosis. The technique has been less widely used in the United Kingdom because of lack of data to support the interruption of perforators in primary superficial venous disorders and lack of clarity about which perforators should be divided in the presence of deep disease.

An operating endoscope is required which provides a light source, imaging and a working channel (for insertion of clipping/diathermy instruments). The instrument should not be too large in diameter (no more than 12–15 mm) and must be long enough to allow access to distal perforators from the upper calf. Dissecting scissors and forceps and a clip applier, which can be passed through the working channel in the endoscope, are also required. Standard laparoscopic equipment will usually suffice but some of the longer, small calibre SEPS endoscopes (e.g., Storz) require their own instruments.

Some surgeons prefer balloon dissection within the subfascial space followed by insufflation using a gas-tight seal around the proximal incision. This variation may also be used with a second instrument port avoiding the need for a working channel in the viewing endoscope. All of the systems require a camera and video monitor.

The patient undergoes duplex scanning immediately prior to surgery in which the number and site of the calf perforators are marked on the skin. Prophylactic heparin is given perioperatively.

A longitudinal incision is made through skin and the deep fascia in the proximal calf. The positioning of the incision is crucial; usually it is placed 2 cm posterior to the medial border of the tibia at a level that avoids diseased calf skin and allows access to the most distal perforators. The operating endoscope is inserted distally, deep to the fascia and the avascular plane developed using blunt dissection with the tip of the instrument under direct vision.

Figure 17

Perforating veins (in fact vascular bundles) can be seen traversing the subfascial plane when the skin and fascia are gently lifted away from the underlying muscles using the tip of the instrument.

Figure 16

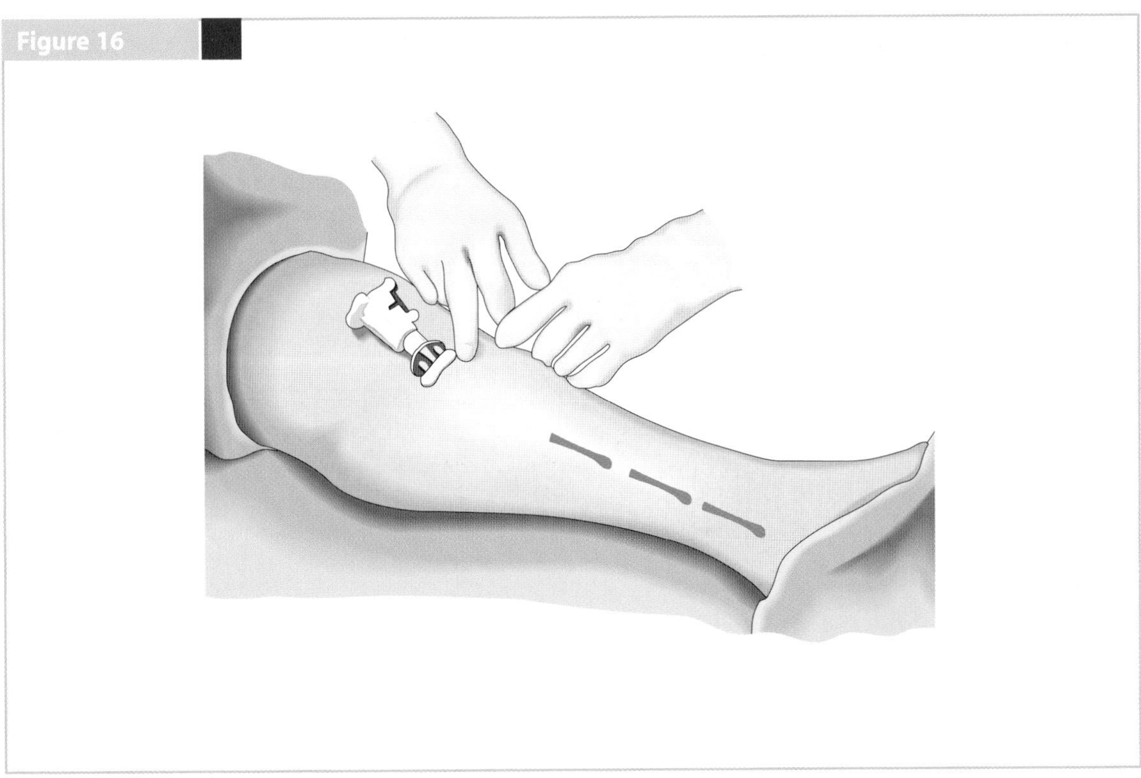

Figure 17

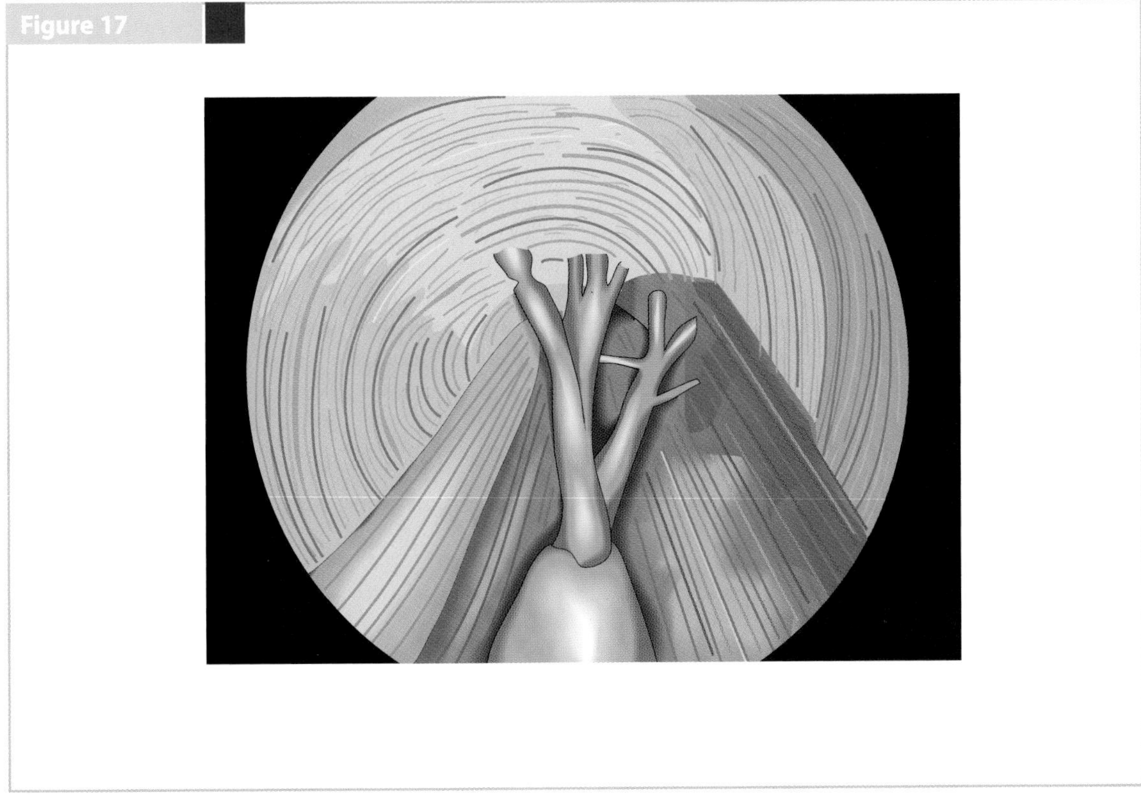

Figure 18

The veins are clipped and then divided serially as the dissection progresses distally in the leg. Clips and sharp division are preferable to diathermy because of the proximity of the posterior tibial neurovascular bundle.

At the end of the procedure the endoscope is removed ensuring there is no bleeding in the subfascial plane. The deep fascia and skin are closed separately.

For division of very distal calf perforators, fasciotomy of the deep posterior compartment may be required during SEPS. The rationale behind this requires understanding of the deep fascial compartments within the leg, which is beyond the scope of this chapter.

Figure 19: Multiple Stab Avulsions

The technique of multiple avulsions is used to remove varicose tributaries of veins. The procedure can be carried out in association with high saphenous ligation and stripping or short saphenous vein ligation.

The varicosities are marked preoperatively using permanent ink tramlines as described earlier in this chapter. A vertical "stab" incision is made into the skin over the vein, using a size 15 blade at right angles to the skin. Vertical incisions produce a better cosmetic appearance when the wound is healed. The length of the incision should not exceed the length of a size 15 blade and care should be taken not to pierce the vein during this manoeuvre.

Multiple incisions are made along the course of each vein to allow the surgeon to locate connecting segments of vein. Using this technique, extensive lengths of vein can be removed.

Figure 20

A vein hook is inserted into the wound and rotated carefully to snare the vein, which is tented up, out of the small incision and grasped with fine-ended mosquito forceps.

Right- and left-handed vein hooks exist, with hooks facing different ways. If the hook is carefully examined, it can be ascertained which direction to rotate the hook in order to snare the vein. There are also various sizes to the hooks. As a general rule the avulsion of small veins should be performed with the smallest of these (size III).

Figure 18

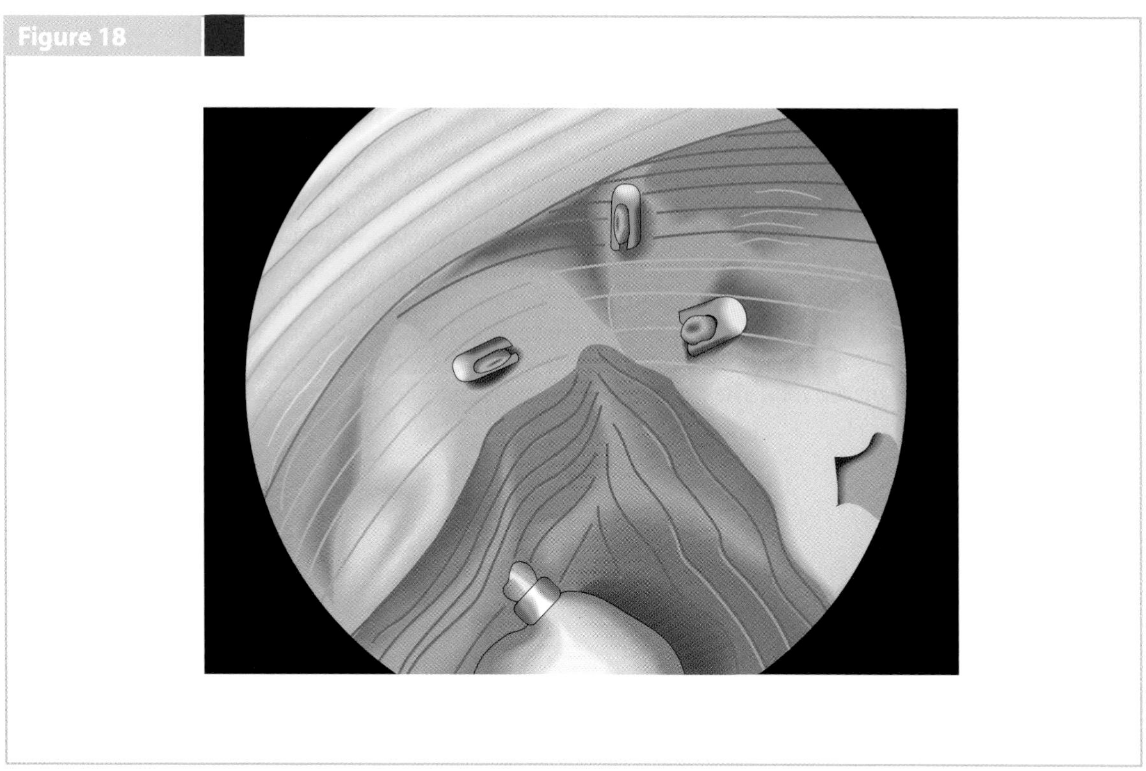

Figure 19

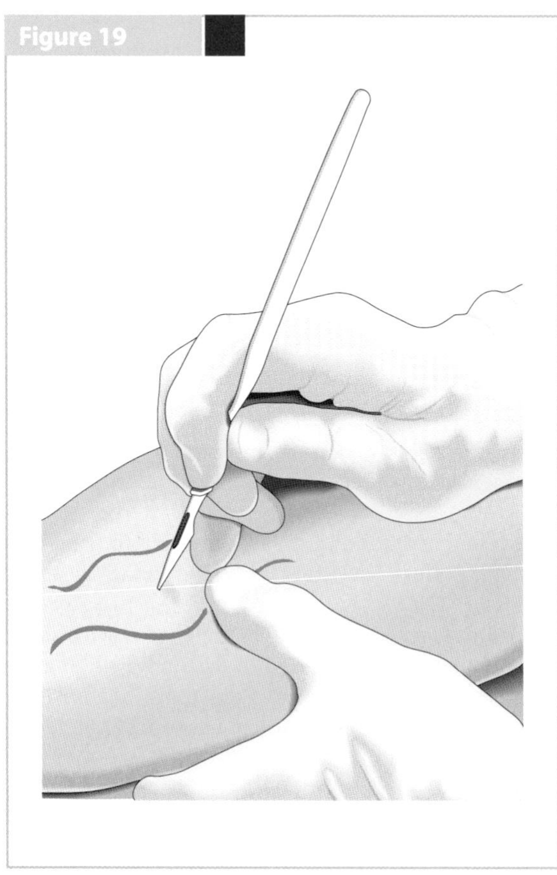

Figure 20

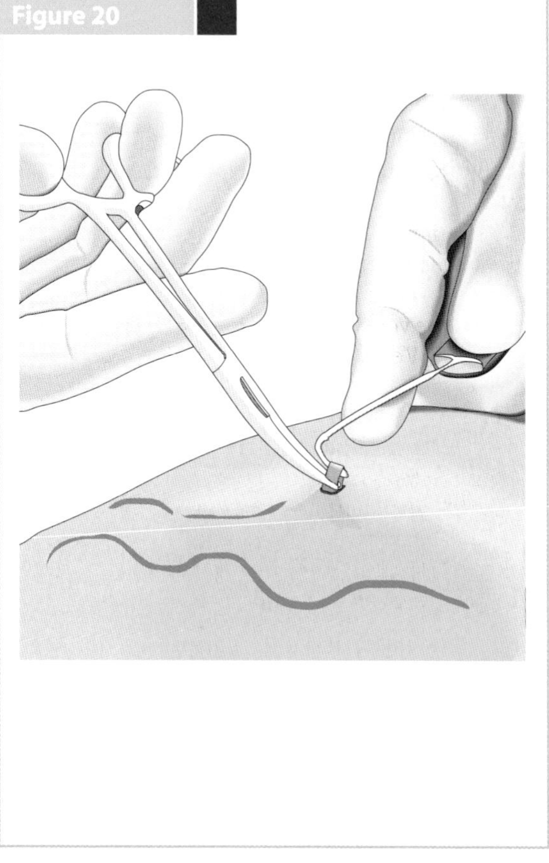

Figure 21

The located vein is gently teased from the wound by applying constant firm tension. As long a length as possible is removed by repeated applications of clips with continued tension. Both proximal and distal segments of the hooked vein should be avulsed separately.

Multiple incisions are used to locate segments of a vein and long segments of vein can be removed by serial avulsions. The course of the vein can be mapped out by exerting traction on the vein. The path of the vein is seen tenting up the skin and the next incision can be made over this. Lengths of vein are removed in this way until the surgeon is confident all the large and troublesome varicosities have been removed.

The surgeon must be aware of the anatomy of the nerves of the leg and avoid avulsions in these areas. The operator should be careful of the common peroneal nerve winding superficially around the head of the fibula. Avulsions are avoided at the foot and ankle also to avoid nervous structures.

Figure 22

Closure of larger avulsion incisions is achieved with a single stitch of a monofilament non-absorbable suture. A Steristrip is applied over the closed wound as a dressing and to improve cosmetic results.

Small wounds are closed with Steristrips, avoiding stretching the skin but adequately closing the wound. Tincture of benzene is used on the skin surrounding the wounds to increase the adhesiveness of the Steristrip.

Figure 23: Dressing of the Leg Following Varicose Vein Surgery

Soft, non-adhesive pad dressings are applied to the leg before application of a crepe bandage. The leg is held clear of the table by a member of the theatre team and the bandage is applied from the foot upwards. The bandage passes underneath the leg at each turn from inside to outside the leg and is applied firmly but care is taken not to constrict the arterial supply. Each turn of the bandage is directed alternately upward and then downward to achieve a crossed pattern in the classical bandaging technique.

The bandage is applied to below the knee for short saphenous vein surgery and to the upper thigh after long saphenous vein surgery to apply haemostatic pressure to avulsion sites and to the tunnel formed in stripping the vein.

Figure 21

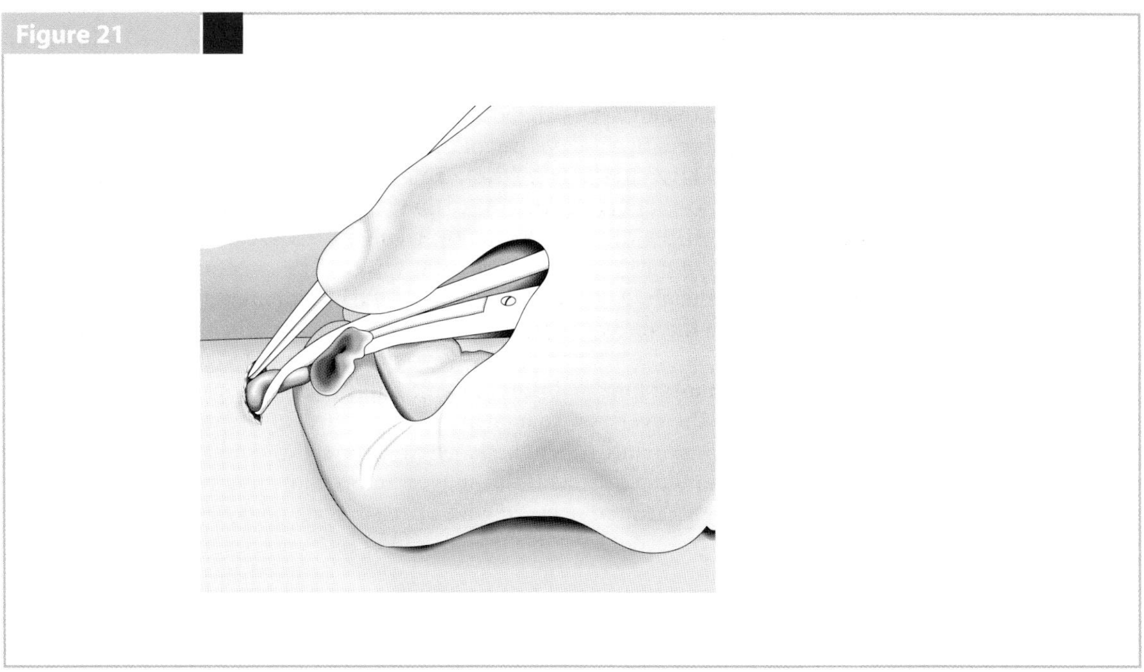

Figure 22

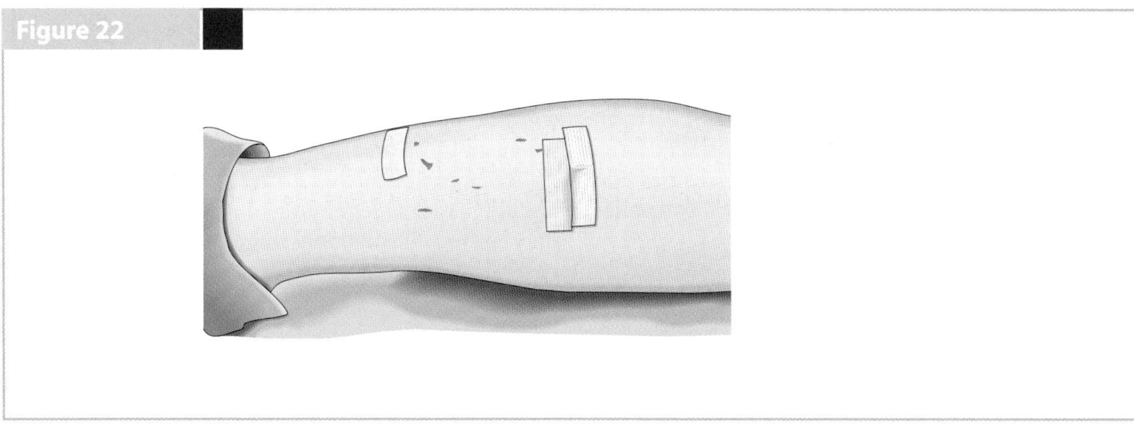

Figure 23

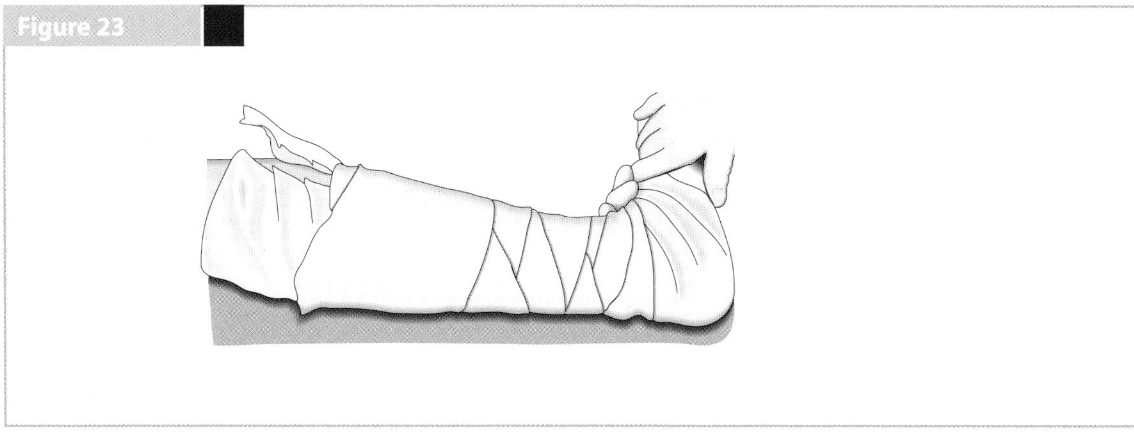

Endovenous Ablation of the Long Saphenous Trunk

Recent technological advances have employed laser or radiofrequency (diathermy) energy sources to ablate the lumen of the LSV in the thigh and thus avoid the groin incision and stripping procedure described above. The technique involves marking of the LSV using duplex ultrasound and cannulation of the vein around knee level with a long 3 or 4F sheath. The energy source fibre is introduced through the sheath such that only the active tip is protruding and followed with ultrasound to the sapheno-femoral junction. In order to avoid thermal injury to the overlying skin, a dilute local anaesthetic solution is infiltrated around the vein again using ultrasound guidance. The local anaesthetic solution infiltrates around the LSV trunk prior to commencing the procedure. The duplex ultrasound gives good images of the spread of the solution. As well as providing anaesthesia (the whole operation can be performed under with the patient under LA), this manoeuvre also protects the overlying skin and any adjacent structures from thermal injury. The subcutanous space is expanded, and the great saphenous vein is contracted, by the effects of the tumescent anasthetic solution. There is debate about the management of proximal branches entering the SFJ, but fear of DVT means that many surgeons leave the most proximal veins open. Isolated case series and small comparative studies suggest improvement in early outcome compared with open surgery. Long-term data is awaited.

POSTOPERATIVE CARE

Following varicose vein surgery, the patient remains in bed with the bandages on overnight, or for the course of the day in the day surgery setting. The bandages are then removed and replaced with elastic compression stockings. Usually class III (TED) stockings are used, to aid venous outflow in the postoperative period. The effect of these stockings is additive and those patients with more severe varicosities may benefit from the use of two pairs of stockings applied to the same leg.

Patients are encouraged to mobilize early the day after surgery, to exercise regularly, to rest with their feet raised and to avoid standing for long periods. The dressings and sutures are removed after 10 days and the patient can return to wearing one pair of compression stockings during the day at all times when standing or sitting with the legs down.

The patient usually returns to work after approximately 2 weeks, depending on their occupation, and may resume driving only when they can comfortably carry out an "emergency stop" procedure.

CONCLUSION

Although often considered a training operation for young surgeons, varicose vein surgery remains the source of a vast number of medical litigation cases. Great care must be taken to avoid damage to surrounding structures and to minimize the chance of future recurrence. In addition, the operation is frequently performed for cosmetic reasons in young people and so the end result of surgery is very important. The surgeon, therefore, should consider carefully the placement and length of each incision and close each wound with care. Following surgery, early mobilization and return to health and work is essential for this population if the operation is to be deemed a success.

REFERENCES

Durkin MT, Turton EP, Scott DJ, Berridge DC (1999) A prospective randomised trial of PIN versus conventional stripping in varicose vein surgery. Ann R Coll Surg Engl 81:171–174

Franks PJ, Wright DD, Moffatt CJ, Stirling J, Fletcher AE, Bulpitt CJ, McCollum CN (1992) Prevalence of venous disease: a community study in West London. Eur J Surg 158:143–147

CHAPTER 35

Endovascular Management of Venous Thrombotic and Occlusive Disease

Melhem J. Sharafuddin, Jamal J. Hoballah, Patricia E. Thorpe

INTRODUCTION

Deep vein thrombosis (DVT) is a common medical condition that can affect both the upper and lower torso and extremities. DVT is associated with high mortality and morbidity rates, and substantial immediate and long-term costs to society. Short-term complications for both upper and lower body DVT include pulmonary embolism (PE) and venous ischemia, while delayed complications include a spectrum of debilitating symptoms referred to as the post-thrombotic syndrome (Carpentier and Priollet 1994).

The classic risk factors for DVT are known as the Virchow's triad: endothelial injury, blood flow abnormalities/stasis, and hypercoagulability. These conditions are frequently met in postoperative, elderly or immobile patients. In addition, acquired and congenital hypercoagulable states have now been recognized as a major risk factor for DVT (Porter and Moneta 1988). Lower extremity DVT, especially recurrent episodes, can be related to underlying occlusive venous disease in the iliofemoral segments that are sequelae of a prior unresolved DVT episode, or extrinsic compression, most commonly at the level of the proximal left iliac vein, which is referred to as the May-Thurner syndrome. The etiology of DVT of the upper torso and extremities is remarkable for its common association with extrinsic compression at the thoracic inlet, acquired intrinsic venous stenosis or intravenous foreign body.

Anticoagulation therapy remains the mainstay of therapy in acute DVT, resulting in improvement of acute symptoms, and protection from PE in the majority of patients (Douketis et al. 1998; Hirsh 1998). It is generally agreed that pharmacologic and/or mechanical thrombolytic therapy can play an important role in patients whose acute symptoms fail to respond to anticoagulation therapy or those who develop limb-threatening venous ischemia (Comerota and Aldridge 1992; Krupski et al. 1990; Markel et al. 1992a). In addition, a more aggressive approach expanding indications for the use of thromboablative therapy has also been advocated by some, based on experimental and clinical studies suggesting a favorable role for early thrombolysis in the preservation of venous valve function and prevention of venous occlusive pathology (Johnson et al. 1995; Markel et al. 1992b; Meissner et al. 1993; O'Shaughnessy and FitzGerald 2001; Rhodes et al. 2000). Currently, the reasonable indications for thromboablative therapy in acute iliofemoral and axillary DVT are listed in Table 1.

Endovascular catheter-directed thrombolysis techniques, using pharmacologic thrombolytic agents alone or in combination with mechanical thrombectomy devices, have been proven highly effective in clearing acute DVT (AbuRahma et al. 2001;

Table 1

Indications for interventional therapy in acute DVT

- Young or highly functional patients with acute iliofemoral or axillary-subclavian DVT (symptoms for less than 14 days)
- Extensive thrombus burden
- Extension to IVC or SVC (especially with floating IVC thrombus)
- Associated findings of venous ischemia
- Phlegmasia dolens
- Symptomatic IVC thrombosis following filter placement
- Propagation of DVT despite conventional therapy
- High likelihood of underlying anatomic abnormality (prior pelvic DVT, compression by pelvic tumor, May-Thurner syndrome, thoracic inlet syndrome)

Bjarnason et al. 1997; Comerota et al. 2000; Mewissen et al. 1999; Semba and Dake 1994; Tarry et al. 1994; Verhaeghe et al. 1997). The combination of catheter-directed pharmaco-thrombolytic therapy, with device-directed mechanical thrombectomy, has become a popular adjunctive technique in patients with a large clot burden or in patients with contraindications to aggressive or prolonged thrombolytic therapy (Sharafuddin et al. 2003). Following clearance of the acute thrombotic component, definitive management of underlying anatomical abnormalities, usually central venous stenosis, should be undertaken. In patients presenting with the post-thrombotic syndrome, management of venous valve dysfunction remains one of the most formidable problems in patients suffering from chronic venous insufficiency (Markel et al. 1992). However, in patients whose chronic symptoms are attributable to venous occlusive pathology, mostly in the iliocaval segments, endovascular stenting can play an important role in alleviating symptoms of venous hypertension (Neglen et al. 2003).

Figure 1: Catheter-Directed Thrombolysis

Catheter-directed thrombolysis techniques are designed to deliver the thrombolytic agent into the direct vicinity of the thrombus, using a variety of specially designed infusion catheters. An ipsilateral retrograde transpopliteal approach is suitable in the majority of cases of iliofemoral DVT (Fig. 1). When extensive popliteal and infrageniculate DVT is present, adjunctive infusion of low-concentration thrombolytic agent via a peripheral pedal vein is generally advocated, which requires placement of tourniquets to force the thrombolytic agent into the crural deep veins.

Figure 1 shows a 28-year-old woman with acute leukemia who developed acute massive swelling of her left lower extremity. Femoropopliteal deep vein thrombosis was diagnosed on ultrasound. She was highly symptomatic and her symptoms did not improve after therapeutic heparinization. **A** Diagnostic ascending venogram was obtained via a superficial pedal vein with tourniquet compression to divert flow into the deep system. There is extensive thrombosis of the popliteal and superficial femoral veins. The iliac venous segment appears patent. **B** Access into the deep system was obtained via direct puncture of the thrombosed popliteal vein in the prone position under ultrasound guidance. A short (5 cm) 5F introducer sheath was placed, through which a multi-side-hole infusion catheter was introduced and positioned across the bulk of the thrombus. Urokinase was infused through both the introduced sheath (to treat the popliteal segment) and through the infusion catheter, at a dose rate of 25,000 IU/h for each. The patient was kept on therapeutic-dose heparin. **C** Completion venogram after 36 h of urokinase infusion. There is complete clearance of the clot burden and restoration of rapid forward flow into the deep venous system.

Upper torso DVT is generally treated in a similar manner to lower torso DVT. Access for catheter-directed techniques is usually accomplished through a single peripherally inserted vascular sheath, usually in the ipsilateral basilic or brachial vein.

Figure 1

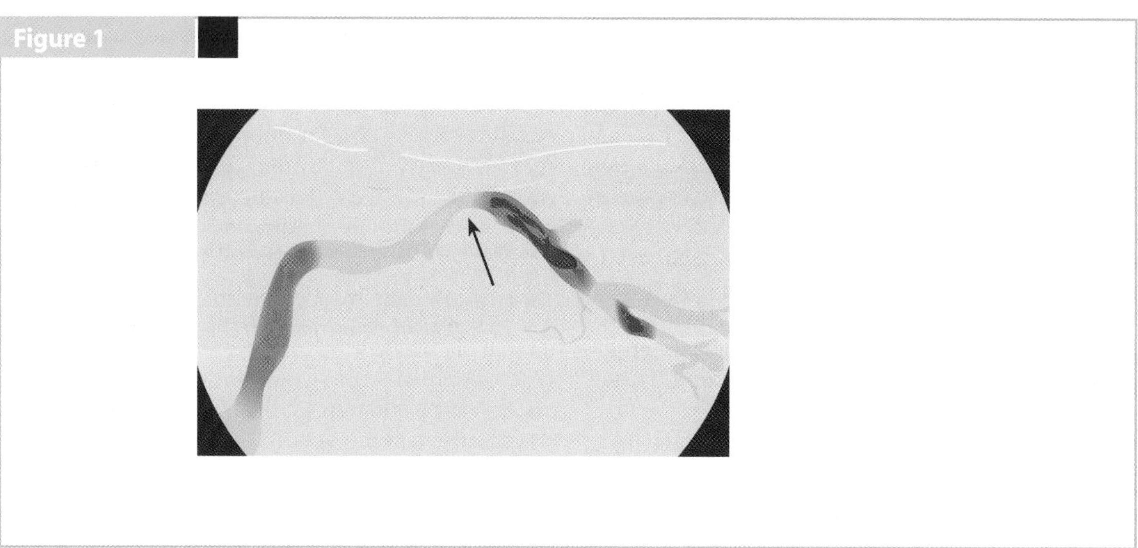

IPSILATERAL TRANSPOPLITEAL RETROGRADE THROMBOLYTIC THERAPY IN ACUTE ILIOFEMORAL DVT

Thrombolytic Therapy Initiation

- The patient is placed in the prone position.
- The popliteal fossa is widely prepped and draped.
- Local anesthetic is administered.
- The popliteal vein is accessed aiming cephalically with a single-wall puncture needle (18–21 gauge), preferably under sonographic guidance.
- A short 5F or 6F vascular introducer sheath is placed.
- An appropriate angiographic catheter-guidewire combination [e.g., multipurpose curve catheter (Cordis, Miami Lakes, FL) with either a straight floppy guidewire (Cook, Bloomington, IN) or a curved tip glidewire (Boston Scientific, Natick, MA) is used to traverse the entire thrombosed segment.
- Once the thrombus is traversed with the catheter, the guidewire is exchanged for a long heavy duty guidewire (e.g., Rosen, Bloomington, IN).
- A 4F or 5F multiple side-hole infusion catheter (e.g., Cragg-McNamara catheter, MTI, Irvine, CA) of an appropriate length is positioned (length of the infusing segment is chosen to cover the entire length of thrombus).
- Delivery of the thrombolytic agent is initiated via the infusion catheter according to one of various accepted protocols (Table 2).
- Systemic heparinization is generally required during the thrombolytic infusion. Heparin is preferably infused through the side-arm of the popliteal sheath. As a rule, full heparinization is used with urokinase or low-dose t-PA infusions. With high dose t-PA and r-PA, subtherapeutic heparinization is used (Table 2).
- The sheath and catheter are secured to the skin (avoid suture), using Steristrips and Tegaderm bandage.
- During the thrombolytic infusion, the patient is observed on a monitored unit that is familiar with the protocols and the recognition of the complications of thrombolytic therapy.

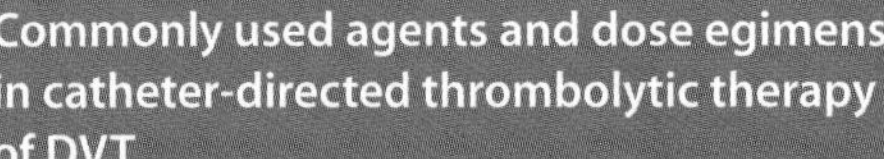
Table 2

Commonly used agents and dose egimens in catheter-directed thrombolytic therapy of DVT

Urokinase (Abbokinase; Abbott, Abbott Park, IL):

- High-dose regimen: continuous infusion at 250,000 IU/h; concomitant therapeutic heparin dosing (PTT 2–2.5 normal)
- Low-dose regimen: 50,000–100,000 IU/h; concomitant therapeutic heparin dosing

Alteplase (recombinant tissue-plasminogen activator [t-PA], Activase; Genentech, South San Francisco, CA):

- Weight-based high-dose regimen: continuous infusion at 0.025–0.05 mg/kg/h; No heparin or subtherapeutic heparin dosing (400–500 IU/h)
- Non-weight-based high-dose regimen: continuous infusion at 3–4 mg/h; No heparin or subtherapeutic heparin dosing (400–500 IU/h)
- High-volume low-dose regimen: continuous infusion at 0.5 mg/h (5 mg alteplase in 500 ml normal saline (0.01 mg/ml) to run at 50 ml/h); concomitant therapeutic heparin dosing is recommended

Reteplase (r-PA; Retavase; Gentocor, Malvern, PA):

- Non-weight-based high-dose regimen: continuous infusion at 0.5–1.0 U/h
- Low-dose regimens: continuous infusion at 0.25 U/h
- Concomitant subtherapeutic heparin dosing (400–500 IU/h)

Thrombolytic Follow-up Check

- The ipsilateral retrograde transpopliteal approach is used.
- Additional access from the right internal jugular or ipsilateral common femoral vein may be used to facilitate adjunctive endovascular interventions such as balloon dilatation and/or stenting.
- Follow-up venography is performed via the transpopliteal sheath. Both the subjective quality of venous flow across the previously thrombosed segment and the extent of residual thrombus are assessed.
- If substantial thrombus (>50%) persists, either the thrombolytic infusion duration is further extended or a trial of percutaneous mechanical thrombectomy can be attempted using an appropriate mechanical thrombectomy device (e.g., Amplatz thrombectomy device, Microvena, Minneapolis, MN). If only minimal residual thrombus persists but the flow remains sluggish, any significant underlying venous stenosis in the femoral or iliac veins is treated. Such intervention can most often be accomplished from the popliteal approach. Alternatively, an ipsilateral antegrade common femoral vein or a retrograde right internal jugular vein approach may be used.
- Completion venography and hemodynamic assessment is obtained.
- The hardware is removed and hemostasis is achieved by manual compression.
- Therapeutic heparinization is continued until long-term thrombolysis is achieved (coumadin or low-molecular weight heparin).

Adjunctive Interventions

- To treat underlying or residual venous stenosis, balloon angioplasty alone is preferred in the femoral segment whereas stent assisted angioplasty is performed in the iliac segments.
- Balloon angioplasty: The infusion catheter is exchanged for a long, heavy duty guidewire to maintain access. An appropriately sized angioplasty balloon is positioned across the stenosis and inflated. Following intervention, the stenosis is assessed by venography and, if needed, pressure gradient measurement. Any significant residual venographic or hemodynamic abnormality (residual stenosis ≥50%, especially in the presence of sluggish forward flow or mean venous pressure gradient ≥10 mmHg), is managed by endovascular stenting.
- Stent-assisted angioplasty: self-expanding stents are typically used (e.g., Smart, Cordis, Miami Lakes, FL). It is crucial that a stent of an appropriate length and diameter is selected (15–20% diameter oversizing, 5–10 mm additional length coverage on each side of the lesion).
- Completion venography and hemodynamic assessment are obtained.
- The hardware is removed and hemostasis is achieved by manual compression.
- Therapeutic heparinization is continued until long-term thrombolysis is achieved (coumadin or low-molecular-weight heparin).

In patients presenting with upper torso DVT associated with an underlying anatomical abnormality, the definitive management following clearance of the acute thrombus largely depends on the etiology of the anatomical obstruction, the presence of malignancy, and other co-morbidities and patient-specific factors (Sharafuddin et al. 2002). In general, underlying primary causes represented by intermittent positional compression at the thoracic outlet are treated with a staged approach with early thrombolytic therapy and anticoagulation, followed by surgical decompression. In the presence of extrinsic compression at the thoracic inlet, stenting should be avoided at all costs before surgical decompression because persistent positional pinching can lead to compression, kinking or fracture of the stent with a high risk of recurrent thrombosis (AbuRahma et al. 2000; Maintz et al. 2001; Phipp et al. 1999). All other secondary causes of central venous obstruction and thrombosis are usually amenable to endovascular treatment with balloon angioplasty and stenting (Schindler and Vogelzang 1999; Yim et al. 2000).

Figure 2

Figure 2A–E shows a 63-year-old man with end-stage renal disease and a functioning left brachiocephalic arteriovenous hemodialysis access. He presented with acute, painful left arm swelling. He had a history of multiple prior central venous hemodialysis accesses. **A** A diagnostic central venogram was obtained via the cephalic vein in the mid-arm. There is occlusion at the level of the subclavian vein with axillo-subclavian thrombus (*arrows*). Note the abundant collaterals. **B** An introducer sheath was placed in the cephalic vein, through which a multi-side-hole infusion catheter was introduced. The infusion length was positioned across the thrombosed segment. Alteplase was infused through the catheter at the rate of 5 mg/h for a duration of 6 h. The patient was also maintained on systemic heparin at 500 IU/h. **C** Final result after thrombolysis and balloon dilatation of a residual stenosis in the central subclavian vein using a 10-mm-diameter balloon. There is restoration of brisk forward flow with complete clearing of contrast and non-opacification of venous collateral. The patient was maintained on therapeutic anticoagulation using enoxaparin. Follow-up venography 1 month later shows maintained patency and forward flow.

Figure 3

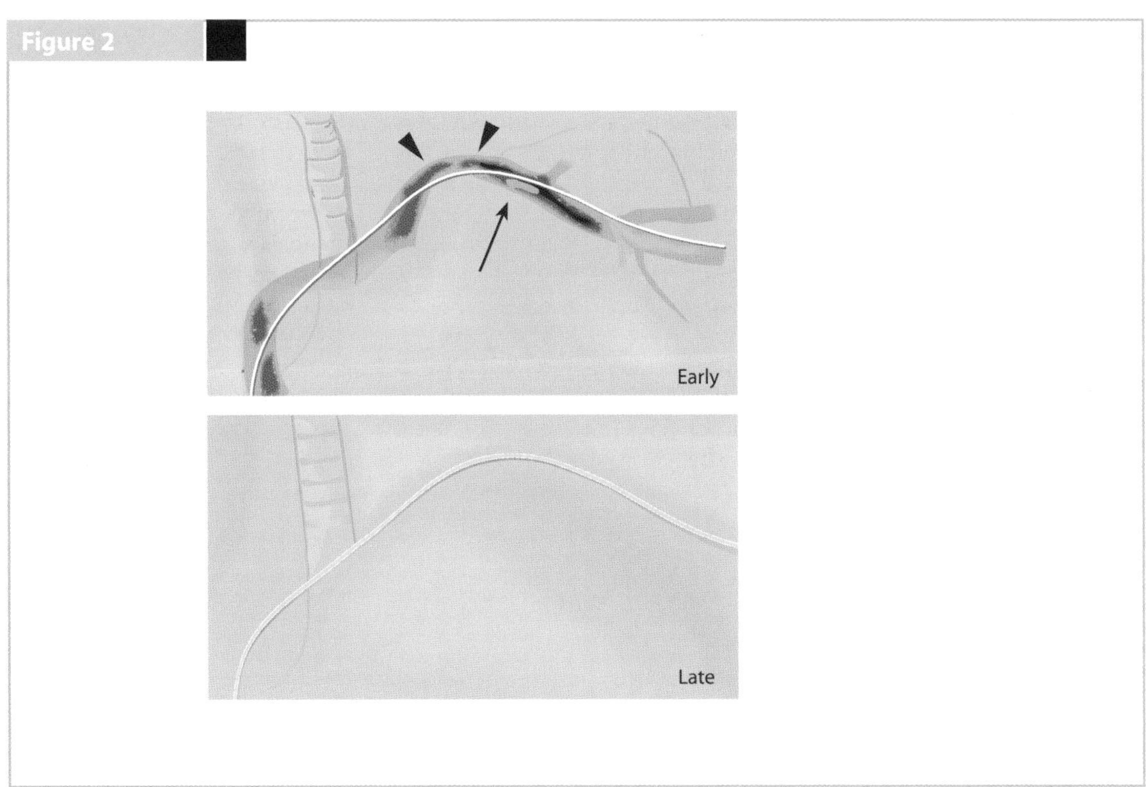
Figure 2
Early
Late

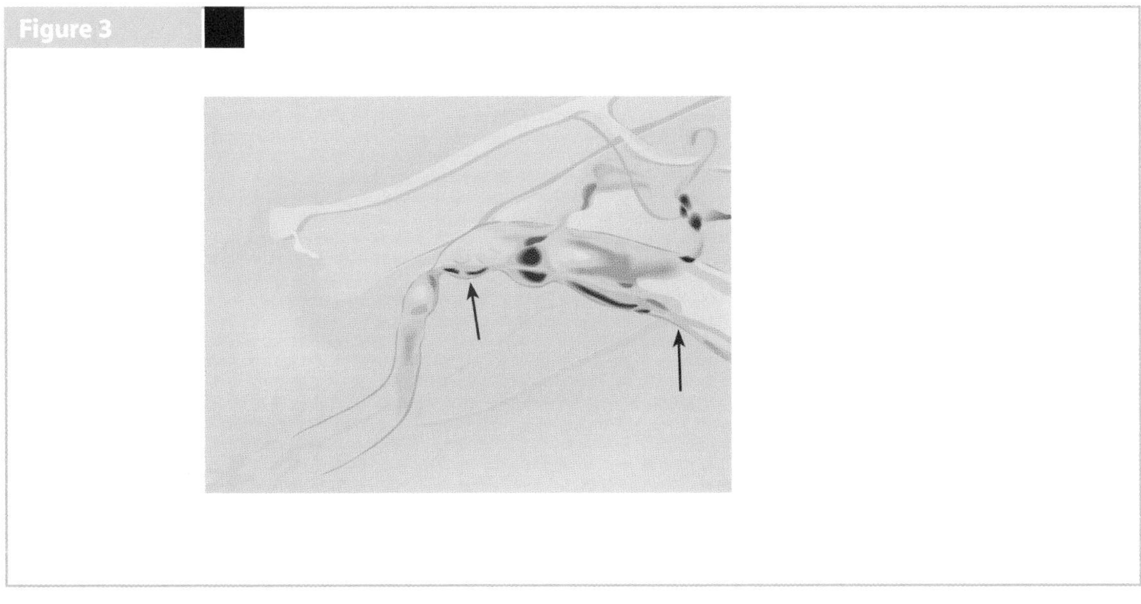
Figure 3

Figure 4

Figure 5

Figure 4

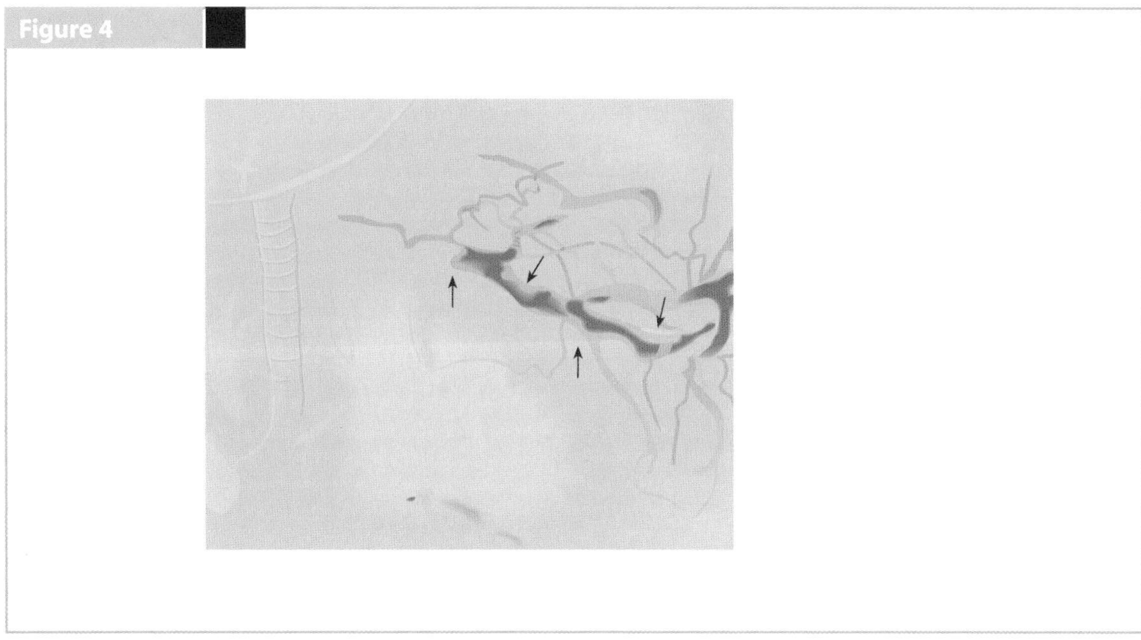

Figure 5

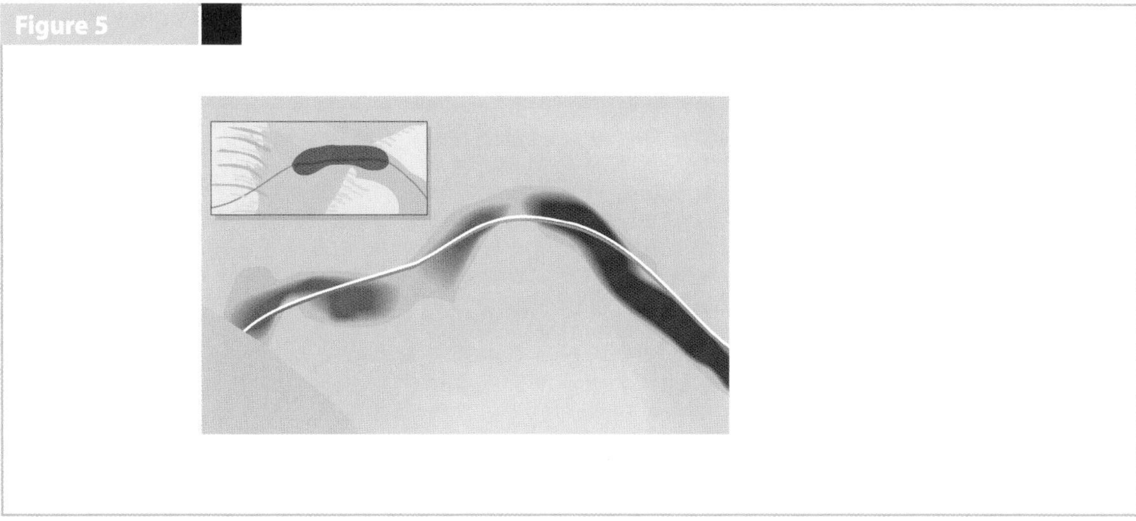

Figure 6

Figure 7

Figure 6

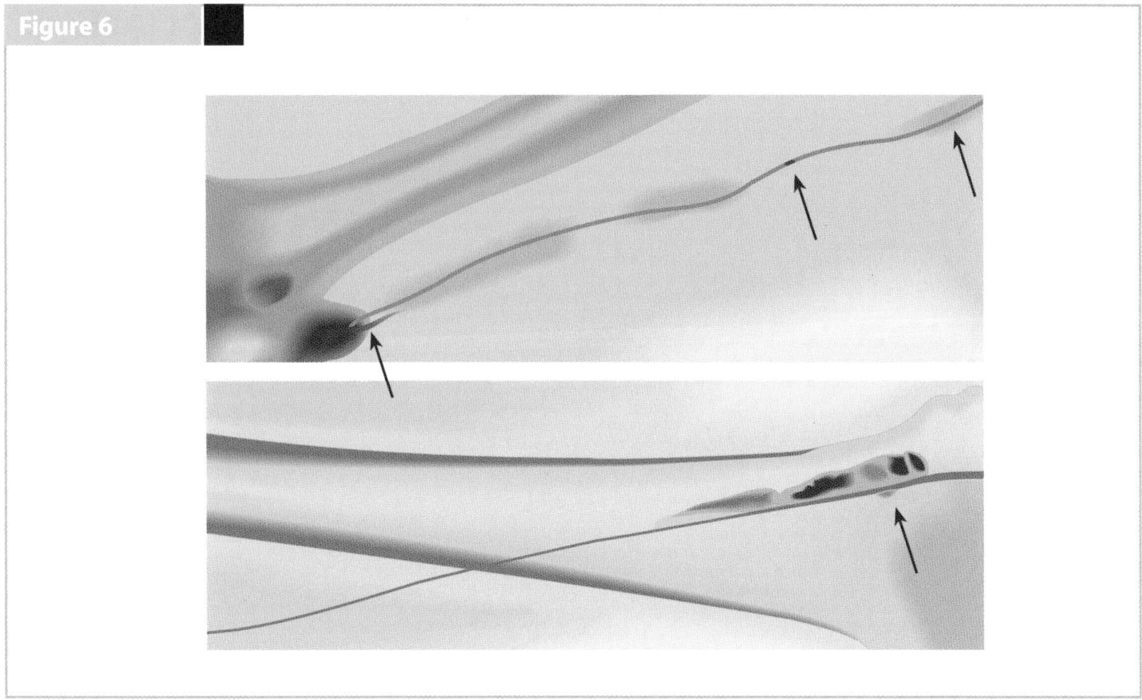

Figure 7

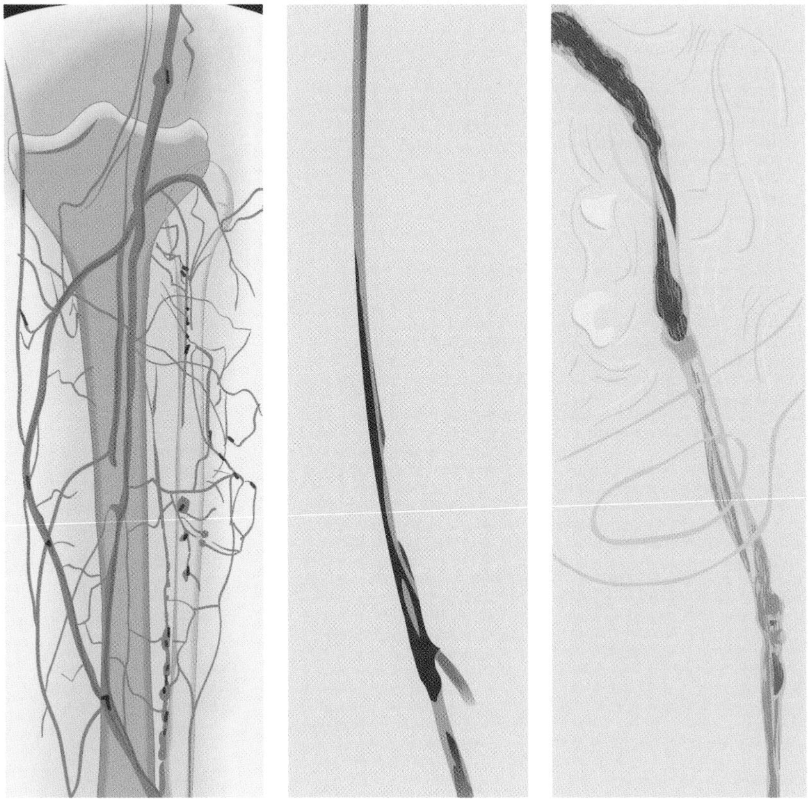

Figure 8

Figure 8

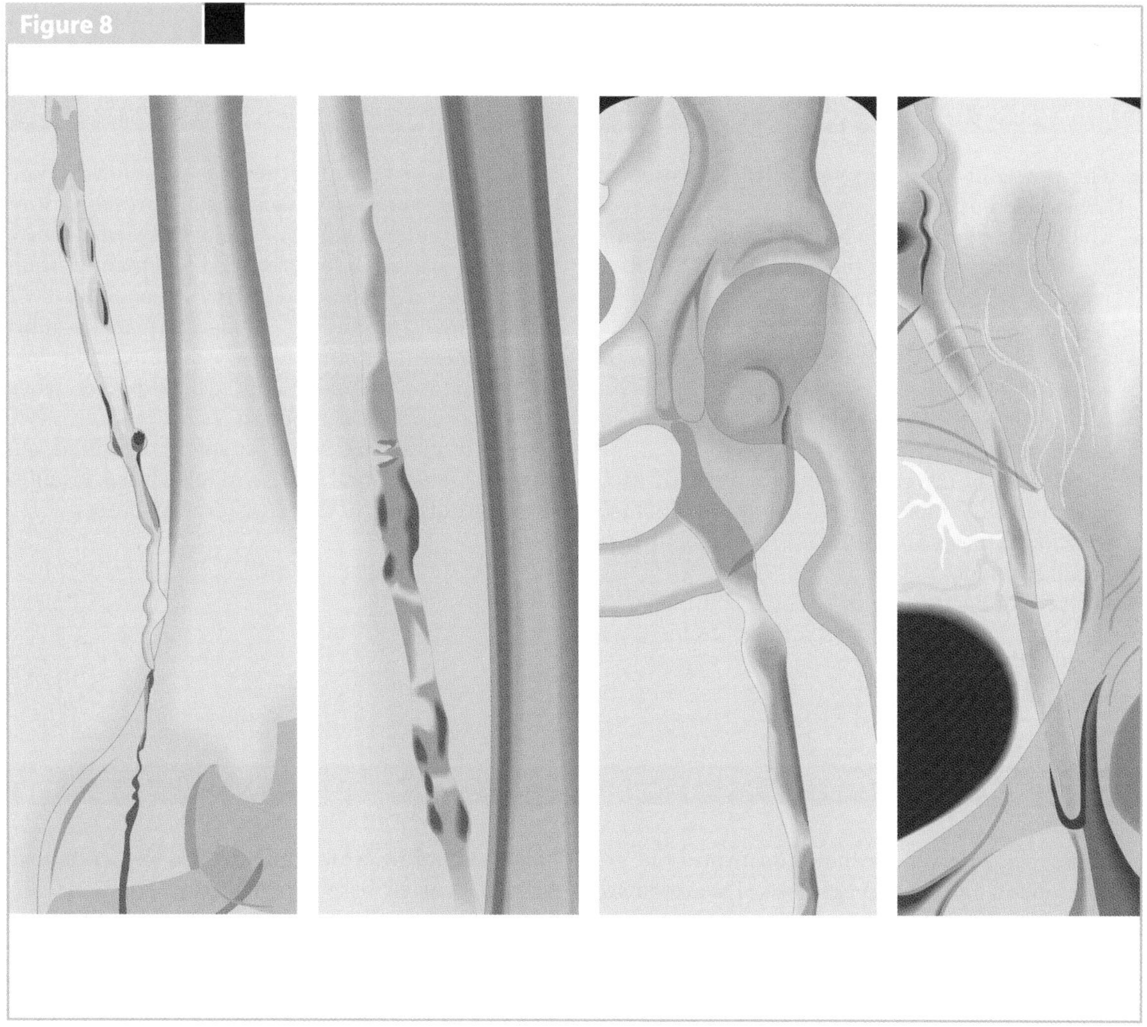

THROMBOLYTIC THERAPY IN ACUTE AXILLARY-SUBCLAVIAN DVT

Thrombolytic Therapy Initiation

- The procedure is performed with the patient in the supine position.
- The basilic or a suitable brachial vein is accessed in the medial aspect of the low arm or, for obese patients, in the antecubital fossa.
- A 5F or 6F vascular sheath is introduced.
- Initial venography is performed to assess the extent and length of thrombus, and the quality of collaterals and forward flow across the thrombosed segment.
- The lesion is traversed with a guidewire as in lower torso DVT and a 4F or 5F multiple side-hole infusion catheter is positioned across the thrombosed segment.
- Delivery of the thrombolytic agent is initiated via the infusion catheter as described under lower torso DVT.

Thrombolytic Check-Adjunctive Interventions

Subsequent to thrombolytic checks, adjunctive interventions such as mechanical thrombectomy, thrombaspiration, balloon angioplasty and, where indicated, stenting are performed in a manner similar to those described under the lower torso DVT section. Again, follow-up venography and adjunct endovascular interventions are best performed from an ipsilateral transbasilic approach. However, when a large-bore access is required, as for example when placement of a large diameter stent is required, additional transfemoral access may be used to allow safer introduction of the necessary hardware.

CONCLUSION

Endovascular intervention now constitutes the primary modality for the management of symptomatic thrombotic venous occlusions both in the upper and lower torso veins. Technical schemes for approaching these procedures are presented above but the procedural details need to be customized to the specific situation in terms of anatomical location, severity and chronicity of thrombus. Adjunctive modalities are often needed to restore acceptable patency. Restoration of forward flow in addition to anatomic patency is crucial and requires optimization of inflow and outflow, which both need to be ascertained. Achievement of these two goals (i.e., anatomic patency and forward flow) often requires adjunctive procedures such as infusions of thrombolytic agents into peripheral veins to restore inflow, aspiration thrombectomy and/or mechanical thrombectomy to manage residual or organizing thrombus, and, where indicated, balloon dilation and stenting. Long-term therapeutic anticoagulation is paramount to maintain patency.

REFERENCES

AbuRahma AF, Robinson PA (2000) Effort subclavian vein thrombosis: evolution of management. J Endovasc Ther 7:302–308

AbuRahma AF, Perkins SE, Wulu JT, Ng HK (2001) Iliofemoral deep vein thrombosis: conventional therapy versus lysis and percutaneous transluminal angioplasty and stenting. Ann Surg 233:752–760

Bjarnason H, Kruse JR, Asinger DA, Nazarian GK, Dietz CA Jr, Caldwell MD et al. (1997) Iliofemoral deep venous thrombosis: safety and efficacy outcome during 5 years of catheter-directed thrombolytic therapy. J Vasc Intervent Radiol 8:405–418

Carpentier P, Priollet P (1994) Epidémiologie de l'insuffisance veineuse chronique. Presse Medicale 23:197–201

Comerota AJ, Aldridge SC (1992) Thrombolytic therapy for acute deep vein thrombosis. Semi Vasc Surg 5:76–81

Comerota AJ, Throm RC, Mathias SD, Haughton S, Mewissen M (2000) Catheter-directed thrombolysis for iliofemoral deep venous thrombosis improves health-related quality of life. J Vasc Surg 32:130–137

Douketis JD, Kearon C, Bates S, Duku EK, Ginsberg JS (1998) Risk of fatal pulmonary embolism in patients with treated venous thromboembolism. JAMA 279:458–462

Hirsh J (1998) Low-molecular-weight heparin: A review of the results of recent studies of the treatment of venous thromboembolism and unstable angina. Circulation 98:1575–1582

Johnson BF, Manzo RA, Bergelin RO, Strandness DE Jr (1995) Relationship between changes in the deep venous system and the development of the postthrombotic syndrome after an acute episode of lower limb deep vein thrombosis: a one- to six-year follow-up. J Vasc Surg 21:307–312; discussion 313

Krupski W, Bass A, Dilley R, Bernstein E, Otis S (1990) Propagation of deep venous thrombosis identified by duplex ultrasonography. J Vasc Surg 12:467–475

Maintz D, Landwehr P, Gawenda M, Lackner K (2001) Failure of wallstents in the subclavian vein due to stent damage. Clin Imag 25:133–137

Markel A, Manzo RA, Bergelin RO, Strandness DE Jr (1992a) Pattern and distribution of thrombi in acute venous thrombosis. Arch Surg 127:305–309

Markel A, Manzo RA, Bergelin RO, Strandness DE Jr (1992b) Valvular reflux after deep vein thrombosis: incidence and time of occurrence. J Vasc Surg 15:377–382; discussion 383–384

Meissner MH, Manzo RA, Bergelin RO, Markel A, Strandness DE Jr (1993) Deep venous insufficiency: the relationship between lysis and subsequent reflux. J Vasc Surg 18:596–605; discussion 606–608

Mewissen MW, Seabrook GR, Meissner MH, Cynamon J, Labropoulos N, Haughton SH (1999) Catheter-directed thrombolysis for lower extremity deep venous thrombosis: report of a national multicenter registry [published erratum appears in Radiology 1999 Dec; 213(3):930]. Radiology 211:39–49

Neglen P, Thrasher TL, Raju S (2003) Venous outflow obstruction: an underestimated contributor to chronic venous disease. J Vasc Surg 38:879–885

O'Shaughnessy A, FitzGerald D (2001) The patterns and distribution of residual abnormalities between the individual proximal venous segments after an acute deep vein thrombosis. J Vasc Surg 33:379–384

Phipp LH, Scott DJ, Kessel D, Robertson I (1999) Subclavian stents and stent-grafts: cause for concern? J Endovasc Surg 6:223–226

Porter JM, Moneta GL (1988) Reporting standards in venous disease: an update. J Vasc Surg 8:172–181

Rhodes JM, Cho JS, Gloviczki P, Mozes G, Rolle R, Miller VM (2000) Thrombolysis for experimental deep venous thrombosis maintains valvular competence and vasoreactivity. J Vasc Surg 31:1193–1205

Schindler N, Vogelzang RL (1999) Superior vena cava syndrome. Experience with endovascular stents and surgical therapy. Surg Clin North Am 79:683–694, xi

Semba CP, Dake MD (1994) Iliofemoral deep venous thrombosis: aggressive therapy with catheter-directed thrombolysis. Radiology 191:487–494

Sharafuddin MJ, Sun S, Hoballah JJ (2002) Endovascular management of venous thrombotic diseases of the upper torso and extremities. J Vasc Interv Radiol 13:975–990

Sharafuddin MJ, Sun S, Hoballah JJ, Youness FM, Sharp WJ, Roh B-S (2003) Endovascular management of venous thrombotic and occlusive diseases of the lower extremities. J Vasc Interv Radiol 14:405–423

Tarry WC, Makhoul RG, Tisnado J, Posner MP, Sobel M, Lee HM (1994) Catheter-directed thrombolysis following vena cava filtration for severe deep venous thrombosis. Ann Vasc Surg 8:583–590

Verhaeghe R, Stockx L, Lacroix H, Vermylen J, Baert AL (1997) Catheter-directed lysis of iliofemoral vein thrombosis with use of rt-PA. Eur Radiol 7:996–1001

Yim CD, Sane SS, Bjarnason H (2000) Superior vena cava stenting. Radiol Clin North Am 38:409–424

Part IX Lymphedema

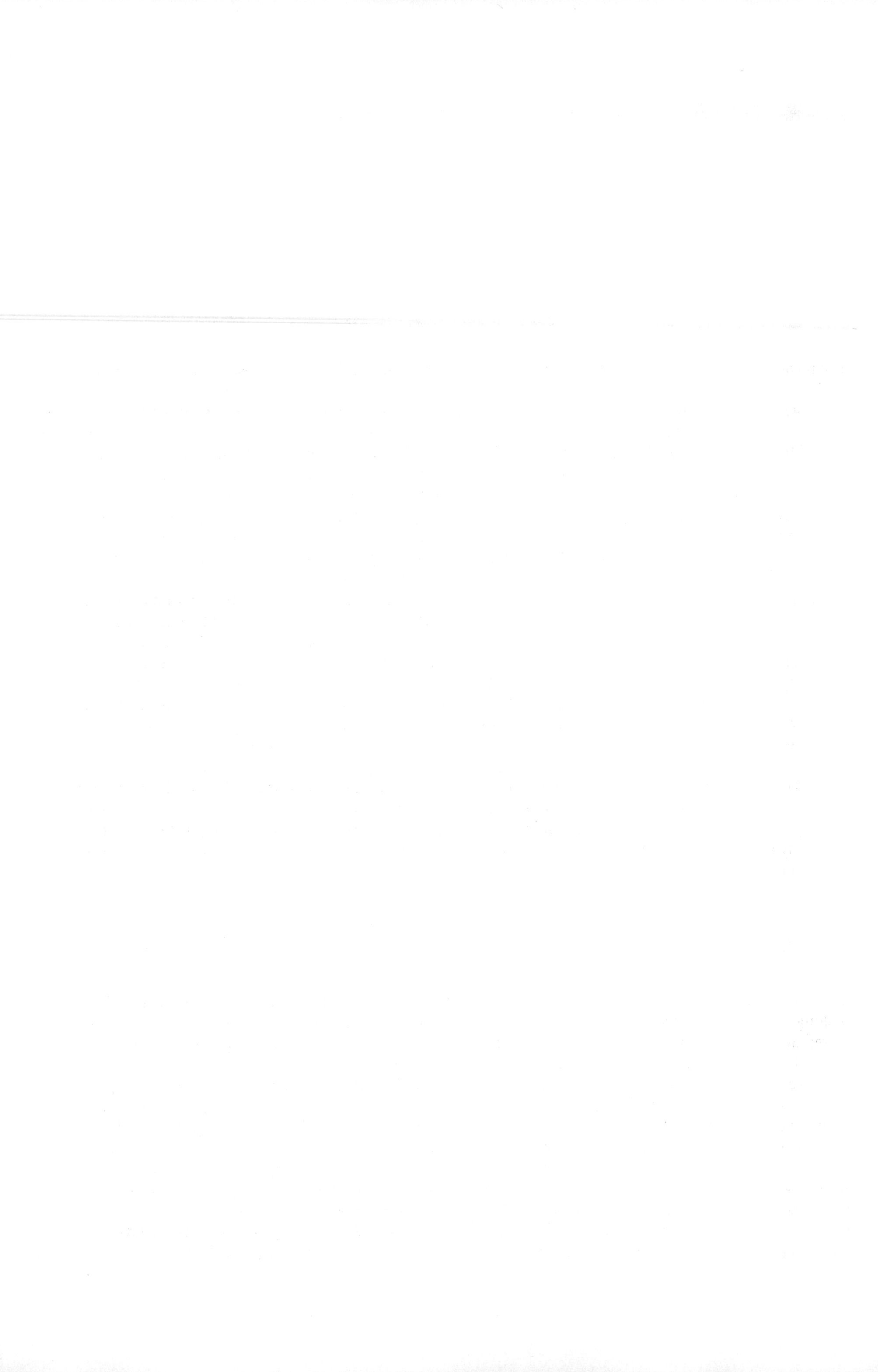

CHAPTER 36

Lymphedema

John Lumley

INTRODUCTION

The term "lymphedema" indicates an abnormal collection of lymph in a region, caused by defective drainage through the lymphatic system. The condition may be primary or secondary. The former is caused by a primary defect in the development of the lymphatic system and the symptoms may present at birth (lymphedema congenita), appear at puberty (lymphedema praecox) or be delayed until adult life (lymphedema tarda). Primary lymphedema may also be familial and in this case it is often termed Milroy's disease. The condition may present as part of a number of congenital syndromes, including Turner's syndrome and generalized vascular malformations. Lymphangiography in these patients may show aplasia, hypoplasia or ectasia of the draining vessels and lymph node abnormalities. Secondary lymphedema follows destruction of lymph nodes and lymphatic channels, usually by inflammatory or neoplastic lesions. The inflammatory varieties may be caused by acute or chronic infections, and in tropical regions filariasis is a common cause. Primary or secondary neoplasia and surgical excision of, or radiotherapy to, such lesions, and the effect of late scarring, may all predispose to lymphedematous changes. In the early stages lymphedema pits on digital pressure, but this characteristic is later lost because of recurrent attacks of cellulitis that give rise to fibrosis, formation of subcutaneous septa and induration. The skin is usually thickened and hyperkeratotic, but ulceration is uncommon and when present is usually associated with direct trauma. Cellulitis and minor trauma may precipitate the onset of primary or secondary lymphedema, and subsequent attacks of cellulitis are a constant feature. Sarcomatous changes are a rare but serious complication. They are usually seen in postmastectomy lymphedema and are characterized by multicentric purple cutaneous raised groups of papular lesions. Differentiation of primary and secondary lymphedema has important prognostic implications. It is usually obvious on clinical grounds but lymphangiography may demonstrate congenital anomalies or secondary lymph node changes. Computerized tomography may be helpful in screening for pelvic and retroperitoneal neoplastic changes. Systemic causes of bilateral lower leg edema from cardiac, renal, hepatic and nutritional disease and myxedema must be excluded, as must lipidemia. Unilateral lymphedema must be differentiated from venous edema and hamartomatous and neoplastic changes of a limb.

TREATMENT

The management of a patient with lymphedema is a lifelong undertaking. Non-surgical measures are directed at controlling the swelling by elevation, firm support and diuretics, and treating and preventing attacks of cellulitis. Regular washing of the skin of the affected area with an antiseptic soap is encouraged, cleaning crevices with cotton wool buds, followed by gentle drying. The patient must lavish great care on the skin of lymphedematous legs, adding appropriate softening creams to dry cracked areas. Fungal infections must be treated and trauma avoided. The latter includes avoidance of severe sunburn and the use of insect repellants when appropriate. In lower limb lymphedema, patients are advised permanently to raise the foot of their beds by 6–9 cm. More vigorous reduction by these means requires hospitalization, with bed elevation, plus a 45° foam wedge placed beneath the mattress. Pneumatic cuffs and massage can be of benefit but are not usually appropriate for long-term management. For upper limb problems high elevation can be achieved in hospital with some form of sling. Supportive stockings need to be specifically fitted and of one-way stretch material to be of value. These are not always acceptable to a patient with a minor degree of swelling, in which case the less effective support tights may be prescribed.

Long-term diuretic therapy, while of some value in fluid reduction, may also be accompanied by unacceptable frequency of micturition. Attacks of cellulitis must be treated immediately with appropriate antibiotics, and in patients with recurrent attacks long-term prophylaxis should be considered. Fibrosis following cellulitic episodes reduces the ease with which swelling can be subsequently reduced. The importance of these conservative measures should be explained to the patient and the relatives, as should the need to accept some disability and to lead an active normal life. They should also be assured that progression of mild lymphedema is not inevitable and that surgical measures are available for severe problems.

The surgery of lymphedema is not a cosmetic procedure and as such must be reserved for progressive enlargement of a limb, for limbs of marked and unmanageable size, progressive skin changes and recurrent infection. The procedures are directed either at excision of large wedges of the involved subcutaneous tissue or creating alternative pathways for lymphatic drainage. The original Charles' procedures involved taking split skin from affected areas and applying it to the deep fascia once the involved subcutaneous tissue had been excised. It produced a not very cosmetically satisfactory 'plus-four' effect and the late cutaneous changes are unsatisfactory. Wedge excision of the involved layers, as described by Homans, has proved more satisfactory. Two- or three-staged resections from the leg and thigh are used. The Thompson procedure, in which subcutaneous excision was combined with an inrolling of a skin flap into the subfascial compartments, with the intention of linking subcuticular and deep lymphatics, has not proved superior to the Homans' procedure, and can be complicated by dermal sinuses.

Attempts to bridge lymphatic defects across the groin and axillae have included anastomosing divided lymph node onto a venotomy, and lymph channels being drawn into the lumen of a vein through a needle passed across both its walls. Omentum or segments of small gut, in which the mucosa has been excised, can be laid across an area with a localized lymphatic defect. These procedures have produced variable and often unpredictable improvement. They are worthy of consideration in secondary lymphedema when there is no likely recurrence of the primary disease. Whatever procedures are undertaken, long-term care of the patient is required and additional excisions and long-term control of skin changes are essential.

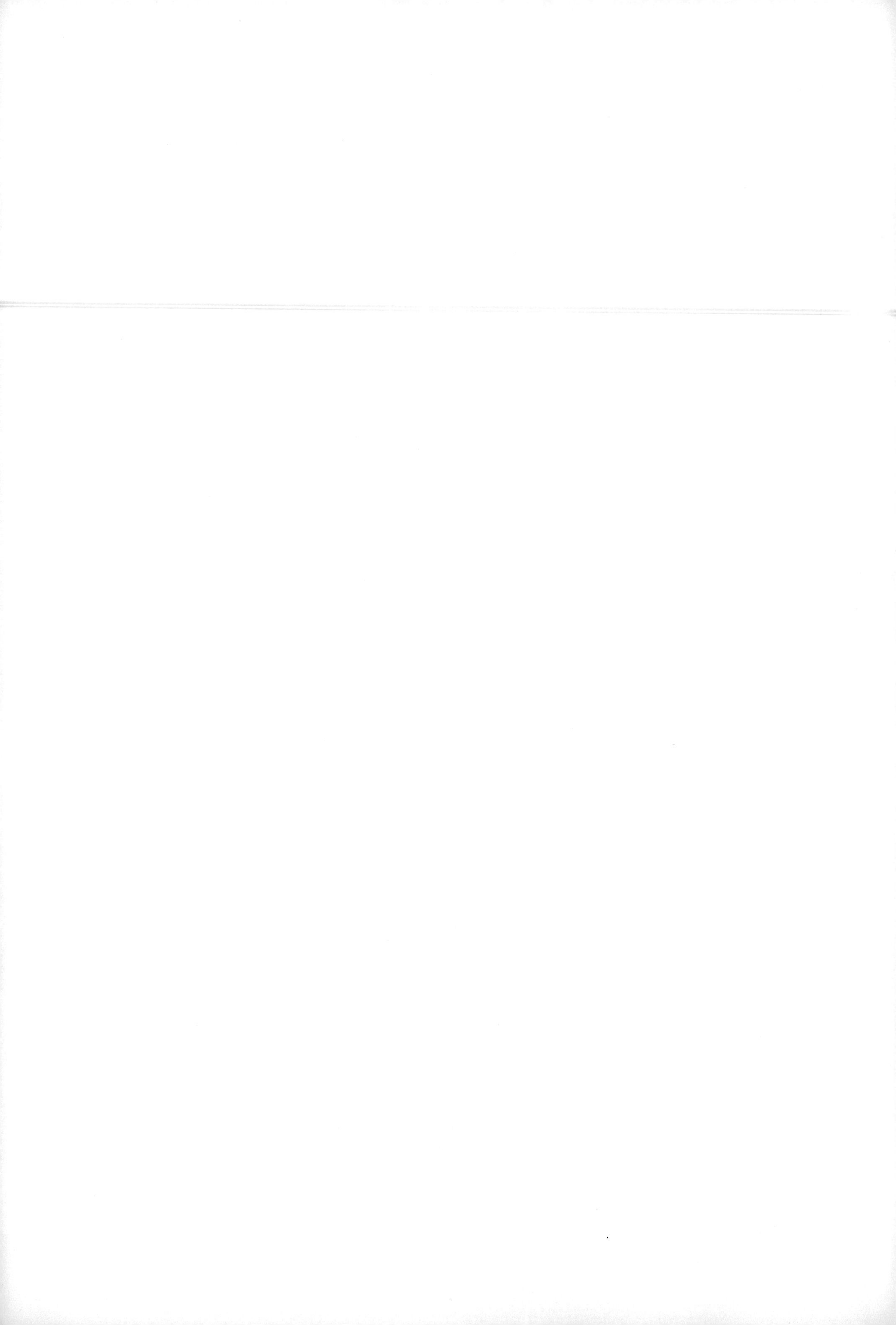

Printing and Binding: Stürtz GmbH, Würzburg